Anesthesia for Pain Management

Anesthesia for Pain Management

Edited by Lily Hunt

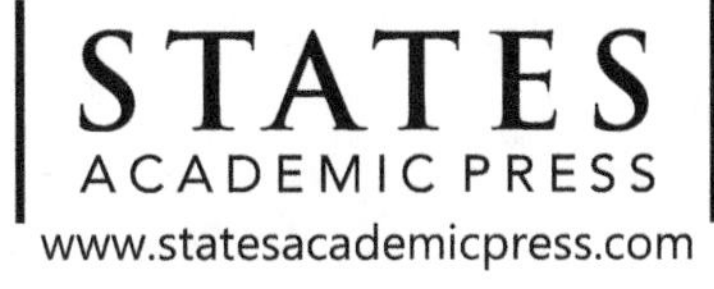

States Academic Press,
109 South 5th Street,
Brooklyn, NY 11249, USA

Visit us on the World Wide Web at:
www.statesacademicpress.com

ISBN: 978-1-63989-783-4

Cataloging-in-Publication Data

Anesthesia for pain management / edited by Lily Hunt.
p. cm.
Includes bibliographical references and index.
ISBN 978-1-63989-783-4
1. Pain medicine. 2. Pain--Treatment. 3. Anesthetics. 4. Anesthesia. I. Hunt, Lily.
RB127 .A54 2023
616.047 2--dc23

Table of Contents

Preface

Every book is initially just a concept; it takes months of research and hard work to give it the final shape in which the readers receive it. In its early stages, this book also went through rigorous reviewing. The notable contributions made by experts from across the globe were first molded into patterned chapters and then arranged in a sensibly sequential manner to bring out the best results.

Anesthesia refers to a state of controlled, short-term loss of awareness or sensation that is induced for medical and veterinary purposes. It may include some or all of the following symptoms such as amnesia, analgesia, unconsciousness and paralysis. There are four main types of anesthesia including general anesthesia, local anesthesia, regional anesthesia and sedation. Anesthesia could also be utilized in various situations such as surgeries, childbirth or other procedures like colonoscopies. It enables people to have procedures that allow them to live lengthier and healthier lives. Pain medicine is a subspecialty of anesthesia that focuses on successfully managing acute and chronic pain caused by a variety of factors. This book is compiled in such a manner, that it will provide in-depth knowledge about the role of anesthesia for pain management. It presents researches and studies performed by experts across the globe. The readers would gain knowledge that would broaden their perspective in this area of medicine.

It has been my immense pleasure to be a part of this project and to contribute my years of learning in such a meaningful form. I would like to take this opportunity to thank all the people who have been associated with the completion of this book at any step.

Editor

1

The intraoperative use of non-opioid adjuvant analgesic agents

Venkatesan Thiruvenkatarajan[1,2*], Richard Wood[1], Richard Watts[1], John Currie[1], Medhat Wahba[1,3] and Roelof M. Van Wijk[1,2]

Abstract

Background: Opioids have long been the mainstay of drugs used for intra-operative analgesia. Due to their well-known short and long term side effects, the use of non-opioid analgesics has often been encouraged to decrease the dose of opioid required and minimise these side effects. The trends in using non-opioid adjuvants among Australian Anaesthetists have not been examined before. This study has attempted to determine the use of non-opioid analgesics as part of an opioid sparing practice among anaesthetists across Australia and New Zealand.

Methods: A survey was distributed to 985 anaesthetists in Australia and New Zealand. The questions focused on frequency of use of different adjuvants and any reasons for not using individual agents. The agents surveyed were paracetamol, dexamethasone, non-steroidal anti-inflammatory agents (NSAIDs), tramadol, ketamine, anticonvulsants, intravenous lidocaine, systemic alpha 2 agonists, magnesium sulphate, and beta blockers. Descriptive statistics were used and data are expressed as a percentage of response for each drug.

Results: The response rate was 33.4%. Paracetamol was the most frequently used; with 72% of the respondents describing frequent usage (defined as usage above 70% of the time); followed by parecoxib (42% reported frequent usage) and dexamethasone (35% reported frequent usage). Other adjuvants were used much less commonly, with anaesthetists reporting their frequent usage at less than 10%. The majority of respondents suggested that they would never consider dexmedetomidine, magnesium, esmolol, pregabalin or gabapentin. Perceived disincentives for the use of analgesic adjuvants varied. The main concerns were side effects, lack of evidence for benefit, and anaesthetists' experience. The latter two were the major factors for magnesium, dexmedetomidine and esmolol.

Conclusion: The uptake of tramadol, lidocaine and magnesium amongst respondents from anaesthetists in Australia and New Zealand was poor. Gabapentin, pregabalin, dexmedetomidine and esmolol use was relatively rare. Most anaesthetists need substantial evidence before introducing a non-opioid adjuvant into their routine practice. Future trials should focus on assessing the opioid sparing benefits and relative risk of using individual non-opioid adjuvants in the perioperative period for specific procedures and patient populations.

Keywords: Opioid analgesia, Non-opioid adjuvants, Opioid sparing, Intraoperative analgesia, Opioid survey

* Correspondence: Venkatesan.Thiruvenkatarajan@sa.gov.au
[1]Department of Anaesthesia, The Queen Elizabeth Hospital, Woodville South 5011, South Australia, Australia
[2]The University of Adelaide, Adelaide 5000, South Australia, Australia

Strengths and limitations

- This is the first survey across Australia and New Zealand of its kind
- The survey was anonymous, and examined diverse sample of anaesthetists in terms of location (public, private practices) and experience
- It included most of the available opioid adjuvants, and examined most of the obstacles for not using them
- A very low response rate of 33.4%, nonetheless, similar to recently published surveys from the ANZCA clinical trials network
- A response bias is possible as the sample is likely to contain practitioners with subspecialty interest. Regional and practice variations (e.g. tertiary vs rural practices, pain service availability) were not investigated in this survey

Background

Opioids have always formed an integral component of a balanced anaesthetic, and remain the most effective drugs for the management of severe pain. Despite their advantages, they come with well-recognised adverse effects such as sedation, nausea and vomiting, constipation and respiratory depression [1–3]. Tolerance and hyperalgesia have been emphasized as adverse effects with longer-term (and occasionally short-term) use [1, 3]. In the community there has also been a general increase in opioid use with social as well as health implications ("the opioid epidemic"). Significant proportion of this epidemic is related to opioid overprescribing in the perioperative context and the anaesthetic implications of this has been discussed in the recent literature [4].

Multimodal analgesic regimens are commonly employed in the intraoperative period. Evidence shows that some adjuvants may enhance analgesic efficacy and facilitate opioid sparing with a reduction in opioid related side effects [3]. Non-opioid multimodal analgesia refers to paracetamol, non-steroidal anti-inflammatory drugs (NSAIDs), regional and local anaesthesia. Non-opioid Adjuvant drugs include N-Methyl-D-aspartate receptor (NMDA) receptor antagonists (e.g. ketamine, nitrous oxide), anticonvulsants (e.g. gabapentinoids), intravenous (IV) lidocaine, systemic alpha 2 agonists, magnesium sulphate, beta blockers, antidepressants (e.g. tricyclics, SNRIs). Their mechanism of action varies, and they act both centrally and peripherally, and the aim is to improve analgesia and reduce side effects [2].

Evidence supporting the use of these agents varies greatly, both with respect to the quality of evidence as well as the number of publications. Adjuvant usage appears to be influenced by patient, anaesthetic and procedure related factors, their availability, and the knowledge base and attitude of anaesthetists. In an earlier survey of anaesthetists, we carried out a cross-sectional questionnaire across the state of South Australia to assess the pattern of analgesic adjuncts used intraoperatively, to better understand their views and preferences [5]. After finding that the non-opioid adjuvants were sparingly used, we decided to survey anaesthetists across Australia and New Zealand to see if this was a pattern reflected across the two countries.

Methods

The survey was approved by the Human Research Ethics Committee of the Central Adelaide Local Health Network (Reference: HREC/18/CALHN/183). The survey was pilot tested within our department (26 specialists), and the questionnaire was enhanced based on the feedback. The survey was reviewed by the Australian and New Zealand College of Anaesthetists (ANZCA) Clinical Trials Network Committee. An email link to the online survey was sent to 1000 randomly selected fellows out of the 5500 ANZCA fellows (specialist anaesthetists) in May 2018. The randomization was done by the ANZCA Clinical Trials Network Committee. The 1000 fellows were randomly extracted from the college's database using a script. This is the standard practice adapted by our college for surveys. The survey was successfully delivered to 985 recipients (867 in Australia and 133 in New Zealand). A reminder email was delivered 2 weeks after the first email and the survey was closed after 4 weeks. The survey monkey (www.surveymonkey.com) platform was used for this anonymous survey. The IP addresses of the respondents were not collected.

The survey explored how frequently an individual agent was used for opioid sparing and the limitations in choosing an individual agent. The list included paracetamol, dexamethasone, NSAIDs, tramadol, NMDA receptor antagonists, anticonvulsants, IV lidocaine, systemic alpha 2 agonists, magnesium sulphate and beta blockers. This list was based on the most commonly used intraoperative agents in our institution, and agents which were previously examined in a cross sectional survey in South Australia [5]. The survey was not aimed at assessing the non-opioid sparing pharmacological properties of these agents.

The participants were questioned using two domains on each non-opioid adjuvant focusing on the frequency of use and any limitations as follows:

1. Frequency of use: a) never b) 10% usage c) 10–30% usage d) 30–50% usage e) 50–70% f) 70–90% g) 90–100%
2. Limiting factors in choosing a particular agent: a) time, b) cost, c) side effects, d) poor efficacy, e) lack of evidence, f) lack of experience with the drug, g)

lack of knowledge about the agent, h) none, and i) other, with the option to free text.

The frequencies were chosen to reflect the usage as rarely (up to 30%), sometimes (30–50%), often (50–70%), very often (70–90%), almost always (90–100%).

A single reply was created for the frequency of use whereas multiple selections were allowed for the limitations. The respondents answered all questions.

Data were analysed using Microsoft Excel 2010. Descriptive statistics were used to present the practitioners demographic and practice characteristics. Data are expressed as a percentage of response for each drug. Percentages reported are based on actual numbers of respondents.

Patient and public involvement

Since this survey was distributed to and was filled by Anaesthetists, there was no direct public or patient involvement in the survey.

Results

Three hundred and twenty nine fellows responded to the survey yielding a response rate of 33.4%. Table 1 describes the demographic profile of the participants. Four out of five respondents were Australian, and this is approximately proportional to the numbers of fellows who were contacted. The majority of the respondents were experienced anaesthetists, with 58% (191) having more than 10 years post fellowship experience. There was also representative spread of private and public work, with just over half (53%) working in both sectors. To simplify the analysis, reported usage of an agent above 70% of the time was categorised as being "frequently used" and usage below 70% deemed as "less frequently" used.

Table 1 Demographics of the respondents. Figures are numbers (percentages) of respondents, $n = 329$

Characteristics	Frequency
Practice location	
Australia	271 (82%)
New Zealand	57 (17%)
Other	1
Specialist practice years	
< 5	63 (19%)
5–10	75 (22%)
> 10	191 (58%)
Practice type	
Public only	93 (28%)
Private only	60 (18%)
Public and private	174 (53%)

Of all the agents, paracetamol was the most frequently used; 72% of the respondents reported frequent usage. This was followed by parecoxib (42% reported frequent usage) and dexamethasone (35% reported frequent usage). There was a steep decline in use of all the remaining adjuvants with less than 10% of anaesthetists reporting their frequent usage. The least used agents were dexmedetomidine, magnesium, esmolol, pregabalin and gabapentin; the vast majority of respondents suggested they would never consider these medications for their opiate sparing properties (Fig. 1).

Concerns which limited the use of individual agents varied and generally no one reason seemed to dominate for each agent.

Across the group, the main concerns were side effects, lack of evidence and experience. While side effect concerns dominated for tramadol, clonidine, ketamine, NSAIDs and gabapentinoids, lack of experience, and paucity of evidence of benefit dominated for magnesium, dexmedetomidine, and esmolol. Cost and time were of least concern to participants (Table 2).

Discussion

The survey provides a "snapshot" of the intraoperative use of non-opioid adjuvants across Australia and New Zealand. We found there were generally less non-opioid adjuvants used than in our earlier local survey across the state of South Australia [5]. Predictably, paracetamol and parecoxib topped the list of commonly used agents, as both have proven opioid sparing properties with a good safety margin. The results of this survey are reviewed below, with reference to the available published evidence. Paracetamol was the most frequently used agent by the respondents; 72% reported frequent use. It is an effective, well tolerated analgesic in the treatment of acute pain and all routes of administration have opioid sparing effects [3, 6, 7]. The convenience and safety of intravenous administration likely accounts for its widespread intraoperative use. A recent Cochrane review supports the safety and the clinical utility of IV paracetamol and pro-paracetamol in postoperative pain settings. However, it failed to reveal a clinically meaningful reduction in opioid-induced adverse events [8].

Parecoxib was the only intravenous selective Cox-2 inhibitor licensed in Australia at the time of this survey [9]. It is widely available in the operative environment and the dosing is convenient. Forty two percent the respondents reported frequent use, with side effects being the main limiting factor to its use. A recent systematic review and meta-analysis of randomized trials has shown that a combination of NSAIDs or Cox-2 inhibitors and paracetamol was superior to the later alone [10]. Based on the evidence and our survey findings, it is highly likely that the combination is often used in the

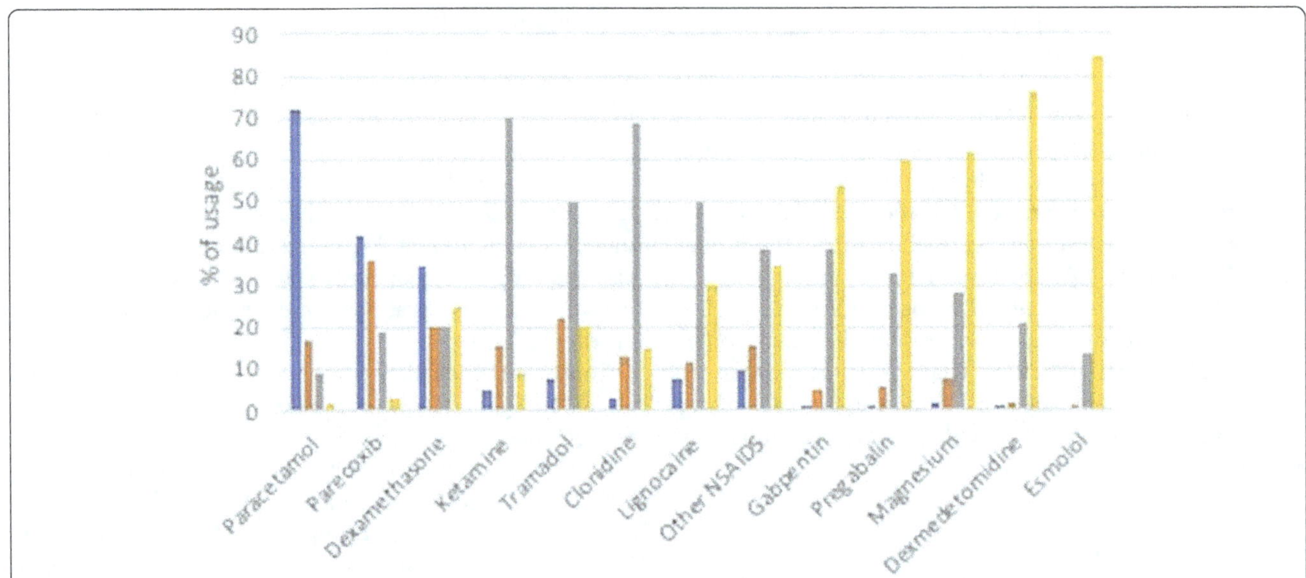

Fig. 1 Use of opioid adjuvants reported as percentage of usage. Use ranked by frequency of administration. Blue: frequently used, usage above 70% of the time; orange: used 30–70% of the time; grey: used up to 30% of the time; yellow: never used. Values on the x-axis represent the proportion of usage of different agents and values on the y-axis represent percentage of responses for each category

perioperative setting. The prescription pattern of NSAIDs in a hospital setting is usually guided by the patients' age as well as gastrointestinal and cardiovascular risk factors [11].

Dexamethasone delivers slight but clinically insignificant analgesic and opioid sparing effects; preoperative administration seems more effective than when given intraoperatively or postoperatively [3, 12]. However, it reduces nausea and vomiting, and improves recovery profile. While it was the third most preferred opioid sparing agent, it is possible that the respondents may have been using dexamethasone predominantly as an anti-emetic. The primary indication of utilising dexamethasone was not specifically asked in the survey, and this is acknowledged as a confounder. It is worth noting that dexamethasone is frequently used in conjunction with opioids in the setting of cancer pain [13].

Table 2 Leading limiting factors identified for the less frequently used opioid adjuvants, Values are percentages of actual responses

Agent	Predominant limiting factor
Tramadol	Side effects (80%)
Clonidine	Side effects (67%)
Ketamine	Side effects (61%)
Other NSAIDs	Side effects (57%)
Gabapentin	Side effects (41%)
Pregabalin	Side effects (37%)
Dexmedetomidine	Lack of experience (49%)
Magnesium	Lack of experience (31%)
Esmolol	Lack of evidence (29%)
Lidocaine	No specific factors identified (37%)

NSAIDs Non-steroidal anti-inflammatory agents

The easy availability and favorable respiratory effects [3] makes tramadol an alternative to opioids in patients with sleep apnoea and in the bariatric population. Yet, its use was poorly reported in this survey, mainly because of potential side effects. This is in contrast to our earlier survey where more than half the respondents reported using it frequently [5]. When used as a single agent, it may be ineffective for moderate to severe acute pain [3].

There is mounting evidence that when administered in sub-anaesthetic doses, both IV and intramuscular ketamine decrease opioid consumption [14, 15]. Surprisingly, the acceptance of ketamine was also poor, in contrast to our earlier survey where almost half the respondents reported using it [5]. Ketamine has well established evidence as a perioperative analgesic and opioid sparing agent, but also has known adverse effects. Concerns about the occurrence of these (61.4% of respondents) might have limited its uptake into mainstream practice, despite that it is generally well tolerated in its analgesic dose range.

A reluctance in using IV lidocaine and magnesium was also observed. Though there is evidence supporting their role as non-opioid adjuvants, no specific limiting factor was reported for IV lidocaine by one-third of the respondents, whereas lack of experience was the foremost limiting factor reported for magnesium. IV lidocaine has proven opioid sparing effects and reduces pain intensity together with reducing the side effects of opioids (nausea and vomiting and ileus) [16, 17]. Perioperative IV lidocaine is particularly effective in abdominal surgery [18]. Indeed, perioperative infusions of lidocaine have been shown to have a preventative analgesic effect (effect lasting > 8 h after cessation of infusion) [19]. Lack of experience was the second major concern expressed in our survey in using lidocaine. Several Enhanced Recovery After Surgery (ERAS) society guidelines have incorporated IV lidocaine regimes; in place of intraperitoneal lidocaine for hysterectomy, and as a substitute to epidural for laparoscopic colorectal surgery [20]. On the other hand, a recent Cochrane review released in June 2018 has concluded that the beneficial effects of perioperative IV lidocaine on reduction of pain, ileus and nausea were uncertain due to limited quality of evidence [21].

Magnesium is an NMDA-receptor antagonist. It improves analgesia and has an opioid-sparing property when employed as an adjunct to IV morphine pain regimens, (meta-analyses and reviews [3, 22–24].). No serious adverse events were identified by the reviews which examined its role as an intraoperative adjunct [22–24]. Respondents' disincentive for magnesium use did not dominate in any particular domain.

Systemic alpha-2 agonists were rarely used by survey respondents, with side effects being the main disincentive for clonidine use, and lack of experience with the use of dexmedetomidine. There is some evidence to suggest that their perioperative use may improve analgesia, reduce opioid consumption, and decrease nausea, without affecting the recovery times [3, 25]. Opioid sparing was reported across ten trials for clonidine and eight for dexmedetomidine [25]. On the other hand, a recent Cochrane review, whilst showing a slight opioid sparing effect in abdominal surgery, was unable to recommend this as a clinically significant finding [26].

Over half of the respondents reported that they have never used gabapentinoids, and the main reported concern was the side effect profile. Although better pain scores can be achieved with these agents, increased risk of dizziness, sedation, and respiratory depression (when given with opioids) were noted, with debatable significance of opioid sparing effect (NNT = 11 to reduce postoperative nausea and vomiting (PONV) with pregabalin) [27–29].

Not surprisingly, esmolol was one of the least preferred of all agents (85% of the respondents had never used it). Recent systematic reviews indicated an opioid sparing effect with esmolol in addition to improving pain intensity [30, 31]. It is worth noting that both these reviews include overlapping RCTs with significant heterogeneity and methodological deficiencies.

Our survey has several limitations. With a response rate of only 33.4%, a non-response bias is a definite possibility. We would have preferred a higher response rate. Regrettably, surveys take time to fill in, and we feel that one questionnaire and one follow up e-mail to a thousand anaesthetists keeps the balance between an acceptable sample size and not harassing our already busy colleagues. Our response rate is similar to recently published surveys from the ANZCA clinical trials network [32–34] and we believe that our results are likely to be representative and are worth reporting. As survey research is vulnerable in that it may deliver socially desirable answers, we have attempted to minimize this by maintaining respondent anonymity [35].

Choosing a non-opioid adjuvant is based on several patient, anaesthetic, and surgical factors such as the presence of neuropathic pain, chronic pain, opioid tolerance, bariatric surgery and sleep apnoea, to name but a few, and it is conceivable that surveying anaesthetists using precise opioid sparing scenarios, e.g.; bariatric surgery or the opioid tolerant patient may have generated different responses. However, it is likely that the respondents would normally care for a significant number of obese and opioid tolerant patients in their routine practice and this would be reflected in their survey responses. Another response bias is possible as the sample is likely to contain practitioners' with subspecialty interest. Regional variations may not be represented in this survey. Also, similar to other surveys, it is likely that our survey would have captured "claimed" behaviour rather than actual behaviour. This survey did not include the use of regional anaesthesia techniques which now form a significant component of opioid sparing strategies, with some respondents alluding to this in their free text response. Further, the survey did not assess the correlation between the respondents age/work experience and the utilization of certain co-analgesics. Choosing a diverse sample in terms of location and experience as well as including most of the available opioid adjuvants were some of the strengths of our study.

The reasons for the reported low usage of non-opioid adjuvants in our study are likely to be multifactorial. Perceived lack of evidence was reported by significant proportion of respondents for agents such as lidocaine, gabapentinoids and magnesium. While this does not reflect the previously presented evidence for the utility of these agents, it may rather reflect the lack of transmission of evidence, and/or 'evidence lag' where there is a period of time before evidence is accepted into practice. It might have been useful if we included the question whether participants felt up-to-date with their knowledge on the topic. Perioperative medicine is increasingly protocol driven in an attempt to standardise practice and improve clinical outcomes. These protocols are normally part of enhanced recovery programs where there is growing evidence of the benefits of pharmacological and regional interventions to decrease opioid requirements [20]. As opioid sparing agents become part of these programs, we may well see an increase in their use in future years.

We feel that our survey has shown that there is a need for further high quality randomised controlled trials in the area of opioid sparing drugs; and specifically there is a need to address the question of whether the adverse effects of some opioid sparing medications are comparable or worse than those of the opioids themselves e.g. gabapentin, alpha 2 agonists, esmolol. Nonetheless, the survey also shows that despite adequate evidence for some adjuvants, the transmission of this evidence to practitioners and/or the translation of this evidence into practice, was still relatively low e.g. ketamine, NSAIDs and magnesium. Indeed a separate survey reports that opioids still constitute the mainstay for acute postoperative pain management in hospitalised patients, and that the need for effective analgesic medications with low adverse risk profile remains unmet [36].

We hope that this type of survey may encourage similar efforts in different geographic regions, and that pooled data regarding current practice and anaesthetists' apprehensions can be used in designing future trials.

Conclusion

This survey demonstrates respondent anaesthetists' preferences and concerns in utilising non-opioid adjuvants for intraoperative opioid sparing across Australia and New Zealand. Most used paracetamol and parecoxib. A notable proportion routinely used dexamethasone though it is considered a weak agent commonly used for PONV. The uptake of tramadol, lidocaine and magnesium despite being supported by evidence was poor. Gabapentin, pregabalin, dexmedetomidine and esmolol use was relatively rare.

Our survey has provided an opportunity to review, and possibly improve, our opioid sparing practice, and given the low usage of some drugs, poses the question of whether there is any real appetite for change. Our results imply that opioids still constitute a major part of the intraoperative analgesic armamentarium. These findings are particularly important, and may indicate that the uptake of the current emerging trend towards "opioid free anaesthesia" would possibly require time. The survey also showed a potential lack of transmission of knowledge possibly implying a need for adequate ongoing education in this regard. Future trials should focus on assessing the clinical utility and the opioid sparing effects of using individual non-opioid adjuvants in the perioperative period for specific procedures and patient populations.

Abbreviations

ANZCA: Australian and New Zealand College of Anaesthetist; Cox-2: Cyclooxygenase 2; ERAS: Enhanced Recovery After Surgery; IV: Intravenous; NMDA: N-Methyl-D-aspartate receptor; NSAIDs: Non-steroidal anti-inflammatory drugs; PONV: postoperative nausea and vomiting; RCTs: Randomised controlled trials; SNRI: Serotonin Noradrenaline Reuptake Inhibitors

Acknowledgements

The authors would like to thank Karen Goulding MPH, ANCZA Clinical Trials Network Manager, Public Health and Preventive Medicine, Monash University, Melbourne, Victoria for her great help and input in facilitating this survey.

Authors contribution

VT Survey design, data analysis and manuscript writing. RWatts Survey design and data analysis. RWood Survey design, data collection, analysis of results and manuscript preparation. JC Data analysis, critical review and drafting of manuscript. MW: Data analysis, manuscript preparation RVW Survey design, results interpretation and manuscript preparation. All the authors have read and approved the manuscript

Author details

[1]Department of Anaesthesia, The Queen Elizabeth Hospital, Woodville South 5011, South Australia, Australia. [2]The University of Adelaide, Adelaide 5000, South Australia, Australia. [3]Pain Management Unit, Flinders Medical Centre, Bedford Park 5042, South Australia, Australia.

References

1. Ramaswamy S, Wilson JA, Colvin L. Non-opioid-based adjuvant analgesia in perioperative care. Continuing Educ Anaesth Crit Care Pain. 2013;13:152–7.
2. Żukowski M, Kotfis K. The use of opioid adjuvants in perioperative multimodal analgesia. Anaesthesiol Intensive Ther. 2012;44:42–6.
3. Schug SA, Palmer GM, Scott DA, et al. Working Group of the Australian and New Zealand College of Anaesthetists and Faculty of Pain Medicine. In: Acute pain management: scientific evidence (4th edition). Melbourne: ANZCA & FPM; 2015.
4. Hah J, Bateman B, Ratliff J, et al. Chronic opioid use after surgery: implications for perioperative Management in the Face of the opioid epidemic. Anesth Analg. 2017;125:1733–40.
5. Thiruvenkatarajan V, Watts R, Barratt A, et al. Intraoperative use of adjuvants for opioid sparing: a cross-sectional survey of anaesthetists in teaching hospitals in South Australia. Anaesth Intensive Care. 2018;46:138–9.
6. Maund E, McDaid C, Rice S, et al. Paracetamol and selective and non-selective non-steroidal anti-inflammatory drugs for the reduction in morphine-related side-effects after major surgery: a systematic review. Br J Anaesth. 2011;106:292–7.
7. Apfel CC, Turan A, Souza K, et al. Intravenous acetaminophen reduces postoperative nausea and vomiting: a systematic review and meta-analysis. PAIN. 2013;154:677–89.
8. McNicol ED, Ferguson MC, Haroutounian S, et al. Single dose intravenous paracetamol or intravenous propacetamol for postoperative pain. Cochrane Database of Systematic Reviews 2016, Issue 5. Art. No.: CD007126. DOI: https://doi.org/10.1002/14651858.CD007126.pub3
9. Mohamad A, McDonnell N, Bloor M, et al. Parecoxib and paracetamol for pain relief following minor day-stay gynaecological surgery. Anaesth Intensive Care. 2014;42:43–50.
10. Martinez V, Beloeil H, Marret E, et al. Non-opioid analgesics in adults after major surgery: systematic review with network meta-analysis of randomized trials. Br J Anaesth. 2017;118(1):22–31.
11. Khalil V, Wang W, Charlson L, Blackley S. Evaluation of prescribing patterns of nonsteroidal anti-inflammatory agents in a tertiary setting. Int J Evid Based Healthc. 2019. https://doi.org/10.1097/XEB.0000000000000173.
12. Waldron N, Jones C, Gan T, et al. Impact of perioperative dexamethasone on postoperative analgesia and side-effects: systematic review and meta-analysis. Br J Anaesth. 2012;110:191–200.
13. Eastman P, Le B. Corticosteroids as co-analgesics with opioids for pain: a survey of Australian and New Zealand palliative care clinicians. Intern Med J. 2015;45(12):1306–10.

14. Rakhman E, Shmain D, White I, et al. Repeated and escalating preoperative subanesthetic doses of ketamine for postoperative pain control in patients undergoing tumor resection: a randomized, placebo-controlled, double-blind trial. Clin Ther. 2011;33:863–73.
15. Laskowski K, Stirling A, McKay WP, et al. A systematic review of intravenous ketamine for postoperative analgesia. Can J Anaesth. 2011;58:911–23.
16. Chaparro LE, Smith SA, Moore RA, et al. Pharmacotherapy for the prevention of chronic pain after surgery in adults. Cochrane Database Syst Rev. 2013;24:CD008307. https://doi.org/10.1002/14651858.Cd008307.pub2.
17. Vigneault L, Turgeon AF, Côté D, et al. Perioperative intravenous lidocaine infusion for postoperative pain control: a meta-analysis of randomized controlled trials. Can J Anaesth. 2011;58:22–37.
18. Sun Y, Li T, Wang N, et al. Perioperative systemic lidocaine for postoperative analgesia and recovery after abdominal surgery: a meta-analysis of randomized controlled trials. Dis Colon Rectum. 2012;55:1183–94.
19. Barreveld A, Witte J, Chahal H, et al. Preventive analgesia by local anesthetics: the reduction of postoperative pain by peripheral nerve blocks and intravenous drugs. Anesth Analg. 2013;116:1141–61.
20. Beverly A, Kaye AD, Ljungqvist O, et al. Essential elements of multimodal analgesia in enhanced recovery after surgery (ERAS) guidelines. Anesthesiol Clin. 2017;35:e115–43.
21. Weibel S, Jelting Y, Pace NL, et al. Continuous intravenous perioperative lidocaine infusion for postoperative pain and recovery in adults. Cochrane Database Syst Rev. https://doi.org/10.1002/14651858.CD009642.pub3.
22. Murphy JD, Paskaradevan J, Eisler LL, et al. Analgesic efficacy of continuous intravenous magnesium infusion as an adjuvant to morphine for postoperative analgesia: a systematic review and meta-analysis. Middle East J Anesthesiol. 2013;22:11–20.
23. De Oliveira GS, Castro-Alves LJ, Khan JH, et al. Perioperative systemic magnesium to minimize postoperative pain. A Meta-analysis of randomized controlled trials. Anesthesiology. 2013;119:178–90.
24. Albrecht E, Kirkham K, Liu S, et al. Peri-operative intravenous administration of magnesium sulphate and postoperative pain: a meta-analysis. Anaesthesia. 2013;68:79–90.
25. Blandszun G, Lysakowski C, Elia N. Effect of perioperative systemicalpha2 agonists on postoperative morphine con-sumption and painintensity: systematic review and meta-analysis of randomized controlled trials. Anesthesiology. 2012;116:1312–22.
26. Jessen Lundorf L, Korvenius Nedergaard H, Møller A. Perioperative dexmedetomidine for acute pain after abdominal surgery in adults. Cochrane Database Syst Rev. 2016;18:CD010358. https://doi.org/10.1002/14651858.CD010358.pub2.
27. Fabritius ML, Geisler A, Petersen PL, et al. Gabapentin for post- operative pain management – a systematic review with meta- analyses and trial sequential analyses. Acta Anaesthesiol Scand. 2016;60:1188–208.
28. Doleman B, Heinink TP, Read DJ, et al. A systematic review and meta-regression analysis of prophylactic gabapentin for postoperative pain. Anaesthesia. 2015;70:1186–204.
29. Eipe N, Penning J, Yazdi F, et al. Perioperative use of pregabalin for acute pain-a systematic review and meta-analysis. Pain. 2015;156:1284–300.
30. Watts R, Thiruvenkatarajan V, Calvert M, et al. The effect of perioperative esmolol on early postoperative pain: a systematic review and meta-analysis. J Anesthesiol Clin Pharmacol. 2017;33:28–39.
31. Gelineau AM, King MR, Ladha KS, et al. Intraoperative Esmolol as an adjunct for perioperative opioid and postoperative pain reduction:ASystematic review, Meta-analysis, and Meta-regression. AnesthAnalg. 2018;126:1035–49.
32. Harrison R, Lee H, Sharma A. A survey of the impact of patient adverse events and near misses on anaesthetists in Australia and New Zealand. Anaesth Intensive Care. 2018;46(5):510–5.
33. Stuetzle KV, Pavlin BI, Smith NA, et al. Survey of occupational fatigue in anaesthetists in Australia and New Zealand. Anaesth Intensive Care. 2018;46: 414–23.
34. Lim A, Braat S, Hiller J, et al. Inhalational versus propofol-based total intravenous anaesthesia: practice patterns and perspectives among Australasian anaesthetists. Anaesth Intensive Care. 2018;46(5):480–7.
35. Durant L, Carey M, Schroder K. Effects of anonymity, gender, and erotophilia on the quality of data obtained from self-reports of socially sensitive behaviors. J Behav Med. 2002;25(5):438–67.
36. Gan TJ, Epstein RS, Leone-Perkins ML, et al. Practice patterns and treatment challenges in acute postoperative pain management: a survey of practicing physicians. Pain Ther. 2018;7(2):205–16.

2

Continuous adductor canal block used for postoperative pain relief after medial unicondylar knee arthroplasty

Fei Lan[1], Yanyan Shen[2], Yanhui Ma[1], Guanglei Cao[3], Nicole Philips[4], Ting Zhang[1] and Tianlong Wang[1*]

Abstract

Background: Peripheral nerve block and local infiltration analgesia (LIA) provide good analgesia after knee replacement. This study evaluated the additional analgesic efficacy of continuous adductor canal block (ACB) added to single-dose LIA after medial unicondylar knee arthroplasty (UKA). We hypothesized ACB would lower pain scores and facilitate postoperative ambulation.

Methods: Forty-six patients were enrolled into this double-blind, randomized, placebo-controlled trial. UKA was performed and all patients received single-dose LIA intraoperatively. Patients were randomized into two groups: Group RP receiving 0.2% ropivacaine or Group Con receiving normal saline. A flow at 6 mL/h was administered for 48 h through a catheter in the adductor canal. Primary outcome was movement pain score at 24 h using the numeric rating scale (NRS-11). Secondary outcomes included serial postoperative pain scores, rate of patients with NRS>3 at rest and movement within 24 and 48 h postoperatively, time to breakthrough pain, quadriceps motor strength, ambulated distance, catheter related infection and patient satisfaction.

Results: Forty-two patients were analyzed. Pain scores with movement at 24 h postoperatively were significantly lower in Group RP than that in Group Con (3 vs. 5 NRS, P<0.001). Compared with Group Con, breakthrough pain occurred later in Group RP (18.5 vs 10.0 h, $P = 0.002$), serial pain scores at rest and with movement and rate of patients with NRS>3 with movement after surgery were significantly lower. Quadriceps motor strength was equivalent, however, ambulated distance on postoperative day 1 and 2 in Group Con was significant less (19.7 vs 37.3 m, $P = 0.046$; 33.4 vs 59.5 m, $P = 0.002$).

Conclusions: Continuous adductor canal block added to single-dose LIA offered better analgesia and facilitated ambulation without motor weakness after medial UKA.

Keywords: Knee, Arthroplasty, Adductor canal block, Local, Analgesia

* Correspondence: w_tl5595@hotmail.com
[1]Department of Anesthesiology Xuanwu Hospital, Capital Medical University, No.45, Changchun Street, Beijing 100053, China

Background

Similar to total knee arthroplasty (TKA), moderate to severe pain caused by surgical trauma and early functional rehabilitation is anticipated after medial unicondylar knee arthroplasty (UKA) [1]. Optimal pain management, while minimizing analgesia-related complications is imperative, as pain after UKA can largely affect early ambulation, rehabilitation, and discharge [2]. Multimodal analgesic regimens, which include pain medications, local infiltration anesthesia (LIA) and peripheral nerve blocks (PNB), may be the most effective way of managing pain after major joint arthroplasty [3, 4]. While each regimen works well following TKA, femoral nerve blockade (FNB) has traditionally been the gold standard for analgesia [5]. The major disadvantages to FNB include, short duration and muscle strength reduction, and as a result, an alternative method is required [6, 7]. Recently, adductor canal block (ACB) has been suggested to be an alternative to FNB and has been shown to provide equivalent analgesia, while preserving quadriceps motor strength [8–10] and facilitating ambulation [11, 12].

The anterior cutaneous branches of the femoral nerve, the saphenous nerve, and branches of the obturator nerve travel through the adductor canal in the medial part of the thigh and innervate the surgical area involved in a medial UKA [13–15]. Previous studies focusing on TKA have suggested that single shot or continuous ACB added to a single-dose LIA can decrease postoperative pain and opioid consumption [16, 17]. Only one study reported that a single shot ACB given preoperatively may provide equivalent analgesia after medial UKA when compared with psoas compartment block [18]. Furthermore, no studies have reported the effect of continuous ACB combined with single-dose local infiltration analgesia (LIA) as a multimodal analgesic regimen after medial UKA.

Therefore, this prospective, randomized, double-blind, placebo-controlled trial compared the effects of continuous ACB added to an intraoperative single-dose LIA after medial UKA. We hypothesized that a continuous infusion ACB, in addition to LIA, would lower pain scores with movement at 24 h after surgery (primary outcome). We also hypothesized that this would improve serial pain scores, preserve quadriceps motor strength during physiotherapy, and facilitate ambulation within 48 h after surgery (secondary outcomes).

Methods

Ethics and registration

Approval was obtained from the Institutional Review Board of Xuanwu Hospital, Capital Medical University, code: 2017(074). The study was prospectively registered at Chictr.org.cn (code: ChiCTR-IOR-16008720) on June 25, 2016, and written informed consent was obtained from all participants before enrollment.

Patient inclusion and exclusion criteria

This prospective, randomized, double-blind, placebo-controlled trial was conducted from March 2017 to February 2018. Patients between 55 and 75 years of age were included if they were scheduled for medial UKA under spinal anesthesia (SA) with the American Association of Anesthesiologists (ASA) physical status of I-II. Patients were excluded if they had a history of opioid addiction, allergy to any of the study medications, a contraindication to ACB (peripheral neuropathy and infection at the procedure site) and/or a contraindication to SA (coagulopathy and recent anti-coagulant medication use).

Randomization and blinding

Randomization was carried out using a computer-generated randomization list. Patients were randomized into two groups; one receiving 0.2% ropivacaine (Group RP), and a control receiving normal saline (Group Con) via the adductor canal. Each patient received a consecutive study number and treatment assigned by the randomization list. The list was stored and only two nurses, who prepared the study medications were allowed access. They had no interaction with the patients. All other medical personnel, participants and outcome assessors were blinded to the interventions.

Administration of anesthesia and surgical procedure

All patients received spinal anesthesia through a median or para- median approach using a 26 or 27 G Whitacre needle with 2.0 ml 0.5% bupivacaine at the L3/4. Sedation with propofol and fluid therapy were administered intraoperatively by an anesthesiologist. Surgical technique was identical for all patients and all procedures were done in a bloodless field by use of a femoral tourniquet. Unless contraindicated, all patients were given oral preoperative multimodal analgesic medications including 400 mg celecoxib and 1000 mg acetaminophen, according to the patients' weight. Ondansetron 4 mg intravenous injections were administered prophylactically to prevent postoperative nausea and vomiting.

LIA and continuous ACB

All patients received LIA, consisting of a total of 100 ml 0.2% ropivacaine, 10 mg oxycodone and 0.5 mg adrenaline. All solutions were prepared under aseptic conditions. This is routinely performed by the surgeon for all medial UKAs before prosthesis implantation and wound closure. Using a similar method described previously [19, 20], 40 mL of the mixture was injected into the posterior capsule and the medial and lateral ligaments before inserting the components, Another 30 ml was injected into the anterior capsule, the synovium and retinacular tissues after insertion of the implants. The remaining mixture was infiltrated into the infrapatellar fat pad and the subcutaneous tissues before the closure of wound.

Upon completion of the surgery, patients were transferred to the post-anesthesia care unit, where standard monitoring was provided and continuous ACB was performed before spinal anesthesia had worn off.

A total of 300 mL (280 ml for infusion and a 20 ml bolus injection) of study solution, either 0.2% ropivacaine or normal saline, was prepared by either of the two unblinded nurses immediately after surgery.

The adductor canal was identified at mid-thigh level under ultrasound guidance and an 18-gauge Pajunk needle was inserted into the canal. A 20 mL bolus of the study drug (0.2% ropivacaine or normal saline) was administered. A bolus injection of 20 mL is required to fill the canal without risking retrograde flow to the femoral triangle [13, 21]. A 22-gauge Pajunk catheter was then placed through the needle and advanced a further 5 cm into the canal. The position was confirmed by ultrasound with a 2–3 mL injection of normal saline. Four hours after bolus injection, a continuous infusion by an electronic pump was activated at 6 mL/h for 48 h. If signs of irritation, allergy, or infection were observed at the catheter site, the intervention was stopped immediately and the patient was excluded from the study. The catheter was removed on postoperative day 2 following the afternoon physiotherapy session.

All patients received a multimodal pain regimen postoperatively: oral acetaminophen 1000 mg and oral celecoxib 200 mg every 12 h. In addition, rescue analgesics were available with oral fast-release oxycodone ≤10 mg every 4 h or as needed. If intolerance of oral medication, the patient was given, IV morphine 2.5 mg every 1 hour or as needed.

Outcome measures

Demographic data were collected preoperatively. The preoperative maximum range of knee motion was assessed. Surgical and spinal block duration, and the length of surgical incision were also recorded. Research personnel blinded to group assignment performed all pre- and postoperative assessments and data collection.

Primary outcome

The primary end point was pain scores with active knee flexion in the operated knee at 24 h after surgery. At the time of the assessment, patients were instructed to record their pain on NRS-11 [22]. The numeric rating scale (NRS) is a tool that allows patients to express their perceived pain, where 0 indicates no pain and 10 indicates the worst possible pain. The NRS-11 was explained to patients in great detail preoperatively.

Secondary outcomes

Pain scores using the NRS-11 and the numbers of patients with NRS>3 at 8, 12, 24, and 48 h after surgery were measured at rest and with movement. Additionally, the investigators recorded the first time point of postoperative pain at rest greater than 3 (NRS > 3), known as breakthrough pain. Opioid consumption during 0–24 h and 24–48 h postoperatively was retrieved from the electronic medical record and oral oxycodone converted to IV morphine equivalents for analysis [23, 24]. As for the ambulation ability assessments, patients were mobilized at least twice on postoperative day (POD) 1 and 2 with physical therapy assistance. During each physical therapy session, patients were asked to ambulate as far as possible. The total ambulated distance, measured in meters, was recorded by blinded outcome assessors. Quadriceps muscle strength was assessed at 4, 8, 12, 24, and 48 h postoperatively by blinded research personnel. Patients were asked to hold the affected limb up with the knee extended against resistance of the examiner and assigned a number using the manual muscle testing (MMT) grading scale (0 = no contraction, 1 = flicker of contraction, 2 = active movement with gravity eliminated, 3 = active movement against gravity but not resistance, 4 = active movement against gravity and some resistance and 5 = normal strength). Moreover, nerve block and catheter related complications and patient satisfaction were also assessed at 24 and 48 h postoperatively and all patients were asked to give a dichotomous verbal assessment ("Satisfied" or "Unsatisfied") of the quality of analgesia.

Statistical analysis

Statistical analysis was performed using IBM SPSS 20 (IBM Corporation, Armonk, New York). According to a pilot study of 12 patients receiving LIA without continuous ACB in our hospital, the mean pain score on movement at 24 h after surgery was NRS = 4.8 [SD, 2.6]. This value has been reported by other, similar studies [19, 25]. Our study intervention was modelled after Andersen (2013), who used combined analgesia after TKA [26]. As a result of combined analgesia, we expected to see a decrease of ≥2 NRS points on movement at 24 h postoperatively in the treatment group. A sample size of 38 patients (19 in each group) was required for a type I error of 0.05 and a power of 90%. Taking into account a potential dropout rate of 20%, we aimed to recruit 46 patients in this study. Unpaired t-tests were used for the statistical analyses and continuous variables are presented as mean (SD). Ordinal and non-normally distributed variables are expressed as median (range), and the Mann-Whitney U test was applied. Dichotomous data (gender, rate of patients with NRS>3 and patient satisfaction) were analyzed using the chi–square test or Fisher's exact test. A $p < 0.05$ was considered to be statistically significant.

Results

Sixty patients were approached for participation in this study. Forty-six patients were finally included and randomized to the treatment group or control group. Forty-two patients completed the study and were analyzed for outcomes. Four subjects were excluded due to protocol violations (Fig. 1). Of the 4 subjects excluded, 3 subjects from both groups requested to withdraw from the study, and 1 subject from Group Con had pump failure during the night. Preoperative measurements and demographic data were similar between groups. Moreover, there was no difference between groups with respect to surgery and spinal block durations, or length of surgical incision ($P > 0.05$, Table 1).

The primary end point of pain scores with active knee flexion in the operated knee at 24 h after surgery was significantly reduced in Group RP compared with Group Con (3 [IQR, 2.75–4.25] vs 5 [IQR, 4–6], $P<0.001$) (Table 2). Furthermore, time until breakthrough pain (NRS > 3) was significantly longer in Group RP than that in Group Con (18.5 [IQR, 4–46] hours vs 10.0 [IQR, 3–24] hours, $P = 0.002$) (Table 2). In addition, NRS pain scores at rest and with movement at 8, 12, 24 and 48 h after surgery (Figs. 2 and 3), and rate of patients with NRS>3 with movement within 24 and 48 h postoperatively were significantly lower in Group RP than in Group Con (Table 2)($P < 0.05$). As for the consumption of IV morphine, there was no significant difference between groups 0–24 h after surgery. However, Group RP consumed significantly less IV morphine at 24–48 h postoperatively compared to Group Con (15.64 ± 10.53 mg vs 27.15 ± 21.46 mg, $p = 0.039$) (Table 3).

There was no difference between groups for quadriceps muscle strength assessed at different postoperative time points ($P > 0.05$) (Fig. 4). However, the treatment group showed a statistically significant improvement in maximum distance ambulated compared with that of the control group on POD 1 and 2: (37.3 ± 32.2 vs 19.7 ± 22.1, $P = 0.046$; 59.5 ± 28.3 vs 33.4 ± 20.8, $P = 0.002$) (Table 2).

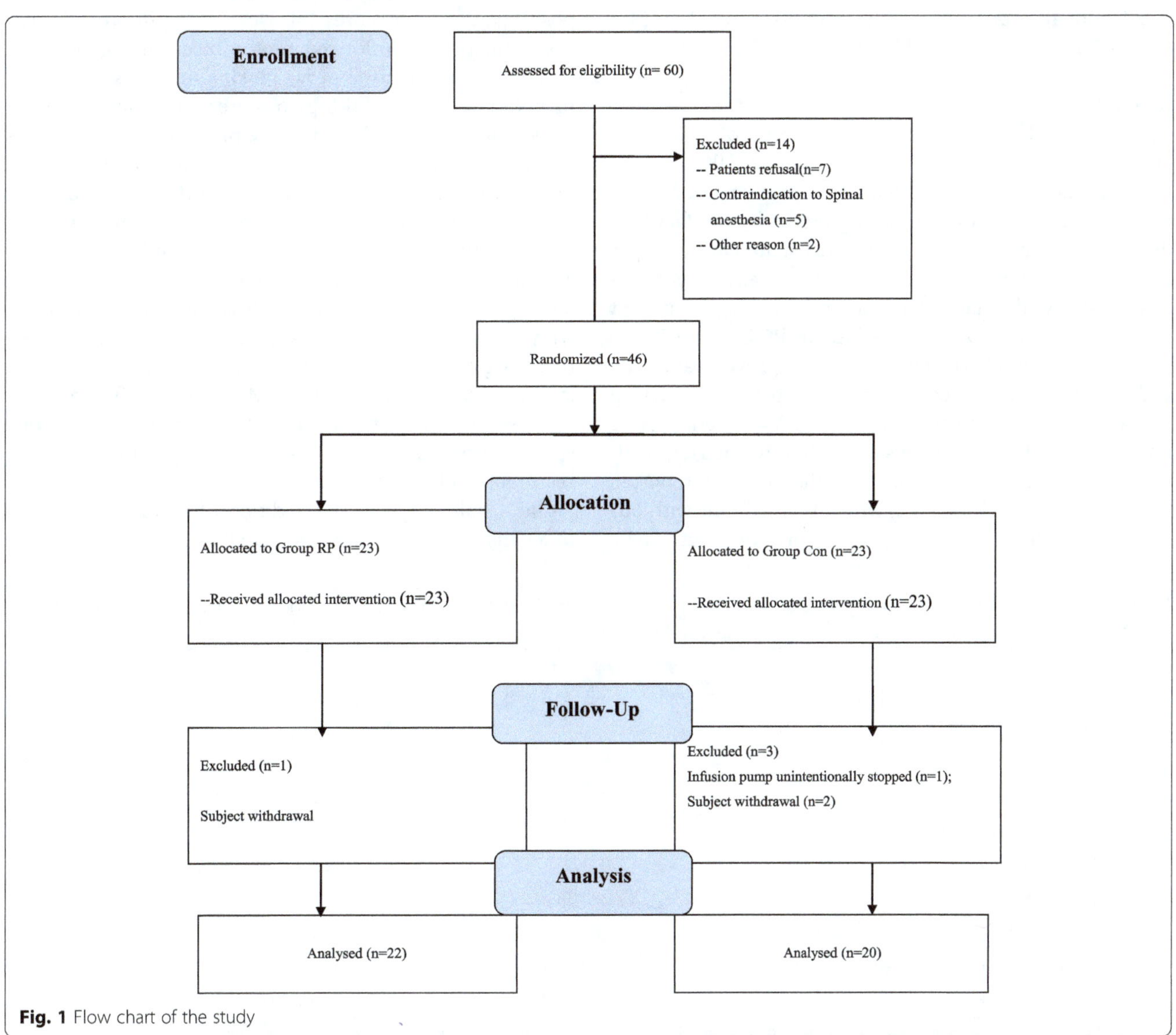

Fig. 1 Flow chart of the study

Table 1 Demographics and baseline characteristics

	Group RP ($n = 22$)	Group Con ($n = 20$)	P value
Age, (y)	66.1 ± 7.2	67.9 ± 6.5	0.397
Weight, (kg)	71.9 ± 9.6	67.3 ± 10.9	0.146
Height, (cm)	162.27 ± 4.92	155.85 ± 4.93	0.221
Body mass index, (kg/m2)	27.3 ± 3.7	27.6 ± 3.8	0.829
Sex, (male)	5	4	0.578
Duration of surgery, (min)	136 ± 22	124 ± 17	0.058
Duration of spinal block, (min)	143 ± 7	140 ± 9	0.215
Surgical incision length, (cm)	13.4 ± 3.0	12.0 ± 3.0	0.097
Range of motion before surgery, (degree)	102 ± 13	102 ± 16	0.667

Values are shown as mean ± SD

In addition, there was no nerve block and catheter related complications to be reported in either groups, and no difference was found in patient analgesia satisfaction at 24 and 48 h postoperatively (86% vs 85%, $P = 0.617$; 81% vs 75%, $P = 0.437$) (Table 3).

Discussion

Our findings demonstrate that the addition of a continuous ACB to single-dose of LIA after medial UKA significantly reduced pain scores with knee movement at 24 h after surgery. This result is strengthened by the fact that the time until breakthrough pain was significantly longer in Group RP. Furthermore, better pain relief was demonstrated by the fact that patients in the treatment group were better able to ambulate on POD 1 and 2.

Previous studies have demonstrated improved pain relief and decreased opioid consumption in patients receiving LIA after knee arthroplasty [27, 28]. However, periarticular infiltration analgesic regimens that infiltrate anterior, medial, and posterior compartments of the knee are reported to only last 6 to 12 h [29, 30], which is consistent with our observation from the time until breakthrough pain. Femoral nerve block when applied as part of multimodal analgesic management for patients undergoing TKA has been reported to decrease opioid consumption and lower postoperative pain scores [5]. Despite the improved analgesic outcomes, prolonged motor block and quadriceps weakness from femoral nerve block inhibit "fast track" rehabilitation [31, 32]. NRS pain scores on movement (knee flexion) at 24 h was chosen as the primary outcome in this study. Assessing pain at this time point is important for determining adequate analgesia for starting physical therapy, as the first physical therapy session was initiated 24 h postoperatively. In addition, previous studies have suggested that movement pain is more important than rest pain [33]. In this study, the duration of spinal anesthesia with 10 mg bupivacaine was approximately 15 min more than surgical duration in Group Con and 6 min more than surgical duration in Group RP. Moreover, the first pain assessment was initiated at 8 h postoperatively. Therefore, spinal anesthesia, which impairs the quality of clinical assessment could be ignored.

Our results support the addition of a continuous ACB to a single-dose LIA after medial UKA to supply sufficient

Table 2 Primary endpoint, percentage of patients with NRS pain score>3 within 24 and 48 h postoperatively, first time point of breakthrough pain and ambulated distance postoperatively

	Group RP $n = 22$	Group Con $n = 20$	p-value
NRS durimg active knee flexion at 24 h postoperatively	3 (2–4)	5 (4–6)	<0.001
Patients with NRS>3 at rest. No. (%)			
within 24 h postoperatively	2 (3)	6 (10)	0.150
within 48 h postoperatively	2 (2)	8 (10)	0.049
Patients with NRS>3 with movement. No. (%)			
within 24 h postoperatively	8 (12)	39 (65)	<0.001
within 48 h postoperatively	17 (19)	54 (68)	<0.001
Time to breakthrough pain (NRS > 3), (hours)	10 (3–24)	18 (4–46)	0.002
Ambulated distance on POD 1, (meters)	37.3 ± 32.2	19.7 ± 22.1	0.046
Ambulated distance on POD 2, (meters)	59.5 ± 28.3	33.4 ± 20.8	0.002

Data are shown as counts, median (interquartile range) or a mean ± SD; NRS = Numeric rating scale (for assessment of pain intensity)

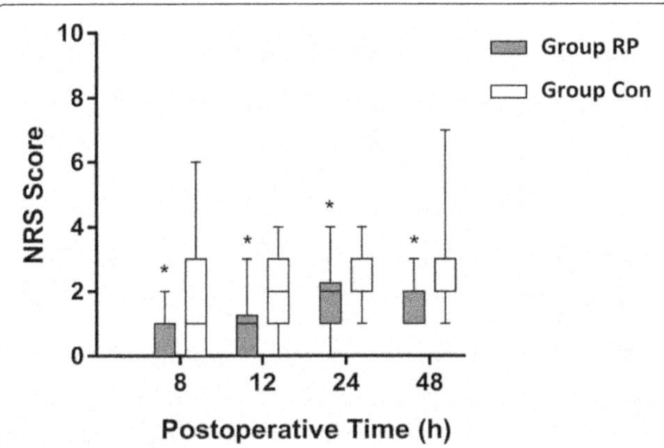

Fig. 2 Pain assessment at different time points postoperatively at rest. Data are expressed as median (horizontal bar) with 25th–75th (box) percentile and minimum to maximum (whiskers). *$P < 0.05$

analgesia, especially with movement, and help with ambulation after the day of surgery. Simple time-by-time comparisons for the repeated pain measurements, strongly inflated the type-I error. As a result, we transformed the data into number of relevant events (NRS>3) and compared the rates after surgery. We found the major difference of pain scores between groups occurred during movement. Similar to this study, previous studies had suggested that continuous ACB combined with single dose LIA can reduce pain scores (at rest and with movement) and opioid consumption after total knee replacement [26, 34]. Andersen et al. reported that saphenous nerve block with single-dose LIA offered better pain relief on the day of surgery than LIA alone after TKA, but no validated physiotherapy testing was used to compare the groups in that study. Conversely, Gudmundsdottir and Franklin reported that there is no pain related benefit to be acquired from adding an ACB to a single-dose LIA during physiotherapy session on POD 1 after TKA [17]. The main reason our results differ relates to the type of knee surgery itself. Total knee arthroplasty is invasive and more painful following surgery, leading to the need for more potent pain relief postoperatively. UKA is characterized by short incisions, less osteotomy and is capable of rapid recovery [35] . However pain is still an important issue in early postoperative functional rehabilitation [1, 36], which was consistent with what we found when comparing the rate of patients with NRS>3 with movement in control group. In this study, the mean surgical incision in both groups was over 12 cm long, similar to conventional surgery. However, it has been reported that even with minimally invasive surgery of UKA (an 8 to 10 cm-long medial parapatellar skin incision), pain scores and functional outcomes were not improve by using LIA alone [37]. Considering the surgical area of nerve innervation in medial UKA, continuous ACB may be uniquely suited to provide postoperative analgesia. Therefore, it is readily explained that continuous ACB plus single shot LIA can reduce pain scores at rest and with movement after surgery, and facilitate ambulation as shown in this study.

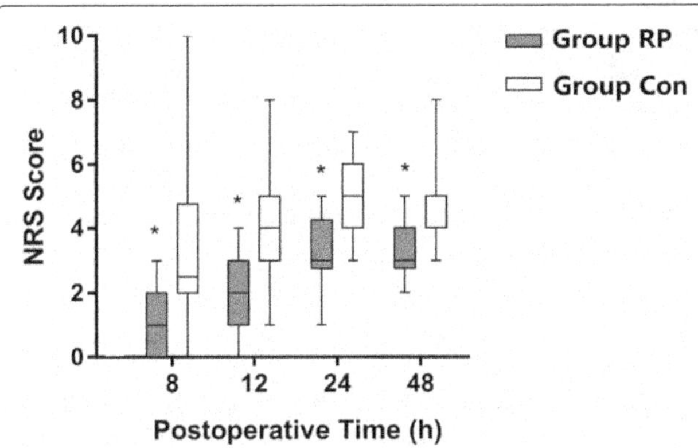

Fig. 3 Pain assessment at different time points postoperatively with movement. Data are expressed as median (horizontal bar) with 25th -75th (box) percentile and minimum to maximum (whiskers). *$P < 0.05$

Patient satisfaction was assessed as "satisfied" or "unsatisfied" at 24 and 48 h postoperatively. Essving (2009) reported that pain scores at rest and with movement were acceptable for patients who underwent medial UKA with intra-articular LIA combined with perioperative oral analgesics within 24 h postoperatively [19]. This is similar to the control group in this study. Therefore we are not surprised that there is no difference in patient satisfaction at 24 h after surgery. Furthermore, there was no difference in IV rescue morphine consumption during 0-24 h postoperatively, although NRS pain scores within 24 h after surgery were significantly lower in Group RP. However, during the 24–48 h postoperative period, intra-articular LIA had completely worn off, leading to an increase in overall pain scores seen in Group Con and likely had negative effects on physiotherapy after post-operative day 1. Increased pain likely led to the increase in IV rescue morphine consumption seen in Group Con during this time period. Therefore, patient satisfaction at 48 h postoperatively in Group Con was lower than in Group RP, although there was no statistical difference.

Motor block caused by peripheral nerve block in the lower extremities is a well-known adverse effect that compromises rehabilitation and even causes a risk of falling [38, 39]. There are case reports to suggest that ACB can affect quadriceps muscle strength, which can limit ambulation abilities [40, 41], however, this seems to be rare. In our study, at 48 h after surgery, there was no difference in quadriceps muscle strength between

Table 3 Morphine consumption, patient satisfaction and catheter related infection after surgery

	Group RP ($n = 22$)	Group Con ($n = 20$)	P value
IV morphine consumption, (mg)			
0–24 h postoperatively	13.82 ± 5.50	17.8 ± 7.41	0.063
24–48 h postoperatively	15.64 ± 10.53	27.15 ± 21.46	0.039
Satisfied patients, No. (%)			
24 h postoperatively	19 (86)	17 (85)	0.617
48 h postoperatively	18 (81)	15 (75)	0.437
Nerve blocking and catheter related complications, No. (%)	0	0	–

Values are shown as mean ± SD or frequency (%)

groups, which likely facilitated patients' early ambulation. From pain evaluation scores at different time points after surgery, it is not difficult to understand why the ambulated distance of patients in the treatment group was much longer compared with the control group. Pain was better managed during the first 48 h after surgery and the quadriceps muscle strength was well maintained.

The use of an invasive placebo may raise ethical concerns for some readers. Although it has been debated that invasive placebos are not consistent with ethical practice [42, 43], there is no consensus on the issue within the research community, nor are there uniform standards between ethics committees. The current study was approved by the Institutional Review Board of Xuanwu Hospital, Capital Medical University and all study participants provided informed consent. We assigned blind investigators to assess complications of nerve block in both groups. No patient in either group experienced temporary or permanent complications from the invasive placebo or treatment.

Although there are limitations to a continuous catheter approach [44, 45], such as patients' unintentional catheter removal, continuous ACB can provide a more prolonged analgesic effect compared with the single-dose method, facilitating rehabilitation on POD 1 and 2. In addition, there was no catheter related complications in either group, and no patient complained of the inconvenience of a portable infusion device.

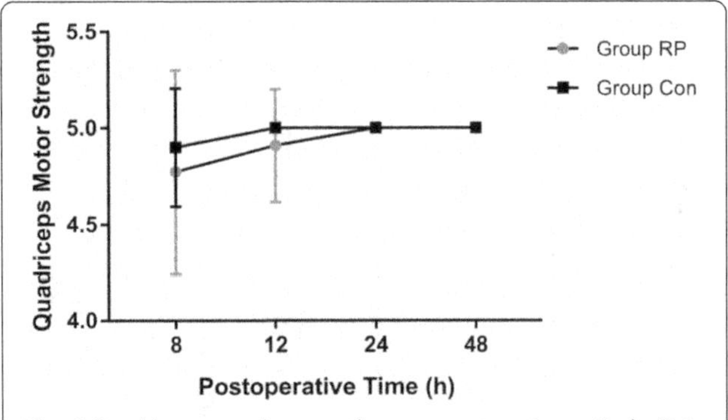

Fig. 4 Quadriceps muscle strength assessment postoperatively. Data are expressed as mean (SD)

In this study, the initial dose of ropivacaine for LIA was less than the maximal dose (225 mg) indicated by drug label [46], however, when combined with ACB bolus, the total dose (240 mg) of ropivacaine was slightly higher than recommended. However, previous studies have shown that injecting a much higher dose of ropivacaine in intra-articular LIA, than used in this study, is safe, with plasma levels below systemic toxic threshold [47–50]. Moreover, there was a 60 min interval between injections, which reduced plasma levels. This procedure is considered safe, while also aiming to maximize the duration of the block as safely as possible.

There are several limitations to this study. In order to guarantee all staff and study participants were blinded to the treatment group, we did not assess the success rate of the block. In that way, we cannot confirm that the blocks were all functioning accurately. However, Saranteas et al. has shown about 95% success rate of ACB using a similar approach [44]. In addition, no professional physiotherapists took part in this study, resulting in the inability to record ambulation ability. However, the strengths of our study include, effective randomization, the successful blinding process, and consistent management in standardizing the pre- and postoperative medication. It also was sufficiently powered for the primary end point. Finally, we did not measure total and free plasma concentrations of ropivacaine following LIA and ACB. This would have allowed us to be certain that systemic toxic thresholds were not reached. Although these values were not measured, patients were monitored closely for signs of toxic symptoms which no patient experienced.

Conclusions

This study suggests that continuous ACB added to single-dose LIA provides sufficient pain treatment after medial UKA and promotes early ambulation. Further studies are needed to address the additional effects that ACB provides to LIA on the day of surgery with a primary focus on ambulation abilities.

Abbreviations

ACB: Adductor Canal Block; ASA: American Association of Anesthesiologists; FNB: Femoral Nerve Blockade; LIA: Local Infiltration Anesthesia; MMT: Manual Muscle Testing; NRS-11: Numeric Rating Scale; PNB: Peripheral Nerve Blocks; SA: Spinal Anesthesia; TKA: Total Knee Arthroplasty; UKA: Unicondylar Knee Arthroplasty

Acknowledgements

We would like to thank Dr. Zheng Li and Dr. Shuai An for their invaluable contributions during this collaboration.

Authors' contributions

FL designed the study, conducted the study, and analyzed the data. YYS analyzed and interpreted the patients' data regarding this study. YHM and TZ performed the patients' anesthesia and continuous adductor canal block, and GLC was a major orthopedist performing surgeries. FL and NP were major contributor in writing the manuscript. TLW helped in designing the study, analyzing the data and revising the manuscript. All authors read and approved the final manuscript.

Author details

[1]Department of Anesthesiology Xuanwu Hospital, Capital Medical University, No.45, Changchun Street, Beijing 100053, China. [2]Department of Anesthesiology, Peking University International Hospital, Beijing, China. [3]Department of Orthopedics Xuanwu Hospital, Capital Medical University, Beijing, China. [4]Department of Critical Care Medicine St. Michael's Hospital, University of Toronto, Toronto, Canada.

References

1. Lygre SH, Espehaug B, Havelin LI, Furnes O, Vollset SE. Pain and function in patients after primary unicompartmental and total knee arthroplasty. J Bone Joint Surg Am. 2010;92:2890–7.
2. Husted H, Lunn TH, Troelsen A, Gaarn-Larsen L, Kristensen BB, Kehlet H. Why still in hospital after fast-track hip and knee arthroplasty? Acta Orthop. 2011; 82:679–84.
3. Vendittoli PA, Makinen P, Drolet P, Lavigne M, Fallaha M, Guertin MC, Varin F. A multimodal analgesia protocol for total knee arthroplasty. A randomized, controlled study. J Bone Joint Surg Am. 2006;88:282–9.
4. Webb CA, Mariano ER. Best multimodal analgesic protocol for total knee arthroplasty. Pain Manag. 2015;5:185–96.
5. Paul JE, Arya A, Hurlburt L, Cheng J, Thabane L, Tidy A, Murthy Y. Femoral nerve block improves analgesia outcomes after total knee arthroplasty: a meta-analysis of randomized controlled trials. Anesthesiology. 2010;113: 1144–62.
6. Zhang Z, Shen B. Effectiveness and weakness of local infiltration analgesia in total knee arthroplasty: a systematic review. J Int Med Res. 2018;46(12): 4874–84. https://doi.org/10.1177/0300060518799616.
7. Johnson RL, Kopp SL, Hebl JR, Erwin PJ, Mantilla CB. Falls and major orthopaedic surgery with peripheral nerve blockade: a systematic review and meta-analysis. Br J Anaesth. 2013;110:518–28.
8. Koh IJ, Choi YJ, Kim MS, Koh HJ, Kang MS, In Y. Femoral nerve block versus Adductor Canal block for analgesia after Total Knee arthroplasty. Knee Surg Relat Res. 2017;29:87–95.
9. Jaeger P, Nielsen ZJ, Henningsen MH, Hilsted KL, Mathiesen O, Dahl JB. Adductor canal block versus femoral nerve block and quadriceps strength: a randomized, double-blind, placebo-controlled, crossover study in healthy volunteers. Anesthesiology. 2013;118:409–15.
10. Kim DH, Lin Y, Goytizolo EA, Kahn RL, Maalouf DB, Manohar A, Patt ML, Goon AK, Lee YY, Ma Y, et al. Adductor canal block versus femoral nerve block for total knee arthroplasty: a prospective, randomized, controlled trial. Anesthesiology. 2014;120:540–50.
11. Machi AT, Sztain JF, Kormylo NJ, Madison SJ, Abramson WB, Monahan AM, Khatibi B, Ball ST, Gonzales FB, Sessler DI, et al. Discharge readiness after Tricompartment Knee arthroplasty: Adductor Canal versus femoral continuous nerve blocks-a dual-center, randomized trial. Anesthesiology. 2015;123:444–56.
12. Grevstad U, Mathiesen O, Valentiner LS, Jaeger P, Hilsted KL, Dahl JB. Effect of adductor canal block versus femoral nerve block on quadriceps strength, mobilization, and pain after total knee arthroplasty: a randomized, blinded study. Reg Anesth Pain Med. 2015;40:3–10.
13. Lund J, Jenstrup MT, Jaeger P, Sorensen AM, Dahl JB. Continuous adductor-canal-blockade for adjuvant post-operative analgesia after major knee surgery: preliminary results. Acta Anaesthesiol Scand. 2011;55:14–9.
14. Burckett-St Laurant D, Peng P, Giron Arango L, Niazi AU, Chan VW, Agur A, Perlas A. The nerves of the Adductor Canal and the innervation of the Knee: an anatomic study. Reg Anesth Pain Med. 2016;41:321–7.
15. Franco CD, Buvanendran A, Petersohn JD, Menzies RD, Menzies LP. Innervation of the anterior capsule of the human Knee: implications for radiofrequency ablation. Reg Anesth Pain Med. 2015;40:363–8.
16. Nader A, Kendall MC, Manning DW, Beal M, Rahangdale R, Dekker R, De Oliveira GS Jr, Kamenetsky E, McCarthy RJ. Single-dose Adductor Canal block with local infiltrative analgesia compared with local infiltrate analgesia after Total Knee arthroplasty: a randomized, double-blind, placebo-controlled trial. Reg Anesth Pain Med. 2016;41:678–84.
17. Gudmundsdottir S, Franklin JL. Continuous adductor canal block added to local infiltration analgesia (LIA) after total knee arthroplasty has no additional benefits on pain and ambulation on postoperative day 1 and 2 compared with LIA alone. Acta Orthop. 2017;88:537–42.
18. Henshaw DS, Jaffe JD, Reynolds JW, Dobson S, Russell GB, Weller RS. An evaluation of ultrasound-guided Adductor Canal blockade for postoperative analgesia after medial Unicondylar Knee arthroplasty. Anesth Analg. 2016;122:1192–201.
19. Essving P, Axelsson K, Kjellberg J, Wallgren O, Gupta A, Lundin A. Reduced hospital stay, morphine consumption, and pain intensity with local infiltration analgesia after unicompartmental knee arthroplasty. Acta Orthop. 2009;80:213–9.
20. Sawhney M, Mehdian H, Kashin B, Ip G, Bent M, Choy J, McPherson M, Bowry R. Pain after unilateral Total Knee arthroplasty: a prospective randomized controlled trial examining the analgesic effectiveness of a combined Adductor Canal peripheral nerve block with periarticular infiltration versus Adductor Canal nerve block alone versus periarticular infiltration alone. Anesth Analg. 2016;122:2040–6.
21. Andersen HL, Andersen SL, Tranum-Jensen J. The spread of injectate during saphenous nerve block at the adductor canal: a cadaver study. Acta Anaesthesiol Scand. 2015;59:238–45.
22. Hjermstad MJ, Fayers PM, Haugen DF, Caraceni A, Hanks GW, Loge JH, Fainsinger R, Aass N, Kaasa S. European palliative care research C: studies comparing numerical rating scales, verbal rating scales, and visual analogue scales for assessment of pain intensity in adults: a systematic literature review. J Pain Symptom Manag. 2011;41:1073–93.
23. Treillet E, Laurent S, Hadjiat Y. Practical management of opioid rotation and equianalgesia. J Pain Res. 2018;11:2587–601.
24. Golembiewski J. Equianalgesic dosing: implications for the perianesthesia setting. J Perianesth Nurs. 2002;17:341–3.
25. Berninger MT, Friederichs J, Leidinger W, Augat P, Buhren V, Fulghum C, Reng W. Effect of local infiltration analgesia, peripheral nerve blocks, general and spinal anesthesia on early functional recovery and pain control in unicompartmental knee arthroplasty. BMC Musculoskelet Disord. 2018;19:249.
26. Andersen HL, Gyrn J, Moller L, Christensen B, Zaric D. Continuous saphenous nerve block as supplement to single-dose local infiltration analgesia for postoperative pain management after total knee arthroplasty. Reg Anesth Pain Med. 2013;38:106–11.
27. Mont MA, Beaver WB, Dysart SH, Barrington JW, Del Gaizo DJ. Local infiltration analgesia with liposomal bupivacaine improves pain scores and reduces opioid use after Total Knee arthroplasty: results of a randomized controlled trial. J Arthroplast. 2018;33:90–6.
28. Sadigursky D, Simoes DP, de Albuquerque RA, Silva MZ, Fernandes RJC, Colavolpe PO. Local periarticular analgesia in Total Knee arthroplasty. Acta Ortop Bras. 2017;25:81–4.
29. Kehlet H, Andersen LO. Local infiltration analgesia in joint replacement: the evidence and recommendations for clinical practice. Acta Anaesthesiol Scand. 2011;55:778–84.
30. Busch CA, Shore BJ, Bhandari R, Ganapathy S, MacDonald SJ, Bourne RB, Rorabeck CH, McCalden RW. Efficacy of periarticular multimodal drug injection in total knee arthroplasty. A randomized trial. J Bone Joint Surg Am. 2006;88:959–63.
31. Sharma S, Iorio R, Specht LM, Davies-Lepie S, Healy WL. Complications of femoral nerve block for total knee arthroplasty. Clin Orthop Relat Res. 2010;468:135–40.
32. Turbitt LR, McHardy PG, Casanova M, Shapiro J, Li L, Choi S. Analysis of inpatient falls after Total Knee arthroplasty in patients with continuous femoral nerve block. Anesth Analg. 2018;127:224–7.
33. Breivik H, Borchgrevink PC, Allen SM, Rosseland LA, Romundstad L, Hals EK, Kvarstein G, Stubhaug A. Assessment of pain. Br J Anaesth. 2008;101:17–24.

34. Hanson NA, Allen CJ, Hostetter LS, Nagy R, Derby RE, Slee AE, Arslan A, Auyong DB. Continuous ultrasound-guided adductor canal block for total knee arthroplasty: a randomized, double-blind trial. Anesth Analg. 2014;118:1370–7.
35. Price AJ, Webb J, Topf H, Dodd CA, Goodfellow JW, Murray DW, Oxford H, Knee G. Rapid recovery after oxford unicompartmental arthroplasty through a short incision. J Arthroplast. 2001;16:970–6.
36. Lum ZC, Lombardi AV, Hurst JM, Morris MJ, Adams JB, Berend KR. Early outcomes of twin-peg mobile-bearing unicompartmental knee arthroplasty compared with primary total knee arthroplasty. Bone Joint J. 2016;98-B(10 Supple B):28–33.
37. Essving P, Axelsson K, Otterborg L, Spannar H, Gupta A, Magnuson A, Lundin A. Minimally invasive surgery did not improve outcome compared to conventional surgery following unicompartmental knee arthroplasty using local infiltration analgesia: a randomized controlled trial with 40 patients. Acta Orthop. 2012;83:634–41.
38. Ilfeld BM, Duke KB, Donohue MC. The association between lower extremity continuous peripheral nerve blocks and patient falls after knee and hip arthroplasty. Anesth Analg. 2010;111:1552–4.
39. Lovald ST, Ong KL, Lau EC, Joshi GP, Kurtz SM, Malkani AL. Readmission and complications for catheter and injection femoral nerve block administration after Total Knee arthroplasty in the Medicare population. J Arthroplast. 2015;30:2076–81.
40. Neal JM, Salinas FV, Choi DS. Local anesthetic-induced myotoxicity after continuous Adductor Canal block. Reg Anesth Pain Med. 2016;41:723–7.
41. Chen J, Lesser JB, Hadzic A, Reiss W, Resta-Flarer F. Adductor canal block can result in motor block of the quadriceps muscle. Reg Anesth Pain Med. 2014;39:170–1.
42. McGuirk S, Fahy C, Costi D, Cyna AM. Use of invasive placebos in research on local anaesthetic interventions. Anaesthesia. 2011;66:84–91.
43. Sites BD, Neal JM. Placebo or intervention? Is it all a sham? Anaesthesia. 2011;66:73–5.
44. Saranteas T, Anagnostis G, Paraskeuopoulos T, Koulalis D, Kokkalis Z, Nakou M, Anagnostopoulou S, Kostopanagiotou G. Anatomy and clinical implications of the ultrasound-guided subsartorial saphenous nerve block. Reg Anesth Pain Med. 2011;36:399–402.
45. Ilfeld BM. Continuous peripheral nerve blocks: an update of the published evidence and comparison with novel, alternative analgesic modalities. Anesth Analg. 2017;124:308–35.
46. Ropivacainehydro chloride Injection. DXY Drugs Information Database. http://drugs.dxy.cn/drug/91500.htm. Accessed 1 June 2016.
47. Bakker SMK, Fenten MGE, Touw DJ, van den Bemt BJF, Heesterbeek PJC, Scheffer GJ, Stienstra R. Pharmacokinetics of 400 mg locally infiltrated Ropivacaine after Total Knee arthroplasty without perioperative tourniquet use. Reg Anesth Pain Med. 2018;43:699–704.
48. Fenten MG, Bakker SM, Touw DJ, van den Bemt BJ, Scheffer GJ, Heesterbeek PJ, Stienstra R. Pharmacokinetics of 400 mg ropivacaine after periarticular local infiltration analgesia for total knee arthroplasty. Acta Anaesthesiol Scand. 2017;61:338–45.
49. Miller RJ, Cameron AJ, Dimech J, Orec RJ, Lightfoot NJ. Plasma Ropivacaine concentrations following local infiltration analgesia in Total Knee arthroplasty: a pharmacokinetic study to determine safety following fixed-dose administration. Reg Anesth Pain Med. 2018;43:347–51.
50. van Haagen MHM, Verburg H, Hesseling B, Coors L, van Dasselaar NT, Langendijk PNJ, Mathijssen NMC. Optimizing the dose of local infiltration analgesia and gabapentin for total knee arthroplasty, a randomized single blind trial in 128 patients. Knee. 2018;25:153–60.

3

The ultrasound-guided proximal intercostal block

Nantthasorn Zinboonyahgoon[1], Panya Luksanapruksa[2], Sitha Piyaselakul[3], Pawinee Pangthipampai[1], Suphalerk Lohasammakul[4], Choopong Luansritisakul[1], Sunsanee Mali-ong[1], Nawaporn Sateantantikul[1], Theera Chueaboonchai[2] and Kamen Vlassakov[5*]

Abstract

Background: The ultrasound-guided proximal intercostal block (PICB) is performed at the proximal intercostal space (ICS) between the internal intercostal membrane (IIM) and the endothoracic fascia/parietal pleura (EFPP) complex. Injectate spread may follow several routes and allow for multilevel trunk analgesia. The goal of this study was to examine the anatomical spread of large-volume PICB injections and its relevance to breast surgery analgesia.

Methods: Fifteen two-level PICBs were performed in ten soft-embalmed cadavers. Radiographic contrast mixed with methylene blue was injected at the 2nd(15 ml) and 4th(25 ml) ICS, respectively. Fluoroscopy and dissection were performed to examine the injectate spread. Additionally, the medical records of 12 patients who had PICB for breast surgery were reviewed for documented dermatomal levels of clinical hypoesthesia. The records of twelve matched patients who had the same operations without PICB were reviewed to compare analgesia and opioid consumption.

Results: Median contrast/dye spread was 4 (2–8) and 3 (2–5) vertebral segments by fluoroscopy and dissection respectively. Dissection revealed injectate spread to the adjacent paravertebral space, T3 (60%) and T5 (27%), and cranio-caudal spread along the endothoracic fascia (80%). Clinically, the median documented area of hypoesthesia was 5 (4–7) dermatomes with 100 and 92% of the injections covering adjacent T3 and T5 dermatomes, respectively. The patients with PICB had significantly lower perioperative opioid consumption and trend towards lower pain scores.

Conclusions: In this anatomical study, PICB at the 2nd and 4th ICS produced lateral spread along the corresponding intercostal space, medial spread to the adjacent paravertebral/epidural space and cranio-caudal spread along the endothoracic fascial plane. Clinically, combined PICBs at the same levels resulted in consistent segmental chest wall analgesia and reduction in perioperative opioid consumption after breast surgery. The incomplete overlap between paravertebral spread in the anatomical study and area of hypoesthesia in our clinical findings, suggests that additional non-paravertebral routes of injectate distribution, such as the endothoracic fascial plane, may play important clinical role in the multi-level coverage provided by this block technique.

Keywords: Nerve block, Paravertebral space, Intercostal space, Intercostal block, Breast surgery

* Correspondence: kvlassakov@bwh.harvard.edu
[5]Department of Anesthesiology, Perioperative and Pain Medicine, Brigham and Women's Hospital, Harvard Medical School, 75 Francis Street, Boston, MA 02115, USA

Background

Regional anesthesia has been consistently associated with superior pain control, lower opioid use and related side effects, when compared to conventional opioid-based analgesia [1–3]. Applicable truncal regional techniques such as paravertebral block and intercostal block have been described [4–7]. The ultrasound-guided thoracic paravertebral block (TPVB) is considered advanced technique [8] due to relative target depth and challenging sonography window, needle visualization [9] and recognized proximity of underlying pleura and lung [10].

The intercostal space (ICS) communicates proximally (medially) with the paravertebral space - as little as 1 ml dye injected into the ICS can spread to the paravertebral space [11]. A larger-volume injection may cause further spread to the paravertebral and/or epidural space, providing multilevel analgesia with 1–2 level injections. The ultrasound-guided proximal intercostal block (PICB) is performed by injecting local anesthetics between the internal intercostal membrane (IIM) and the endothoracic fascia/parietal pleura (EFPP), closely lateral to the tip of the transverse process (TP). While the PICB has been utilized as an alternative technique to TPVB for breast anesthesia/analgesia in our institutions, the exact mechanism of the block has not been elucidated.

The goals of this study were to examine the anatomical spread of PICB injectate and explore its translation into clinical analgesia after breast surgery. The anatomy part of the study assessed the spread of methylene blue and radiographic contrast injection into the IIM-EFPPC plane of cadavers with both fluoroscopy and anatomical dissection. The clinical part consisted of a retrospective medical records review of patients who had undergone breast surgery under general anesthesia (GA) with and without PICB, examining the dermatomal analgesia/hypoesthesia distribution and the analgesic effect of the PICB.

Methods

Anatomy study

After IRB review and exemption, ten cadavers were prepared for the study by soft embalming technique [12]. The cadavers were legally donated to Mahidol University and the donors and their next of kin provided informed consent for the use the cadavers for academic and research purposes during the donation process, all following strictly the institutional and the national protocols and guidelines. Two anesthesiologists trained in regional anesthesia performed PICBs at the 2nd and 4th ICS under real-time ultrasound guidance (SonoSite M-Turbo, linear 38 mm 10–12 MHz transducer, Fujifilm SonoSite, Bothell, WA) and with echogenic needles (22G 50mm, Pajunk® GmbH, Geisingen, Germany The paramedian sagittal scan started by identifying the first rib, then proceeded caudally, to identify the 2nd and the 4th intercostal spaces. The ultrasound probe was then moved medially to identify the tips of the corresponding transverse processes and then moved back laterally to the proximal part of the ICS till optimal sagittal views of ribs, intercostal muscles and parietal pleura were obtained. The needle was inserted in-plane in a caudal-to-cranial direction until its tip was located under the IIM; then, anterior (downward) displacement of EFPP by the injectate provided confirmation of correct needle tip position and satisfactory injection.

The injectate was prepared by mixing a radiographic contrast agent (Ultravist240; Iopromide 240 mg iodine/ml) 30 ml with methylene blue 2 ml and diluted with water to 80 ml. After the needle was in satisfactory position by ultrasound imaging, 15 ml of injectate was injected at the 2nd proximal ICS and 25 ml at the 4th proximal ICS over 1–2 min. Real-time fluoroscopy was performed and recorded immediately after each injection to evaluate the spread of contrast (Fig. 1). The cadavers were then dissected within 1 h to examine the spread of methylene blue in the intercostal, paravertebral and epidural spaces and along the endothoracic fascia plane. The dissection started from the 2nd and 4th ribs and continued towards the corresponding thoracic levels, then extended from the lower cervical spine to the mid-thoracic spine (Figs. 2, 3, 4). The interpretation of the spread of radiographic contrast [13] and methylene blue was determined in consensus by 3 clinicians (NZ, PP, PL). Challenging anatomical spread from the dissection were interpreted by an expert anatomist (SP). Significant spread to the intercostal neurovascular bundle, the paravertebral space or the epidural space was interpreted as coverage of the corresponding vertebral segment. All fluoroscopic and dissection images were deposited in an encrypted computer for subsequent review.

Clinical study

With IRB approval, the research team identified and reviewed the medical records of 12 consecutive patients who had undergone breast surgery under general anesthesia (GA) and PICB retrospectively, in order to compare the documented dermatomal levels of analgesia and hypoesthesia with the block to the results of the anatomical study. As the PICB technique had been introduced to our institution shortly before our study, the effects of the blocks, including dermatomal spread, were being assessed and documented in great detail for quality assurance. In order to compare the analgesic effect to the GA group, we performed sample size calculations, aiming to detect a 50% decrease of pain scores in the PICB group. Kim et al. [14] showed average pain score after mastectomy to be 5/10 with SD of 2/10. Using the software tool nQuery Advisor MTT0–1 (Informer Technologies, Inc., Los Angeles, CA, USA) a sample size of 12 patients per

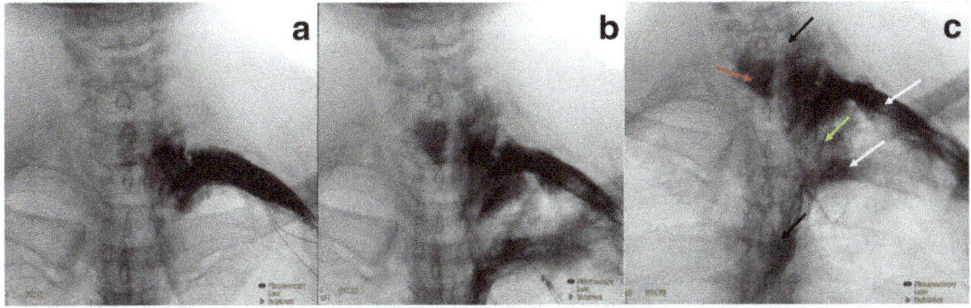

Fig. 1 **a** Fluoroscopic image of 2nd proximal intercostal space injection; **b** Fluoroscopic image after the subsequent 4th proximal intercostal space injection; **c** The final image illustrates the distal (lateral) spread to the left 2nd and 4th intercostal spaces (white arrows), the corresponding ipsilateral paravertebral spread from C6 to T6 (black arrows), contralateral epidural spread (red arrow) and endothoracic plane spread (green arrow)

group was calculated with alpha error of 0.05 and power of 80%.

The PICBs were performed using a SonoSite X-Porte US machine with a linear 38 mm 10–12 MHz ultrasound probe (Fujifilm SonoSite, Bothell, WA) and the 21G 80 mm Sonoplex needle (Pajunk® GmbH, Geisingen, Germany). Blocks were performed with standard ASA monitoring. The scanning and needling techniques were identical as in the anatomical study (Fig. 5). Once the needle was in correct position by US imaging, 10–15 ml and 20–25 ml of 0.25% bupivacaine (bupivacaine is the most affordable and most commonly used long-acting local anesthetic in Thailand), were injected into the 2nd and 4th proximal ICS, respectively (adjusted to the maximum allowable dose per body weight) to produce anterior (downward) displacement of EFPP in confirmation of optimal needle tip position and satisfactory injection.

The research team matched other 12 patients who had had the same operation with the same surgeon under general anesthesia without blocks to compare pain scores and opioids consumption. The statistical analysis included T test for normal distribution and Mann-Whitney U test for non-normal distribution, utilizing PASW statistics software (SPSS) 18.0 (SPSS Inc., Chicago, IL, USA).

All patients received general anesthesia (controlled ventilation with endotracheal tube or laryngeal mask airway). The medication choices were at the discretion of the anesthesiologist including administration of perioperative muscle relaxant, sedative and analgesics. Recorded perioperative opioid administration included all opioids given in the pre-, intra-, and post- operative periods up until discharge from the recovery room, converted to mg morphine equivalent (MME) IV units.

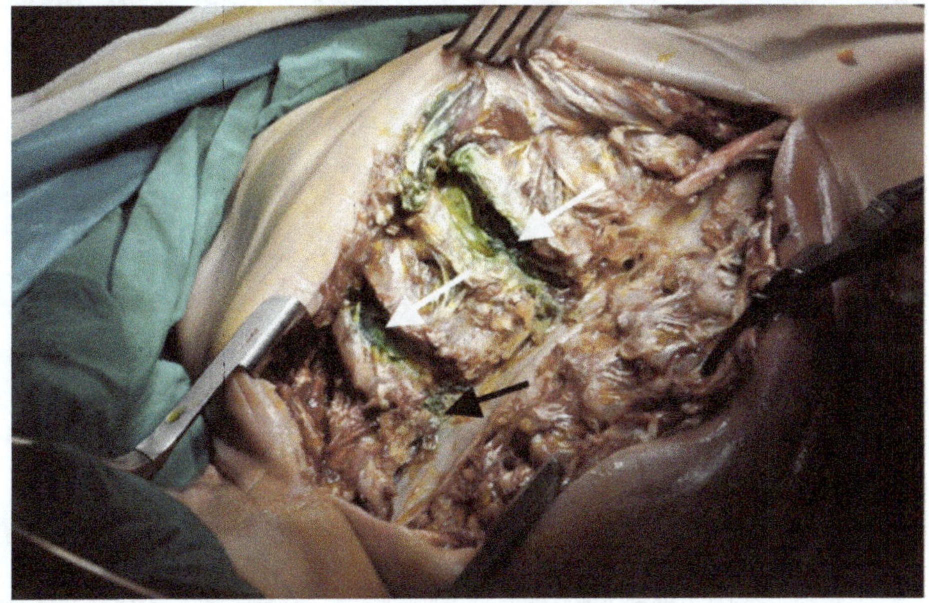

Fig. 2 Dissection revealing 2nd and 4th intercostal space spread (white arrows) and paravertebral spread (black arrow)

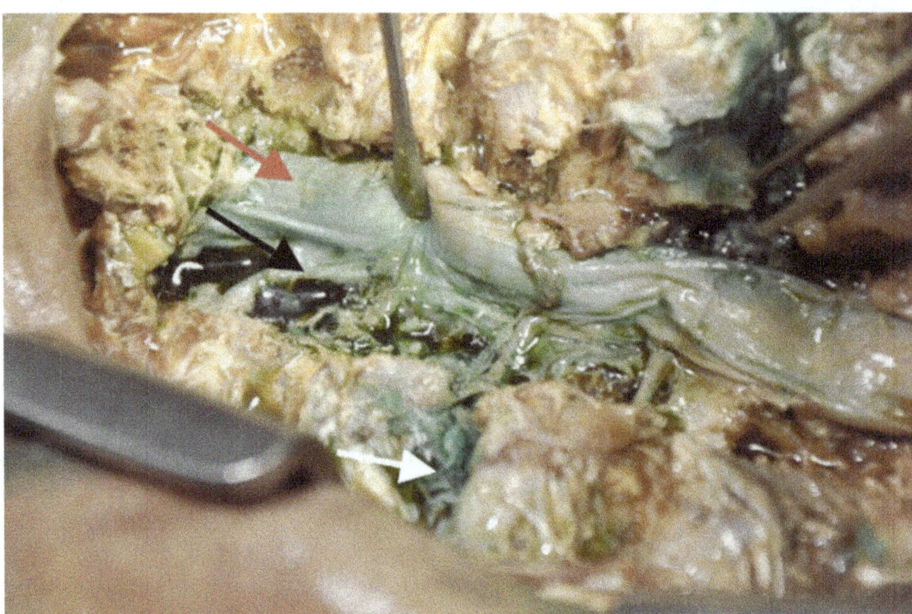

Fig. 3 Dissection demonstrating intercostal neurovascular spread (white arrow), paravertebral spread (black arrow) and staining of the dura mater (epidural spread - red arrow)

Results

Anatomy part

PICB injections were performed in 10 cadavers. Two level injections at 2nd and 4th ICS were performed in 15 chest walls. (The trial injection at other different level (T3 and T5) or TPVBs were excluded). Demographic data and injectate spread interpretation are shown in Table 1. Spinal segments coverage was assessed, separately by fluoroscopy and dissection, for an evidence of intercostal, paravertebral or/and epidural spread. As the contrast spread was interpreted with real-time fluoroscopy, whereas the anatomical dissection was performed 1 h later, discrepancies between fluoroscopic and anatomical findings could be due in part to this time gap. The median PICB coverage was 4 (range 2–8) vertebral segments by fluoroscopy and 3 (range 2–5) segments by dissection (Table 1).

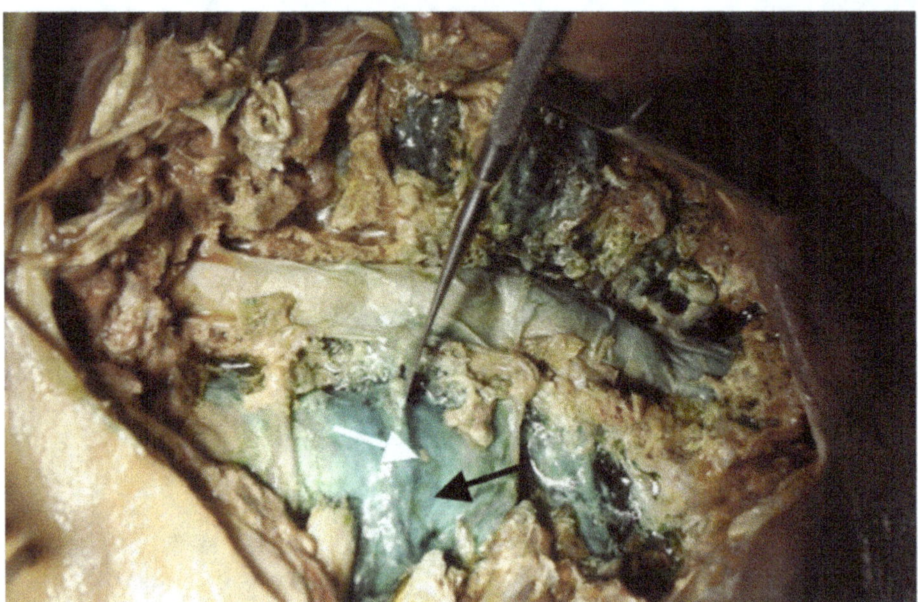

Fig. 4 Dissection revealing trans-segmental EFPP spread (black arrow); the underlying visceral pleura showed no methylene blue staining as seen via the small opening deliberately created during the dissection (white arrow)

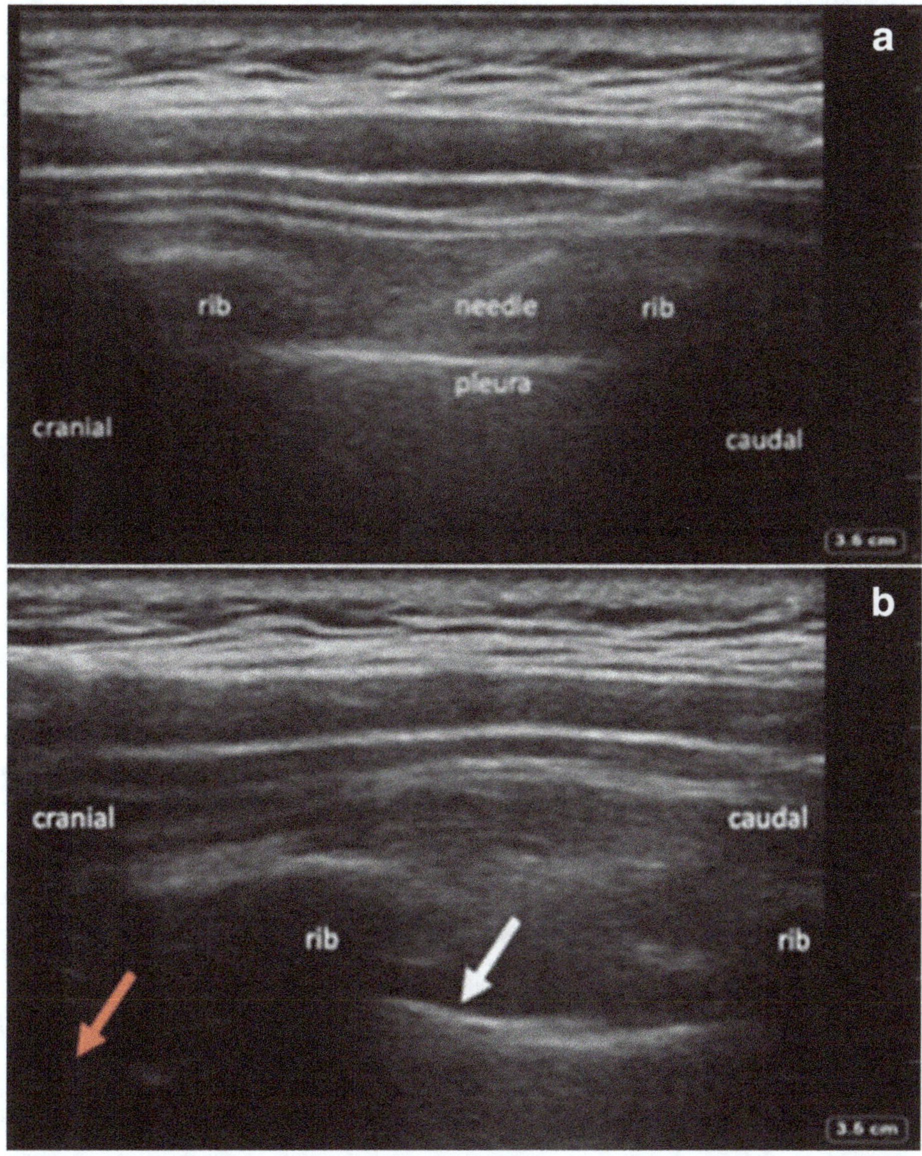

Fig. 5 Saved ultrasound images of PICB in one of the patients from the clinical study. **a** Upper image shows the needle tip near the caudal border of the 4th rib, and just underneath the internal intercostal membrane. **b** Image below shows the anterior displacement of endothoracic fascia and parietal pleura at the level of injection (white arrow) and the next level cranially (red arrow)

T2 and T4 levels were covered 100% by intercostal spread, by both fluoroscopy and dissection. However, adjacent T3 paravertebral/epidural spread was 53% (fluoroscopy) and 60% (dissection), whereas adjacent T5 level coverage was 67% (fluoroscopy) and 27% (dissection) (Fig. 6).

Eighty percent (12 of 15 specimens) of the dissections showed methylene blue staining of the endothoracic fascia at least from 2nd to 5th ICS, without any staining of the visceral pleura (Fig. 4). Three specimens revealed no endothoracic or ICS spread, but extensive paraspinal muscle staining.

The average distances from midline (spinous processes) to needle entry points were 4.35+/− 1.06 cm at the 2ndICS and 3.8+/− 1.13 cm at the 4thICS. The average depth (measured by ultrasound perpendicularly from skin to the tip of the needle in final position) was 2.01+/− 0.56 cm at the 2ndICS and 1.72+/− 0.40 cm at the 4thICS. The average needle visualization, by needle visualization score was fair. (Graded by 0 = poor needle visualization, 1 = fair needle visualization, 2 = good needle visualization. The scores were 1.00+/− 0.71 for the 2ndICS and 1.15+/− 0.80 for the 4thICS).

Clinical part

The demographic data and the dermatomal hyposesthesia/analgesia distribution in the 12 patients who underwent

Table 1 Demographic data of cadaver and injectate spread observed by fluoroscopy and dissection

Body	Injection number	Sex	Age (years)	Height (cm)	Side	Intercostal, paravertebral or epidural spread by fluoroscopy (segment)	Intercostal, paravertebral or epidural spread by dissection (segment)	Endothoracic spread from dissection
1	1	M	67	160	Right	C7-T6 (7)	T1-T4 (4)	yes
2	2	M	70	162	Right	T2-T6 (5)	T1-T5 (5)	yes
3	3	F	84	146	Left	C7-T6 (7)	T2-T5 (3)	yes
3	4	F	84	146	Right	T2-T5 (4)	T2-T4 (3)	yes
4	5	M	47	175	Left	T2-T5 (4)	T2, T4 (2)	yes
4	6	M	47	175	Right	T2, T4-T5 (3)	T2-T4 (3)	yes
5	7	M	77	174	Left	T2, T4 (2)	T2-T4 (3)	yes
5	8	M	77	174	Right	T2, T4 (2)	T2-T4 (3)	yes
6	9	M	57	162	Left	T2, T4-T5 (3)	T2, T4 (2)	no
6	10	M	57	162	Right	T2, T4 (2)	T2, T4 (2)	no
7	11	M	72	153	Left	T2, T4-T6 (4)	T2, T4-T6 (4)	yes
7	12	M	72	153	Right	T2-T4 (3)	T2-T4 (3)	yes
8	13	M	65	110	Left	T2, T4 (2)	T2, T4 (2)	no
9	14	NA	NA	NA	Right	C6-T6 (8)	T1, T2, T4 (3)	yes
10	15	NA	NA	NA	Left	T2-T5 (4)	T2-T5 (4)	yes

breast surgeries with PICB are presented in Table 2. There were no observed and reported procedure-related complications in the patients who received PICB.

The documented median hypoesthesia area was 5 dermatomes (range 4–7 dermatomes) and the distribution is shown in Fig. 7.

Table 3 presents demographic data of matched patients without PICB. There were no statistically significant differences in age, weight, height and BMI between the patient groups (*P* values = 0.63, 0.11, 0.57 and 0.14 respectively).

The comparison of pain scores and opioid consumption between 12 patients receiving PICB and general anesthesia (GA) and 12 matched patients receiving GA alone (same operation performed by the same surgeon), is presented in Table 4.

Discussion

Truncal regional anesthesia techniques such as TPVB and the classic intercostal blocks have been utilized for anesthesia and/or analgesia for patients undergoing breast surgery [2, 4, 5]. Recent evidence also suggests that regional anesthesia techniques could potentially reduce the incidence of chronic postsurgical pain and even influence cancer recurrence [1, 15, 16]. However, TPVB is considered advanced regional anesthetic technique [8]

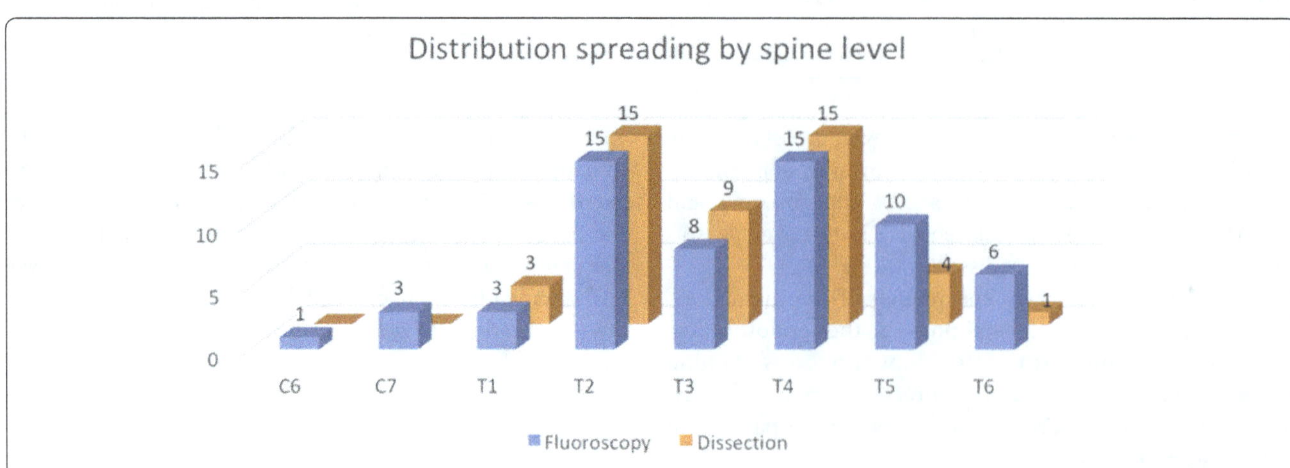

Fig. 6 Distribution of radiographic contrast by fluoroscopy (blue) and of methylene blue by dissection (orange) from 15 two-level injections in cadavers, by spine segmental level

Table 2 Demographic data, type of operation, amount of local anesthetic and dermatomal level after proximal intercostal space block

Patient	Age (years)	BMI (kg/m^2)	Operation	Dermatomal level	Amount of 0.25% bupivacaine (2nd/4th ICB, ml)
1	47	22	MRM	T1-T5	10/20
2	51	21	WE with SLNB	T2-T6	15/20
3	60	27	WE with needle localize	T2-T6	15/25
4	48	28	TM with SLNB	T2-T5	15/25
5	49	27	TM with ALND	T1-T6	15/25
6	53	28	TM	T1-T6	15/25
7	44	25	TM with SLNB	T1-T6	15/25
8	61	23	lumpectomy with ALND	T1-T5	10/20
9	50	17	MRM	T1-T5	10/20
10	77	27	TM with SLNB	T2-T5	15/25
11	52	32	lumpectomy with SLNB	C6-T3	15/25
12	63	28	TM with SLNB	C8-T6	15/25

TM total mastectomy, *MRM* modified radical mastectomy, *WE* wide excision, *SLNB* sentinel lymph node biopsy, *ALND* axillary lymph node dissection. In order to maintain the patients' anonymity, we present BMI rounded to the nearest whole number, instead of individual weight and height in exact numbers

and technically challenging due to difficulties with needle visualization [9] and identification of important collateral structures such as pleura, lung [10]. The classic intercostal nerve block is performed by landmark technique along the mid-axillary line and is considered an intermediate-difficulty technique [8]. Usually, it provides only single-dermatome analgesia per injection, therefore necessitating multiple injections to achieve analgesia for breast surgery [5]. This can be time-consuming and associated with more patient discomfort and procedural risks.

The proximal portion of the ICS (between the tip of the transverse process medially and the costal angle laterally) contains the intercostal nerves and communicates with the paravertebral space medially. Paraskeuopoulos et al. have demonstrated that as little as 1 ml methylene blue injected into the ICS 5 cm lateral to the spinous processes can spread to the paravertebral space [11]. Therefore, a larger volume PICB may result in spread into the paravertebral space and even the epidural space, providing multilevel analgesia with 1–2 level injections [17] offering alternative to TPVB.

As the breast is mainly innervated by T2-T5 spinal nerves [3] and the axilla (intercostobrachial nerve, T2) is a common site of persistent pain after axillary node dissection [18]; we utilize a combined 2nd/4th PICB technique for analgesia after breast surgery. Since pilot single-level cadaver injections demonstrated only 1–3 level spread per injection, the subsequent injections were performed with combined two-level injections, reflected in our current clinical practice. Hypothesizing that the ICSs are smaller cranially, we arbitrarily chose 15 and 25 ml for 2nd and 4th PICB, respectively. Real-time fluoroscopy demonstrated contrast consistently spreading beyond the ICS after the first 5 ml, concordant with the anatomy findings by Moorthy et al. [19] that intercostal injectate of 5 ml

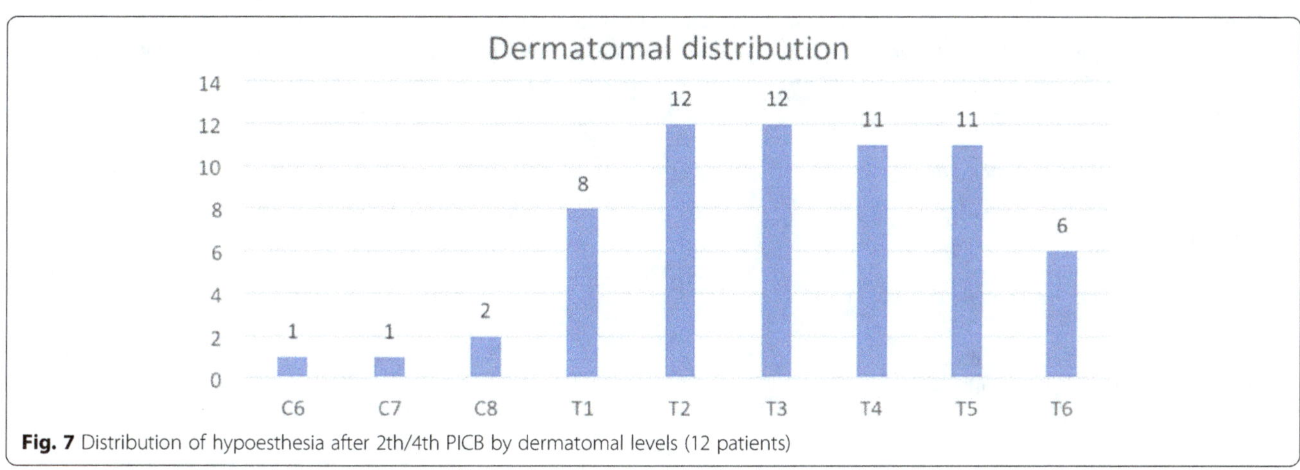

Fig. 7 Distribution of hypoesthesia after 2th/4th PICB by dermatomal levels (12 patients)

Table 3 Demographic data and type of operation of matched patients

Patient	Age (years)	BMI (kg/m^2)	Operation
1	56	27	MRM
2	63	30	WE with SLNB
3	43	26	WE with needle localize
4	38	20	TM with SLNBx
5	31	35	TM with ALND
6	74	36	TM
7	68	33	TM with SLNBx
8	46	28	Lumpectomy with SLNB with ALND
9	55	25	MRM
10	64	33	TM with SLNBx
11	41	24	lumpectomy with SLNB
12	49	22	TM with SLNB with ALND

TM total mastectomy, *MRM* modified radical mastectomy, *WE* wide excision, *SLNB* sentinel lymph node biopsy, *ALND* axillary lymph node dissection. In order to maintain the patients' anonymity, we present BMI rounded to the nearest whole number, instead of individual weight and height in exact numbers

is confined to one ICS, whereas 10 ml spread outside the injected ICS via the potential space between the pleura and the internal intercostal muscle.

The PICBs produced consistent distribution within the injected intercostal space (100% at 2nd and 4th intercostal space) but demonstrated great variability in paravertebral spread (0–7 segments), similar to the variability of paravertebral spread in TPVB described in previous studies [20, 21]. In our results, the discrepancy between paravertebral spread by anatomy dissection (60% in T3 and 27% in T5) and area of hypoesthesia in clinical finding (100% in T3 and 92% in T5 dermatome) leaves many questions. First, the sensory block area in clinical practice and the methylene blue and contrast media distribution in cadavers, may not be comparable due to different injectate viscosities and solubilities, different injection rates and pressures, and different tissue density in vivo and postmortem. Second, the ability to assess separately T3 or T5 dermatome sensation, especially when T2 and T4 dermatomes are anesthetized, is limited. Finally, while we originally hypothesized that the PICB causes multi-level analgesia through medial communication with the paravertebral space, it is plausible to consider additional non-paravertebral route(s) of distribution.

Our dissections revealed methylene blue spread inside the respective intercostal spaces and along the investing tissues around the injection sites in 80% of the specimens. The endothoracic fascia is interposed between the parietal pleura and the superior costotransverse ligament and extends laterally as an intervening fascia between pleura and internal intercostal membrane. The absence of dye on the visceral pleura and the underlying lung surface (Fig. 4) suggests that the injectate spreads above the parietal pleura and the investing layer is the endothoracic fascia. Since the confirmatory sign of a successful ultrasound-guided PICB injection is the anterior displacement of the pleura, the injectate spreads most likely in the IIM-EFPP plane. Moorthy et al. [19] demonstrated that a 10 ml of intercostal injection can cause multilevel spread (average area of spread of 51.1+/ 19 cm^2) through the potential space between the pleura and the internal intercostal muscle, which supports this hypothesis. The three dissections which revealed no endothoracic or adjacent ICS spread, but extensive paraspinal muscle staining might be explained with inadvertently shallow needle placement causing injectate spread into muscle instead of endothoracic fascia plane. Predictable 2nd and 4th intercostal distribution combined with paravertebral and endothoracic fascia plane spread may present a plausible complex model for reliable dermatomal coverage of PICB in the clinical finding. The multiple anatomical routes of injectate distribution with PICB, influenced particularly by the block needle tip position relative to the internal intercostal membrane, may provide

Table 4 Postoperative analgesic effects of Proximal intercostal block (PICB); a comparison between PICB plus general anesthesia versus general anesthesia alone. Peri-operative opioids consumption includes opioids used during the intraoperative period and in the recovery room. Short-acting opioids include intravenous fentanyl. Long-acting opioids include intravenous morphine and meperidine

Pain scores, opioids consumption and PACU stay	GA with PICB (median/ percentile; P25, P75)	GA without PICB (median/ percentile; P25, P75)	*P* value
Initial numeric rating pain score in PACU (0–10)	0 (0,2.50)	0 (0,7.50)	0.671
Numeric rating pain score before discharge from PACU (0–10)	2.5 (0,3)	3.0 (2,4)	0.143
Total peri-operative opioids consumption (short and long acting opioids; intravenous morphine equivalent, mg)	7 (3.13,10.13)	11 (10,14.75)	0.004
Total peri-operative opioids consumption (long acting opioids; intravenous morphine equivalent, mg)	1 (0,2)	6 (2.50, 9.75)	0.003
PACU stay (minutes)	80 (71.25,105.00)	75 (71.25,90)	0.671

possible explanations to the inter-individual variability in segmental spread and ultimately, in clinical coverage.

Potential advantages of the PICB over TPVB (both with paramedian sagittal US scanning), include superior US-visualization of pleura and block needle due to shorter skin-to-target distance and more perpendicular US beam-to-pleura/needle orientation (unpublished data). Additionally, the longer distance of block needle from spinal canal may hypothetically convey improved safety, especially in patients who are at increased risk of bleeding complications.

Our clinical findings suggest that high-volume two-level PICBs consistently produce sensory block in dermatomes relevant to adequate analgesia after breast surgery, and could logically decrease pain and opioid consumption after mastectomy and lumpectomy. The surprisingly low median pain scores on arrival to recovery room in both groups are likely due to a combination of residual general anesthetic effect, the effect of other analgesics administered in the operating room and even individual pain thresholds. Our study was not designed and powered to examine differences in pain scores and only demonstrated a trend towards lower pain scores in the PICB group. As the shortcomings of our clinical study stem from its retrospective design with no anesthetic/analgesic standardization, well-controlled prospective trials are needed to further evaluate the analgesic, anesthetic and recovery profiles of PICB.

The discrepancy between the observed segmental spread by fluoroscopy (2–8 vertebral segments) and dissection (2–5 vertebral segments) may also seem surprising. Among the logical explanations, two appear most plausible: [1] while the contrast spread was interpreted with real-time fluoroscopy, the anatomical dissections were performed 1 h later, therefore discrepancies between fluoroscopic and anatomical findings could be due in part to this time gap; [2] it is also possible that some of the contrast spread in the paraspinous musculature could have been overinterpreted by antero-posterior fluoroscopy as "clinically useful" distribution in the paravertebral, intercostal and endothoracic fascia planes.

Conclusions

Large-volume ultrasound-guided proximal intercostal blocks, performed at the 2nd and 4th intercostal spaces, produced a predictable lateral injectate spread along the corresponding intercostal neurovascular bundle, a less consistent medial spread to the adjacent paravertebral/epidural spaces and a contiguous endothoracic fascia plane distribution in the anatomy study. The incomplete overlap of anatomical paravertebral spread and dermatomal distribution of clinical hypoesthesia suggests additional non-paravertebral route of injectate spread, including the endothoracic fascia plane, confirmed by the staining patterns in the anatomy specimens.

Abbreviations

ASA: American Society of Anesthesiologists; BMI: Body Mass Index; EFPP: Endothoracic fascia/parietal pleura; GA: General anesthesia; ICS: Intercostal space; IIM: Internal intercostal membrane; PICB: Ultrasound-guided proximal intercostal block; T: Thoracic (referring to vertebral/segmental or dermatomal level); TP: Transverse process; TPVB: Ultrasound-guided thoracic paravertebral block

Acknowledgements

The authors would like to thank Ms. Natnicha Sriburiruk for her contributions to statistical analysis, manuscript editing, and journal submission.

Authors' contributions

NZ: study design, cadaveric injections, analysis, manuscript preparation, principal investigator; PL: dissections; SP: body preparation, major contributions to and discussion of anatomical part; PP: cadaveric injections, contribution to regional anesthesia technique and clinical cases; SL: data collection; CL: cadaveric injections, contribution to regional anesthesia technique and clinical cases; SM: data analysis; NS: data collection (retrospective clinical data) and analysis; TC: dissections; KV: study design, manuscript preparation, major contributions to overall project. All authors have read and approved the manuscript.

Author details

[1]Department of Anesthesiology, Siriraj Hospital, Mahidol University, 2 Phranok road, Bangkoknoi 10700, Thailand. [2]Department of Orthopedic Surgery Siriraj Hospital, Mahidol University, 2 Phranok road, Bangkoknoi 10700, Thailand. [3]Department of Anatomy, Siriraj Hospital, Mahidol University, 2 Phranok road, Bangkoknoi 10700, Thailand. [4]Department of Surgery, Siriraj Hospital, Mahidol University, 2 Phranok road, Bangkoknoi 10700, Thailand. [5]Department of Anesthesiology, Perioperative and Pain Medicine, Brigham and Women's Hospital, Harvard Medical School, 75 Francis Street, Boston, MA 02115, USA.

References

1. Amaya F, Hosokawa T, Okamoto A, et al. Can acute pain treatment reduce postsurgical comorbidity after breast Cancer surgery? A literature review. Biomed Res Int. 2015;2015:Article ID 641508.
2. Schnabel A, Reichl SU, Kranke P, et al. Efficacy and safety of paravertebral blocks in breast surgery: a meta-analysis of randomized controlled trials. Br J Anaesth. 2010;105(6):842–52.
3. Woodworth G, Ivie R, Nelson S, Walker C, Maniker R. Perioperative breast analgesia, a qualitative review of anatomy and regional techniques. Reg Anesth Pain Med. 2017;42:609–31.
4. Abdallah FW, Morgan PJ, Cil T, et al. Ultrasound-guided multilevel paravertebral blocks and total intravenous anesthesia improve the quality of recovery after ambulatory breast tumor resection. Anesthesiology. 2014;120(3):703–13.
5. Kolawole IK, Adesina MD, Olaoye IO. Intercostal nerves block for mastectomy in two patients with advanced breast malignancy. J Natl Med Assoc. 2006;98(3):450–3.
6. Shibata Y, Nishiwaki K. Ultrasound-guided intercostal approach to thoracic paravertebral block. Anesth Analg. 2009;109(3):996–7.
7. Ben-Ari A, Moreno M, Chelly JE, Bigeleisen PE. Ultrasound-guided paravertebral block using an intercostal approach. Anesth Analg. 2009;109(5):1691–4.
8. Hargett MJ, Beckman JD, Liguori GA, Neal JM. Education Committee in the Department of anesthesiology at Hospital for Special Surgery. Guidelines for regional anesthesia fellowship training. Reg Anesth Pain Med. 2005;30(3):218–25.
9. O'Riain SC, Donnell BO, Cuffe T, et al. Thoracic paravertebral block using real-time ultrasound guidance. Anesth Analg. 2010;110(1):248–51.
10. Karmakar MK. Ultrasound guided thoracic paravertebral block. In: Karmakar MK, editor. Musculoskeletal ultrasound for regional anesthesia and pain medicine. 2nd ed. Hong Kong: Department of anaesthesia and intensive care the Chinese university of Hong Kong; 2016. p. 345–69.
11. Paraskeuopoulos T, Saranteas T, Kouladouros K, et al. Thoracic paravertebral spread using two different ultrasound-guided intercostal injection techniques in human cadavers. Clin Anat. 2010;23(7):840–7.
12. Thiel W. The preservation of the whole corpse with natural color [article in

German]. Ann Anat. 1992;174(3):185–95.

13. Marhofer P, Kettner SC, Hajbok L, et al. Lateral ultrasound-guided paravertebral blockade: an anatomical-based description of a new technique. Br J Anaesth. 2010;105(4):526–32.
14. Kim SH, Oh YJ, Park BW, Sim J, Choi YS. Effects of single-dose dexmedetomidine on the quality of recovery after modified radical mastectomy: a randomized controlled trial. Minerva Anestesiol. 2013;79(11):1248–58.
15. Exadaktylos AK, Buggy DJ, Moriarty DC, Mascha E, Sessler DI. Can anesthetic technique for primary breast cancer surgery affect recurrence or metastasis? Anesthesiology. 2006;105(4):660–4.
16. Deegan CA, Murray D, Doran P, Ecimovic P, Moriarty DC, Buggy DJ. Effect of anaesthetic technique on oestrogen receptor-negative breast cancer cell function in vitro. Br J Anaesth. 2009;103(5):685–90.
17. Hadzic A. Intercostal block. In: Hadzic A, editor. Hadzic's peripheral nerve blocks and anatomy for ultrasound-guided regional anesthesia, vol. 303-310. New York: McGrawHill Medical; 2012. p. 303–10.
18. Bruce J, Thornton AJ, Scott NW, Marfizo S, Powell R, Johnston M, Wells M, Heys SD, Thompson AM. Chronic preoperative pain and psychological robustness predict acute postoperative pain outcomes after surgery for breast cancer. Br J Cancer. 2012;107(6):937–46.
19. Moorthy SS, Dierdorf SF, Yaw PB. Influence of volume on the spread of local anesthetic-methylene blue solution after injection for intercostal block. Anesth Analg. 1992;75(3):389-91.
20. Cheema SP, Ilsley D, Richardson J, Sabanathan S. A thermographic study of paravertebral analgesia. Anaesthesia. 1995;50:118–21.
21. Karmakar MK, Critchley LA, Ho AM, et al. Continuous thoracic paravertebral infusion of bupivacaine for pain management in patients with multiple fractured ribs. Chest. 2003;123(2):424–31.

4

Effect of baseline cognitive impairment on association between predicted propofol effect site concentration and bispectral index or sedation score

Frederick Sieber[1*], Karin Neufeld[2], Esther S. Oh[3], Allan Gottschalk[4] and Nae-Yuh Wang[5]

Abstract

Background: This study determined whether the relationship between predicted propofol effect site concentration (Ce) and observer's assessment of alertness/sedation scale (OAA/S) or Bispectral Index (BIS) was similar comparing cognitively intact vs impaired patients undergoing hip fracture repair with spinal anesthesia and sedation.

Methods: Following informed consent baseline mini-mental status exam (MMSE), Clinical Dementia Rating (CDR) and geriatric depression scale (GDS) were obtained. Intraoperatively OAA/S, BIS, and propofol (timing and exact amounts) administered were recorded. Cerebrospinal fluid was collected for Alzheimer's (AD) biomarkers. Mean Ce level (AvgCe) during surgery was calculated using the area under the Ce measurement series from incision to closure, divided by surgical time. Average OAA/S (AvgOAA/S), and BIS (AvgBIS) were similarly calculated. Pearson correlations of AvgCe with AvgOAA/S and AvgBIS were calculated overall and by CDR. Nonparametric locally weighted scatterplot smoothing (LOWESS) fits of AvgOAA/S and AvgBIS on AvgCe were produced, stratified by CDR. Multivariable regression incorporating baseline cognitive measurements or AD biomarkers assessed AvgOAA/S or AvgBIS associations with AvgCe.

Results: In 186 participants AvgBIS and AvgOAA/S correlated with AvgCe (Pearson $\rho = -0.72$; $p < 0.0001$ and Pearson $\rho = -0.81$; $p < 0.0001$, respectively), and remained unchanged across CDR levels. Association patterns of AvgOAA/S or AvgBIS on AvgCe guided by LOWESS fits and modeled through regression, were similar when stratified by CDR ($p = 0.16$). Multivariable modeling found no independent effect on AvgBIS or AvgOAA/S by MMSE, CDR, GDS, or AD biomarkers after accounting for AvgCe.

Conclusions: When administering sedation in conjunction with spinal anesthesia, cognitive impairment does not affect the relationship between predicted propofol AvgCe and AvgOAA/S or AvgBIS.

Keywords: Propofol, Deep sedation, Conscious sedation, Cognitive dysfunction, Hip fractures, Bispectral index, observer's assessment of alertness and sedation (OAA/S), Geriatric anesthesia

* Correspondence: fsieber1@jhmi.edu
[1]Department of Anesthesiology and Critical Care Medicine, Johns Hopkins Bayview Medical Center, 4940 Eastern Avenue, Baltimore, MD 21224, USA

Background

As the population ages, the prevalence of dementia is increasing. Alzheimer's disease (AD), the most common form of dementia in the United States (U.S.), is estimated to affect 5.7 million individuals in 2018, and the annual incidence is expected to double by 2050 [1]. Nearly one third of all people 85 years and older have AD, and it is thought that a large fraction of those that remain undiagnosed possess varying degrees of subclinical AD pathology [2]. In adults≥65 years of age undergoing surgery, preoperative cognitive dysfunction, including dementia, is common [3–5]. For instance, in the hip fracture population, dementia prevalence has been reported to be 33% [6]. Despite the increasing numbers of patients with cognitive impairment undergoing surgery, the literature provides little guidance concerning their anesthetic management. Specifically, it is unclear whether during maintenance of sedation cognitive impairment alters the relationship between predicted effect site concentration and clinically observed Bispectral Index number or sedation score.

Previous investigations examining maintenance anesthetic requirements studied general anesthesia and report no difference in sensitivity to inhalational agents [7] or infusion rate requirements with total intravenous anesthesia [8] comparing patients with and without cognitive dysfunction. While general anesthesia is certainly important to study, the number of procedures utilizing propofol as the primary means of providing procedural sedation or sedation in conjunction with regional anesthesia is enormous. However, there is little information concerning clinical anesthetic dosing requirements in patients with cognitive dysfunction during propofol sedation. We therefore performed a secondary analysis of the STRIDE (A Strategy to Reduce the Incidence of Postoperative Delirium in Elderly Patients) trial data to test the hypothesis that the clinical anesthetic dosing requirements during propofol sedation are similar comparing patients with and without cognitive impairment. The aim of this study was to determine if the relationship between predicted propofol effect site concentration (Ce) and the modified observer's assessment of alertness/sedation scale (OAA/S) [9] or Bispectral index ((BIS) Brain Monitoring System, http://www.medtronic.com/covidien/products/brainmonitoring) number was similar during maintenance of sedation comparing cognitively intact versus cognitively impaired participants.

Methods

Study design and participants

The STRIDE trial was a randomized, two-group, parallel, superiority trial whose principal objective was to assess the effectiveness of lighter versus heavier sedation during spinal anesthesia in elderly patients undergoing hip fracture repair. The trial was first registered at ClinicalTrials.gov under registration number NCT00590707 on 1/2008. Johns Hopkins IRB approval was obtained for the prospective STRIDE trial on 9/27/2010 (NA_00041873). All participants provided their written informed consent.

The primary outcome of the STRIDE trial was the impact of the intervention on the incidence of delirium during postoperative Day 1 to Day 5 or to hospital discharge, whichever occurs first. These results have been previously reported [10, 11]. In short, no overall difference in the incidence of postoperative in-hospital delirium was found between the intervention groups, but a significant effect modification by level of comorbidity was observed, where lighter sedation imparts lower in-hospital delirium risk in patients with low pre-operative comorbidity [10]. In addition, when comparing lighter versus heavier sedation, there is no difference in mortality or functional outcomes of elderly hip fracture patients 1 year after surgery [11]. STRIDE was conducted at a single clinical center. A detailed description of the entire trial protocol was published previously in the supplemental material of Li et al. [12].

Briefly, patients ≥65 years old who were undergoing hip fracture repair with spinal anesthesia and propofol sedation and who did not have preoperative delirium or severe dementia were randomized to receive either heavier (OAA/S 0–2) or lighter (OAA/S 3–5) intraoperative sedation. The inclusion criteria were 1) admission to Johns Hopkins Bayview Medical Center for surgical repair of traumatic hip fracture; 2) 65 years of age or older; 3) a preoperative mini-mental status exam (MMSE) [13] score of 15 or higher; and 4) receiving spinal anesthesia. The exclusion criteria included 1) receiving general anesthesia; 2) inability to speak or understand English; 3) severe chronic obstructive pulmonary disease or congestive heart failure; 4) refusal to give informed consent; 5) non-participating attending surgeon; 6) hip fractures in both hips on same admission; 7) repair of another fracture concurrently with the hip fracture; 8) prior hip surgery on the same hip to be repaired in the current surgery; and 9) preoperative delirium.

Data collection at baseline prior to surgery

Prior to surgery, baseline MMSE, modified Clinical Dementia Rating (CDR) as previously described [14], geriatric depression scale (GDS) [15], and Charlson comorbidity index (CCI) [16] were obtained, in addition to demographic information. CDR was adjudicated by a consensus diagnosis panel [10]. CDR scores were classified as follows: 0 = normal, 0.5 = mild cognitive impairment, ≥1 = dementia. Evaluations using Confusion Assessment Method (CAM) [17], Delirium Rating Scale-R-98 (DRS-R-98) [18], and abbreviated digit span test (DST) were also collected at baseline and used to confirm absence of preoperative delirium.

Intervention

After satisfactory administration of spinal anesthesia, the patient was randomly assigned to one of two groups in blocks with equal allocation, stratified by age and MMSE at baseline. Intra-operatively, one group had the depth of sedation maintained at an OAA/S score of 0–2. This was the heavier sedation group. Patients in the other group had the depth of sedation maintained at an OAA/S score of 3–5. This was the lighter sedation group.

Data collection during surgery

The propofol was titrated individually for each participant to achieve and maintain the depth of sedation required by that participant's assigned treatment group (lighter or heavier sedation). The depth of sedation for all participants was measured by the OAA/S, administered every 15 min intra-operatively. During the intraoperative study period, the BIS was also recorded. The BIS monitor readout was covered throughout the surgery so that the Study Anesthesiologist/Anesthetist remained masked to the BIS values while administering propofol. The BIS readings served as an independent measure of the level of adherence to the trial interventions. Mean arterial blood pressure (MAP) was measured via oscillotonometry every 5 min, and automatically recorded in the electronic medical record. After surgery, the MAP values were abstracted and entered into the database. After surgery, the BIS values were abstracted, matched in time to their corresponding MAP values, and entered into the database at 5 min intervals. During surgery propofol was administered intravenously using the Alaris PC 8100 series infusion pump which gives continuous output of total volume (ml) infused. A continuous download of total propofol volume infused was obtained for each study case. From this data, the predicted propofol Ce was calculated on a minute by minute basis using the method of Schnider et al. [19]. Ce values were then matched in time to their corresponding MAP values and entered into the database at 5-min intervals.

Mean predicted Ce level (AvgCe) during surgery for each participant was calculated based on the area under the Ce measurement series from incision to end of surgery, divided by the surgery time --- the length of time between incision and end of surgery. Average OAA/S (AvgOAA/S), BIS (AvgBIS) and MAP (AvgMAP) levels during surgery were calculated using the same approach. The Ce values matched in time to the corresponding MAP values were used in the calculation of avgCe. Similarly, the BIS and OAA/S values matched in time to the corresponding MAP values were used in the calculation of avgBIS and avgOAA/S, respectively.

Prior to the administration of spinal anesthesia, approximately 6 cc of cerebrospinal fluid (CSF) was collected and stored for later analysis of AD biomarkers [14].

Statistical analysis

Distributions of baseline characteristics before surgery and measurements during surgery were described. Mean and standard deviations (SDs) were calculated for continuous variables and frequency distributions (n and %) were reported for categorical variables. Potential level of systematic bias in using AvgOAA/S and AvgBIS as proxy measures of AvgCe during surgery were assessed using Bland-Altman (B-A) plots. Given that AvgOAA/S and AvgBIS were both significantly correlated with AvgCe with negative correlations, reversed variables (5-AvgOAA/S and 100-AvgBIS, respectively) were used in the B-A analysis. Due to the differences in range of score for these 3 variables, all three variables were also standardized to have mean = 0 and SD = 1 to produce the B-A plots. Pearson correlations were calculated overall and by CDR and CCI levels. To explore whether the associations between AvgOAA/S or AvgBIS and AvgCe were influenced by cognitive measurement or comorbidity, nonparametric locally weighted scatterplot smoothing (LOWESS) fits of AvgOAA/S and AvgBIS on AvgCe were produced, stratified by the CDR score levels (0, 0.5, and ≥ 1). Similar LOWESS fits were also derived according to the CCI levels (0, 1, 2, and > 2). For ease of interpretation, nonlinear associations suggested by the LOWESS fit were approximated by linear or segmental linear models, as appropriate, in subsequent regression analyses. To better understand the relationship between AvgOAA/S or AvgBIS and AvgCe, multivariable regression analyses incorporating baseline cognitive measurements or CSF biomarkers as potential effect modifiers were performed to assess potential differentiation of associations of AvgOAA/S and AvgBIS with AvgCe by levels of these variables. Analyses were carried out using SAS 9.4, and an estimated association or interaction with p-value < 0.05 was considered statistically significant.

Results

Table 1 shows the baseline characteristics for this patient group. Exact timing of propofol change in infusion rates and boluses was recorded in 186/200 participants. Thus, we focused the analyses on these 186 participants. BIS data was not recorded in $n = 3$ and baseline CDR was not completed in $n = 2$ patients. As an ancillary study to the main STRIDE trial, cerebrospinal fluid biomarkers were obtained in $n = 178$ patients. No statistically significant difference in baseline characteristics between these 186 participants and those 14 patients who did not have predicted Ce measurement was noted (Table 1).

Systematic bias of OAA/S and BIS measurements against Ce

Over the observed range of AvgOAA/S or AvgBIS, no systematic bias in using them as proxy measures of AvgCe during surgery was found (Fig. 1). The mean

Table 1 Patient characteristics in Mean (SD) or n (%) at baseline and measurements during surgery

Baseline characteristics	With Ce (*n* = 186)	Without Ce (*n* = 14)
Before surgery		
Age	81.9 (7.8)	79.8 (7.0)
Mini-Mental Status Examination (MMSE)	24.2 (3.7)	25.1 (3.4)
Geriatric depression scale score	3.9 (3.6)	3.0 (2.0)
Clinical Dementia Rating (*n* = 184/14)		
0	75 (41%)	7 (50%)
0.5	88 (48%)	6 (43%)
≥ 1.0	21 (11%)	1 (7%)
Charlson Comorbidity Score	1.5 (1.7)	2.0 (2.4)
0	66 (35%)	6 (43%)
1	83 (45%)	3 (21%)
2	26 (14%)	3 (21%)
> 2	11 (6%)	2 (14%)
Alzheimer's cerebrospinal fluid biomarkers		
Total Tau, pg/ml (*n* = 164/6)	490.8 (275.1)	617.7 (435.7)
Phosphorylated Tau (pg/ml (*n* = 163/6)	56.7 (25.1)	63.0 (32.9)
Amyloid Beta 42 (pg/ml (n = 164/6)	298.3 (164.1)	281.2 (106.7)
Amyloid Beta 42/Total Tau(n = 164/6)	0.71 (0.38)	0.61 (0.32)
Amyloid Beta 42/Phosphorylated Tau (n = 163/6)	5.75 (2.83)	5.16 (2.29)
During surgery		
Observers Assessment Alertness/Sedation score	2.2 (2.1)	1.4 (2.1)
Bispectral Index number (*n* = 183/13)	69.1 (18.1)	75.0 (13.7)
Brain Effect Site Concentration, ug/ml	1.26 (0.79)	--- (---)
Mean Arterial Pressure	73.4 (10.5)	77.1 (11.8)

CDR, Clinical Dementia Rating (0 = normal, 0.5 = mild cognitive impairment, ≥1 = dementia); MMSE, Mini-Mental Status Examination (maximum score of 30 points)

difference of AvgOAA/S and AvgBIS from AvgCe were both 0, with 95.2% of the observed differences within the range of +/− 1.96SD.

BIS determinants

AvgBIS was strongly correlated with AvgCe during surgery (Pearson ρ = − 0.72; $p < 0.0001$), and the correlation remained strong across CDR levels (Table 2).

The correlation seemed the strongest in patients with CDR = 0, with a trend toward weaker correlation as cognitive decline measured by CDR worsened. The strong correlation between AvgBIS and AvgCe was also maintained throughout the range of preoperative Charlson co-morbidity scores observed in the STRIDE population (Table 3).

There was no statistically significant differentiation on the level of association between AvgBIS and AvgCe by CDR or CCI levels.

Linear regression modeling demonstrated that AvgBIS was strongly predicted by AvgCe ($p < .0001$) and less so by avgMAP ($p = 0.01$). AvgBIS and AvgMAP correlated at CCI = 0 (r = 0.37; $p = 0.002$). However, at higher CCI scores correlations were statistically not significant between AvgBIS and AvgMAP (Table 4).

Modest correlations existed between AvgBIS and AvgMAP at mild cognitive impairment (MCI, CDR = 0.5) level only.

OAA/S determinants

AvgOAA/S was strongly correlated with AvgCe during surgery (Pearson ρ = − 0.81; $p < 0.0001$), and the correlation remained strong across CDR levels (Table 2). The correlation seemed the strongest in patients with CDR = 0, with a trend toward slightly weaker correlation as cognitive decline measured by CDR worsen. The overall correlation between AvgOAA/S and AvgCe was strong and maintained throughout the range of preoperative Charlson co-morbidity scores observed in the STRIDE population (Table 3). AvgOAA/S and AvgMAP did not correlate throughout the range of preoperative CCI and CDR scores observed in the STRIDE population. Results from linear regression modeling also demonstrates that AvgOAA/S level is strongly predicted by AvgCe ($p < .0001$), but not by AvgMAP.

Effect of baseline cognition or comorbidity

Regression analyses based on association patterns suggested by nonparametric LOWESS fits of AvgOAA/S on AvgCe showed no statistically significant difference between association patterns when stratified by either the CDR score levels (0, 0.5, and ≥ 1; $p = 0.16$) or the CCI score levels (0, 1, 2, and ≥ 3; $p = 0.37$) (Fig. 2, A and C). Similarly, association patterns suggested by LOWESS fits of AvgBIS on AvgCe were not statistically different when stratified by either the CDR score levels (0, 0.5, and ≥ 1) or the CCI score levels (0, 1, 2, and ≥ 3) (Fig. 2, B and D). AvgOAA/S and avgBIS were highly correlated. At CDR 0, 0.5, and 1 or 2, the Pearson correlation was 0.81 ($p < 0.0001$), 0.76 ($p < 0.0001$), and 0.63 ($p = 0.002$), respectively. Multivariable modeling found no independent effect on AvgBIS by either MMSE, CDR, CDR sum of boxes, GDS, or any cerebrospinal fluid AD biomarker (data not shown). Other variables tested without independent effect on AvgBIS included age, BMI, and CCI. Regression modeling found no association between AvgOAA/S and either MMSE, CDR, CDR sum of boxes, or any cerebrospinal fluid AD biomarker. Two interactions independently predicted AvgOAA/S. AvgOAA/S was predicted by an age-AvgCe interaction as well as an

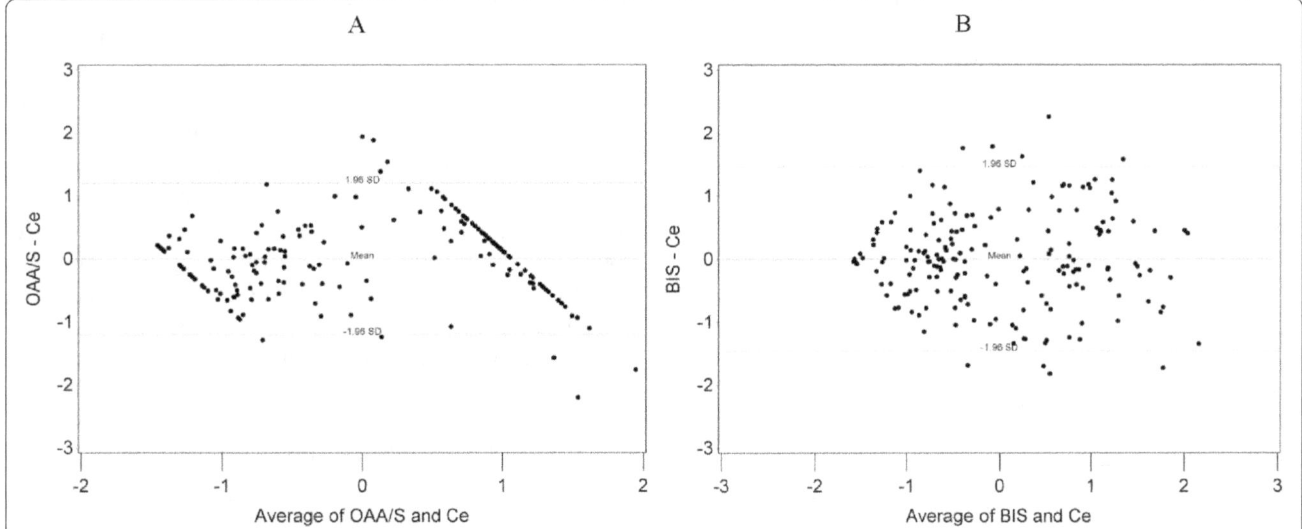

Fig. 1 Bland-Altman plots. **a** shows Bland-Altman plot for OAA/S and Ce. Y-axis is calculated difference between OAA/S and Ce; X-axis is mean of OAA/S and Ce. OAA/S values were reversed in order (i.e., 5 – OAA/S was used). OAA/S and Ce values were then standardized to have respective distributions both with mean of 0 and standard deviation of 1. **b** shows Bland-Altman plot for BIS number and Ce. Y-axis is calculated difference between BIS number and Ce; X-axis is mean of BIS number and Ce. BIS values were reversed in order (i.e., 100 – BIS was used). BIS and Ce values were then standardized to have respective distributions both with mean of 0 and standard deviation of 1

age-GDS interaction (Table 5), where the same level of increase in AvgCe was observed with greater decrease in AvgOAA/S score in older patients than in younger patients, and that patients with more severe depressive symptoms before surgery were observed with lower AvgOAA/S score during surgery than patients with less severe depressive symptoms with greater magnitude in this sedation score differences among older patients than in younger patients. Other variables tested without independent effect on AvgOAA/S included BMI, and CCI.

Discussion

This study did not find evidence to support that the associations between predicted propofol AvgCe and both AvgOAA/S and AvgBIS during sedation among elderly patients undergoing hip fracture repair were significantly altered by baseline CDR or any of the other baseline cognitive variables analyzed.

The current study reports that during sedation, the predicted propofol AvgCe and to a lesser extent AvgMAP affect AvgBIS. The literature reports that BIS, blood propofol concentration [20], Ce [21], and blood pressure are closely related [22]. However, in clinical circumstances where blood pressure decreases occur independent of anesthetic cardiovascular effects, decreases in brain perfusion may be associated with lower BIS numbers independent of anesthetic depth [23–25]. Even less dramatic changes in blood pressure have been associated with BIS modifications. For instance, during stable anesthetic maintenance, blood pressure and BIS are independently correlated (r = 0.696) during positional change from supine to beach chair in preparation for shoulder surgery [26]. The mean BIS level during sedation was not independently affected by any of the baseline cognitive measurements including CDR and CDR sum of boxes, MMSE, or CSF AD biomarker levels. Previous investigations examining the effects of cognitive dysfunction on maintenance anesthetic dosing requirements studied only general anesthesia, used multiple agents and analyzed either retrospective data [7] or

Table 2 Correlations between AvgCe and AvgBIS or Avg OAA/S, overall and by clinical dementia rating

	Avg BIS		Avg OAA/S	
	Pearson	P	Pearson	P
Overall	−0.72	<.0001	−0.81	<.0001
Clinical Dementia Rating				
0	−0.81	<.0001	− 0.86	<.0001
0.5	−0.67	<.0001	−0.80	<.0001
≥ 1	−0.58	0.0070	−0.78	<.0001

Table 3 Correlations between AvgCe and AvgBIS or Avg OAA/S by level of Charlson co-morbidity scores

	Avg BIS		Avg OAA/S	
	Pearson	P	Pearson	P
Charlson Co-Morbidity Index				
0	−0.80	<.0001	−0.86	<.0001
1	−0.68	<.0001	−0.81	<.0001
2	−0.76	<.0001	−0.73	<.0001
> 2	−0.61	0.05	−0.94	<.0001

Table 4 Correlations between AvgBIS and AvgMAP, overall and by Charlson score and clinical dementia rating

	Pearson	P
Overall	0.21	0.004
Charlson Co-Morbidity Index		
0	0.37	0.002
1	0.12	0.29
2	0.14	0.50
> 2	0.27	0.42
Clinical Dementia Rating		
0	0.18	0.12
0.5	0.31	0.004
≥ 1	−0.11	0.66

lacked adequate power [8]. In addition, the severity of dementia was incompletely characterized using either baseline MMSE [8] or history of dementia to establish diagnosis [7]. These studies reported no difference in sensitivity to inhalational agents (as defined by BIS only) [7] or infusion rate requirements using the total intravenous combination of remifentanil and propofol [8] during maintenance of general anesthesia when comparing patients by presence or absence of cognitive dysfunction. Our study is unique in its focus on sedation, using more than simply BIS to assess sedation depth, and careful classification of preoperative cognitive state. In addition, the use of a single anesthetic agent is pertinent to procedural sedation which in actual practice is often accomplished with only the single agent propofol.

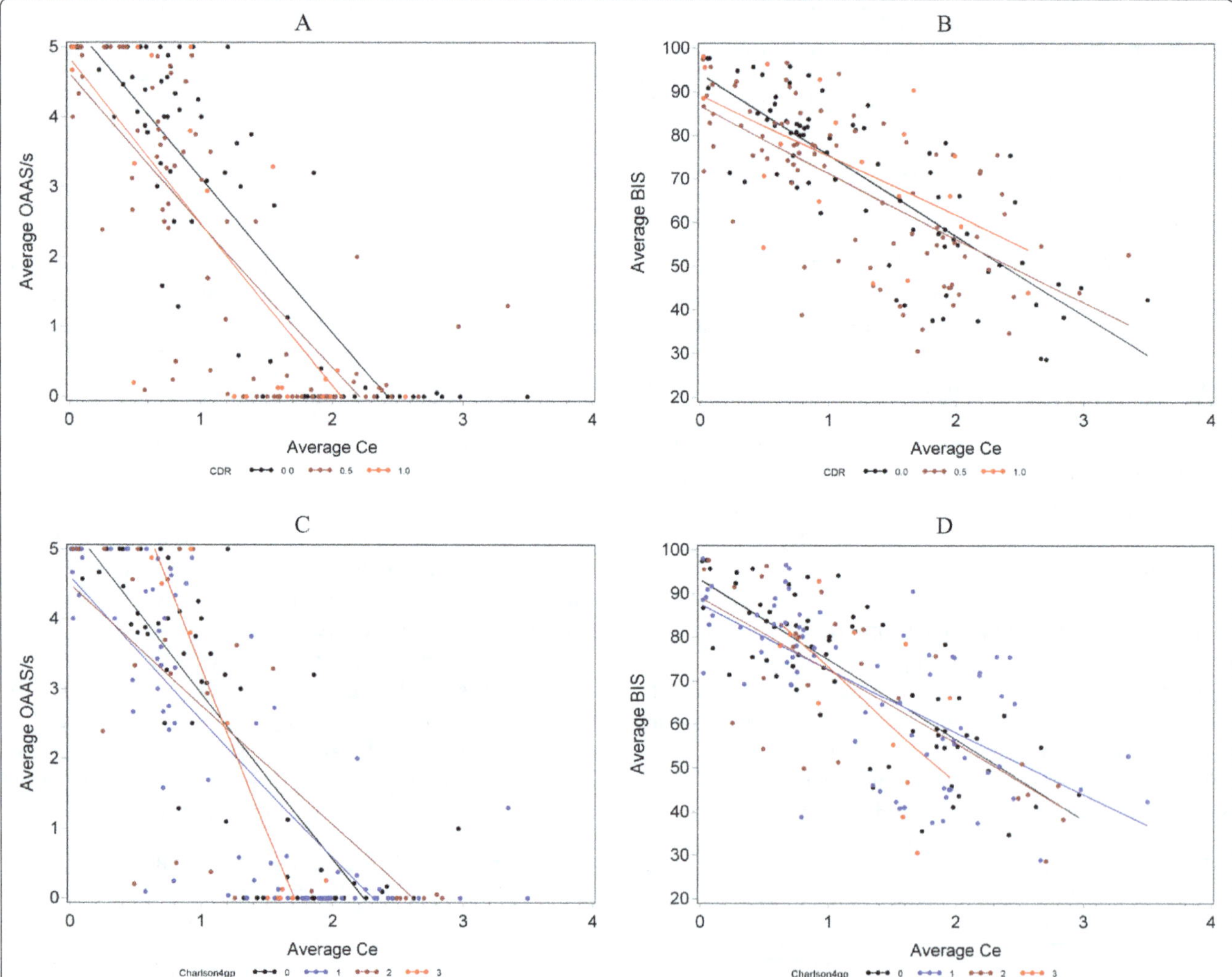

Fig. 2 Nonparametric locally weighted scatterplot smoothing (LOWESS) fits of AvgOAA/S and AvgBIS on AvgCe stratified by the Clinical Dementia Rating (CDR) score levels and Charlson Co-morbidity Index (CCI) score levels. **a**: Nonparametric LOWESS fit of AvgOAA/S on AvgCe stratified by the CDR score levels (0, 0.5, and ≥ 1) with fitted lines for each CDR score level. **b**: Nonparametric LOWESS fit of AvgBIS on AvgCe stratified by the CDR score levels (0, 0.5, and ≥ 1) with fitted lines for each CDR score level. **c**: Nonparametric LOWESS fit of AvgOAA/S on AvgCe when stratified by the CCI score levels (0, 1, 2, and ≥ 3) with fitted lines for each CCI score level. **d**: Nonparametric LOWESS fit of AvgBIS on AvgCe when stratified by the CCI score levels (0, 1, 2, and ≥ 3) with fitted lines for each CCI score level

Table 5 Multivariate Regression Analysis for Predictors of AvgOAA/S

Parameter	Estimate	Standard Error	t Value	P
Intercept	0.39	0.699	0.56	0.57
AvgCe	−1.55	0.137	−11.36	<.0001
AvgMAP	0.01	0.007	1.69	0.09
AvgBIS	0.04	0.006	7.15	<.0001
Age	0.02	0.021	0.83	0.41
AvgCe and Age Interaction	−0.03	0.011	−2.83	0.005
Geriatric Depression Score (GDS)	−0.02	0.021	−1.07	0.29
GDS and Age Interaction	−0.01	0.002	−2.34	0.020

The current study reports that during sedation, the predicted propofol AvgCe affects AvgOAA/S in confirmation of previous reports demonstrating correlations between the blood propofol concentration and OAA/S [27]. AvgOAA/S was affected by an age-AvgCe interaction such that the same level of increase in AvgCe would observe greater decrease in AvgOAA/S score in older patients than in younger patients. This is consistent with Schnider et al. [19] who observed increasing sensitivity to propofol in elderly patients for loss of consciousness. Both age and level of spinal anesthesia have been reported to modify sedation scores [28]. In the current study, age is the more important modifying factor of OAA/S as the overall level of spinal anesthesia demonstrated little variation among participants (T9 ± 1.5 dermatomes). AvgOAA/S was also predicted by age-GDS interaction such that higher GDS scores in conjunction with age were associated with lower AvgOAA/S score at the same Ce. The GDS is a tool to assess symptoms of depression, and there is evidence to suggest that depression and cognitive impairment may be due to related brain dysfunction [29]. As the interaction between GDS and age in determining OAA/S score have not previously been reported, it will require confirmation. Similar to AvgBIS, AvgOAA/S score was not influenced by any of the baseline cognitive measures performed in the STRIDE study.

Strengths

Exact amounts and administration time of propofol was recorded allowing for calculation of predicted Ce. Multiple assessments of baseline cognition were performed in this study and all were able to be tested to verify the robustness of our conclusions. Level of sedation was assessed both behaviorally as well as with BIS. Little systematic bias was observed for both means of assessing sedation depth defined by predicted Ce.

Limitations

Fourteen patients were not included in analysis. However, the baseline characteristics of these 14 patients are comparable to the 186 participants included in this report, and sensitivity analysis demonstrates that the study results would not have been affected by these additional 14 patients on analyses not involving predicted Ce. Only the surgical period was analyzed, and no conclusions can be made concerning hysteresis during induction or emergence which might occur in states of cognitive dysfunction. Reporting the predicted propofol Ce is better than reporting the dose and helps refine our clinical observations. However, without blood concentrations predicted Ce is subject to bias and inaccuracies which limits the ability to make definitive conclusions concerning pharmacodynamic interactions between cognition and sedation requirements. Although ignoring the variability of individual measurements around the mean level over time during surgery, using the mean levels of Ce, OAA/S and BIS during surgery to study their interrelationship with other variables reflects the common practice of maintaining the sedation around a goal level, whether implicitly or not, in clinical management. Lastly, this study performed secondary analysis using existing trial data, with fixed sample size not specifically powered to confirm any hypotheses tested in this study. Although age was identified as significantly modifying the association between Ce and OAA/S, we were not able confirm similar effect modification by pre-operative cognitive state measured by CDR score or other baseline cognitive variables using the STRIDE data.

Conclusion

In summary, during sedation under spinal anesthesia, AvgBIS and AvgOAA/S score are good proxies of predicted AvgCe during surgery in routine clinical practices, as evident in the high correlation and 0 systematic bias demonstrated in the results. Furthermore, the relationships between the predicted AvgCe and both AvgBIS and AvgOAA/S score do not appear to be altered by baseline cognitive impairment. None of the baseline cognitive variables studied in STRIDE independently exerted an effect on either the AvgBIS number or AvgOAA/S score.

Abbreviations

AD: Alzheimer's Disease; AvgBIS: Average Bispectral Index; AvgCe: Mean Predicted Ce Level; AvgMAP: Average Mean Arterial Blood Pressure; AvgOAA/S: Average Observer's Assessment of Alertness/Sedation Scale; B-A: Bland-Altman; BIS: Bispectral Index; CAM: Confusion Assessment Method; CCI: Charlson Comorbidity Index; CDR: Clinical Dementia Rating; Ce: Predicted Propofol Effect Site Concentration; CSF: Cerebrospinal Fluid; DRS-R-98: Delirium Rating Scale-R-98; DST: Digit Span Test; GDS: Geriatric Depression Scale; LOWESS: Locally Weighted Scatterplot Smoothing; MAP: Mean Arterial Blood Pressure; MMSE: Mini-mental Status Exam; OAA/S: Observer's Assessment of Alertness/Sedation Scale; SD: Standard Deviations; STRIDE: A Strategy to Reduce the Incidence of Postoperative Delirium in Elderly Patients

Acknowledgments

The authors would like to thank the assessment team (Kori Kindbom, Rachel Burns, Michael Sklar) for their excellent follow-up of patients, the DSMB members: Jeffery Carson, M.D., Chair; Lee Fleisher, M.D.; Steve Epstein, M.D.; Jay Magaziner, PhD; Anne Lindblad, PhD; and Safety Officer: Sarang Kim, M.D. for their time, effort, and oversight, and Linda Sevier for her expert preparation of the manuscript.

Authors' contributions

FES – Conception, design, acquisition, analysis, interpretation of data, and drafted and revised the work. KN – Acquisition, interpretation of data, revised the work. ESO- Acquisition, interpretation of data, revised the work. AG – Conception, acquisition, analysis, data interpretation, drafted and revised work. NYW - Conception, design, acquisition, analysis, interpretation of data, and drafted and revised the work. All authors approved the submitted version and have agreed to be personally accountable for their contributions and to ensure that questions related to the accuracy or integrity of any part of the work,' even ones in which the author was not personally involved, are appropriately investigated, resolved, and the resolution documented in the literature.

Author details

[1]Department of Anesthesiology and Critical Care Medicine, Johns Hopkins Bayview Medical Center, 4940 Eastern Avenue, Baltimore, MD 21224, USA. [2]Department of Psychiatry and Behavioral Sciences, Johns Hopkins University School of Medicine, A4Center Suite 457, 4940 Eastern Ave, Baltimore, USA. [3]Division of Geriatric Medicine and Gerontology, Psychiatry and Behavioral Sciences & Neuropathology, Johns Hopkins University School of Medicine, Mason F. Lord Building, Center Tower, 5200 Eastern Avenue, 7th Floor, Baltimore, MD 21224, USA. [4]Departments of Anesthesiology and Critical Care Medicine and Neurosurgery, Johns Hopkins Hospital, 1800 Orleans St, Baltimore, MD 21287, USA. [5]Medicine, Biostatistics and Epidemiology, The Johns Hopkins University, 2024 E. Monument Street, Suite 2-500, Baltimore, MD 21287, USA.

References

1. Alzheimer's Association. 2018 Alzheimer's disease facts and figures 2018.
2. Alzheimer's disease facts and figures. Alzheimer's & dementia: the journal of the Alzheimer's Association 2017; 13:325–373.
3. Robinson TN, Wu DS, Pointer LF, Dunn CL, Moss M. Preoperative cognitive dysfunction is related to adverse postoperative outcomes in the elderly. J Am Coll Surg. 2012;215(1):12–7 discussion 17-8.
4. Styra R, Larsen E, Dimas MA, Baston D, Elgie-Watson J, Flockhart L, et al. The effect of preoperative cognitive impairment and type of vascular surgery procedure on postoperative delirium with associated cost implications. J Vasc Surg. 2019;69(1):201–9.
5. Evered LA, Silbert BS, Scott DA, Maruff P, Ames D, Choong PF. Preexisting cognitive impairment and mild cognitive impairment in subjects presenting for total hip joint replacement. Anesthesiology. 2011;114(6):1297–304.
6. Lee HB, Mears SC, Rosenberg PB, Leoutsakos JM, Gottschalk A, Sieber FE. Predisposing factors for postoperative delirium after hip fracture repair in individuals with and without dementia. J Am Geriatr Soc. 2011;59(12):2306–13.
7. Perez-Protto S, Geube M, Ontaneda D, Dalton JE, Kurz A, Sessler DI. Sensitivity to volatile anesthetics in patients with dementia: a case-control analysis. Can J Anaesth. 2014;61(7):611–8.
8. Erdogan MA, Demirbilek S, Erdil F, Aydogan MS, Ozturk E, Togal T, et al. The effects of cognitive impairment on anaesthetic requirement in the elderly. Eur J Anaesthesiol. 2012;29(7):326–31.
9. Glass PS, Bloom M, Kearse L, Rosow C, Sebel P, Manberg P. Bispectral analysis measures sedation and memory effects of propofol, midazolam, isoflurane, and alfentanil in healthy volunteers. Anesthesiology. 1997;86(4): 836–47.
10. Sieber FE, Neufeld KJ, Gottschalk A, Bigelow GE, Oh ES, Rosenberg PB, et al. Effect of depth of sedation in older patients undergoing hip fracture repair on postoperative delirium: the STRIDE randomized clinical trial. JAMA Surg. 2018;8.
11. Sieber F, Neufeld KJ, Gottschalk A, Bigelow GE, Oh ES, Rosenberg PB, et al. Depth of sedation as an interventional target to reduce postoperative delirium: mortality and functional outcomes of the strategy to reduce the incidence of postoperative delirium in elderly patients randomized clinical trial. Br J Anaesth. 2019;122(4):480–9.
12. Li T, Wieland LS, Oh E, Neufeld KJ, Wang NY, Dickersin K, et al. Design considerations of a randomized controlled trial of sedation level during hip fracture repair surgery: a strategy to reduce the incidence of postoperative delirium in elderly patients. Clin Trials 2017 Jan 01:1740774516687253-supplemental material.
13. Folstein MF, Folstein SE, McHugh PR. "Mini-mental state". A practical method for grading the cognitive state of patients for the clinician. J Psychiatr Res. 1975;12(3):189–98.
14. Oh ES, Blennow K, Bigelow GE, Inouye SK, Marcantonio ER, Neufeld KJ, et al. Abnormal CSF amyloid-beta42 and tau levels in hip fracture patients without dementia. PLoS One. 2018;13(9):e0204695.
15. Yesavage JA, Sheikh JI. 9/Geriatric Depression Scale (GDS). Clin Gerontol 1986 11/18; 5(1–2):165–173.
16. Charlson ME, Pompei P, Ales KL, MacKenzie CR. A new method of classifying prognostic comorbidity in longitudinal studies: development and validation. J Chronic Dis. 1987;40(5):373–83.
17. Inouye SK, van Dyck CH, Alessi CA, Balkin S, Siegal AP. RI. H. Clarifying confusion: the confusion assessment method. A new method for detection of delirium. Ann Intern Med. 1990;113(12):941–8.
18. Trzepacz PT, Mittal D, Torres R, Kanary K, Norton J, Jimerson N. Validation of the delirium rating scale-revised-98: comparison with the delirium rating scale and the cognitive test for delirium. J Neuropsychiatry Clin Neurosci. 2001;13(2):229–42.
19. Schnider TW, Minto CF, Shafer SL, Gambus PL, Andresen C, Goodale DB, et al. The influence of age on propofol pharmacodynamics. Anesthesiology. 1999;90(6):1502–16.
20. Rasmussen LS, Christiansen M, Rasmussen H, Kristensen PA, JT M. Do blood concentrations of neurone specific enolase and S-100 beta protein reflect cognitive dysfunction after abdominal surgery? ISPOCD Group Br J Anaesth. 2000;84(2):242–4.
21. Liu SH, Wei W, Ding GN, Ke JD, Hong FX, Tian M. Relationship between depth of anesthesia and effect-site concentration of propofol during induction with the target-controlled infusion technique in elderly patients. Chin Med J. 2009;122(8):935–40.
22. Kazama T, Ikeda K, Morita K, Kikura M, Doi M, Ikeda T, et al. Comparison of the effect-site k (eO) s of propofol for blood pressure and EEG Bispectral index in elderly and younger patients. Anesthesiology. 1999;90(6):1517–27.
23. Myles PS. Bispectral index monitoring in ischemic-hypoxic brain injury. J Extra Corpor Technol 2009; 41(1):P15–9.
24. Merat S, Levecque JP, Le Gulluche Y, Diraison Y, Brinquin L, Hoffmann JJ. BIS monitoring may allow the detection of severe cerebral ischemia. Can J Anaesth. 2001;48(11):1066–9.
25. Win NN, Kohase H, Miyamoto T, Umino M. Decreased bispectral index as an indicator of syncope before hypotension and bradycardia in two patients with needle phobia. Br J Anaesth. 2003;91(5):749–52.
26. Lee SW, Choi SE, Han JH, Park SW, Kang WJ, Choi YK. Effect of beach chair position on bispectral index values during arthroscopic shoulder surgery. Korean J Anesthesiol. 2014;67(4):235–9.
27. Casati A, Fanelli G, Casaletti E, Colnaghi E, Cedrati V, Torri G. Clinical assessment of target-controlled infusion of propofol during monitored anesthesia care. Can J Anaesth. 1999;46(3):235–9.
28. Roh GU, Kim Y, Ha SH, Jeong KH, Choi S, Han DW. Modelling of the sedative effects of Propofol in patients undergoing spinal Anaesthesia: a Pharmacodynamic analysis. Basic Clin Pharmacol Toxicol. 2016;118(6):480–6.
29. Morimoto SS, Alexopoulos GS. Cognitive deficits in geriatric depression: clinical correlates and implications for current and future treatment. Psychiatr Clin North Am. 2013;36(4):517–31.

5

Efficacy of non-opioid analgesics to control postoperative pain

John A. Carter[1*], Libby K. Black[2], Dolly Sharma[3], Tarun Bhagnani[3] and Jonathan S. Jahr[4]

Abstract

Background: The aim of this network meta-analysis (NMA) was to evaluate the safety and efficacy of intravenous (IV) Meloxicam 30 mg (MIV), an investigational non-steroidal anti-inflammatory drug (NSAID), and certain other IV non-opioid analgesics for moderate-severe acute postoperative pain.

Methods: We searched PubMed and CENTRAL for Randomized Controlled Trials (RCT) (years 2000–2019, adult human subjects) of IV non-opioid analgesics (IV NSAIDs or IV Acetaminophen) used to treat acute pain after abdominal, hysterectomy, bunionectomy or orthopedic procedures. A Bayesian NMA was conducted in R to rank treatments based on the standardized mean differences in sum of pain intensity difference from baseline up to 24 h postoperatively (sum of pain intensity difference: SPID 24). The probability and the cumulative probability of rank for each treatment were calculated, and the surface under the cumulative ranking curve (SUCRA) was applied to distinguish treatments on the basis of their outcomes such that higher SUCRA values indicate better outcomes. The study protocol was prospectively registered with by PROSPERO (CRD42019117360).

Results: Out of 2313 screened studies, 27 studies with 36 comparative observations were included, producing a treatment network that included the four non-opioid IV pain medications of interest (MIV, ketorolac, acetaminophen, and ibuprofen). MIV was associated with the largest SPID 24 for all procedure categories and comparators. The SUCRA ranking table indicated that MIV had the highest probability for the most effective treatment for abdominal (89.5%), bunionectomy (100%), and hysterectomy (99.8%). MIV was associated with significantly less MME utilization versus all comparators for abdominal procedures, hysterectomy, and versus acetaminophen in orthopedic procedures. Elsewhere MME utilization outcomes for MIV were largely equivalent or nominally better than other comparators. Odds of ORADEs were significantly higher for all comparators vs MIV for orthopedic (gastrointestinal) and hysterectomy (respiratory).

Conclusions: MIV 30 mg may provide better pain reduction with similar or better safety compared to other approved IV non-opioid analgesics. Caution is warranted in interpreting these results as all comparisons involving MIV were indirect.

Keywords: Analgesia, Meloxicam, Opioid, Pain assessment, Postoperative Pain

* Correspondence: jcarter@bluepointllc.org
[1]Blue Point LLC, 711 Warrenville Road, Wheaton, IL 60189, USA

Background

Management of postoperative pain remains a significant issue, including providing adequate pain control beyond immediate postsurgical recovery [1–3]. Poorly managed acute postoperative pain may have a significant impact on clinical and economic outcomes and is a consistent risk factor for persistent or chronic postoperative pain [3–5]. Opioid analgesics are the foundation of treatment for moderate-to-severe postsurgical pain and are among the most effective agents for the management of pain in many settings [6]. However, opioids are associated with the potential risks of opioid-related adverse drug events (ORADEs), (such as respiratory and gastrointestinal related events) and abuse or dependence, which can significantly increase the cost of medical care [7–9].

Multimodal pain management guidelines have been developed that provide guidance on reducing opioid monotherapy and the doses of opioids used to treat acute pain, while still providing effective pain management [10–12] This approach involves the administration of various opioid and non-opioid agents that act on different sites, resulting in a synergistic and additive effect [10–12]. The goal of multimodal pain management is to reduce ORADEs and their costs, as well as the risks of opioid abuse or dependence [13].

Non-opioid pharmacologic therapies for potential use in the multimodal regimen include acetaminophen and/or non-steroidal anti-inflammatory drugs (NSAIDs). Recent practice guidelines have recommended that unless contraindicated, all patients should receive around-the-clock treatment with acetaminophen or NSAIDs as part of multimodal analgesia for post-operative pain management [14]. When NSAIDs and/or acetaminophen are included in treatment regimens with opioids for pain relief, an opioid-sparing effect has been demonstrated [15]. Intravenous use of NSAIDs can achieve a faster onset of action and peak plasma concentrations compared to oral treatment regimens [10]. Parenteral formulations of ketorolac and ibuprofen were the only IV NSAIDs currently approved for postoperative pain management in the United States (US) at the time this study was conducted [16]. Studies have found that ketorolac reduces opioid consumption by 25–45% and provides additional benefits such as improving bowel function after colorectal surgery and epidural pain after cesarean delivery [17–19]. Intravenous ibuprofen is approved for the management of mild to moderate pain and for the management of moderate to severe pain as an adjunct to opioid analgesics [20]. Another non-opioid analgesic, acetaminophen, has an onset of action of 15 min when given as IV which is faster than the oral formulation and is associated with opioid-sparing effects [21].

NSAIDs act by inhibiting prostaglandin production through acetylation of cyclooxygenase (COX-1 and/or COX-2). Most NSAIDs are non-selective (i.e. they inhibit the activity of both COX-1 and COX-2). Inhibition of COX-1 activity is considered as a major contributor to NSAID gastrointestinal toxicity [22]. Non-selective NSAIDs are associated with an increased risk of gastrointestinal bleeding, cardiotoxicity, hepatotoxicity, renal dysfunction, and drug induced asthma [20, 23]. Ketorolac, the most widely used IV NSAIDs, has demonstrated a higher risk of gastro-toxicity and gastroduodenal lesions [24]. NSAIDs that selectively inhibit COX-2 are associated with fewer gastrointestinal effects [25, 26]. However, studies have linked selective COX-2 inhibitor to higher risk of myocardial infarction, stroke, and death [27].

A formulation of intravenous meloxicam (meloxicam IV; Anjeso™) (MIV) that utilizes a novel nanocrystal formulation has been approved by the U.S. Food and Drug Administration for the management of moderate-to-severe pain alone or in combination with other analgesics [28]. It belongs to the oxicam family of chemicals and blocks COX-2 more than it does COX-1, thus having fewer gastrointestinal side effects compared to non-selective NSAIDs, and without interfering with platelet function [29, 30]. Its efficacy and safety have been evaluated in seven Phase 2/3 randomized controlled clinical trials (RCTs) following procedures including dental surgery, abdominal hysterectomy, bunionectomy, abdominoplasty, and other major procedures [31–37]. Since these trials did not allow concomitant NSAID use and were placebo controlled, MIV has not yet been compared to other non-opioid IV analgesics. Hence, we conducted a network-meta-analysis (NMA) to assess the safety and efficacy of MIV relative to other IV non-opioid analgesics for moderate-severe postoperative pain. The study was conducted according to the Preferred Reporting Items for Systematic Reviews and Meta-Analyses (PRISMA) guidelines, Cochrane Handbook for Systematic Review of Interventions, and the International Society for Pharmacoeconomics and Outcomes Research (ISPOR) task force on Indirect Comparisons and Good Research Practices.

Methods

Search strategy

Using a pre-specified protocol, which was registered with PROSPERO (CRD42019117360), a systematic search was conducted in PubMed, Medline, EBSCO, Web of Science, Scopus, ClinicalTrials.gov, and Cochrane CENTRAL to identify randomized clinical trials from 2000 to 2019 and involving at least one of the following procedures or procedure groups: open abdominal (excluding hysterectomy), bunionectomy, open hysterectomy, orthopedic (joint replacement including knee, ankle, hip, shoulder). The literature search included publications on RCTs that reported clinical effectiveness, tolerability/safety, in adult patients receiving post-operative pain treatment. The search had no limits with respect to language or country.

Study selection and eligibility criteria

In the first round of screening, all titles and abstracts were screened by a single investigator against the inclusion and exclusion criteria, using the PICOT criteria (population, interventions, comparators, outcomes, time period). The inclusion criteria for this NMA were: Studies that were conducted between 2000 and 2019 and that were RCTs; studies with adult patients (≥ 18 years) treated for post-operative pain involving one of the following procedures including, open abdominal (excluding hysterectomy), bunionectomy, open hysterectomy, orthopedic (joint replacement including knee, ankle, hip, shoulder); post-operative treatment with at least one non-opioid pain medication; and studies with the outcomes of ORADEs, opioid utilization, and pain intensity. Studies were eligible only if they included these comparators in at least one treatment group administered as follows: product was not administered continuously or as an infiltration, patients were randomized to product postoperatively in response to objectively measured moderate-severe pain (i.e., no preemptive administration), follow-up was conducted ≥12 h postoperatively.

A senior investigator validated 10% of the rejected abstracts to confirm accuracy. Abstracts with insufficient information were included. Full-text articles for the included abstracts were retrieved for in-depth review in the second round of screening, conducted by a single investigator using the same inclusion and exclusion criteria applied at the abstract level. A second investigator confirmed all excluded studies; any discrepancies were resolved by both the investigators together. Throughout the process, discrepancies were addressed by consensus between the two investigators. All screenings, extractions and validations were conducted in a shared Covidence database.

Two types of study selection criteria, restrictive and broad, were used to conduct this NMA. Under the restrictive study selection criteria, the studies were required to have waited until patients reached moderate-severe pain before they were administered the study analgesic. No such criteria were used for the broader analysis. The current study focuses on the results from the restrictive analysis as it better aligns with the clinical conditions in which MIV has been evaluated (i.e., postoperative moderate-severe pain). Results from the broader analysis are not reported here but may be available upon request.

Data extraction

Full data extraction was performed on all studies included following the second round of screening. Extracted data included study descriptors, patient characteristics, treatment-level information, and outcomes (pain intensity, ORADEs). Data was extracted by two independent reviewers. Any discrepancies were resolved by agreement and consensus of the two investigators. Adjudication and extractions were made in a shared Covidence database (data held in a commonly shared Review Manager database). Where not reported, original confidence intervals were imputed based on information from the study reporting the point estimate combined with information from the literature regarding variability in the given endpoints.

Outcomes and statistical analysis

Bayesian NMA was conducted using the netmeta and GeMTC packages in R to pool effect sizes of direct and indirect comparisons. The main outcomes analyzed were sum of pain intensity difference (SPID), total morphine milligram equivalents (MME) used, and ORADE frequency. SPID 24 (i.e., up to 24 h postoperatively) was chosen as the target pain outcome because it was expected that reporting beyond this timeframe would not be consistent across studies and we required a common timeframe to make comparisons across procedure groups. Two types of ORADEs were included in the analysis: respiratory (e.g. pulmonary congestion & hypostasis, pulmonary insufficiency following surgery and trauma, respiratory complications, other pulmonary insufficiency, bradypnea, acute respiratory failure, hypoxemia, hypoxia, mechanical ventilator) and gastrointestinal (e.g., paralytic ileus, postoperative ileus, constipation, nausea/vomiting). Sample-weighted mean differences were used for data measured on the same scale, and standardized mean differences (SMDs) were used where scales were not the same. Continuous outcomes (i.e., SPID and MMEs) were evaluated as mean differences versus placebo and dichotomous outcomes (i.e., ORADEs) as odds ratios (ORs). Where not otherwise reported, standard deviations were imputed using methods specified in the Cochrane guidelines (Section 16.1.3.2) [38]. A fixed effect approach was chosen for pain and MME outcomes due to the homogeneity of the study designs for those outcomes at the procedure level. Mixed-effects was used for ORADE outcomes given the heterogeneous compositions of the constituent adverse event categories [39].

Markov chain Monte Carlo methods were used to derive 95% credible intervals (CrIs). Credible intervals of the posterior distribution represented estimates for effect sizes, which can be interpreted similarly to confidence intervals [40]. The probability and the cumulative probability of rank for each treatment were calculated, and the surface under the cumulative ranking curve (SUCR A) was applied to distinguish each treatment by efficacy and safety where higher SUCRA values indicated better outcomes.

Results

Study selection

A total of 2313 unduplicated study abstracts identified through literature search were screened for eligibility. Full text articles of 472 abstracts that met the inclusion/exclusion criteria were further screened, to identify 27 RCTs included in the analysis (Fig. 1). Eighty-six of the 445 excluded full-text studies were used in various capacities for generating informative priors. Informative priors were used to dictate the appropriate probability distributions for the Bayesian analysis.

The characteristics of the 27 included studies are described in Table 1 [32–36, 41–62]. The network evaluated for all drugs and procedure types in this study is shown in Fig. 2. MIV was indirectly compared with only those IV treatments that were available at the time in the US (acetaminophen, ibuprofen and ketorolac). Studies for other non-opioid analgesics such as parecoxib and diclofenac were used for indirect comparison with the placebo arms in those studies.

Outcomes from NMA

Pain

A total of sixteen studies contributed to the analysis for pain for abdominal, bunionectomy, and hysterectomy procedure categories: Orthopedic procedures were excluded for the pain outcome category because pain outcomes were not reported for MIV for this category. Among abdominal procedures, MIV was associated with significantly greater pain reductions versus acetaminophen, ketorolac, other medications, and placebo (Fig. 3a). MIV was nominally more effective in reducing pain versus ibuprofen, but the confidence intervals overlapped (Fig. 3a). However, the SUCRA ranking table indicated an 89.6% probability that MIV was the most effective treatment for abdominal

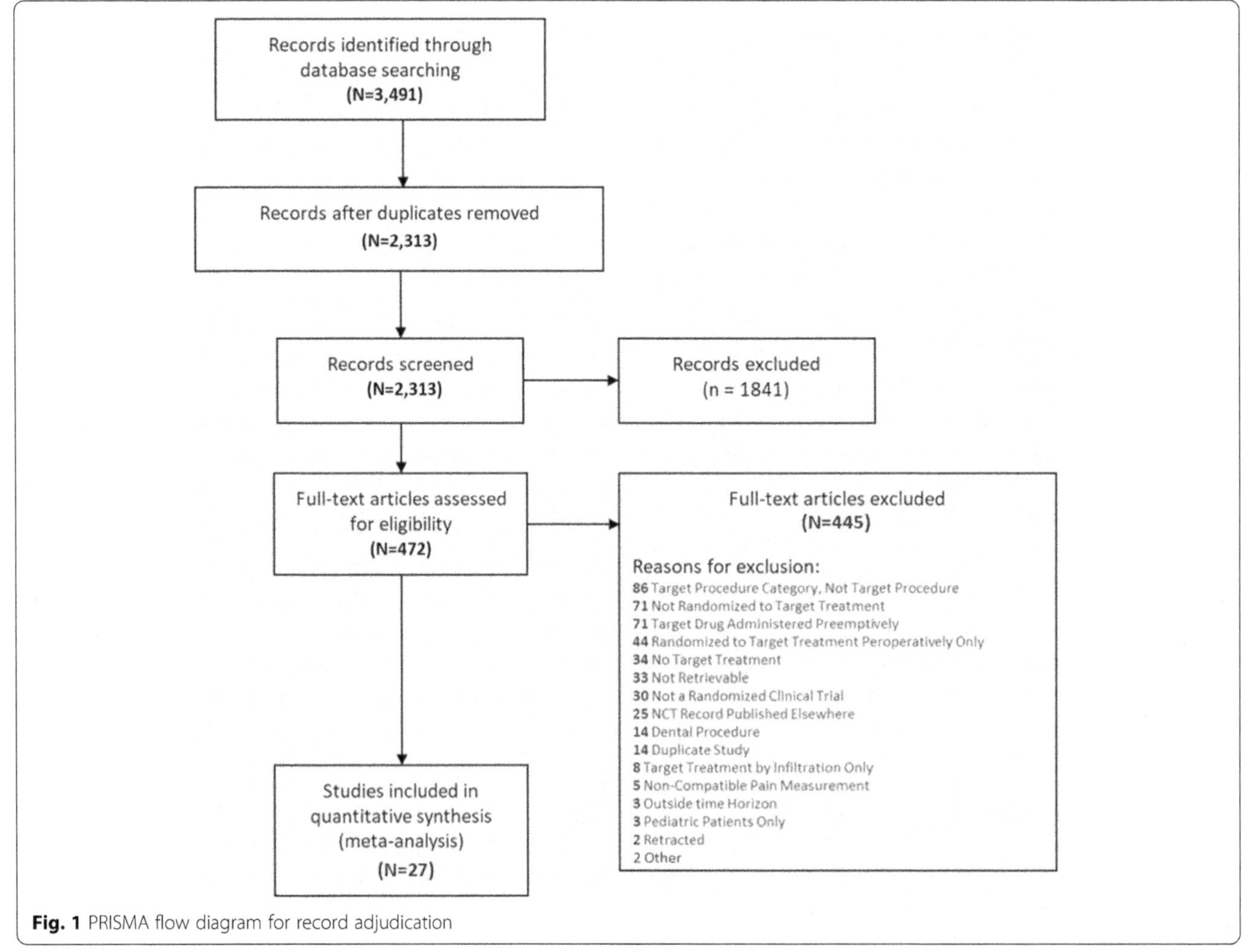

Fig. 1 PRISMA flow diagram for record adjudication

Table 1 Characteristics of the RCTs included in this study ($N = 27$)

Author, Year (Procedure)	Sample Size	Treatments	Pain		MMEs Consumed				ORADEs		
			Included	SPID	Included	Hour 24	Hour 48	Hour 72	Included	GI	Respiratory/ Cardiovascular
Apfelbaum 2008 [41] (Bunionectomy)	255	Parecoxib (60 mg)	Yes	−50.64	No	–	–	–	Yes	0.21	–
		Parecoxib (40 mg)		−62.69		–	–	–		0.24	–
		Placebo		−65.22		–	–	–		0.38	–
Bakhsha 2016 [42] (Cesarean)	60	Diclofenac (suppository)[A] / Placebo	Yes	−19.26	No	–	–	–	No	–	–
		Acetaminophen		−21.01		–	–	–		–	–
Bangash 2018 [43] (Multiple, Elective)	220	Ketorolac + Acetaminophen	Yes	−47.95	No	–	–	–	No	–	–
		Ketorolac + Placebo		−41.74		–	–	–		–	–
Bergese 2017 [36][B] (Multiple)	720	MIV	No	–	Yes	–	26.3	28.4	Yes	0.39	0.00
		Placebo		–		–	34.3	37.4		0.49	0.00
Berkowitz 2017 [44] (Orthopedic)[B]	379	MIV	No	–	Yes	22.1	33.5	35.45	Yes	0.43	0.01
		Placebo		–		31.1	46.3	47.84		1.34	0.02
Bikhazi 2004 [45] (Hysterectomy)	329	Parecoxib (60 mg)	Yes	−18.2	No	–	–	–	Yes	0.71	–
		Parecoxib (40 mg)		−71.04		–	–	–		0.61	–
		Ketorolac (30 mg)		−91.28		–	–	–		0.55	–
		Placebo		−14.8		–	–	–		0.44	–
		Morphine (4 mg)		−45.24		–	–	–		0.66	–
Castro 2000 [46] (Abdominal)	230	Tramadol (100 mg)	Yes	−31.73	No	–	–	–	No	–	–
		Metamizol (2000 mg)		−58.93		–	–	–		–	–
		Ketorolac (30 mg)		−3.08		–	–	–		–	–
Daniels 2019 [47] (Bunionectomy)	276	Acetaminophen	Yes	−9.6	Yes[E]	–	45.00	–	No	–	–
		Ibuprofen		−8.6		–	37.50	–		–	–
		Placebo		1.5		–	61.50	–		–	–
Daniels 2013 [48] (Orthopedic)	277	Diclofenac	No	–	Yes	27.96	33.49	35.42	Yes	0.46	–
		Ketorolac (15–30 mg)		–		34.41	46.27	53.97		0.52	–
		Placebo		–		47.82	56.94	61.27		0.71	–
Essex 2018 [49] (Orthopedic)	116	Acetaminophen	No	–	No	–	–	–	Yes	–	0.02
		Placebo		–		–	–	–		–	0.07
Gago Martinez 2016 [50] (Abdominal)[D]	135	Ibuprofen	Yes	−24.5	Yes	17.36	26.32	–	No	–	–
		Placebo		−18.11		32.18	38.53	–		–	–
Gan 2012 [51] (Abdominal)	132	Placebo	Yes	−17.64	Yes	11.20	15.60	15.90	Yes	0.96	0.07
		Ketorolac (30 mg)		−27.56		6.70	8.53	8.50		0.79	0.05
		Diclofenac (18,75 mg)		−24.4		6.80	8.54	8.80		0.86	0.02
		Diclofenac (37.5 mg)		−61.08		–	–	–		–	–
Gottlieb 2018 [33] (Bunionectomy)[B]	96	MIV	Yes	−21.4	Yes[E]	–	57.40	–	No	–	–
		Placebo		10.32		–	77.00	–		–	–
Hynes 2006 [52] (Orthopedic)	120	Acetaminophen	No	–	No	–	–	–	Yes	0.05	0.00
		Diclofenac		–		–	–	–		0.05	0.075
Kim 2001 [53] (Abdominal)[D]	22	Ketorolac	Yes	−33.71	Yes	10.00	20.67	–	No	–	–
		Placebo		−26.95		28.00	34.88	–		–	–
Kroll 2010 [54] (Hysterectomy)[D]	319	Ibuprofen (800 mg)	Yes	−26.82	Yes	47.3	71.72	–	Yes	0.64	0.04
		Placebo		−20.09		55.9	66.92	–		0.70	0.02

Table 1 Characteristics of the RCTs included in this study (*N* = 27) *(Continued)*

Author, Year (Procedure)	Sample Size	Treatments	Pain		MMEs Consumed				ORADEs		
			Included	SPID	Included	Hour 24	Hour 48	Hour 72	Included	GI	Respiratory/ Cardiovascular
Pareek 2011 [55] (Orthopedic)	158	Etodolac	No	–	No	–	–	–	Yes	0.05	–
		Diclofenac		–		–	–	–		0.05	–
Pollak 2018 [35] (Bunionectomy)[B]	120	MIV	Yes	−50.4	Yes	–	27.25	–	Yes	0.29	0.00
		Placebo		−34.52		–	37.45	–		0.40	0.00
Rechberger 2018 [32] (Hysterectomy)[B,D]	215	MIV	Yes	−19.47	Yes	15.90	31.80	–	Yes	0.00	0.00
		Morphine		0.77		28.80	–	–		0.10	0.00
		Placebo		4.61		48.00	96.00	–		0.00	0.00
Reinhart 2000 [56] (Bunionectomy)	38	Ketorolac	Yes	2.86	No	–	–	–	No	–	–
		Placebo [C]		4.87		–	–	–		–	–
Rindos 2019 [57] (Hysterectomy)	183	Acetaminophen	Yes	2.38	No	–	–	–	No	–	–
		Placebo		2.86		–	–	–		–	–
Singla 2018 [34] (Abdominal)[B]	219	MIV	Yes	−1.1	Yes	18.30	26.90	–	Yes	0.35	0.04
		Placebo		−0.91		21.90	35.35	–		0.51	0.02
Singla 2010 [58] (Orthopedic)	185	Ibuprofen	No	–	Yes	41.10	–	–	Yes	0.27	–
		Placebo		–		59.50	–	–		0.19	–
Takeda 2019 [59] (Orthopedic)	97	Acetaminophen	No	–	Yes	80.01	–	–	No	–	–
		Placebo		–		81.31	–	–		–	–
Thybo 2019 [60] (Orthopedic)	281	Acetaminophen	No	–	Yes	36.00	–	–	Yes	0.04	0.03
		Ibuprofen		–		26.00	–	–		0.01	0.04
Wilson 2018 [61] (Cesarean)	141	Acetaminophen	No	–	Yes	20.00	47.00	–	No	–	–
		Placebo		–		32.00	48.00	–		–	–
Wong 2010 [62] (Abdominal)	66	Parecoxib	No	–	Yes	26.00	–	43.50	Yes	0.00	–
		Ketorolac		–		29.40	–	55.50		0.12	–

Abbreviations: *RCT* Randomized Clinical Trial, *MME* Morphine milligram equivalent, *ORADE* Opioid-related adverse drug events, *SPID* Sum of pain intensity differences, *GI* Gastrointestinal

[a]Assumes diclofenac suppositories are common practice for pain control in Cesarean sections

[b]Uses the 2-h windowed last observation carried forward (W2LOCF) value

[c]Used group KIV versus group L from the original report

[d]MME values at week 48 were extrapolated from MME values in the given study reported before hour 48 based on a regression using data from the other reatined studies for the relationships betwwen time and MME utilization

[e]MME at 48 weeks for was calculated from the median or median oxycodone use, which was converted to MMEs using a conversion factor of 1.4 per the guidance from the Centers for Medicare and Medicaid Services

procedures versus a 10.4% probability for ibuprofen (Table 2).

For bunionectomy, MIV was significantly more effective for pain reduction versus all other treatment options (as represented by SPID 24). As indicated in the forest plot (Fig. 3b) and the SUCRA ranking table (Table 2), the order of treatments with respect to efficacy for the pain outcome (SPID 24, best to worst) was MIV, acetaminophen, ibuprofen, ketorolac, placebo, and other. In the hysterectomy procedure category, MIV was again the most effective treatment option for reducing pain for up to 24 h postoperatively (Fig. 3c, Table 2). The order of treatments with respect to efficacy for the pain outcome (SPID 24, best to worst) was MIV, ibuprofen, ketorolac, other, acetaminophen, and placebo.

Morphine milligram equivalents

Seventeen studies contributed to the analysis for MME across all procedures. Overall, MIV was associated with significant reduction in MME in all procedure categories (Fig. 4) versus placebo. For abdominal procedures (Fig. 4a), MIV was associated with a 38% higher, significant reduction (– 8.7 [– 9.1, – 8.3] vs -6.3 [-7.3, -5.3]) in MME used for rescue treatment up to 48 h postoperatively compared with ibuprofen, a 23% higher, significant reduction (– 8.7 [– 9.1, – 8.3] vs -7.1 [-7.7, -6.5]) compared with ketorolac, and a 778% higher, significant reduction (-8.7 [-9.1, -8.3] vs -1.0 [-3.3, 1.4]) versus acetaminophen. For bunionectomy, the treatment options were statistically equivalent (Fig. 4b). For hysterectomy, MIV was associated with a >1,000% higher

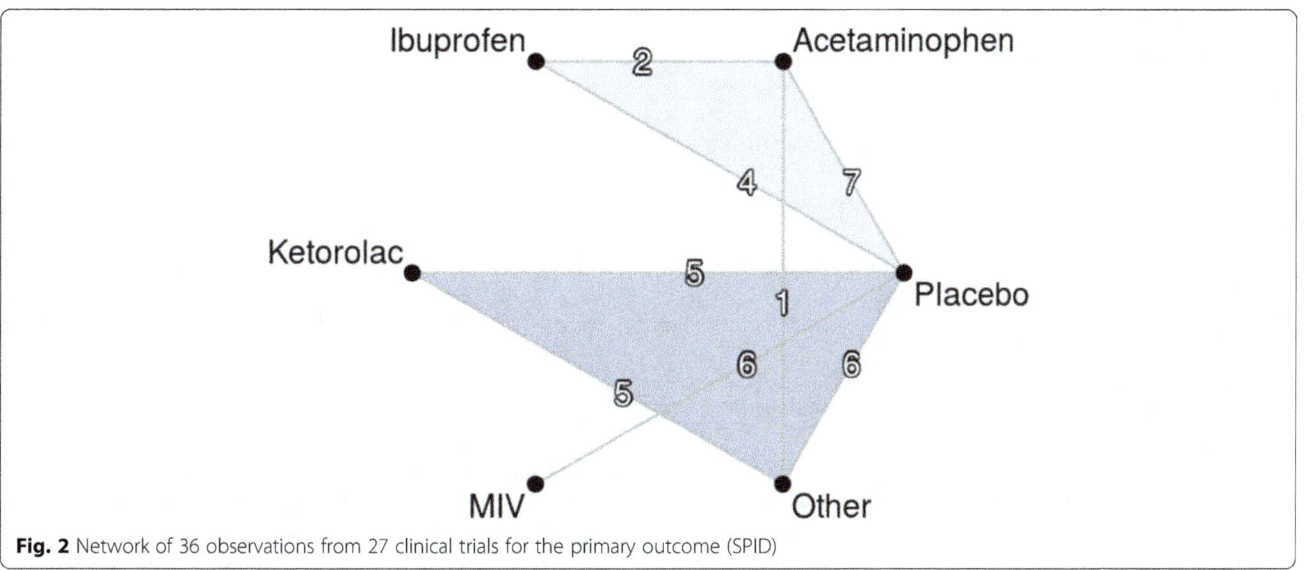

Fig. 2 Network of 36 observations from 27 clinical trials for the primary outcome (SPID)

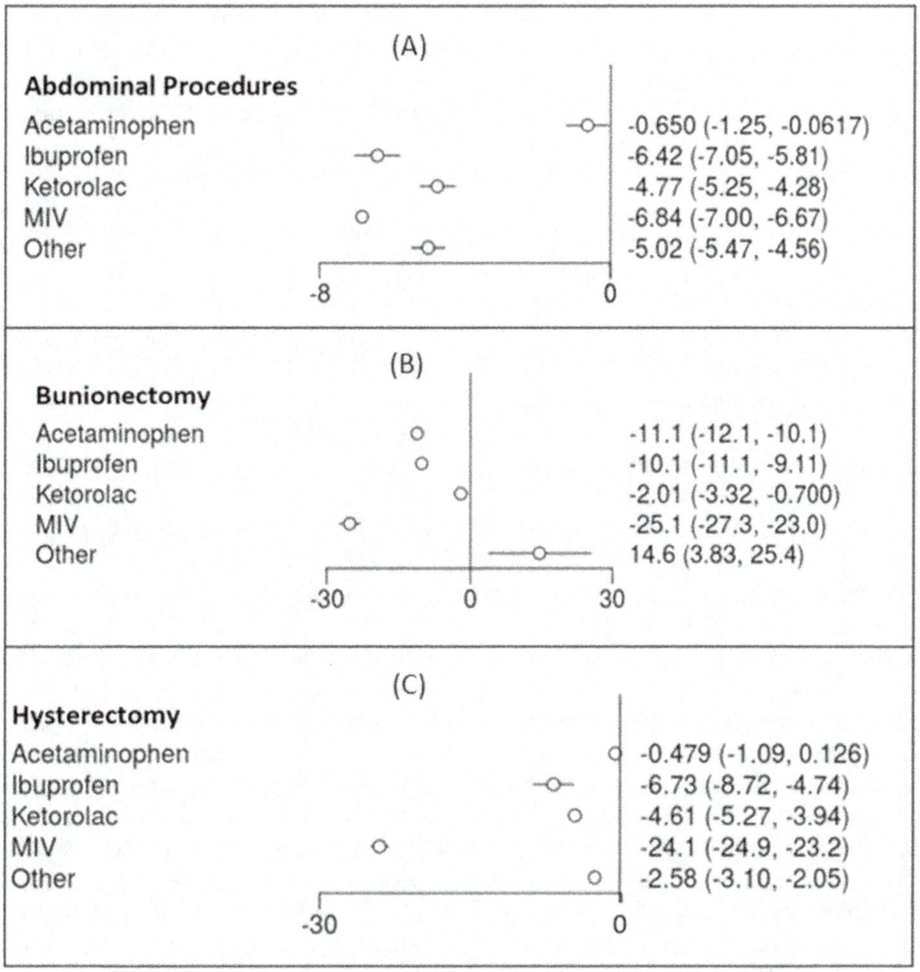

(A)

Abdominal Procedures

Treatment	Estimate (95% CI)
Acetaminophen	-0.650 (-1.25, -0.0617)
Ibuprofen	-6.42 (-7.05, -5.81)
Ketorolac	-4.77 (-5.25, -4.28)
MIV	-6.84 (-7.00, -6.67)
Other	-5.02 (-5.47, -4.56)

-8 0

(B)

Bunionectomy

Treatment	Estimate (95% CI)
Acetaminophen	-11.1 (-12.1, -10.1)
Ibuprofen	-10.1 (-11.1, -9.11)
Ketorolac	-2.01 (-3.32, -0.700)
MIV	-25.1 (-27.3, -23.0)
Other	14.6 (3.83, 25.4)

-30 0 30

(C)

Hysterectomy

Treatment	Estimate (95% CI)
Acetaminophen	-0.479 (-1.09, 0.126)
Ibuprofen	-6.73 (-8.72, -4.74)
Ketorolac	-4.61 (-5.27, -3.94)
MIV	-24.1 (-24.9, -23.2)
Other	-2.58 (-3.10, -2.05)

-30 0

Fig. 3 Summed pain intensity difference up to postoperative hour 24 (SPID 0–24) **a** Abdominal procedures **b** Bunionectomy **c** Hysterectomy

Table 2 Treatment Ranks Pooled Across Procedures for SPID 24 (Hours 0–24)[a]

Rank	Abdominal [b]	Bunionectomy	Hysterectomy [b]	Orthopedic
1	MIV (89.6%)	MIV (100%)	MIV (99.8%)	Results not included here because pain scores for MIV patients who underwent orthopedic procedures were not reported.
2	Ibuprofen	Acetaminophen	Ibuprofen	
3	Other	Ibuprofen	Other	
4	Ketorolac	Other	Ketorolac	
5	Acetaminophen	Ketorolac	Acetaminophen	
6	Placebo	Placebo	Placebo	

Note: Probabilities of top ranking are given in parentheses
Abbreviations: *MIV* Investigational IV meloxicam 30 mg
[a.] The 24-h period was the longest common follow-up time among procedure categories
[b.] Abdominal procedures and hysterectomy were included only open procedures

significant reduction (−32.1 [−33.9, − 30.3%] vs - <0.1 [-0.1, 0.1]) in MME used for rescue treatment up to 48 h postoperatively compared with acetaminophen and 117% higher significant reduction (−32.1 [−33.9, −30.3] vs -14.8 [-19.3 vs -10.2]) compared with ketorolac. MIV was also associated with a 170% higher significant reduction (−32.1 [−33.9, -30.3] vs -11.9 [-12.9, -11.0]) in MME used for rescue treatment up to 48 h compared with ibuprofen (Fig. 4c). Finally, for orthopedic procedures, MIV was associated with a significant reduction (−12.1 [−15.0 , −8.8] vs 9.6 [2.3, 12.9]) in MMEs used for rescue treatment up to 48 h postoperatively compared with acetaminophen. No significant results were found for ketorolac or ibuprofen (Fig. 4).

ORADE

Overall, the odds of ORADE were lower with MIV than with the other comparators (including all comparisons regardless of postoperative pain threshold; additional data available upon request). Across the abdominal procedure category, the odds of having either respiratory or gastrointestinal ORADE for Hours 0–48 associated with both ibuprofen and ketorolac were significantly higher compared with MIV (OR, Random Effects [95% CrI]: Ibuprofen (Respiratory): 1.3 [1.1, 1.5]; Ibuprofen (Gastrointestinal): 2.1 [1.6, 2.6]; Ketorolac (Respiratory): 1.6 [1.3, 1.9]; Ketorolac (Gastrointestinal): 1.4 [1.1, 1.7]). For bunionectomy, the odds of having both respiratory (OR, Random Effects [95% CrI]: 1.6 [1.3, 1.9]) or gastrointestinal (OR, Random Effects [95% CrI]: 1.4 [1.1, 1.7]) ORADE for Hours 0–48 associated with ketorolac were significantly higher compared with MIV. The findings, however, were not significant for acetaminophen compared with MIV (OR, Random Effects [95% CrI], Respiratory: 1.1 [0.8, 1.4]; Gastrointestinal: 0.8 [0.5, 1.1]). For hysterectomy, the odds of having both respiratory or gastrointestinal ORADE for Hours 0–48 associated with both ibuprofen and acetaminophen were significantly higher compared with MIV (OR, Random Effects [95% CrI]: acetaminophen (Respiratory): 1.8 [1.1, 2.5]; acetaminophen (Gastrointestinal): 1.3 [1.1, 1.5]; Ibuprofen (Respiratory): 1.4 [1.3, 1.5]; Ibuprofen (Gastrointestinal): 1.9 [1.4, 2.4]) (Fig. 3c). Significantly higher odds of respiratory ORADE (OR, Random Effects [95% CrI]: 2.2 [1.6,2.8] were found to be associated with ketorolac in comparison with MIV with no significant finding for gastrointestinal ORADE (OR, Random Effects [95% CrI]: 0.9 [0.7,1.1]. For miscellaneous orthopedic procedures, the odds of having a respiratory or gastrointestinal ORADE for Hours 0–48 associated with both ibuprofen and ketorolac were significantly higher compared with MIV except for ketorolac (respiratory), (OR, Random Effects [95% CrI]: Ibuprofen (Respiratory): 1.6 [1.4, 1.8]; Ibuprofen (Gastrointestinal): 2.1 [1.4, 2.8]; Ketorolac (Respiratory): 1.2 [0.7, 1.7]; Ketorolac (Gastrointestinal): 2.4 [1.8, 3.0]) (Fig. 5).

Discussion

Meloxicam, a NSAID, was first approved in the US in 2000 for oral use [28]. Oral meloxicam has been marketed to treat symptoms of osteoarthritis and rheumatoid arthritis but has a slow onset of action largely caused by its poor water solubility [63]. Intravenous meloxicam is an approved product that utilizes the NanoCrystal™ platform, a technology designed to enable enhanced bioavailability of poorly water-soluble drug compounds [63]. Based on the results of multiple clinical trials, MIV has been found to provide relief of moderate to severe acute pain, alone or in combination with other analgesics within the first 15 min after dosing and up to 24 h after dosing compared to placebo. The current study assessed the safety and efficacy of MIV relative to other IV non-opioid analgesics for managing moderate-severe postoperative pain by conducting an NMA. The outcomes associated with pain, MME and ORADEs (respiratory and gastrointestinal) were indirectly compared with non-opioid IV analgesics comparators including acetaminophen, ibuprofen and ketorolac.

In reducing pain intensity (SPID 24), MIV was significantly more effective than all comparators for all

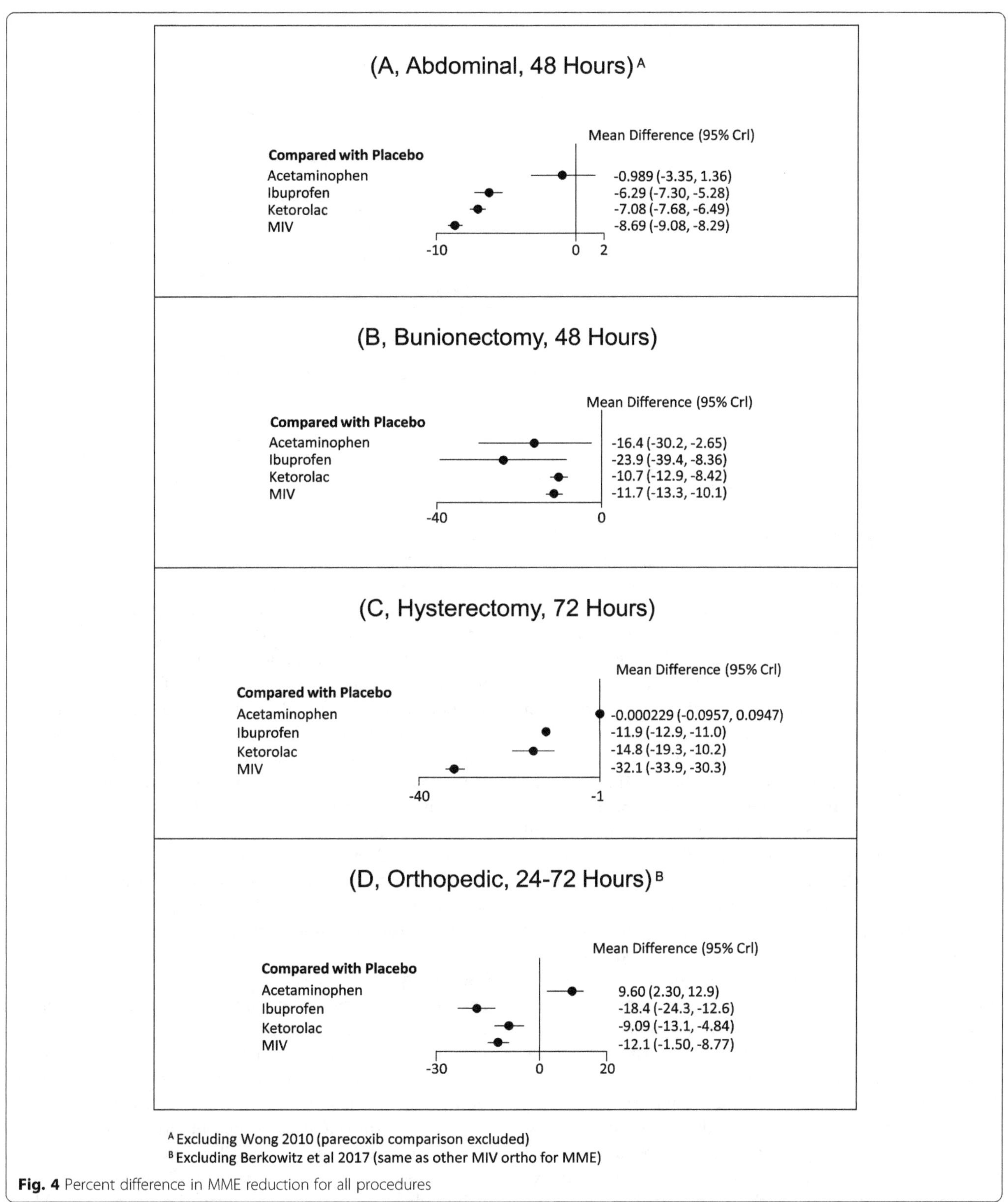

Fig. 4 Percent difference in MME reduction for all procedures

procedure categories. In the case of MME, similar findings were observed, where MIV was associated with significant reduction in MME for most comparisons at 48- and 72-h postoperatively. Among MME comparisons for abdominal procedures and hysterectomy, a significant reduction in MME was observed with MIV compared to all comparators (acetaminophen, ibuprofen, and ketorolac). Mixed results were observed among other

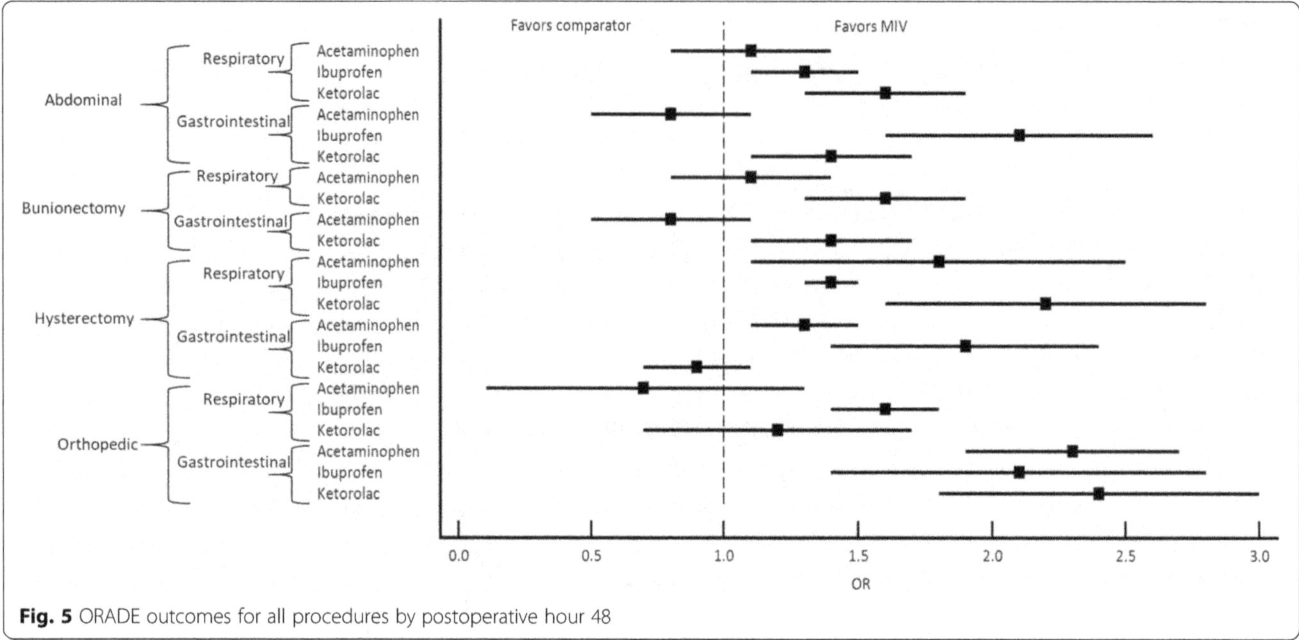

Fig. 5 ORADE outcomes for all procedures by postoperative hour 48

procedure categories, wherein, MIV was equivalent to other comparators in bunionectomy and orthopedic procedures, except versus acetminophen where a significant reduction in MME was observed with MIV in comparison. MIV was also observed to be associated with lower odds of ORADEs compared to other NSAIDs and acetaminophen for most procedures and comparators. Compared with ketorolac, MIV resulted in lower odds of ORADE for all procedures except hysterectomy (gastrointestinal ORADE) and orthopedic (respiratory ORADE) procedures. In case of acetaminophen, MIV did not show a reduction in ORADEs for most procedure categories including abdominoplasty (respiratory and gastrointestinal), bunionectomy (respiratory and gastrointestinal) and orthopedic (respiratory) except for hysterectomy and orthopedic (gastrointestinal).

This study has several limitations. First, the outcomes evaluated in this study were not controlled for dose-dependent effects as there were not enough number of studies to stratify by doses and consider variable dosing. However, this could have impacted outcomes if in some studies there were treatment groups with extremely higher/lower dosing, which was not found in our case. The doses were found to be within a narrow range. Secondly, outcomes are highly sensitive to underlying assumptions. For example, assumptions regarding what constituted a similar procedure to abdominoplasty affected which studies were chosen for that comparison. Since these were not abdominoplasties, there is some uncertainty regarding the external validity of the comparison. Also, confidence intervals for continuous data extracted from the literature were imputed when not reported in the original reports. This imputation requires assumptions regarding the shape of the probability distribution for those confidence intervals, which in turn affects the confidence intervals around the outcomes we produced. Third, some trials were not powered for evaluating the extracted outcomes. Fourth, few studies in the postoperative pain literature reported moderate-severe pain after surgery as inclusion criterion. Since the focus of the study was to compare (indirectly) MIV with other non-opioid analgesics, it was important that we included studies that had similar inclusion and exclusion criteria as MIV studies. Given that only limited number of current studies had the same inclusion criteria as MIV studies, relatively older studies were included in analysis to maintain homogeneity within the selected studies. Fifth, MIV trials were unique due to the two-hour window analysis of pain. Sixth, comparisons were not controlled for timing of pain assessment relative to rescue administration.

Conclusion

The current study found that among patients reporting moderate to severe postoperative pain MIV was superior in pain reduction for abdominoplasty, bunionectomy and hysterectomy when compared with acetaminophen, ibuprofen, and ketorolac. In reducing MME, MIV was superior or equivalent to all comparators and among all procedure categories except ibuprofen (bunionectomy and hysterectomy) and ketorolac (bunionectomy and orthopedic). Finally, MIV reduced the odds of ORADEs in most comparisons except ketorolac for hysterectomy (gastrointestinal ORADE) and orthopedic (respiratory ORADE) procedures, and acetaminophen for abdominoplasty (respiratory and gastrointestinal), bunionectomy (respiratory and gastrointestinal) and orthopedic (respiratory). Results should be interpreted with caution due to the indirect nature of the comparisons to approved IV non-opioid analgesics. Nevertheless, these results suggest MIV 30 mg may provide better pain reduction with similar or better safety to approved IV non-opioid analgesics.

Abbreviations

CrI: Credible interval; COX-1 and/or COX-2: Cyclooxygenase; MIV: IV meloxicam 30 mg; MME: Morphine milligram equivalent; NMA: Network-meta-analysis; NSAID: Non-steroidal anti-inflammatory drug; OR: Odds ratio; ORADE: Opioid-related adverse drug event; PICOT: Population, interventions, comparators, outcomes, time period; RCT: Randomized controlled clinical trial; SMD: Standardized mean difference; SPID: Sum of pain intensity difference; SUCRA: Surface under the cumulative ranking curve

Acknowledgements

Not applicable.

Authors' contributions

All authors conceived and designed the study. LB, JC, DS and TB participated in manuscript writing, data collection and data analysis. LB and JJ critically reviewed and edited the manuscript. All authors read and approved the final manuscript.

Author details

[1]Blue Point LLC, 711 Warrenville Road, Wheaton, IL 60189, USA. [2]Baudax Bio Inc, Malvern, PA, USA. [3]EPI-Q, Inc, Oak Brook, IL, USA. [4]Department of Anesthesiology and Perioperative Medicine, UCLA, Los Angeles, CA, USA.

References

1. Jahr JS, Bergese SD, Sheth KR, et al. Current perspective on the use of opioids in perioperative medicine: an evidence-based literature review, national survey of 70,000 physicians, and multidisciplinary clinical appraisal. Pain Med. 2018;19(9):1710–9. https://doi.org/10.1093/pm/pnx191.
2. Lovich-Sapola J, Smith CE, Brandt CP. Postoperative Pain control. Surg Clin North Am. 2015;95(2):301–18. https://doi.org/10.1016/j.suc.2014.10.002.
3. Sinatra R. Causes and consequences of inadequate management of acute pain. Pain Med. 2010;11(12):1859–71. https://doi.org/10.1111/j.1526-4637.2010.00983.x.
4. Warfield CA, Kahn CH. Acute pain management. Programs in U.S. hospitals and experiences and attitudes among U.S. adults. Anesthesiology. 1995; 83(5):1090–4. https://doi.org/10.1002/14651858.CD003348.pub2.
5. Janssen SA, Spinhoven P, Arntz A. The effects of failing to control pain: an experimental investigation. Pain. 2004;107(3):227–33. https://doi.org/10.1016/j.pain.2003.11.004.
6. Schumacher MA, Basbaum AI, Naidu RK. Opioid agonists & antagonists. In: Weitz M, Lebowitz H, editors. Basic & Clinical Pharmacology. 13th ed. New York City: McGraw-Hill Education; 2015.
7. McAdam-Marx C, Roland CL, Cleveland J, Oderda GM. Costs of opioid abuse and misuse determined from a medicaid database. J Pain Palliat Care Pharmacother. 2010;24(1):5–18. https://doi.org/10.3109/15360280903544877.
8. Oderda GM, Evans RS, Lloyd J, et al. Cost of opioid-related adverse drug events in surgical patients. J Pain Symptom Manag. 2003;25(3):276–83. https://doi.org/10.1016/S0885-3924(02)00691-7.
9. Oderda GM, Said Q, Evans RS, et al. Opioid-related adverse drug events in surgical hospitalizations: impact on costs and length of stay. Ann Pharmacother. 2007;41(3):400–7. https://doi.org/10.1345/aph.1H386.
10. Berry PH et al. National Pharmaceutical Council. Pain: Current Understanding of Assessment, Management, and Treatments. 2001. Available from: https://www.npcnow.org/publication/pain-current-understanding-assessment-management-and-treatments.
11. Rana MV, Desai R, Tran L, Davis D. Perioperative Pain control in the ambulatory setting. Curr Pain Headache Rep. 2016;20(3):18. https://doi.org/10.1007/s11916-016-0550-3.
12. Jahr JS, Donkor KN, Sinatra RS. Non-Selective Non-Steroidal Anti-Inflammatory Drugs (NSAIDs), Cyclooxygenase-2 Inhibitors (COX-2Is), and Acetaminophen in Acute Perioperative Pain: Analgesic efficacy, opiate-sparing effects, and adverse effects. In: Sinatra R, de Leon-Cassola O, Ginsberg B, Viscusi ER, editors. Acute Pain Management. 2nd ed. New York: Cambridge University Press; 2009. p. 332–65.
13. Bollinger AJ, Butler PD, Nies MS, Sietsema DL, Jones CB, Endres TJ. Is scheduled intravenous acetaminophen effective in the pain management protocol of geriatric hip fractures? Geriatr Orthop Surg Rehabil. 2015;6(3): 202–8. https://doi.org/10.1177/2151458515588560.
14. Chou R, Gordon DB, de Leon-Casasola OA, et al. Management of Postoperative Pain: a clinical practice guideline from the American Pain society, the American Society of Regional Anesthesia and Pain Medicine, and the American Society of Anesthesiologists' committee on regional anesthesia, Executive Commi. J Pain. 2016;17(2):131–57. https://doi.org/10.1016/j.jpain.2015.12.008.
15. Elia N, Lysakowski C, Tramèr M. Does multimodal analgesia with acetaminophen, nonsteroidal anti-inflammatory drugs, or selective cyclooxygenase-2 inhibitors and patient-controlled analgesia morphine offer advantages over morphine alone? meta-analyses of randomized trials. Anesthesiology. 2005;103(6):1296–304 doi: 0000542–200512000-00025.
16. Conway SL, Mattews ML, Pesaturo KA. The role of parenteral NSAIDs in postoperative pain control. US Pharm. 2010;35(5):HS16.
17. Garimella VCC. Postoperative Pain control. Clin Colon Rectal Surg. 2013; 26(3):191–6. https://doi.org/10.1016/j.suc.2014.10.002.
18. Chapman SJ, Garner JJ, Drake TM, Aldaffaa M, Jayne DG. Systematic review and meta-analysis of nonsteroidal anti-inflammatory drugs to improve gi recovery after colorectal surgery. Dis Colon Rectum. 2019;62(2):248–56. https://doi.org/10.1097/DCR.0000000000001281.
19. Pavy TJG, Paech MJ, Evans SF. The effect of intravenous ketorolac on opioid requirement and pain after cesarean delivery. Anesth Analg. 2001;92(4): 1010–4. https://doi.org/10.1097/00000539-200104000-00038.
20. Cumberland Pharmaceuticals Inc. CALDOLOR (ibuprofen) Injection; 2016. p. 1–15. http://www.caldolor.com/. Accessed 17 Apr 2019.
21. Moller PL, Sindet-Pedersen S, Petersen CT, Juhl GI, Dillenschneider A, Skoglund LA. Onset of acetaminophen analgesia: comparison of oral and intravenous routes after third molar surgery. Br J Anaesth. 2005;94(5):642–8. https://doi.org/10.1093/bja/aei109.
22. McGettigan P, Henry D. Current problems with non-specific COX inhibitors. Curr Pharm Des. 2000;6(17):1693–724. https://doi.org/10.2174/1381612003398690.
23. Stephens J. The burden of acute postoperative pain and the potential role of the COX-2-specific inhibitors. Rheumatology. 2003;42(suppl3):iii40–52. https://doi.org/10.1093/rheumatology/keg497.
24. Polomano BRC, Fillman M, Giordano NA, Vallerand AH, Pain T. Multimodal analgesia for acute postoperative and trauma-related Pain. Am J Nurs. 2017; 117(3 Suppl 1):S12–26.
25. Schoenfeld P. Gastrointestinal safety profile of meloxicam: a meta-analysis and systematic review of randomized controlled trials. Am J Med. 1999; 107(6A):48S–54S. https://doi.org/10.1016/S0002-9343(99)00367-8.
26. Hunt RH, Harper S, Watson DJ, et al. The gastrointestinal safety of the COX-2 selective inhibitor etoricoxib assessed by both endoscopy and analysis of upper gastrointestinal events. Am J Gastroenterol. 2003;98(8):1725–33. https://doi.org/10.1111/j.1572-0241.2003.07598.x.
27. Mukherjee D, Nissen SE, Topol EJ. Risk of cardiovascular events associated with selective COX-2 inhibitors. JAMA. 2001;286(8):954–9. https://doi.org/10.1001/jama.286.8.954.
28. MOBIC (meloxicam) tablet. [package insert]. Ridgefield, CT: Boehringer Ingelheim Pharmaceuticals I. MOBIC Product Information; 2018. p. 1–30. https://docs.boehringer-ingelheim.com/Prescribing%20Information/PIs/Mobic/MobicTabs7-5-15mg.PDF. Accessed 17 Apr 2019.
29. Dannhardt G, Kiefer W. Cyclooxygenase inhibitors - current status and future prospects. Eur J Med Chem. 2001;36(2):109–26. https://doi.org/10.1016/S0223-5234(01)01197-7.
30. Wright JM. The double-edged sword of COX-2 selective NSAIDs. CMAJ. 2002;167(10):1131–7.
31. Christensen SE, Cooper SA, Mack RJ, McCallum SW, Du W, Freyer A. A randomized double-blind controlled trial of intravenous meloxicam in the treatment of Pain following dental impaction surgery. J Clin Pharmacol. 2018;58(5):593–605. https://doi.org/10.1002/jcph.1058.
32. Rechberger T, Mack RJ, Mccallum SW, Du W, Freyer A. Analgesic efficacy and safety of intravenous meloxicam in subjects with moderate-to-severe Pain after open abdominal hysterectomy: a phase 2 randomized clinical trial. Anesth Analg. 2019;128(6):1309–18. https://doi.org/10.1213/ANE.0000000000003920.

33. Gottlieb IJ, Tunick DR, Mack RJ, et al. Evaluation of the safety and efficacy of an intravenous nanocrystal formulation of meloxicam in the management of moderate-to-severe pain after bunionectomy. J Pain Res. 2018;11:383–93. https://doi.org/10.2147/JPR.S149879.
34. Singla N, Bindewald M, Singla S, et al. Efficacy and safety of intravenous meloxicam in subjects with moderate-to-severe Pain following Abdominoplasty. Plast Reconstr Surg Glob Open. 2018;6(6):e1846. https://doi.org/10.1097/GOX.0000000000001846.
35. Pollak RA, Gottlieb IJ, Hakakian F, et al. Efficacy and safety of intravenous meloxicam in patients with moderate-to-severe Pain following Bunionectomy. Clin J Pain. 2018;34(10):918–26. https://doi.org/10.1097/AJP.0000000000000609.
36. Bergese SD, Melson TI, Candiotti KA, et al. A phase 3 , randomized , placebo- controlled evaluation of the safety of intravenous meloxicam following major surgery. Clin Pharmacol Drug Dev. 2019;8(8):1062–72. https://doi.org/10.1002/cpdd.666.
37. Singla N, Mccallum SW, Mack RJ, Freyer A, Hobson S. Safety and efficacy of an intravenous nanocrystal formulation of meloxicam in the management of moderate to severe pain following laparoscopic abdominal surgery. J Pain Res. 2018;11:1901–3. https://doi.org/10.2147/JPR.S163736.
38. Higgins JPT, Thomas J, Chandler J, Cumpston M, Li T, Page MJ, Welch VA (editors). Cochrane handbook for systematic reviews of interventions version 6.0 (updated July 2019). Cochrane, 2019. Available from: www.training.cochrane.org/handbook.
39. Higgins JP, Thompson SG. Quantifying heterogeneity in a meta-analysis. Stat Med. 2002;21(11):1539–58. https://doi.org/10.1002/sim.1186.
40. Ghosh M, Kim YH. The behrens-fisher problem revisited: a bayes-frequentist synthesis. Can J Stat. 2001;29(1):5–17. https://doi.org/10.2307/3316047.
41. Apfelbaum JL, Desjardins PJ, Brown MT, Verburg KM. Multiple-day efficacy of parecoxib sodium treatment in postoperative bunionectomy pain. Clin J Pain. 2008;24(9):784–92. https://doi.org/10.1097/AJP.0b013e31817a717c.
42. Bakhsha F, Niaki AS, Jafari SY, Yousefi Z, Aryaie M. The Effects of Diclofenac Suppository and Intravenous Acetaminophen and their Combination on the Severity of Postoperative Pain in Patients Undergoing Spinal Anaesthesia During Cesarean Section. J Clin Diagn Res. 2016;10(7):UC09–12. https://doi.org/10.7860/JCDR/2016/15093.8120.
43. Bangash AA, Durrani Z. Effectiveness of acetaminophen in control of breakthrough pain: randomized controlled trial. J Pak Med Assoc. 2018;68(7):994–1001.
44. Berkowitz RD, Sharpe K, Mack RJ, McCallum S, Gomez A, Freyer A, Du W. A Phase 3, Placebo-Controlled Study of Meloxicam IV Following Major Surgery: Safety and Opioid Use Following Major Orthopedic Procedures. Poster 5174 presented at the 2018 World Congress on Regional Anesthesia & Pain Medicine. April 19-21, 2018. New York City, New York, United States of America.
45. Bikhazi GB, Snabes MC, Bajwa ZH, et al. A clinical trial demonstrates the analgesic activity of intravenous parecoxib sodium compared with ketorolac or morphine after gynecologic surgery with laparotomy. Am J Obstet Gynecol. 2004;191(4):1183–91. https://doi.org/10.1016/j.ajog.2004.05.006.
46. Castro F, Pardo D, Mosquera G, Peleteiro R, Camba MA. Management of postoperative pain with PCA in upper abdominal surgery. Comparative study: tramadol versus metamizol and kerotolac [Tratamiento del dolor postoperatorio con PCA en cirugia del abdomen superior. Estudio comparativo, tramadol versus metamizol]. Rev la Soc Esp del Dolor. 2000;7:12–6.
47. Daniels SE, Playne R, Stanescu I, Zhang J, Gottlieb IJ, Atkinson HC. Efficacy and Safety of an Intravenous Acetaminophen/Ibuprofen Fixed-dose Combination After Bunionectomy: a Randomized, Double-blind, Factorial, Placebo-controlled Trial. Clin Ther. 2019;41(10):1982–1995.e8. https://doi.org/10.1016/j.clinthera.2019.07.008.
48. Daniels S, Melson T, Hamilton DA, Lang E, Carr DB. Analgesic efficacy and safety of a novel injectable formulation of diclofenac compared with intravenous ketorolac and placebo after orthopedic surgery: a multicenter, randomized, double-blinded, multiple-dose trial. Clin J Pain. 2013;29(8):655–63. https://doi.org/10.1097/AJP.0b013e318270f957.
49. Essex MN, Choi HY, Bhadra Brown P, Cheung R. A randomized study of the efficacy and safety of parecoxib for the treatment of pain following total knee arthroplasty in Korean patients. J Pain Res. 2018;11:427–33. https://doi.org/10.2147/JPR.S147481.
50. Gago Martínez A, Escontrela Rodriguez B, Planas Roca A, Martínez RA. Intravenous ibuprofen for treatment of post-operative pain: a multicenter, double blind, placebo-controlled, randomized clinical trial. PLoS One. 2016;11(5):e0154004. https://doi.org/10.1371/journal.pone.0154004.
51. Gan TJ, Daniels SE, Singla N, Hamilton DA, Carr DB. A novel injectable formulation of diclofenac compared with intravenous ketorolac or placebo for acute moderate-to-severe pain after abdominal or pelvic surgery: a multicenter, double-blind, randomized, multiple-dose study. Anesth Analg. 2012;115(5):1212–20. https://doi.org/10.1213/ANE.0b013e3182691bf9.
52. Hynes D, McCarroll M, Hiesse-Provost O. Analgesic efficacy of parenteral paracetamol (propacetamol) and diclofenac in post-operative orthopaedic pain. Acta Anaesthesiol Scand. 2006;50(3):374–81. https://doi.org/10.1111/j.1399-6576.2006.00971.x.
53. Kim MH, Hahm TS. Plasma levels of interleukin-6 and interleukin-10 are affected by ketorolac as an adjunct to patient-controlled morphine after abdominal hysterectomy. Clin J Pain. 2001;17(1):72–7. https://doi.org/10.1097/00002508-200103000-00010.
54. Kroll PB, Meadows L, Rock A, Pavliv L. A multicenter, randomized, double-blind, placebo-controlled trial of intravenous ibuprofen (IV-ibuprofen) in the management of postoperative Pain following abdominal hysterectomy. Pain Pract. 2011;11(11):23–32. https://doi.org/10.1111/j.1533-2500.2010.00402.x.
55. Pareek A, Chandurkar N, Gupta A, et al. Comparative evaluation of efficacy and safety of etodolac and diclofenac sodium injection in patients with postoperative orthopedic pain. Curr Med Res Opin. 2011;27(11):2107–15. https://doi.org/10.1185/03007995.2011.619179.
56. Reinhart DJ, Stagg KS, Walker KG, et al. Postoperative analgesia after peripheral nerve block for podiatric surgery: clinical efficacy and chemical stability of lidocaine alone versus lidocaine plus ketorolac. Reg Anesth Pain Med. 2000;25(5):506–13. https://doi.org/10.1053/rapm.2000.7624.
57. Rindos NB, Mansuria SM, Ecker AM, Stuparich MA, King CR. Intravenous acetaminophen vs saline in perioperative analgesia with laparoscopic hysterectomy. Am J Obstet Gynecol. 2019;2220(4):373.e1–8. https://doi.org/10.1016/j.ajog.2019.01.212.
58. Singla N, Rock A, Pavliv L. A multi-center, randomized, double-blind placebo-controlled trial of intravenous-ibuprofen (IV-ibuprofen) for treatment of pain in post-operative orthopedic adult patientspme. Pain Med. 2010;11(8):1284–93. https://doi.org/10.1111/j.1526-4637.2010.00896.x.
59. Takeda Y, Fukunishi S, Nishio S, Yoshiya S, Hashimoto K, Simura Y. Evaluating the effect of intravenous acetaminophen in multimodal analgesia after Total hip Arthroplasty: a randomized controlled trial. J Arthroplast. 2019;34(6):1155–61. https://doi.org/10.1016/j.arth.2019.02.033.
60. Thybo KH, Hägi-Pedersen D, Dahl JB, et al. Effect of combination of Paracetamol (acetaminophen) and ibuprofen vs either alone on patient-controlled morphine consumption in the first 24 hours after Total hip Arthroplasty: the PANSAID randomized clinical trial. JAMA. 2019;321(6):562–71. https://doi.org/10.1001/jama.2018.22039.
61. Wilson SH, Wolf BJ, Robinson SM, Nelson C, Hebbar L. Intravenous vs Oral acetaminophen for analgesia after cesarean delivery: a randomized trial. Pain Med. 2019;20(8):1584–91. https://doi.org/10.1093/pm/pny253.
62. Wong JON, Tan TDM, Cheu NW, et al. Comparison of the efficacy of parecoxib versus ketorolac combined with morphine on patient-controlled analgesia for post-cesarean delivery pain management. Acta Anaesthesiol Taiwanica. 2010;48(4):174–7. https://doi.org/10.1016/j.aat.2010.09.001.
63. Weyna DR, Cheney ML, Shan N, et al. Improving solubility and pharmacokinetics of meloxicam via multiple-component crystal formation. Mol Pharm. 2012;9(7):2094–102. https://doi.org/10.1021/mp300169c.

6

Wound infiltration with ropivacaine as an adjuvant to patient controlled analgesia for transforaminal lumbar interbody fusion

Kunpeng Li, Changbin Ji, Dawei Luo, Hongyong Feng, Keshi Yang and Hui Xu*

Abstract

Background: Surgical procedure usually causes serious postoperative pain and poor postoperative pain management negatively affects quality of life, function and recovery time. We aimed to investigate the role of wound infiltration with ropivacaine as an adjuvant to patient controlled analgesia (PCA) in postoperative pain control for patients undergoing transforaminal lumbar interbody fusion.

Methods: One hundred twelve patients undergoing lumbar fusion were retrospectively reviewed and divided into two groups (ropivacaine and control groups) according to whether received wound infiltration with ropivacaine or not. Visual Analogue Scale (VAS) score, analgesics consumption, number of patients requiring rescue analgesic, hospital duration and incidence of complications were recorded. Surgical trauma was assessed using operation time, intraoperative blood loss and incision length.

Results: The amount of sufentanil consumption in ropivacaine group at 4 h postoperatively was lower than that of control group (24.5 ± 6.0 μg vs 32.1 ± 7.0 μg, $P < 0.001$) and similar results were observed at 8, 12, 24, 48 and 72 h postoperatively($P < 0.001$). Fewer patients required rescue analgesia within 4 to 8 h postoperatively in ropivacaine group (10/60 vs 19/52, $P = 0.017$). Length of postoperative hospital durations were shorter in patients receiving ropivacaine infiltration compared to control cohorts (6.9 ± 0.9 days vs 7.4 ± 0.9 days, $P = 0.015$). The incidence of PONV in ropivacaine group was lower than that in control group (40.4% vs 18.3%, $P = 0.01$). However, VAS scores were similar in two groups at each follow-up points postoperatively, and no difference was observed($P > 0.05$).

Conclusion: Wound infiltration with ropivacaine effectively reduces postoperative opioid consumption and PONV and may be a useful adjuvant to PCA to improve recovery for patients undergoing lumbar spine surgery.

Keywords: Wound infiltration, Ropivacaine, Pain management, PCA, Transforaminal lumbar interbody fusion

* Correspondence: xuhspine@163.com
Department of Orthopaedics, Liaocheng People's Hospital, No 67 Dongchang West Road, Liaocheng City 252000, Shandong Province, China

Background

Transforaminal lumbar interbody fusion (TLIF) has been widely used in treatment of lumbar degenerative spine disorders, and achieved good clinical results and high patient satisfaction [1, 2]. It can decompress the nerve roots, immobilize the instrumented segments and provide stability of spine. Despite its good outcome, surgical procedure usually causes serious postoperative pain and poor pain management negatively affects quality of life, function, and recovery [3].

Traditionally, patient-controlled analgesia (PCA) has been identified as effective in postoperative pain management and is the most frequently used analgesic method for spine surgery [4, 5]. However, the main drug used is opioid analgesics, which have severe side effects including nausea or vomiting, confusion, urinary retention, sedation, respiratory depression, and pruritus [6]. Therefore, finding other analgesic strategies with fewer potentially adverse effects will be beneficial for patients suffering from postoperative pain.

In recent years, wound infiltration with local anesthetics has become an attractive method in postoperative analgesia because of its safety, simplicity and low-cost [7, 8]. As a local anesthetic, ropivacaine is a propyl analog of bupivacaine with longer duration of action and much safer cardiotoxicity profile. Several reports [9, 10] have confirmed that wound infiltration with ropivacaine could significantly reduce postoperative pain, mitigate supplemental analgesic demand as well as curtail hospital stay following some surgeries, such as joint replacement, abdominal surgeries, and cesarean deliveries.

With the ideal analgesic modality for lumbar fusion surgery still unknown and possibly simpler alternatives to local infiltration analgesia gaining popularity, it is imperative to clarify the role of wound infiltration with ropivacaine in managing postoperative pain after this procedure. We hypothesized that wound infiltration with ropivacaine as an adjuvant to PCA for patients undergoing TLIF is more effective than PCA alone, resulting in lower postoperative pain scores, less consumption of opioid medications and lower incidence of postoperative nausea and vomiting (PONV) compared with PCA alone.

Methods

Patient population

This retrospective cohort study was conducted in Liaocheng People's Hospital. All patients were identified to undergo single-level TLIF procedure with a single surgeon between January 2016 and December 2018. The inclusion criteria were as follow: age 18–65 years, primary diagnosis of lumbar disc herniation, lumbar spinal stenosis and lumbar degenerative spondylolisthesis (grade 1), single level TLIF (L3/4, L4/5 or L5/S1), American Society of Anesthesiologists (ASA) grade I to II. Patients were excluded according to the exclusion criteria: allergic to ropivacaine, preoperative opioid consumption in last 3 months, and history of spine surgery.

Enrolled patients were divided into two groups, ropivacaine group and control group. Each patient provided written informed consent before enrollment. The study was approved by the Ethics Committee of Liaocheng People's Hospital.

Surgical procedure

The procedure was performed as described by Ge [11]. All procedures were carried out under controlled general anesthesia with endotracheal intubation. Each patient was positioned prone on a radiolucent operating table after induction of general anesthesia. Radiographs were used to check the operation level. A midline approach was used to expose the lamina and spinous processes. Bilateral pedicle screws were placed and a rod was sited using special persuaders. The laminectomy and facetectomy were then performed at the level. The cartilaginous material was removed from the endplates using the scraper. The autogenous morselized bone from the laminae and processus articularis was placed into the anterior intervertebral space. This was followed by the implantation of cage plus autogenous bone. The wound was copiously irrigated and closed in layers. Routine monitoring included electrocardiography, pulse oximetry, blood pressure, and arterial blood gas analysis. All patients received general anesthesia with 0.1% propofol, dexmethetomedine, fentanyl, remifentanil and cisatracurium. No preemptive scheduled analgesic regimen was employed.

Wound infiltration with ropivacaine

Just before closure, 10 ml ropivacaine (concentration: 0.75%) was infiltrated in paravertebral muscles, subcutaneous, and cutaneous tissue along each side of the wound edges. At the end of surgery, patients were turned to supine position, and extubated successfully on the table. Once awake and responded to verbal commands, patients were transferred to the post-anesthesia care unit (PACU). After PACU, patients were transferred to spine ward for further monitoring and recovery care.

Postoperative management

All patients received intravenous PCA with 0.8 μg/ml of sufentanil for 72 h. The sufentanil was administrated via PCA pump at a bolus of 2 ml (1.6μg) with a 5 min lockout time and the maximum dosage was 12.8μg per hour. Flurbiprofen axetil was injected as a rescue analgesic when requested by patients with visual analogue scale (VAS) scores≥5.

Patients were routinely administered prophylactic antibiotics for 24 h and encouraged to start out-of-bed activities with braces within 3 days after surgery. Mechanical thomboprophylaxis was given to prevent phlebothrombosis of both legs. Since discharge from the hospital, all patients were clinically and radiologically assessed in outpatient clinic every 3 months.

Observation index

Primary outcome was total sufentanil consumption over the first 72 h. The sufentanil consumption can be calculated by multiplying the volume by the concentration (0.8μg/ml, total 200μg sufentanil in 250 ml saline). The volume of saline was shown in the PCA pump. Secondary outcome measures were VAS scores, number of patients requiring flurbiprofen axetil as analgesic rescue and incidence of complications including PONV and wound infection. Operation time, intraoperative blood loss, incision length and length of postoperative hospital duration were also recorded in the data.

Sample size and statistical analyses

The sample size was determined for the primary outcome measure. According to previous study [12], a difference of more than10ug in sufentanil consumption at 24 h after surgery between groups was considered clinically relevant. Under the assumption that the standard deviation is 16μg, a sample size of 41 per group was determined (power = 80%, $p = 0.05$). For the secondary outcome of VAS score, sample size estimates were also considered. On the basis of the data from clinical practice and the study by Elder et al. [13], the standard deviation for the VAS was assumed to be 2.0 and a sample size of 38 patients per group would provide statistical power of 80% to detect a difference between groups of 1.3. Additionally, we reviewed several similar reports [14, 15] and found that the number of treated subjects was approximately 40 to 50. Therefore, we determined that a total of 50 patients per group were enrolled. The power was 0.872 according to primary outcome data mentioned above ($n = 50$, $\sigma = 16$, $\delta = 10$, $\alpha = 0.05$). The sample size and power analysis were performed using Power and Sample Size Calculation version 3.1.6.

The SPSS 22.0 statistical package (SPSS, Chicago, IL, U.S.A.) was used for statistical analyses. Continuous data were presented as the mean ± standard deviation and analyzed using two-sample t test and ANOVA analysis. Chi square test was performed to analyze count data. For all analyses, a P value < 0.05 was considered statistically significant.

Results

This clinical trial enrolled 112 patients undergoing single-level TLIF procedure, 60 patients who received wound infiltration with ropivacaine in ropivacaine group and 52 without ropivacaine infiltration in control group.

Table 1 Characteristics of the patient cohort in two groups

Parameter	Ropivacaine group	Control group	*P* value
Number of patients	60	52	
Age (years)	57.9 ± 7.7 (41–73)	56.9 ± 7.5 (42–72)	0.529
Gender, males/females	39/21	35/17	0.799
Weight (kg)	67.2 ± 8.2	66.3 ± 8.9	0.581
Height (cm)	167.9 ± 6.5	168.8 ± 6.5	0.472
BMI (kg/m^2)	23.8 ± 2.0	23.2 ± 2.1	0.134
Diagnosis			0.775
LDH	26	32	
LSS	17	16	
LDS	9	12	
Operation level			0.790
L3/4	6	5	
L4/5	25	32	
L5/S1	21	23	
Operation time (min)	103.1 ± 15.2	106.5 ± 17.1	0.260
Intraoperative blood loss (ml)	250.6 ± 38.6	258.1 ± 39.7	0.314
Incision length (cm)	6.2 ± 0.7	6.1 ± 0.8	0.299
Postoperative hospital duration (day)	6.9 ± 0.9	7.4 ± 0.9	0.015

LDH Lumbar disc herniation, *LSS* Lumbar spinal stenosis, *LDS* Lumbar degenerative spondylolisthesis

Patients' demographics and basic characteristics, including age, gender, weight, height, body mass index (BMI), primary diagnosis and operation level were shown in the Table 1, and no significant difference was observed between two groups.

Operation index and hospital duration

The mean operation time was 103.1 ± 15.2 min and 106.5 ± 17.1 min in ropivacaine and control groups respectively, and no difference was found ($P = 0.26$). There was also no difference in incision length and intraoperative blood loss between two groups ($P = 0.299$ and $P = 0.314$) (Table 1).

For patients receiving ropivacaine infiltration, length of postoperative hospital duration was 6.9 ± 0.9 days, which was shorter than that of control cohort (7.4 ± 0.9 days), and significant difference was detected between two groups ($P = 0.015$) (Table 1).

Postoperative analgesics consumption

The amount of sufentanil consumption at 4 h postoperatively in ropivacaine group was lower than that in control group ($P < 0.001$). Significant difference was also found in the cumulative sufentanil consumption between two groups at 8, 12, 24, 48 and 72 h after surgery ($P < 0.001$).

Patients in the ropivacaine group consumed less sufentanil than those in the control group within 4 to 8 h postoperatively ($P < 0.001$). Similar results were observed within 8 to12 hours and 12 to 24 h postoperatively ($P < 0.001$ and $P = 0.001$). However, no difference was detected within 24 to 48 h and 48 to 72 h postoperatively ($P = 0.276$ and $P = 0.547$) (Fig. 1).

There were five patients who required flurbiprofen axetil as rescue in the ropivacaine group and eight in the control group within first 4 h postoperatively, and no difference was found($P = 0.245$). However, fewer patients in ropivacaine group needed analgesic rescue within 4 to 8 h postoperatively compared to control group ($P = 0.017$). Within 8 to 12 h postoperatively, no difference was found between two groups ($P = 0.101$) (Table 2).

Table 2 The administration of flurbiprofen axetil in two groups

Period	Ropivacaine group	Control group	*P* value
First 4 h	5/60	8/52	0.245
From 4 to 8 h	10/60	19/52	0.017
From 8 to 12 h	6/60	11/52	0.101

Pain evaluation

Average VAS scores at 4 h postoperatively was 3.7 ± 1.5 points in ropivacaine group and 3.7 ± 1.3 points in control group, and no difference was observed ($P = 0.808$). Similar results were shown between the ropivacaine and control groups at 8 h (4.1 ± 1.3 vs 4.3 ± 1.1, $P = 0.568$), 12 h (4.3 ± 1.3 vs 4.4 ± 1.2, $P = 0.655$), 24 h (3.3 ± 1.1 vs 3.4 ± 1.0, $P = 0.822$), 48 h (2.4 ± 0.6 vs 2.3 ± 0.5, $P = 0.700$)

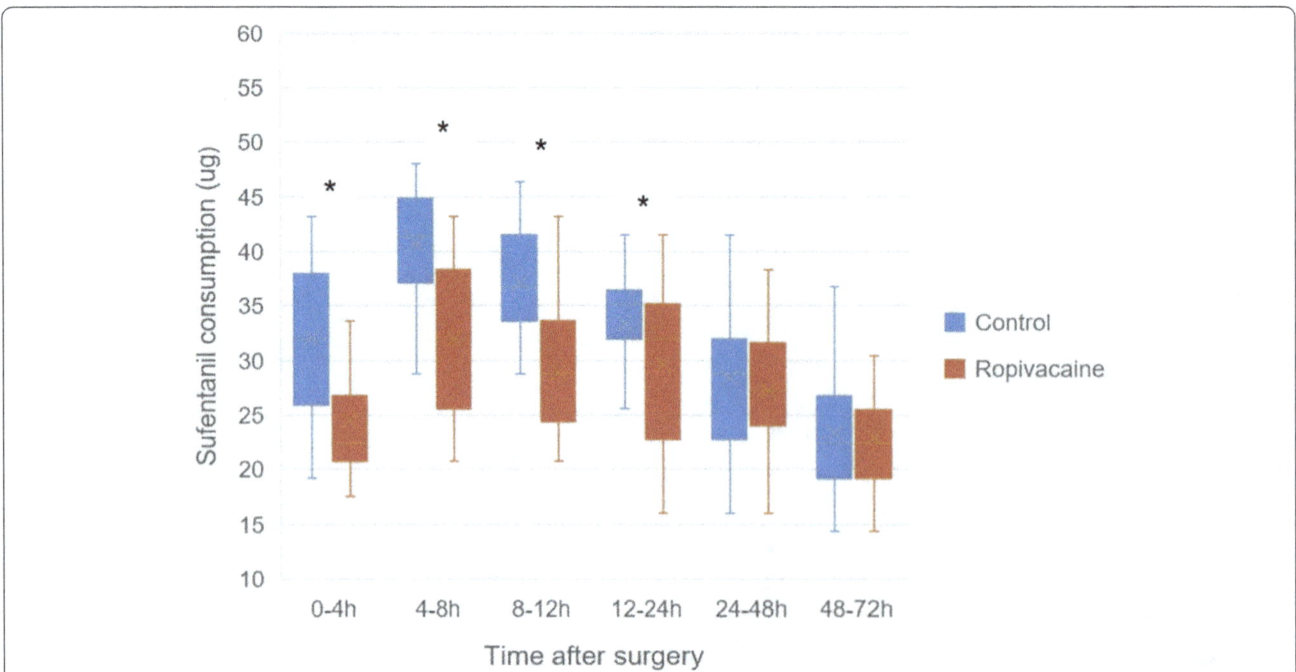

Fig. 1 Boxplot showing sufentanil consumption in the postoperative period for two groups. The boxes indicate the interquartile range, the crosses within the boxes indicate the median, and the whiskers indicate the range. The asterisks indicate significance($P < 0.05$). h = hours postoperatively

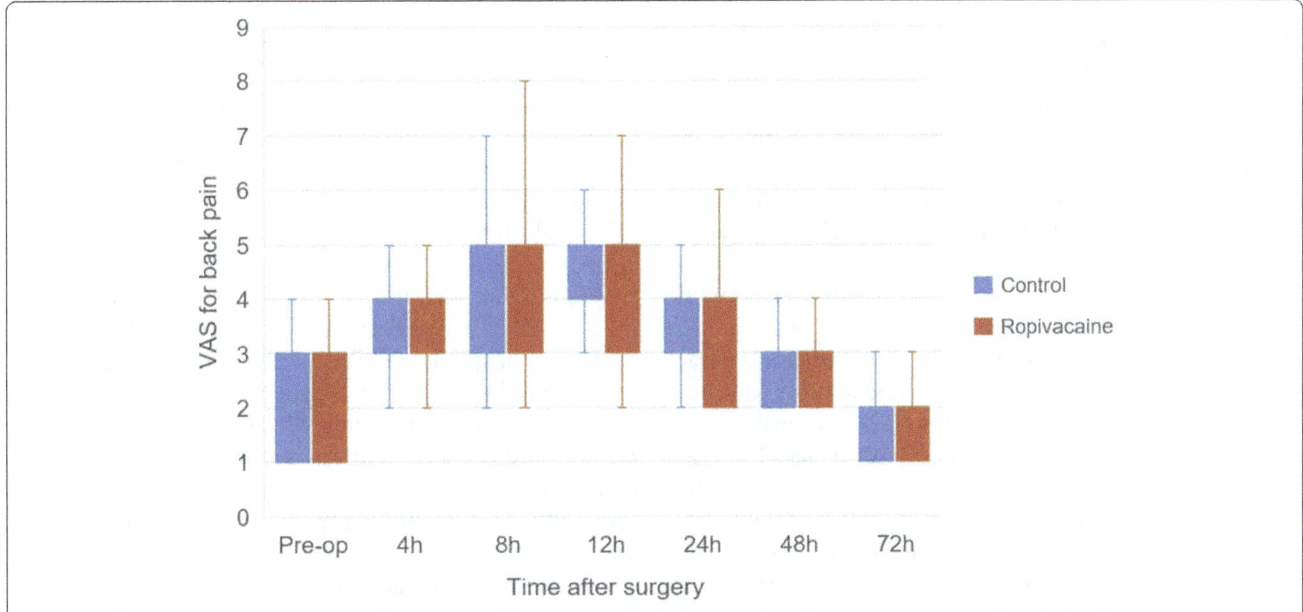

Fig. 2 Boxplot showing VAS scores for back pain over the first 72 h postoperatively for two groups. The boxes indicate the interquartile range, the crosses within the boxes indicate the median, and the whiskers indicate the range. No significant difference was observed at each time between two groups($P > 0.05$). h = hours postoperatively

and 72 h (1.8 ± 0.6 vs 1.8 ± 0.6, $P = 0.964$) postoperatively (Fig. 2).

Complications

The incidence of PONV in the ropivacaine group was lower than that in the control group (18.3% vs 40.4%, $P = 0.010$). Only one patient had wound infection in each group and no difference was detected ($P = 0.919$, Table 3). These two patients recovered after routine antibiotic treatment and dressing change. No clinical deterioration, permanent morbidity or mortality occurred in this study. There was also no hardware failure, nerve root injury, cerebrospinal fluid leakage, and adjacent segment disc herniation over the follow-up.

Discussion

In this study, we adopted wound infiltration with ropivacaine as an adjuvant to PCA in TLIF procedure to assess its efficacy in postoperative pain management. Results showed better outcomes in patients who received the wound infiltration with ropivacaine. It reduced the consumption of opioid drugs via PCA after TLIF procedure and decreased the number of patients who required rescue analgesia, while achieving similar pain relief. The data further indicated a lower incidence of PONV and a shorter hospital duration in the ropivacaine group.

Table 3 The incidence of complications in two groups

Complication	Ropivacaine group	Control group	*P* value
PONV	11/60	21/52	0.010
wound infection	1/60	1/52	0.919

Currently, PCA is the most widely used approach to manage postoperative pain after spine surgery. However, the use of opioids in PCA is often associated with adverse effects. So multimodal pain management is recommended in order to reduce opioid-related adverse effects. Since Mullen and Cook first demonstrated the use of wound infiltration with local anesthetics in spine surgery in 1979 [16], a few literatures reported the application of wound infiltration with local anesthetics in several surgical procedures. Koehler [15] performed a randomized controlled trial and reported that surgical-site injection with a multimodal cocktail could reduce narcotic utilization and provide improved pain control, with no adverse effects attributable to the local injection. Similarly, in a retrospective study of patients undergoing thoracolumbar junction fracture surgery, Swennen [17] found that local infiltration analgesia had a reduction of VAS and morphine consumption in postoperative pain control. Another two studies [13, 18] on the continuous analgesic infusion also demonstrated better outcomes in managing postoperative pain with less opioid use and lower pain scores.

The main outcome measures in this study were visual analogue pain score and opioid usage. In the current study, results showed patients receiving ropivacaine infiltration reported similar VAS scores and less sufentanil consumption via PCA at each follow-up point within 72 h after surgery, which was not completely consistent with previous reports. Although similar VAS score was reported in two groups, less opioid use was another important indicator that reflected the decreased postoperative pain in ropivacaine group. We further found that periodic consumption of sufentanil in the ropivacaine patients was less than that of the control group only within 24 h postoperatively. We attributed this to that the single dose of ropivacaine was injected in our study and its duration acted within 24 h [19]. This also indicated that the decreased opioid consumption would be associated with the use of wound infiltration with ropivacaine.

There are multiple choices for local anesthetic. Bupivacaine and ropivacaine are commonly used after surgery, but ropivacaine is reported to have a lower risk of cardiovascular or central nervous system toxicity [20]. Elder [18] used an elastomeric pump to infuse 0.5% bupivacaine into the wound for pain control in lumbar spinal fusion and data showed that continuous bupivacaine infusion resulted in lower pain scores and narcotic use with lower incidence of nausea and vomiting and decreased times to mobility and functional independence. He also considered that a single intraoperative dose of local anesthetic does not provide adequate postoperative pain control because of the short period of analgesic effect inherent to local anesthetics. But Sun's study reported that local wound infiltration with single dose of ropivacaine after open hepatectomy could improve postoperative pain relief, reduce surgical stress response, and accelerate postoperative recovery. Our study confirmed that intraoperative wound infiltration with single dose of ropivacaine could provide pain relief and reduce opioid use within postoperative 24 h. However, a small number of studies have demonstrated contrary results showing wound infiltration with ropivacaine does not offer significant postoperative pain relief [21, 22]. Kakagia [23] compared local infiltration of ropivacaine with levobupivacaine in a randomized controlled trial and found that in terms of intensity and duration of analgesia, ropivacaine was less effective than levobupivacaine in reducing postoperative pain associated with mini abdominoplasty.

PONV is a common side effect of opioid-based intravenous PCA. Previous studies reported that a logarithmic dose response relationship between the use of postoperative opioids and PONV [24, 25]. The decreased rate of PONV that was observed in ropivacaine group may be related to less opioid consumption consumed by patients receiving wound infiltration with ropivacaine, which was similar to Li's report from a randomized controlled trial [26]. PONV was also an unpleasant side effect feared by many patients during acute postoperative course, which can also cause dehydration, electrolyte imbalance, postoperative bleeding, wound dehiscence, and pulmonary aspiration [27, 28]. Hence, in addition to improving patient experience, the lower rate of PONV may also contribute to shorter length of hospital duration.

Effective pain management is now recognized as one of the three fundamental aspects of enhanced recovery after surgery [29]. In this trial, we investigated the role of wound infiltration with ropivacaine in postoperative hospital duration, which was reported to be a better indicator of patient recovery [30]. Patients who received wound infiltration with ropivacaine as an adjuvant to PCA had shorter length of postoperative hospital duration compared to those receiving PCA alone. These suggested that the use of ropivacaine infiltration may promote enhanced recovery and further decrease postoperative hospital stay in patients undergoing TLIF, which may be attributed to the decreased opioid use of PCA after wound infiltration with ropivacaine.

There are some limitations to this study, which may impair the ability to assess the effect of wound infiltration with ropivacaine on postoperative pain management. First, this was a retrospective cohort study in a single center, not randomized and blind, which may introduce the possibility of selection bias. Second, we did not analyze the difference of time to administrate rescue analgesic. Moreover, this study enrolled a small patient population. In the future, prospectively randomized controlled study, including more patients in multicenter will be performed to properly evaluate the role of wound infiltration with ropivacaine as an adjuvant to PCA in postoperative pain management.

Conclusion

Results of this study indicate that wound infiltration with ropivacaine effectively reduces postoperative opioid consumption and PONV and may be a useful adjuvant to PCA to improve recovery for patients undergoing lumbar spine surgery.

Abbreviations

TLIF: Transforaminal lumbar interbody fusion; PCA: Patient-controlled analgesia; ASA: American Society of Anesthesiologists; PACU: Post-anesthesia care unit; VAS: Visual analogue scale; PONV: Postoperative nausea and vomiting

Acknowledgments

No

Authors' contributions

LKP and XH contributed to study design, data collection and analysis, drafting of manuscript and revised the manuscript. CBJ and FHY contributed to the data analysis and interpretation. LDW and YKS data collection and analysis. All authors have read and approved the final manuscript.

References

1. Qin R, Liu B, Zhou P, et al. Minimally invasive versus traditional open transforaminal lumbar interbody fusion for the treatment of single-level spondylolisthesis grades 1 and 2: a systematic review and meta-analysis. World Neurosurg. 2018. https://doi.org/10.1016/j.wneu.2018.10.202.
2. de Kunder SL, van Kuijk SMJ, Rijkers K, et al. Transforaminal lumbar interbody fusion (TLIF) versus posterior lumbar interbody fusion (PLIF) in lumbar spondylolisthesis: a systematic review and meta-analysis. Spine J. 2017;17:1712–21. https://doi.org/10.1016/j.spinee.2017.06.018.

3. Kehlet H, Dahl JB. Anaesthesia, surgery, and challenges in postoperative recovery. Lancet (London, England). 2003;362:1921–8. https://doi.org/10.1016/s0140-6736(03)14966-5.
4. Gessler F, Mutlak H, Tizi K, et al. Postoperative patient-controlled epidural analgesia in patients with spondylodiscitis and posterior spinal fusion surgery. J Neurosurg Spine. 2016;24:965–70. https://doi.org/10.3171/2015.8.Spine15415.
5. Toktas ZO, Konakci M, Yilmaz B, et al. Pain control following posterior spine fusion: patient-controlled continuous epidural catheter infusion method yields better post-operative analgesia control compared to intravenous patient controlled analgesia method. A retrospective case series. European Spine J. 2016;25:1608–13. https://doi.org/10.1007/s00586-016-4507-3.
6. Bohl DD, Louie PK, Shah N, et al. Multimodal Versus Patient-Controlled Analgesia After an Anterior Cervical Decompression and Fusion. Spine. 2016; 41:994–8. https://doi.org/10.1097/brs.0000000000001380.
7. Mont MA, Beaver WB, Dysart SH, Barrington JW, Del Gaizo DJ. Local Infiltration Analgesia With Liposomal Bupivacaine Improves Pain Scores and Reduces Opioid Use After Total Knee Arthroplasty: Results of a Randomized Controlled Trial. J Arthroplasty. 2018;33:90–6. https://doi.org/10.1016/j.arth.2017.07.024.
8. Affas F. Local infiltration analgesia in knee and hip arthroplasty efficacy and safety. Scand J Pain. 2016;13:59–66. https://doi.org/10.1016/j.sjpain.2016.05.041.
9. Cha SM, Kang H, Baek CW, et al. Peritrocal and intraperitoneal ropivacaine for laparoscopic cholecystectomy: a prospective, randomized, double-blind controlled trial. J Surg Res. 2012;175:251–8. https://doi.org/10.1016/j.jss.2011.04.033.
10. O'Neill P, Duarte F, Ribeiro I, Centeno MJ, Moreira J. Ropivacaine continuous wound infusion versus epidural morphine for postoperative analgesia after cesarean delivery: a randomized controlled trial. Anesthesia Analgesia. 2012; 114:179–85. https://doi.org/10.1213/ANE.0b013e3182368e87.
11. Ge DH, Stekas ND, Varlotta CG, et al. Comparative Analysis of Two Transforaminal Lumbar Interbody Fusion Techniques: Open TLIF Versus Wiltse MIS TLIF. Spine. 2018. https://doi.org/10.1097/brs.0000000000002903.
12. Li K, Li H, Luo D, et al. Efficacy of local infiltration analgesia with ropivacaine for postoperative pain management in cervical laminoplasty: a retrospective study. Sci Rep. 2020;10:4217. https://doi.org/10.1038/s41598-020-61229-2.
13. Elder JB, Hoh DJ, Liu CY, Wang MY. Postoperative continuous paravertebral anesthetic infusion for pain control in posterior cervical spine surgery: a case-control study. Neurosurgery. 2010;66:99–106; discussion 106–107. https://doi.org/10.1227/01.Neu.0000349208.87863.B3.
14. Johnson RL, Amundson AW, Abdel MP, et al. Continuous Posterior Lumbar Plexus Nerve Block Versus Periarticular Injection with Ropivacaine or Liposomal Bupivacaine for Total Hip Arthroplasty: A Three-Arm Randomized Clinical Trial. J Bone Joint Surg Am Vol. 2017;99:1836–45. https://doi.org/10.2106/jbjs.16.01305.
15. Koehler D, Marsh JL, Karam M, Fruehling C, Willey M. Efficacy of Surgical-Site, Multimodal Drug Injection Following Operative Management of Femoral Fractures: A Randomized Controlled Trial. J Bone Joint Surg Am Vol. 2017;99:512–9. https://doi.org/10.2106/jbjs.16.00733.
16. Mullen JB, Cook WA Jr. Reduction of postoperative lumbar hemilaminectomy pain with Marcaine. Technical note. J Neurosurg. 1979;51: 126–7. https://doi.org/10.3171/jns.1979.51.1.0126.
17. Swennen C, Bredin S, Eap C, Mensa C, Ohl X, Girard V. Local infiltration analgesia with ropivacaine in acute fracture of thoracolumbar junction surgery. Orthopaedics Traumatol Surg Res. 2017;103:291–4. https://doi.org/10.1016/j.otsr.2016.11.012.
18. Elder JB, Hoh DJ, Wang MY. Postoperative continuous paravertebral anesthetic infusion for pain control in lumbar spinal fusion surgery. Spine. 2008;33:210–8. https://doi.org/10.1097/BRS.0b013e318160447a.
19. Riff C, Guilhaumou R, Marsot A, et al. Ropivacaine Wound Infiltration for Pain Management After Breast Cancer Mastectomy: A Population Pharmacokinetic Analysis. Clin Pharmacol Drug Dev. 2018. https://doi.org/10.1002/cpdd.452.
20. Zink W, Graf BM. Benefit-risk assessment of ropivacaine in the management of postoperative pain. Drug Safety. 2004;27:1093–114. https://doi.org/10.2165/00002018-200427140-00003.
21. Braito M, Dammerer D, Schlager A, Wansch J, Linhart C, Biedermann R. Continuous wound infiltration after hallux Valgus surgery. Foot Ankle Int. 2018;39:180–188.10.1177/1071100717736292.
22. Beaussier M, Parc Y, Guechot J, Cachanado M, Rousseau A, Lescot T. Ropivacaine preperitoneal wound infusion for pain relief and prevention of incisional hyperalgesia after laparoscopic colorectal surgery: a randomized, triple-arm, double-blind controlled evaluation vs intravenous lidocaine infusion, the CATCH study. Colorectal Dis. 2018;20:509–19. https://doi.org/10.1111/codi.14021.
23. Kakagia DD, Fotiadis S, Tripsiannis G, Tsoutsos D. Postoperative analgesic effect of locally infiltrated levobupivacaine in fleur-de-Lys abdominoplasty. Aesthetic Plastic Surg. 2007;31:128–32. https://doi.org/10.1007/s00266-006-0187-4.
24. Yi MS, Kang H, Kim MK, et al. Relationship between the incidence and risk factors of postoperative nausea and vomiting in patients with intravenous patient-controlled analgesia. Asian J Surg. 2018;41:301–6. https://doi.org/10.1016/j.asjsur.2017.01.005.
25. Gan TJ. Risk factors for postoperative nausea and vomiting. Anesthesia Analgesia. 2006;102:1884–98. https://doi.org/10.1213/01.Ane.0000219597.16143.4d.
26. Li J, Yang JS, Dong BH, Ye JM. The Effect of Dexmedetomidine Added to Preemptive Ropivacaine Infiltration on Postoperative Pain after Lumbar Fusion Surgery: A Randomized Controlled Trial. Spine. 2019. https://doi.org/10.1097/brs.0000000000003096.
27. Chae D, Kim SY, Song Y, et al. Dynamic predictive model for postoperative nausea and vomiting for intravenous fentanyl patient-controlled analgesia. Anaesthesia. 2020;75:218–26. https://doi.org/10.1111/anae.14849.
28. Singh K, Bohl DD, Ahn J, et al. Multimodal Analgesia Versus Intravenous Patient-Controlled Analgesia for Minimally Invasive Transforaminal Lumbar Interbody Fusion Procedures. Spine (Phila Pa 1976). 2017;42:1145–50. https://doi.org/10.1097/brs.0000000000001992.
29. Nimmo SM, Foo ITH, Paterson HM. Enhanced recovery after surgery: Pain management. J Surg Oncol. 2017;116:583–91. https://doi.org/10.1002/jso.24814.
30. Rao Z, Zhou H, Pan X, et al. Ropivacaine wound infiltration: a fast-track approach in patients undergoing thoracotomy surgery. J Surg Res. 2017;220: 379–84. https://doi.org/10.1016/j.jss.2017.05.082.

7

The analgesic efficacy and safety of peri-articular injection versus intra-articular injection in one-stage bilateral total knee arthroplasty

Kai-Yuan Cheng[1,2], Bin Feng[1], Hui-Ming Peng[1], Yan-Yan Bian[1], Lin-Jie Zhang[2], Chang Han[2], Gui-Xing Qiu[1] and Xisheng Weng[1*]

Abstract

Background: As an essential component of multimodal analgesia approaches after total knee arthroplasty (TKA), local infiltration analgesia (LIA) can be classified into peri-articular injection (PAI) and intra-articular injection (IAI) according to administration techniques. Currently, there is no definite answer to the optimal choice between the two techniques. Our study aims to investigate analgesic efficacy and safety of PAI versus IAI in patients receiving simultaneous bilateral TKA.

Methods: This randomized controlled trial was conducted from February 2017 and finished in July 2018. Sixty patients eligible for simultaneous bilateral total knee arthroplasty were randomly assigned to receive PAI on one side and IAI on another. Primary outcomes included numerical rating scale (NRS) pain score at rest or during activity at 3 h, 6 h, 12 h, 24 h, 48 h, and 72 h following surgery. Secondary outcomes contained active or passive range of motion (ROM) at 1, 2, and 3 days after surgery, time to perform straight leg raise, wound drainage, operation time, and wound complications.

Results: Patients experienced lower NRS pain scores of the knee receiving PAI compared with that with PAI during the first 48 h after surgery. The largest difference of NRS pain score at rest occurred at 48 h (PAI: 0.68, 95%CI[0.37, 0.98]; IAI: 2.63, 95%CI [2.16, 3.09]; $P < 0.001$); and the largest difference of NRS pain score during activity also took place at 48 h (PAI: 2.46, 95%CI [2.07, 2.85]; IAI: 3.90, 95%CI [3.27, 4.52]; $P = 0.001$). PAI group had better results of range of motion and time to perform straight leg raise when compared with IAI group. There were no differences in operation time, wound drainage, and wound complication.

Conclusion: PAI had the superior performance of pain relief and improvement of range of motion to IAI. Therefore, the administration technique of peri-articular injection is recommended when performing local infiltration analgesia after total knee arthroplasty.

Level of evidence: Therapeutic Level I.

Keywords: Peri-articular injection, Intra-articular injection, Total knee arthroplasty, Pain management

* Correspondence: xshweng@medmail.com.cn
[1]the Department of Orthopaedic Surgery, Peking Union Medical College Hospital, Beijing 100730, China

Background

Although total knee arthroplasty (TKA) has been recognized as the optimal treatment method for the end stage of knee osteoarthritis, over 50% patients experienced moderate to severe postoperative pain after receiving the surgery [1]. Perioperative pain management in TKA may be insufficient and hinders the process of fast recovery [2]. Multimodal analgesia regimen gains popularity in recent years, encompassing patient-controlled analgesia [3], epidural analgesia [4], femoral nerve block [5], and local infiltration analgesia [6]. However, every single method has its pros and cons: patient-controlled analgesia (PCA) is quite useful for severe pain, but it could also result in sequent side effects such as nausea, vomiting, constipation, and respiratory depression [7]; the epidural analgesia involving intrathecal injection raised the risk of nausea, hypotension, and respiratory depression [8]; despite adequate analgesia of femoral nerve block, it has been associated with quadriceps weakness and increased risk of in-hospital falls [9]. In recent years, local infiltration analgesia (LIA) is becoming more commonly applied in TKA for its convenience, splendid analgesic efficacy, and fewer side effects [10–12].

LIA is commonly performed as direct injection of a cocktail solution containing local anaesthetic, opioids, adrenaline, glucocorticoids, and nonsteroidal anti-inflammatory drugs (NSAIDs) into the surgical area to relieve inflammation and pain [13, 14]. Administration techniques of LIA could be classified into peri-articular injection (PAI) and intra-articular injection (IAI). It is well-known that exogenous IAI of hyaluronate is valid as a treatment for the symptoms of knee osteoarthritis [15]. IAI of the novel, microsphere-based, extended-release formation of triamcinolone acetonide leads to a prolonged reduction in symptoms of osteoarthritis [16]. Deducted from studies above, IAI of analgesic cocktail may also play a role in pain relief after TKA. In addition, PAI could increase the risk of paralysis of common peroneal nerve, while IAI may consume less operation time and have no increased risks. Therefore, although most surgeons perform LIA in TKA as PAI, and never just IAI, we are curious about the comparison within LIA administration techniques, between PAI and IAI. In 2015, Perret published an article comparing PAI and IAI in TKA in Australia [17]. The study failed to show statistically significant benefit in either technique. Besides, the study is not a prospective randomized controlled trial (RCT). At present, there is no RCT existing towards the comparison between PAI and IAI of analgesic cocktail in TKA.

This randomized study aimed at determining the effect of administration techniques of LIA on pain relief and postoperative rehabilitation. We compared analgesics efficacy and safety of PAI versus IAI in patients receiving simultaneous bilateral TKA during the in-hospital period.

Methods

Trial design and ethics approval

This single-centre, prospective randomized controlled trial (RCT) was performed at the Department of Orthopedic Surgery, Peking Union Medical College Hospital, following the Consolidated Standards of Reporting Trials (CONSORT) statement guidelines for reporting parallel-group randomized controlled trial [18]. The eligible patients were supposed to receive simultaneous bilateral total knee arthroplasty, in which one side of the knees underwent PAI and another one underwent IAI. The details of randomized allocation were described in the following 'Randomization and Blinding' part. The study was approved by the institutional review board of Peking Union Medical College Hospital (25th Oct, 2016) and performed in accordance with the standards of 1964 Declaration signed in Helsinki. All patients participating in this trial signed informed consent. The trial was registered on Chinese Clinical Trial Registry as ChiCTR1800020420 (respectively registered on 29th December, 2018).

Eligibility

Patients were identified on the day before scheduled surgery and evaluated for eligibility. Patients will be enrolled in the study if they meet the criteria: 1) older 18 years old; 2) receive simultaneous bilateral total knee arthroplasty during the same anaesthesia session; 3) diagnosed with osteoarthritis or rheumatoid arthritis. Exclusion criteria are:1) a history of allergy to any of the injectable drug ingredients or excipients; 3) severe deformity of genu varum or valgum (change of femoral-tibial angle $> 20°$); 4) comorbid with bronchospasm, acute rhinitis, nasal polyps, angioneurotic edema, urticaria, and other allergic reactions after taking aspirin or NSAIDs (including COX-2 inhibitors); 5) severe liver injury (serum albumin< 25 g/L or Child-Pugh score ≥ 10), inflammatory bowel disease, opioids abuse, a body mass index (BMI) of > 35 kg/m^2; 6) American Society of Anesthesiologists (ASA) category of > 3, or physical, emotional, or neurological conditions that would compromise compliance with postoperative rehabilitation and assessment.

Randomization and blinding

The LIA administration technique and the order of the operations for the two knees of each participant were randomly allocated using a computer-generated table, which was conducted by investigators not involving in the whole trial protocol except for this randomization and blinding procedure. For each participant, a sealed

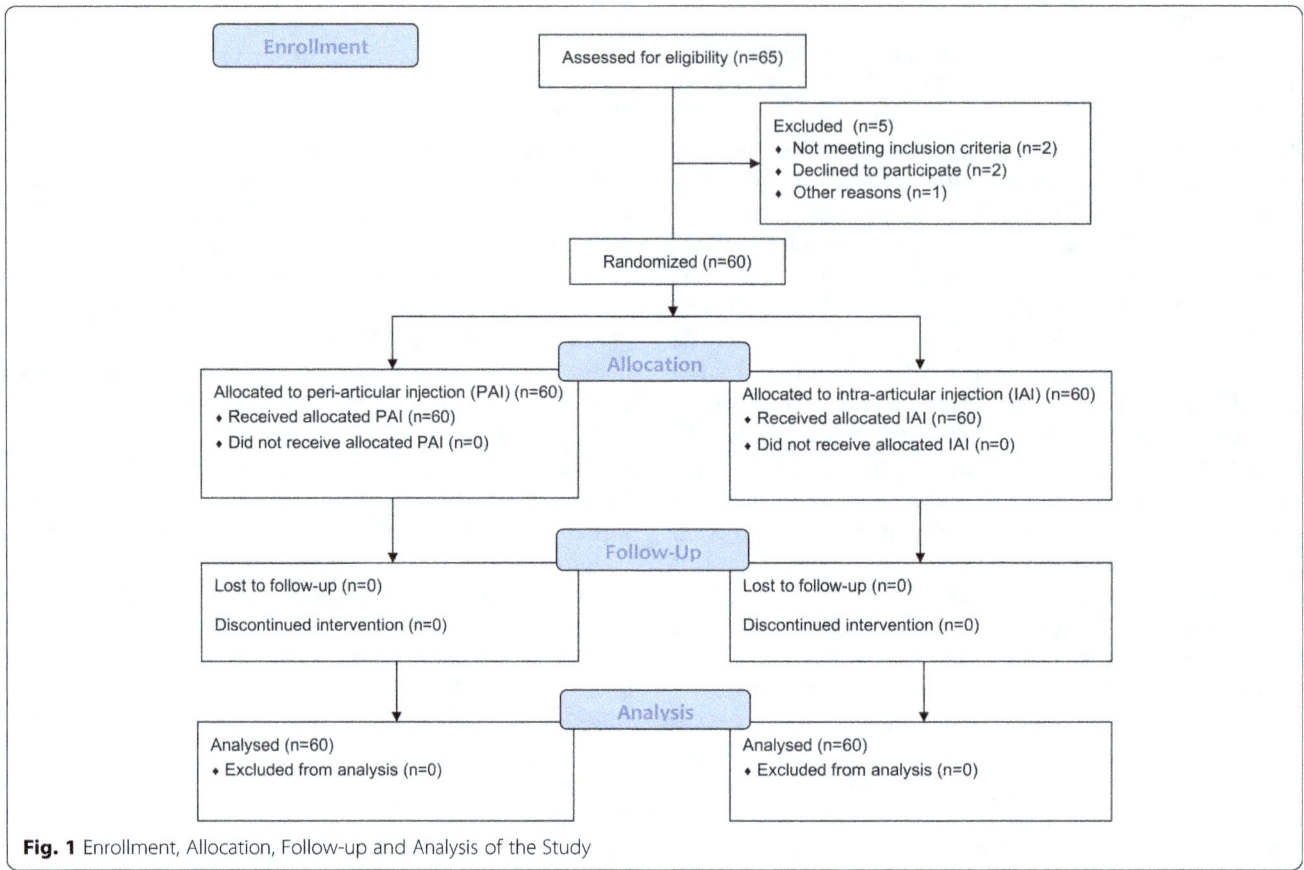

Fig. 1 Enrollment, Allocation, Follow-up and Analysis of the Study

envelope was opened in the operating room to identify the treatment assignment. The patient received PAI on one side and IAI on another. The orthopaedic surgeon was informed about the administration allocation before skin incision. The patients, data collectors, and analysts were blinded during the entire trial.

Interventions procedure

All the surgeries were performed through medial parapatellar approach by the corresponding author (Xisheng Weng) with 250 mmHg tourniquet under general anaesthesia. The constituent of administered cocktail solution in our study combined the components in previous studies [19–22], consisting of 200 mg ropivacaine, 100μg fentanyl, 0.25 mg adrenaline, 50 mg flurbiprofen axetil, and 1 mg diprospan, with addition of normal saline to a 60 mL soliton. A drainage tube was placed laterally to the prosthesis components in every joint, clamped for 3 h [23] and then unlocked, and removed in the second morning after surgery. The drainage tube has 6 orifices and all of them were located inside the articular cavity.

Intervention procedure was conducted according to the randomized allocation. In PAI group, before prosthesis installation, 20 mL of cocktail solution was injected into the posterior capsule, including femoral attachments of anterior cruciate ligament and posterior cruciate ligament, posteromedial and posterolateral capsules. After prosthesis installation, the residual 40 mL was injected into the medial and lateral collateral ligament, quadriceps tendon, patellar tendon, pes anserinus, fat pad and subcutaneous tissues. In IAI group, after closure of deep fascia, the cocktail solution was injected into the articular cavity through the drainage tube. It is the watertight test that we perform after suturing the deep fascia in every joint to check the watertight condition of the area. If fluids were leaking in somewhere, we would make more sutures to ensure the articular cavity was watertight. Both PAI and IAI were single-shot administrations. No participants received any regional nerve blocks or epidural block during the whole perioperative period. Participants were free to choose the use of PCA according to their wills.

After surgery, participants routinely received 40 mg of parecoxib in every 12 h and 650 mg of acetaminophen in every 8 h. The rescue analgesia treatment included morphine, oxycodone or pethidine. The consumption of overall opioids of every participant was documented.

Outcome measurements

The primary outcome was pain intensity at rest or during activity assessed by NRS pain score at 3, 6, 12, 24, 36, 48, and 72 h after surgery. Secondary outcome

Table 1 Baseline Characteristics of the Patients*

Characteristic	Peri-articular Injection	Intra-articular Injection	*P* value
Female, n (%)	55 (91.6)		
Age—yr mean [95%CI]	65.8 [64.0, 67.6]		
Body mass index† – -kg/m^2 mean [95%CI]	27.7 [26.7, 28.8]		
Ethnics, n (%)			
Han	56 (93.3)		
Minority‡	4 (6.7)		
Diagnosis, n (%)			
Osteoarthritis	56 (93.3)		
Rheumatoid arthritis	4 (6.7)		
ASA grade, n (%)			
I	3 (5.0)		
II	53 (88.3)		
III	4 (6.7)		
IV	0		
Numerical rating scale at rest mean [95%CI]	0.16 [0.04, 0.28]	0.20 [0.04, 0.35]	0.855
Numerical rating scale during activity mean [95%CI]	5.25 [4.87, 5.62]	4.98 [4.51, 5.45]	0.317
Range of motion actively§ mean [95%CI]	94.8 [93.3, 96.2]	94.0 [92.7, 95.4]	0.453
Range of motion passively ¶ mean [95%CI]	115.9 [114.2, 117.5]	114.0 [112.4, 115.6]	0.103

* No significant differences between groups in the reported characteristics were found at baseline
† The body-mass index is the weight in kilograms divided by the square of the height in meters
‡ Four patients are Chinese minorities, including two Manchu and two Mongols
§ Range of motion actively is patients bending knees by themselves
¶ Range of motion passively is physicians bending patients' knees

included active and passive range of motion at 1, 2 and 3 days after surgery, volume of wound drainage, postoperative days required to perform straight leg raise, length of hospital stay and opioids use in morphine equivalents. Range of motion (ROM) was calculated as the sum of angles of knee flexion and extension measured by a long-arm goniometer without removing outside dressing. In our study, active ROM means patients bend their knee joints freely without enforcement, and passive ROM means investigators bend their knee joints as most under their tolerance. The operation time was counted from skin incision to wound dressing. Morphine consumption was calculated as the sum of morphine equivalents divided by the weight of the patient.

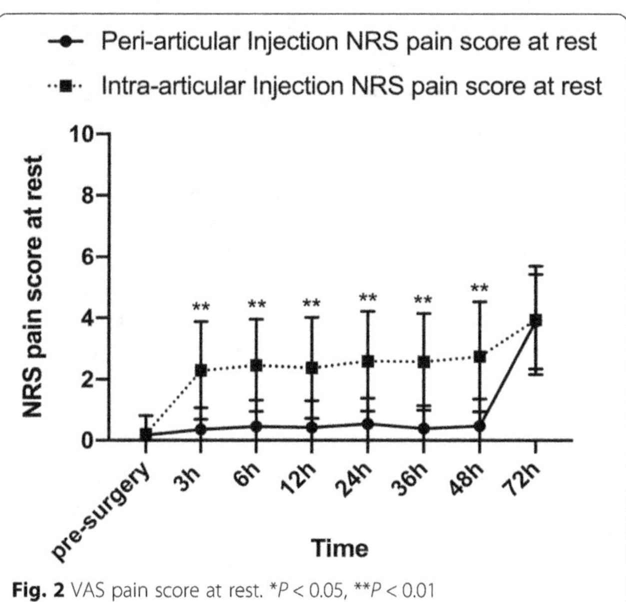

Fig. 2 VAS pain score at rest. *$P < 0.05$, **$P < 0.01$

Sample size

Our hypothesis was to substantiate the non-inferiority of IAI compared with PAI. The sample size was calculated according to the following formula [24]:

$$n = 2^*[(u_{1-\alpha/2} + u_{1-\beta})\ \sigma/\delta]^2.$$

To show a clinically important difference of 1.3 [25] in NRS pain score between PAI group and IAI group, with a standard deviation of 2.0 according to the published article [17], a power 0.90 and a two-tailed significance of <0.05, each group required 49 subjects.

Statistical analysis

Measurement data were expressed as mean and 95% confidence interval (95% CI). Shapiro–Wilk test and Levene test were performed to evaluate normality and

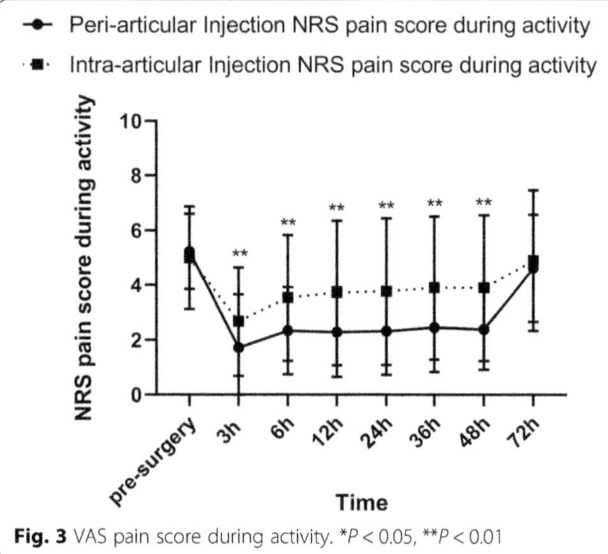

Fig. 3 VAS pain score during activity. *$P < 0.05$, **$P < 0.01$

homogeneity of variance of the data, respectively. If data did not comply with normal distribution or equal variance, a non-parametric test (Mann-Whitney) was applied; if else, student t-test was undertaken to analyse the difference between the two groups. The dichotomous data were analysed by Fisher's exact test, in that 50% of cells have expected count less than 5. SPSS version 25.0 software was used during the analysis process.

Results

Baseline characteristics

Between February 2017 and July 2018, 65 patients were enrolled in the study, among which 5 patients were excluded for violating criteria (severe deformity with more than 5 mm bone defect of tibia plateau inspected during surgery, refusal to participate and incoordination to respond) (Fig. 1). A total of 60 patients participated in the study. All of them finished the process of randomization, allocation, trial administration and postoperative assessment. Baseline characteristics of the participants are illustrated in Table 1, including gender, age, body mass index, ethnics, diagnosis, and ASA grade. There were no differences in NRS pain score and ROM between two groups before the surgery and intervention.

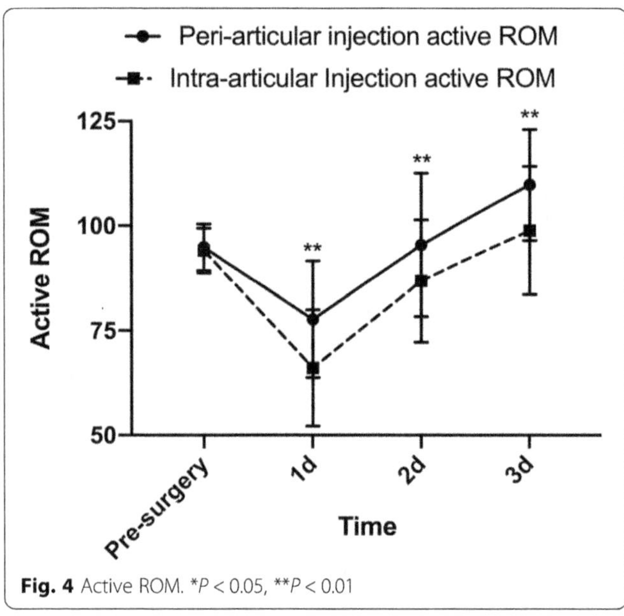

Fig. 4 Active ROM. *$P < 0.05$, **$P < 0.01$

Primary outcome

During the first 48 h after surgery, NRS pain score in PAI group was significantly lower than that in IAI group (Fig. 2, Fig. 3 and Additional file 1: Table S1). The difference of NRS pain score between the two groups was larger at rest compared with that during activity. The differences of NRS pain score at 3 h, 6 h, 12 h, 24 h, 36 h, 48 h at rest and at12h, 24 h, 36 h and 48 h during activity were over 1.3 with a clinically important difference. The largest difference in NRS pain score occurred in 48 h after surgery at rest (PAI: 0.68 [0.37, 0.98]; IAI: 2.63 [2.16, 3.09], $P < 0.001$; Between-group difference: − 1.95 [− 2.50, − 1.39]) or during activity (PAI: 2.46 [2.07, 2.85]; IAI: 3.90 [3.27, 4.52], $P = 0.001$; Between-group difference in change: − 1.43 [− 2.16, − 0.70]). There were no differences between two groups in NRS pain score at 72 h after the surgery at rest ($P = 0.426$) or during activity ($P = 0.287$).

Secondary outcome

PAI group had better results of active ROM and passive ROM in the first 3 days after surgery compared with IAI group (Fig. 4, Fig. 5, and Additional file 2: Table S2). The largest difference in active ROM (PAI: 77.6 [74.0, 81.2]; IAI: 66.0 [62.4, 69.6], $P < 0.001$; Between-group difference in change: 11.5 [6.5, 16.6]) and passive ROM (PAI: 91.7 [88.8, 94.7]; IAI: 84.9 [82.0, 87.9], $P = 0.001$; Between-group difference in change: 6.8 [2.6, 10.9]) between two groups took place at day 1 after surgery. There were no significant differences in operation time ($P = 0.614$) and wound drainage volume ($P = 0.607$) (Table 2). PAI group consumed less time to perform straight leg raise postoperatively (PAI: 1.08 [0.90, 1.25]; IAI: 1.45 [1.21, 1.68], $P = 0.012$; Between-group difference in change: − 0.36 [− 0.65, − 0.08]). The length of hospital day was 5.53 [4.98, 6.07] and morphine consumption was 1.23 mg/kg [1.15, 1.31].

Complication

In PAI group, there was one case complicated with deep venous thrombus, one with nerve palsy and one with fat liquefaction. In IAI group, there was one case complicated with deep venous thrombus. Generally, there were no differences in wound complications between the two

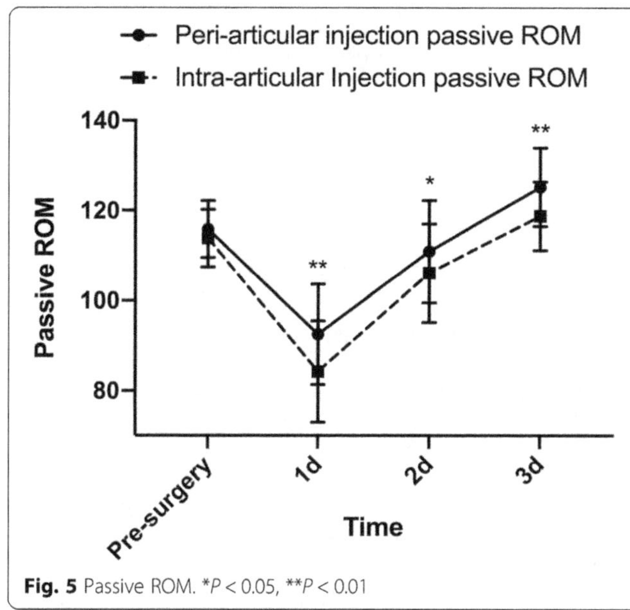

Fig. 5 Passive ROM. *$P < 0.05$, **$P < 0.01$

groups (Table 3). The overall wound complication rate was 3/60 in PAI group and 1/60 in IAI group (Relative risk, 1.526 [0.842, 2.768], $P = 0.619$).

Discussion

Our results demonstrate that PAI provides superior analgesic benefit to IAI in patients receiving TKA. The advantage of PAI over IAI on NRS pain score faded off after 48 h, while ROM was continuously better in PAI group than IAI group during the first 3 days after the surgery. In addition, it took less time for PAI group to perform straight leg raise postoperatively. There were no differences in operation time, volume of wound drainage and wound complications between two groups. Our study substantiated the superiority of PAI to IAI in analgesia after total knee arthroplasty. Therefore, PAI technique was recommended for performing LIA in TKA.

PAI group showed a statistically significant reduction in postoperative VAS pain scores in a previous study [17], which positively correlated with NRS pain scores in our study [26]. In a retrospective study [27], Tietje demonstrated that patients receiving PAI of local anaesthetics in TKA had a noticeable decrease in length of hospital stay and incidence of postoperative nausea and vomiting when compared to patients receiving IAI. In the early period after surgery, it is pain that mainly accounts for patients hospitalization [2]. Besides, the occurrence of nausea and vomiting in patients after surgery may vary from the usage of opioids [7]. Therefore, it could be deducted from the results of Tietje that the analgesic benefit of PAI may underlie the decreased length of hospital stay and incidence of postoperative nausea and vomiting. In the current study, PAI had advantages of pain relief over IAI, corresponding with our deduction from Tietje study.

There are several mechanisms underlying the analgesic benefit of PAI over IAI. According to a previous cadaveric study [28], the outer capsule is more abundant of innervation such as saphenous nerve and genicular nerves, while the inner synovium and articular cavity have fewer nerve distribution. Another histologic survey of human cadaveric knees performed by Jiranek et al. [29] elucidated the distribution of free nerve endings after hematoxylin and eosin staining. High concentrations of nociceptors were found in the medial and lateral retinacula, patellar tendon, pes anserinus, and meniscofemoral ligaments. The lowest concentration was seen in the central portion of the anterior cruciate ligament. Thus, the conduct of PAI could be more effective than IAI because of denser innervation of the outside capsule and soft tissues in the knee joint. Besides, since we placed a drainage tube in every joint, solution in the articular cavity was more likely to be drained out and solution in the soft tissues around the knee joint could continue to work out. It would be more difficult for cocktail solution of PAI group to escape from the joint than that of IAI. It also might be the persistent effect of cocktail solution in PAI group that contributes to the analgesic benefits. The volume of cocktail solution was the same in both groups, and according to our previous

Table 2 Secondary Outcomes

Characteristic	Mean [95%CI]			*P* Value
	Peri-Articular Injection	Intra-Articular Injection	Between-Group Difference in Change [95%CI]	
Operation time (min)	70.0 [68.4, 71.6]	69.8 [67.9, 71.7]	0.2 [−2.2, 2.6]	0.614
Wound drainage volume day 1 (mL)	85.7 [66.1, 105.4]	82.8 [65.1, 100.4]	2.9 [− 23.1, 29.1]	0.992
Wound drainage volume day 2 (mL)	95.9 [74.3, 117.5]	87.6 [68.3, 107.0]	8.2 [−20.4, 36.9]	0.731
Wound drainage volume in total (mL)	181.7 [148.5, 214.9]	170.4 [138.0, 202.8]	11.2 [−34.6, 57.1]	0.607
Postoperative days required to perform straight leg raise	1.08 [0.90, 1.25]	1.45 [1.21, 1.68]	−0.36 [−0.65, −0.08]	0.026
Morphine consumption (mg/kg)	1.23 [1.15, 1.31]		–	–
Length of hospital stay	5.53 [4.98, 6.07]		–	–

Table 3 Wound Complications

Complications	Peri-Articular Injection, n (%)	Intra-Articular Injection, n (%)	Relative risk of PAI [95% CI]	*P* value
Deep venous thrombus	1 (1.6)	1 (1.6)	1.000 [0.247, 4.045]	1.000
Nerve palsy	1 (1.6)	0	2.017 [1.683.2.418]	1.000
Fat liquefaction	1 (1.6)	0	2.017 [1.683.2.418]	1.000
Overall infection	0	0	–	–
Articular hematoma	0	0	–	–
Overall complications	3 (5.0)	1 (1.6)	1.526 [0.842, 2.768]	0.619

assumptions, the volume of wound drainage of IAI group was supposed to outnumber that of PAI group. However, there was no difference in the volume of wound drainage in our study. This paradox requires more substantive evidence to explain. For the further investigation to uncover the potential mechanism, a biocompatible and undegraded detector could be included in the cocktail solution to detect the real-time concentration and volume of the solution constituents in the articular cavity and soft tissues around the knee joint.

To our knowledge, this is the first RCT study comparing analgesic efficacy and safety of PAI with that of IAI in patients receiving simultaneous bilateral TKA. The highlight of our study is the self-control design, where participants received PAI on one side and IAI on another. Owing to the homogeneity inside one participant, the only possible explanation for the remarkable differences in outcomes may lay in distinctive interventions. The conclusion of our study is confirmative.

However, there is no exception for limitations in our study. Firstly, the ceiling effect makes it impossible to distinguish the differences in systemic adverse effects, ambulation mobility and morphine consumption between two groups. In addition, one pain could increase or reduce the other. Thus, the difference in our study could be overestimated or underestimated. Despite the qualitative conclusion in the study, further research is required to determine the exact difference between the two groups. Besides, the outcomes were only limited to in-hospital data without long-term follow-up data and the long-term effect needs to be further evaluated.

Conclusion

Generally, we conducted a randomized controlled trial to compare the analgesic efficacy and safety of PAI versus IAI in patients receiving simultaneous total knee arthroplasty. PAI had more analgesic benefits than IAI after the surgery. There were no differences between PAI and IAI in wound drainage, operation time, and wound complications. The administration technique of PAI is recommended when performing LIA in TKA.

Supplementary information

Additional file 1: Table S1. Numerical Rating Scale (NRS) at rest or during activity

Additional file 2: Table S2. Range of Motion

Abbreviations

ASA: American Society of Anesthesiologists; BMI: Body mass index; CI: Confidence interval; CONSORT: Consolidated standards of reporting trials; IAI: Intra-articular injection; LIA: Local infiltration analgesia; NRS: Numerical rating scale; NSAIDs: Nonsteroidal anti-inflammatory drugs; PAI: Peri-articular injection; PCA: Patient-controlled analgesia; RCT: Randomized controlled trial; ROM: Range of motion; TKA: Total knee arthroplasty

Acknowledgements

No special acknowledgements.

Authors' contributions

KYC drafted and revised the manuscript, analysed the data, collected the original study data and reviewed the data analysis. BF conducted the intervention procedure and helped to draft the manuscript. HMP conceived of the study and analysed the data. YYB conducted the intervention procedure and helped to draft the manuscript. LJZ collected the original data, interpreted the comments on the manuscript and revised the manuscript. CH collected the original data, interpreted the comments on the manuscript and revised the manuscript. GXQ participated the design of the study and reviewed the data analysis. XW conceived of the study, participated the design of the study, reviewed the data analysis and revised the manuscript. All authors read and approved the final manuscript.

Author details

[1]the Department of Orthopaedic Surgery, Peking Union Medical College Hospital, Beijing 100730, China. [2]Chinese Academy of Medical Sciences and Peking Union Medical College, Beijing 100730, China.

References

1. Buvanendran A, Fiala J, Patel KA, Golden AD, Moric M, Kroin JS. The incidence and severity of postoperative pain following inpatient surgery. Pain Med. 2015;16(12):2277–83.
2. Husted H, Lunn TH, Troelsen A, Gaarn-Larsen L, Kristensen BB, Kehlet H. Why still in hospital after fast-track hip and knee arthroplasty? Acta Orthop. 2011; 82(6):679–84.
3. Ferrante FM, Orav EJ, Rocco AG, Gallo J. A statistical model for pain in patient-controlled analgesia and conventional intramuscular opioid regimens. Anesth Analg. 1988;67(5):457–61.
4. Mahoney OM, Noble PC, Davidson J, Tullos HS. The effect of continuous epidural analgesia on postoperative pain, rehabilitation, and duration of hospitalization in total knee arthroplasty. Clin Orthop Relat Res. 1990;260: 30–7.
5. Sakai N, Inoue T, Kunugiza Y, Tomita T, Mashimo T. Continuous femoral versus epidural block for attainment of 120 degrees knee flexion after total knee arthroplasty: a randomized controlled trial. J Arthroplast. 2013;28(5): 807–14.
6. Essving P, Axelsson K, Kjellberg J, Wallgren O, Gupta A, Lundin A. Reduced morphine consumption and pain intensity with local infiltration analgesia (LIA) following total knee arthroplasty. Acta Orthop. 2010;81(3):354–60.

7. Dart RC, Surratt HL, Cicero TJ, Parrino MW, Severtson SG, Bucher-Bartelson B, Green JL. Trends in opioid analgesic abuse and mortality in the United States. N Engl J Med. 2015;372(3):241–8.
8. Choi PT, Bhandari M, Scott J, Douketis J. Epidural analgesia for pain relief following hip or knee replacement. Cochrane Database Syst Rev. 2003;3: CD003071.
9. Feibel RJ, Dervin GF, Kim PR, Beaule PE. Major complications associated with femoral nerve catheters for knee arthroplasty: a word of caution. J Arthroplast. 2009;24(6 Suppl):132–7.
10. Fan L, Zhu C, Zan P, Yu X, Liu J, Sun Q, Li G. The comparison of local infiltration analgesia with peripheral nerve block following Total knee Arthroplasty (TKA): a systematic review with meta-analysis. J Arthroplast. 2015;30(9):1664–71.
11. Uesugi K, Kitano N, Kikuchi T, Sekiguchi M, Konno S. Comparison of peripheral nerve block with periarticular injection analgesia after total knee arthroplasty: a randomized, controlled study. Knee. 2014;21(4):848–52.
12. Tanikawa H, Sato T, Nagafuchi M, Takeda K, Oshida J, Okuma K. Comparison of local infiltration of analgesia and sciatic nerve block in addition to femoral nerve block for total knee arthroplasty. J Arthroplast. 2014;29(12): 2462–7.
13. Vendittoli PA, Makinen P, Drolet P, Lavigne M, Fallaha M, Guertin MC, Varin F. A multimodal analgesia protocol for total knee arthroplasty. A randomized, controlled study. J Bone Joint Surg Am. 2006;88(2):282–9.
14. Kehlet H. Synergism between analgesics. Ann Med. 1995;27(2):259–62.
15. Hunter DJ. Viscosupplementation for osteoarthritis of the knee. N Engl J Med. 2015;372(11):1040–7.
16. Conaghan PG, Cohen SB, Berenbaum F, Lufkin J, Johnson JR, Bodick N. Brief report: a phase IIb trial of a novel extended-release microsphere formulation of triamcinolone Acetonide for Intraarticular injection in knee osteoarthritis. Arthritis Rheum. 2018;70(2):204–11.
17. Perret M, Fletcher P, Firth L, Yates P. Comparison of patient outcomes in periarticular and intraarticular local anaesthetic infiltration techniques in total knee arthroplasty. J Orthop Surg Res. 2015;10:119.
18. Moher D, Hopewell S, Schulz KF, Montori V, Gotzsche PC, Devereaux PJ, Elbourne D, Egger M, Altman DG. CONSORT 2010 explanation and elaboration: updated guidelines for reporting parallel group randomised trials. BMJ. 2010;340:c869.
19. Ikeuchi M, Kamimoto Y, Izumi M, Fukunaga K, Aso K, Sugimura N, Yokoyama M, Tani T. Effects of dexamethasone on local infiltration analgesia in total knee arthroplasty: a randomized controlled trial. Knee Surg Sports Traumatol Arthrosc. 2014;22(7):1638–43.
20. Bhutta MA, Ajwani SH, Shepard GJ, Ryan WG. Reduced blood loss and transfusion rates: additional benefits of local infiltration Anaesthesia in knee Arthroplasty patients. J Arthroplast. 2015;30(11):2034–7.
21. van Haagen MHM, Verburg H, Hesseling B, Coors L, van Dasselaar NT, PNJ L, NMC M. Optimizing the dose of local infiltration analgesia and gabapentin for total knee arthroplasty, a randomized single blind trial in 128 patients. Knee. 2018;25(1):153–60.
22. Mullaji A, Kanna R, Shetty GM, Chavda V, Singh DP. Efficacy of periarticular injection of bupivacaine, fentanyl, and methylprednisolone in total knee arthroplasty:a prospective, randomized trial. J Arthroplast. 2010;25(6):851–7.
23. Jeon YS, Park JS, Kim MK. Optimal release timing of temporary drain clamping after total knee arthroplasty. J Orthop Surg Res. 2017;12(1):47.
24. Kadam P, Bhalerao S. Sample size calculation. Int J Ayurveda Res. 2010;1(1): 55–7.
25. Chang AK, Bijur PE, Esses D, Barnaby DP, Baer J. Effect of a single dose of Oral opioid and nonopioid analgesics on acute extremity pain in the emergency department: a randomized clinical trial. JAMA. 2017;318(17): 1661–7.
26. Breivik EK, Björnsson GA, Skovlund E. A comparison of pain rating scales by sampling from clinical trial data. Clin J Pain. 2000;16(1):22–8.
27. Tietje T, Davis AB, Rivey MP. Comparison of 2 methods of local anesthetic-based injection as part of a multimodal approach to pain management after Total knee Arthroplasty. J Pharm Pract. 2015;28(6):523–8.
28. Kennedy JC, Alexander IJ, Hayes KC. Nerve supply of the human knee and its functional importance. Am J Sports Med. 1982;10(6):329–35.
29. Ross JA, Greenwood AC, Sasser P 3rd, Jiranek WA. Periarticular injections in knee and hip Arthroplasty: where and what to inject. J Arthroplast. 2017; 32(9S):S77–80.

8

Ropivacaine infiltration analgesia of the drainage exit site enhanced analgesic effects after breast cancer surgery

Baona Wang[1†], Tao Yan[1†], Xiangyi Kong[2†], Li Sun[3], Hui Zheng[1*] and Guohua Zhang[1*]

Abstract

Background: Postoperative pain after breast cancer surgery remains a major challenge in patient care. Local infiltration analgesia is a standard analgesic technique used for pain relief after surgery. Its application in patients who underwent mastectomy requires more clear elucidation. This study aimed to investigate the effect of ropivacaine infiltration of drainage exit site in ameliorating the postoperative pain after mastectomy.

Methods: A prospective randomized controlled study was conducted in 74 patients who were scheduled for unilateral mastectomy by standardized general anesthesia. Both intervention group and control group were given infiltration of the two entry points of drainage catheters with 10 ml 0.5% ropivacaine (Group A) ($n = 37$) or 10 ml normal saline (Group B) ($n = 37$). Pain scores were recorded in post-anesthesia care unit (PACU), at 6 h, 12 h, 24 h and 36 h after operation by using a visual analogue scale (VAS). Postoperative nausea and vomiting (PONV) incidence, postoperative analgesic and antiemetic requirements, the incidence of chronic pain, as well as the quality of recovery were recorded.

Results: The patients in Group A showed a significant reduction in postoperative pain in PACU ($p < 0.0005$), at 6 h ($p < 0.0005$), 12 h ($p < 0.0005$), and 24 h after surgery ($p < 0.05$) when compared to those in Group B. There were more postoperative analgesic requirements in Group B ($p < 0.05$). With regard to the quality of recovery, Group A was shown to be much superior over Group B ($p < 0.05$).

Conclusions: Ropivacaine infiltration of the two drainage exit sites decreased the degree of postoperative acute pain after mastectomy, and this approach improved patients' quality of recovery.

Keywords: Local infiltration analgesia, Ropivacaine, Drainage exit site, Postoperative pain, Breast cancer

* Correspondence: zhenghui0715@hotmail.com; d1974@163.com
†Baona Wang, Tao Yan and Xiangyi Kong contributed equally to this work.
[1]Department of Anesthesiology, National Cancer Center/National Clinical Research Center for Cancer/Cancer Hospital, Chinese Academy of Medical Sciences and Peking Union Medical College, Beijing 100021, China

Background

Postoperative pain is one of the most common challenges in women following breast cancer surgeries, which impairs rehabilitation and increases the length of hospital stay. About 50% of patients who receive mastectomy might experience persistent postoperative pain [1, 2]. Sensory disturbances such as burning or sensory loss caused from the wound are commonly observed as sequelae of mastectomy, and this might be due to intraoperative nerve injury [3]. However, complaints of acute postoperative pain in patients who received mastectomy are also frequently observed. After mastectomy, a drainage tube is routinely placed, which assists in monitoring bleeding, and fluid or air removal. The wound is infiltrated or irrigated with local anesthetic to reduce acute postoperative pain, and is widely used in surgeries [4, 5]. However, few studies have paid much attention in investigating whether postoperative pain could be effectively alleviated by infiltrating anesthesia at the drainage exit site after mastectomy. Based on our clinical experiences, the major location of the acute pain might be at the insertion sites of the two drainage catheters, which were placed below the skin flap at the end of the surgical procedure. For the firm anchorage of the drain to the skin and sealing of the space around the drain, the two entry points of catheter insertion were chosen over healthy skin below the inframammary fold of the breast, wherein most of the subcutaneous nerves were not damaged, meaning that they were still sensitive to pain. Park's study [6] reported that surgical drains are associated with high postoperative opioid use after breast cancer surgery, and this supported our observation.

Although multimodal analgesic strategies including opioids, acetaminophen, non-steroidal anti-inflammatory drugs (NSAIDs), peripheral regional techniques, patient-controlled modalities as well as local anesthetic techniques such as wound infiltration are available, postoperative pain still has been poorly managed. Analgesia-related side-effects such as nausea and vomiting, dizziness, constipation and itching are commonly observed, impairing patients' satisfaction and delaying their discharge time [7, 8]. Postoperative pain after breast cancer surgery can be effectively alleviated by regional nerve block techniques, for example the thoracic paravertebral nerve block (PVB) [9]. But a long learning cycle and invasive nature of the method limited the implementation of PVB in breast cancer surgery.

This prospective randomized controlled study aimed to investigate if infiltration of ropivacaine at the insertion sites of the two drain catheters in mastectomy would reduce postoperative acute pain, postoperative nausea and vomiting (PONV), and chronic pain.

Methods

Study design

This prospective, randomized controlled trial was designed in adherence to the CONSORT guidelines and was registered in Chictr.org.cn registry system on 24 February 2020 (ChiCTR2000030139). This study was conducted in Cancer Hospital, Chinese Academy of Medical Sciences between September and November 2019, and has been approved by the institutional ethics committee (IRB Approval Number: 20/351–2135). All patients were followed up until 3 months after discharge from the hospital.

Participants

Patients who underwent unilateral mastectomy with axillary lymph node dissection (ALND) or sentinel lymph node biopsy (SLNB) were enrolled in this study. Written informed consent was obtained from patients. The patients aged 20 ~ 70 years, and with the American Society of Anesthesiologists physical status of I to III were included. Patients with the following conditions were excluded from the study: history of severe cardiovascular or pulmonary, hepatic, renal, neurologic, and psychiatric or metabolic diseases; history of allergy to any of the potential study medications; active drug abuse; intake of NSAIDs, opioids, or other analgesics in the 24 h before surgery; pregnancy; breastfeeding, active menstruation.

Randomization

Prior to study initiation, 80 sequentially numbered envelopes containing the allocation were prepared. The involved patients were randomly assigned to 10 ml 0.5% ropivacaine infiltration (Group A) or 10 ml normal saline infiltration (Group B) groups. A physician independent of the study randomly inserted 40 anesthesia strategies for each group into the envelopes. The random allocation sequence was generated using computer-generated random numbers. The researchers opened the envelope to determine as to which anesthesia strategy to implement before the induction of general anesthesia. All perioperative data were collected by an investigator who was blinded to the patient's allocation, and was responsible for measuring the outcome.

Interventions

Standard general anesthesia was induced using sufentanil 0.3 ~ 0.6 μg/kg, propofol 1 ~ 2 mg/kg and cis-Atracurium 0.2 ~ 0.4 mg/kg in the two groups. After laryngeal mask airway insertion, the patients were mechanically ventilated to maintain the end-tidal carbon dioxide concentration at 35 ~ 45 mmHg with a fresh gas flow of 2 L/min 60% oxygen. Anesthesia was maintained by constant inhalation of 1.5 ~ 2.5% sevoflurane and constant infusion of remifentanil at a rate of 0.1 ~

0.2 μg/kg/min. Sufentanil 0.1 μg/kg was added intraoperatively as required. At the end of the surgery all patients received 100 mg of flurbiprofen (an NSAID). Dexamethasone 8 mg (given after induction) and ondansetron 4 mg (given at the end of surgery) were used for prevention of postoperative nausea and vomiting (PONV). All surgical procedures were finished by the same surgical team with the same standardized technique. The two drainage catheters were placed by the surgeon before closing the surgical incision. Before the placement, the subcutaneous tissue of the two entry points of the catheters received local infiltration, which included intervention group (Group A) by 10 ml 0.5% ropivacaine and control group (Group B) by 10 ml normal saline (5 ml for each point). After operation, all patients were extubated and transferred to the post-anesthesia care unit (PACU). Flurbiprofen 100 mg was provided by intravenous injection daily to control the postoperative pain within 3 days after operation. If the pain visual analogue scale (VAS) was ≥3, 100 mg tramadol was administered as a rescue analgesic. For postoperative antiemetic treatment, metoclopramide was intravenously administrated if the nausea VAS was ≥5 or episodes of vomiting ≥2. All patients received standard postoperative therapies according to the pathological characteristics.

Outcomes

The primary outcomes

The pain was immediately assessed after returning to PACU and at 6 h, 12 h, 24 h, and 36 h after operation using a VAS (0 = no pain to 10 = most severe pain). The incidence of PONV was recorded simultaneously, using a three-point ordinal scale (0 = none, 1 = nausea, 2 = retching, 3 = vomiting), and nausea was evaluated by VAS. The number of patients who received postoperative analgesic or antiemetic drugs was recorded.

Secondary outcomes

The status of chronic pain in patients was collected using the breast cancer pain questionnaire, which was first developed by Gartner et al. [3]. A Pain Burden Index (PBI) can be calculated according to the data collected by the questionnaire surveys. It was calculated by adding the pain severity scale (0 ~ 10) from anatomic locations of breast, axilla, chest wall and arm, and multiplied by the frequency of pain at each site (constantly—5 points, daily—4 points, occasionally—3 points, weekly—2 points, monthly—1 point, and never—0 points).

The quality of recovery including 40 questions (QoR-40), which is used as a measure of quality of recovery, was distributed to patients for collecting data 24 h after operation. This included five factors of emotional state, physical comfort, psychological support, physical independence, and pain. In all, the highest score was 200 while the lowest being 40 and the more score, the better the results.

Also the remaining data, including the consumption of sufentanil during the surgery, types of surgical procedures, operation and anesthesia time, age, body mass index (BMI), history of smoking and PONV were collected,

Sample size and statistical analysis

The sample size was calculated based on our preliminary experiment that enrolled 10 cases in each group. The mean pain VAS at 12 h after the surgery was 1.2 ± 2.1 for Group A and 2.9 ± 2.2 for Group B. Using standard sample size calculation formula to achieve a power of 0.8 at $\alpha = 0.05$, there should be at least 29 patients included in each group to detect a significant difference. Considering the possibility of data censored, a total of 40 patients in each group were recruited to guarantee the sample size. SPSS 23.0 for windows (SPSS, Inc., Chicago, IL, USA) was used for data analysis. Normally distributed continuous data were expressed as means (SD), and were analyzed using analysis of variance (ANOVA), independent-sample t-test or paired t-test. Nonparametric data were analyzed by Mann-Whitney and Wilcoxon text. Two-sided tests were performed to declare statistical significance at $p < 0.05$.

Results

The random assignment of the participants into the two groups and analysis of the outcome was presented in Fig. 1. Finally, a total of 74 patients were included in this study. Demographic characteristics, including age, body weight, body height, BMI, smoking status, and history of PONV were comparable in both groups (Table 1). In addition, no significant differences were found in the consumption of sufentanil during surgery, the durations of anesthesia and surgery, and the types of surgical procedures used (Table 1).

Surgical drains were reported to be associated with high postoperative opioid use after breast-conserving surgery[6]. Although whether surgical drains increase opioid consumption after mastectomy has not been investigated, pain originating from the insertion sites of the two drainage catheters constitutes a major part of acute postoperative pain. In this study, we found that ropivacaine infiltration of the two drainage exit sites have significantly reduced the postoperative pain in PACU (VAS score, 0.54 ± 1.07 vs. 1.97 ± 1.48, $p < 0.0005$), at 6 h (VAS score, 0.49 ± 1.12 vs. 2.24 ± 1.36, $p < 0.0005$), 12 h (VAS score, 0.86 ± 1.29 vs. 2.30 ± 1.35, $p < 0.0005$), and 24 h after operation (VAS score, 1.35 ± 1.27 vs. 1.97 ± 1.32, $p < 0.05$) (Fig. 2). However, at 36 h after operation, a significant difference was not observed any more (1.51 ± 1.15 vs. 1.68 ± 1.23, $p > 0.05$) (Fig. 2). More number of

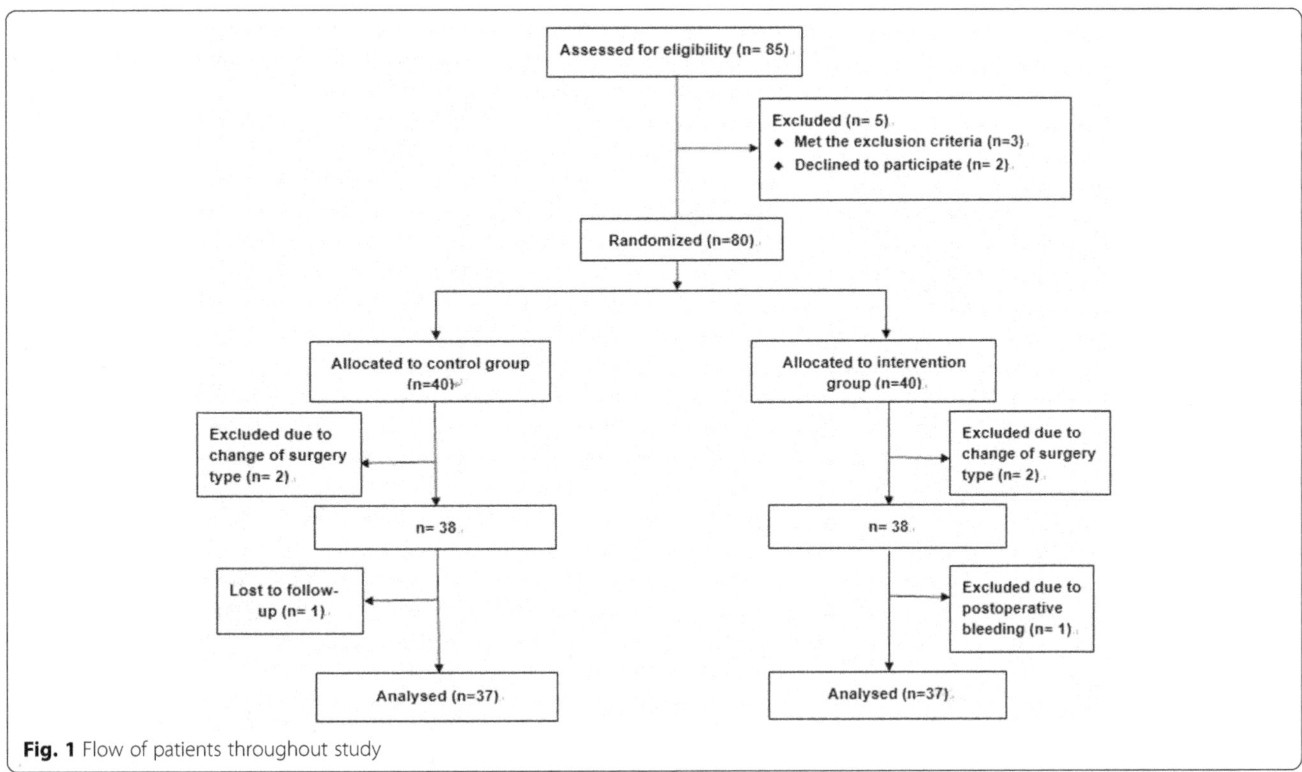

Fig. 1 Flow of patients throughout study

patients required for postoperative rescue analgesic in Group B than in Group A (17 vs. 7, $p < 0.05$).

We did not collect pain scores of restricted movement of the shoulder and values of arm abduction angle. Because the operated arm was tightly bound and forbidden to move by surgeons within 3 days after the operations, in case of wound dehiscence, subcutaneous effusion and hematoma.

The intervention showed no effect on the incidence of chronic pain within 3 months, and PBI in the two groups showed similar results (Table 2). No significant differences were found between the two groups in terms of PONV incidence (Table 3) and the requirements for postoperative antiemetic treatment. The QoR-40 score of Group A was significantly higher than Group B (185.8 ± 8.3 vs 179.7 ± 11.2, $p < 0.05$).

Discussion

To our knowledge, this is the first prospective randomized controlled study to reveal ropivacaine infiltration of

Table 1 Baseline characteristics of patients in the study and the control groups

	Group A(n = 37)	Group B(n = 37)	P value
Age (years)[a]	52.1 ± 9.0	49.1 ± 9.9	0.17
Weight (kg)[a]	61.8 ± 8.7	59.8 ± 8.4	0.32
Height (cm)[a]	160.3 ± 5.5	159.4 ± 5.0	0.44
Body mass index[a]	24.0 ± 3.6	23.9 ± 3.1	0.82
Smoking (%)	0	0	–
History of PONV (%)	5 (13.5%)	4 (10.8%)	0.48
Surgical procedure			0.41
mastectomy + axillary dissection (%)	30 (80.1%)	27 (73.0%)	
mastectomy + SNLB (%)	7 (19.9%)	10 (27.0%)	
Surgery time (min)[a]	98.1 ± 31.3	111.0 ± 28.8	0.07
Length of anesthesia (min)[a]	113.5 ± 30.1	125.5 ± 27.9	0.08
Consumption of Sufentanil (μg)[a]	24.8 ± 5.7	23.8 ± 5.0	0.42

[a]Values are expressed as the mean ± standard deviation; *PONV* postoperative nausea and vomiting; *SNLB* sentinel lymph node biopsy

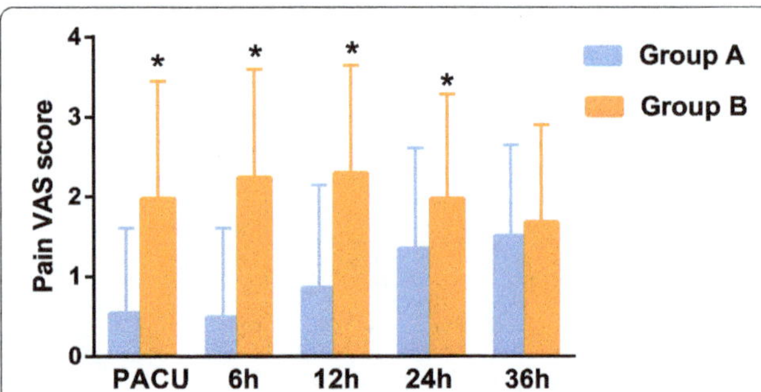

Fig. 2 Pain VAS score of patients in the study and control groups. Compared with Group B, postoperative pain in Group A was significantly reduced in PACU (VAS score, 0.54 ± 1.07 vs. 1.97 ± 1.48, $p < 0.0005$), at 6 h (VAS score, 0.49 ± 1.12 vs. 2.24 ± 1.36, $p < 0.0005$), 12 h (VAS score, 0.86 ± 1.29 vs. 2.30 ± 1.35, $p < 0.0005$), and 24 h after operation (VAS score, 1.35 ± 1.27 vs. 1.97 ± 1.32, $p < 0.05$). *$p < 0.05$; Group A: intervention group (ropivacaine infiltration); Group B: control group (normal saline infiltration); PACU: Post-anesthesia care unit; VAS: Visual analogue scale

the two drainage exit sites, which significantly reduced postoperative pain and analgesic requirements and improved the quality of recovery after mastectomy.

Park's study [10] reported that compared with other breast surgical procedure types, mastectomy required consumption of more opioids during the first week postoperatively. Opioid consumption plays an important role in postoperative pain control after mastectomy. However, opioid-related adverse effects led to other problems that delay the recovery, and so novel analgesics or strategies with less side-effects are urgently needed. Kairaluoma et al. [11] have found that PVB could improve postoperative pain and reduce opioid consumption after modified radical mastectomy. Nevertheless, compared with local infiltration anesthesia, the regional block technique is considered more challenging technically, and needs a longer learning period. According to our results, ropivacaine infiltration of the two drainage exit sites during mastectomy is a simple, easy, and economical approach for pain relieving, without any opioid-related adverse effects. Correspondingly, postoperative analgesic requirements were reduced, and the quality of recovery was improved.

Table 2 Incidence of chronic pain in the study and the control groups

	Group A (*n* = 37)	Group B (*n* = 37)	*p* value
Location			
Chest wall	8 (21.6%)	12 (32.4%)	0.30
Axillary	9 (24.3%)	7 (18.9%)	0.58
arm	5 (13.5%)	4 (10.8%)	0.72
Total	19 (51.4%)	16 (43.2%)	0.49
PBI[a]	7.3 ± 9.7	7.3 ± 9.0	0.75

[a]Values are expressed as the mean ± standard deviation; *PBI* Pain Burden Index

Table 3 Incidence of PONV in the study and the control groups

	Group A (*n* = 37)	Group B (*n* = 37)	*p* value
In the PACU			
PONV	9 (24.3%)	11 (29.7%)	0.93
Asymptomic	28 (75.7%)	26 (70.3%)	
PACU-6 h			
PONV	8 (21.6%)	8 (21.6%)	0.90
Asymptomic	29 (78.4%)	29 (78.4%)	
6 h–12 h			
PONV	6 (16.2%)	12 (32.4%)	0.12
Asymptomic	31 (83.8%)	25 (67.6%)	
12 h–24 h			
PONV	3 (8.1%)	5 (13.5%)	0.46
Asymptomic	34 (91.9%)	32 (86.5%)	
24 h–36 h			
PONV	0 (0%)	1 (2.7%)	0.31
Asymptomic	37 (100%)	36 (97.3%)	

PONV postoperative nausea and vomiting; *PACU* post-anesthesia care unit

To compare with the previous similar studies, in Table 4 we summarized 8 randomized controlled trials that evaluated the efficacy of local analgesic for pain relief in breast cancer surgery, in which the local analgesic was either injected into the wound preoperatively or instilled through the drainage tube into the wound postoperatively. However, in this study, we chose to perform local infiltration anesthesia of the two drainage exit sites with ropivacaine, based on the evidence that pain caused by the drainage plays a vital role in postoperative pain. Five of the above mentioned trials [12–16] showed no differences between the control and experimental groups, in which Baudry et al.'s studies [12] enrolled patients who received breast-conserving surgery with or without ALND. However, the postoperative pain of different types of surgical technique remained different. The breast-conserving surgeries are susceptible to acute pain of the wound. In contrast, mastectomy surgeries are susceptible to burning, sensory loss or other abnormal sensations due to nerve damage, while acute pain is not reported as the main complaint [20]. Thus, it is not precise to compare the pain score between these two types of surgery due to the different mechanisms of pain. Our study is designed by including patients who received mastectomy, which provided comparable results. Nirmala et al. [17–19] have found that the local analgesic group showed significant reduction in the postoperative pain within 90 min, 6 h, and 15 h, respectively. Although the infiltration location in our study was different from theirs, local infiltration anesthesia showed effective results for patients who received mastectomy, and had a longer effective duration (24 h).

Table 4 Characteristics of the selected randomized controlled trials

Study	Research aim	Surgical technique	Intervention	Infiltration locations	Result	Ref
Baudry [2008]	evaluate the effect of R wound infiltration	MRM or partial mastectomy with ALND	R: 4.75 mg/mL R 40 mL C: NS 40 mL	The wound	no differences	[12]
Johansson [2003]	whether infiltration with R + fentanyl improves PP	Partial mastectomy with or without ALND	R1: 0.375% R R2: 0.375% R + Fentanyl 0.5 μg/kg C: Nil	The wound	no differences	[13]
Johansson [2000]	whether infiltration with R improves PP	Partial mastectomy with or without ALND	R: R 3.75 mg/mL C: NS 0.3 mL/kg	The wound of breast and axilla	no differences	[14]
Rica [2007]	if infiltration with R could improve PP	Mastectomy and ALND	R1: Preoperative 0.2% R 20 mL + NS to 80 mL R2: Postoperative 0.2% R 20 mL + NS to 80 mL	The wound	no differences	[15]
Talbot [2004]	determine the influence of B irrigation on PP	MRM	B: 0.5% B 20 mL C: NS	Through the axillary drain into the axillary wound	no differences	[16]
Nirmala [2019]	Whether wound instillation with B improve PP	MRM	R: 0.25% B 40 ml C: 40 ml normal saline	through chest and axillary drains into the wound	providing better analgesia within 15 h	[17]
Vigneau [2011]	document the effect of R infiltration	Mastectomy or lumpectomy with ALND	R: R 7.5 mg/mL solution 20 mL C: NS 20 mL	The wound	PP was lower at 2, 4 and 6 h after surgery	[18]
Albi-Feldzer [2013]	evaluate the influence of R wound infiltration	Conservative surgery with ALND, MRM with or without ALND	R: 0.375% R 3 mg/kg mixed with saline C: Saline solution	the wound, the 2nd & 3rd intercostal spaces and the humeral insertion of major pectoralis	decreased immediate PP (≤90 min)	[19]

ALND axillary lymph node dissection; *B* bupivacaine; *C* control; *MRM* modified radical mastectomy; *NS* normal saline; *R* ropivacaine; *PP* postoperative pain

The incidence of PONV in the two groups remained similar. However, from 6 h to 12 h after operation, PONV occurred in 6 patients in Group A and 12 in Group B. This difference might due to the side-effects of higher tramadol requirement in Group B. At 3-months follow-up, no significant differences were discovered with regard to the incidence of chronic pain. The mechanism of chronic pain is complicated, and it is still poorly controlled. Although our intervention decreased the postoperative pain more effectively, no surgical, demographic, and psychosocial factors that influenced chronic pain after breast surgery considered [21]. It has been reported that 30% ~ 51% of patients suffered from persistent pain after breast cancer surgery [2]. In our study, 51.35% of patients in Group A and 43.24% in Group B suffered from chronic pain. Nearly half of the patients are tortured by chronic pain. Therefore, it is still regarded as a great challenge to explore the reduction and treatment of chronic pain after breast cancer surgery. Furthermore, combined with the other pain-control methods, local infiltration anesthesia might further reduce the occurrence of postoperative acute pain, and even have positive effects on chronic pain.

However, there are certain limitations in this study that require consideration. Firstly, the sample size is small, and so it is not sufficient to perform subgroup analysis. Secondly, follow-up of the patient's pain after 3-months was not evaluated.

Conclusions

In conclusion, ropivacaine infiltration of two drainage exit sites effectively decreased the degree of postoperative acute pain and analgesic requirements within 24 h, and meanwhile improved patients' quality of recovery. Further large scale studies are warranted to study the outcomes in the future, and explore efficient approach that relieve pain after mastectomy in long run.

Abbreviations

PACU: Post-anesthesia care unit; PONV: Postoperative nausea and vomiting; VAS: Visual analogue scale; NSAIDs: Nonsteroidal anti-inflammatory drugs; BMI: Body mass index; SD: Standard deviation; ANOVA: Analysis of variance; PBI: Pain burden index; PVB: Paravertebral nerve block; ALND: Axillary lymph node dissection; SLNB: Sentinel lymph node biopsy

Acknowledgements

We thank our colleagues at the Department of Anesthesiology, National Cancer Center/National Clinical Research Center for Cancer/Cancer Hospital, Chinese Academy of Medical Sciences and Peking Union Medical College, Beijing, 100021, China.

Authors' contributions

WBN contributed to study design, data collection and analysis, drafting of manuscript. GHZ and ZH contributed to study design, data collection and analysis, drafting of manuscript. YT and KXY contributed to the study design, data analysis and interpretation, and revised the manuscript. SL contributed to data analysis, and revised the manuscript. All authors have read and approved the final manuscript.

Author details
[1]Department of Anesthesiology, National Cancer Center/National Clinical Research Center for Cancer/Cancer Hospital, Chinese Academy of Medical Sciences and Peking Union Medical College, Beijing 100021, China.
[2]Department of Breast Surgery, National Cancer Center/National Clinical Research Center for Cancer/Cancer Hospital, Chinese Academy of Medical Sciences and Peking Union Medical College, Beijing 100021, China.
[3]Department of Anesthesiology, National Cancer Center/National Clinical Research Center for Cancer/Cancer Hospital & Shenzhen Hospital, Chinese Academy of Medical Sciences and Peking Union Medical College, Shenzhen 518116, China.

References

1. Apfelbaum JL, Chen C, Mehta SS, Gan TJ. Postoperative pain experience: results from a National Survey Suggest Postoperative Pain Continues to be undermanaged. Anesth Analg. 2003;97:534–40.
2. Wang L, Gordon GH, Sean SA, Romerosa B, Kwon HY, Kaushal A, et al. Predictors of persistent pain after breast cancer surgery: a systematic review and meta-analysis of observational studies. CMAJ. 2016;188:352–61.
3. Gartner R, Jensen MB, Nielsen J, Ewertz M, Kroman N, Kehlet H. Prevalence of and factors associated with persistent pain following breast cancer surgery. JAMA. 2009;302:1985–92.
4. Nadeem M, Sahu A. Ultrasound guided surgery under Dilutional local anesthesia and no sedation in breast cancer patients. Surgeon. 2020;18:91–4.
5. Rao KV, Ludbrook G, van Wijk RM, Hewett PJ, Moran JL, Thiruvenkatarajan V, et al. Comparison of ultrasound-guided transmuscular quadratus lumborum block catheter technique with surgical pre-peritoneal catheter for postoperative analgesia in abdominal surgery: a randomised controlled trial. Aneasthesia. 2019;74:1381–8.
6. Park KU, Kyrish K, Yi M, Bedrosian I, Caudle AS, Kuerer HM, et al. Opioid use after breast-conserving surgery: prospective evaluation of risk factors for high opioid use. Ann Surg Oncol. 2020;27:730–5.
7. Del Vecchio G, Spahn V, Stein C. Novel opioid analgesics and side effects. ACS Chem Neurosci. 2017;8:1638–40.
8. Duthie DJ, Nimmo WS. Adverse effects of opioid analgesic drugs. Br J Anaesth. 1987;59:61–77.
9. Naja ZM, Naccache N, Ziade F, El-Rajab M, Itani T, Baraka A. Multilevel nerve stimulator-guided paravertebral block as a sole anesthetic technique for breast cancer surgery in morbidly obese patients. J Anesth. 2011;25:760–4.
10. Park KU, Kyrish K, Terrell J, Yi M, Caudle AS, Hunt KK, et al. Surgeon perception versus reality: opioid use after breast cancer surgery. Surg Oncol. 2019;119:909–15.
11. Kairaluoma PM, Bachmann MS, Korpinen AK, Rosenberg PH, Pere PJ. Single-injection paravertebral block before general anesthesia enhances analgesia after breast cancer surgery with and without associated lymph node biopsy. Anesth Analg. 2004;99:1837–43.
12. Baudry G, Steghens A, Laplaza D, Koeberle P, Bachour K, Bettinger G, et al. Ropivacaine infiltration during breast cancer surgery: postoperative acute and chronic pain effect. Ann Fr Anesth Reanim. 2008;27:979–86.
13. Johansson A, Kornfält J, Nordin L, Svensson L, Ingvar C, Lundberg J. Wound infiltration with ropivacaine and fentanyl: effects on postoperative pain and PONV after breast surgery. J Clin Anesth. 2003;15:113–8.
14. Johansson A, Axelson J, Ingvar C, Luttropp H-H, Lundberg J. Preoperative ropivacaine infiltration in breast surgery. Acta Anaesthesiology Scand. 2000; 44:1093–8.
15. Rica MA, Norlia A, Rohaizak M, Naqiyah I. Preemptive ropivacaine local anesthetic infiltration versus postoperative ropivacaine wound infiltration in mastectomy: postoperative pain and drain outputs. Asian J Surg. 2007;30: 34–9.
16. Talbot H, Hutchinson SP, Edbrooke DL, Wrench I, Kohlhardt SR. Evaluation of a local anaesthesia regimen following mastectomy. Anesthesia. 2004;59: 664–7.
17. Nirmala J, Harsh K, Padmaja D, Gopinath R. Role of wound instillation with bupivacaine through surgical drains for postoperative analgesia in modified radical mastectomy. Indian J Anesthesia. 2015;59:15–20.
18. Vigneau A, Salengro A, Berger J, Rouzier R, Barranger E, Marret E, et al. A double blind randomized trial of wound infiltration with ropivacaine after breast cancer surgery with axillary nodes dissection. BMC Anesthesiol. 2011; 11:23.
19. Albi-Feldzer A, Mouret-Fourme EE, Hamouda S, Motamed C, Dubois PY, Jouanneau L, et al. A double-blind randomized trial of wound and intercostal space infiltration with ropivacaine during breast cancer surgery: effects on chronic postoperative pain. Anesthesiology. 2013;118:318–26.
20. Kehlet H, Jensen TS, Woolf CJ. Persistent postsurgical pain: risk factors and prevention. Lancet. 2006;367:1618–25.
21. Tara L, Emily D, Nantthasorn Z, Tari A, Laura D, Rob R, et al. Chronic pain after breast surgery: a prospective, observational study. Ann Surg Oncol. 2018;25:2917–24.

9

Postpartum cerebral venous thrombosis misdiagnosed as postdural puncture headache

Mi K. Oh[1], Jae H. Ryu[2], Woo J. Jeon[3], Chang W. Lee[4] and Sang Y. Cho[5*]

Abstract

Background: Cerebral venous thrombosis can be a fatal complication of the postpartum period. Pregnancy is known to be a risk factor for thromboembolism in itself.

Case presentation: A normal spontaneous vaginal delivery was planned for a 20-year-old primigravida patient with patient-controlled epidural analgesia. Next morning, the patient complained of an occipital headache. An epidural blood patch was performed for diagnostic and therapeutic purpose with 10 ml of autologous blood. That night, she had an episode of seizures. Endotracheal intubation was done to secure the airway. She was transferred to an intensive care unit. Brain CT angiography and MRI showed superior sagittal sinus thrombosis with acute infarct and mild subarachnoid haemorrhage. For cerebral venous thrombosis treatment, heparin was injected and for intracranial pressure control, a hypertonic solution was injected. Despite this medical treatment, intracranial pressure continued to rise. The next day, her mental state changed to stupor. Emergency decompressive craniectomy was performed. Her mental state improved rapidly after surgery. A week later, she was transferred to a general ward. Her health recovered and she was discharged.

Conclusions: We experienced postpartum cerebral venous thrombosis misdiagnosed as postdural puncture headache. We hope that this case report would be helpful in situation which a postpartum young woman complains severe headache in spite of management for headache including autologous epidural blood patch.

Keywords: Cerebral venous thrombosis, Postdural puncture headache, Pregnancy

Background

Cerebral venous thrombosis (CVT) can be a fatal complication of the postpartum period [1]. Pregnancy is known to be a risk factor for thromboembolism in itself. Because the most common symptom of CVT is a nonspecific headache, it is difficult to diagnose. We report a case of a CVT patient who was misdiagnosed with postdural puncture headache.

* Correspondence: chosy@hanyang.ac.kr
[5]Department of Anesthesiology and Pain Medicine, Hanyang University Guri Hospital, 249-1, Gyomun-dong, Guri-si, Gyeonggi-do 471-701, Republic of Korea

Case presentation

A 20-year-old primigravida patient was referred to our hospital with premature rupture of membrane at 35 weeks of gestation. She has no other medical history except that she was a hepatitis B virus carrier. In the blood test on admission, coagulation profile including prothrombin time (INR) (0.98), activated partial thromboplastin time (25 s) and platelet count (295,000/mm^3) were within normal limit. A normal spontaneous vaginal delivery was planned with patient-controlled epidural analgesia. With the patient in the left lateral decubitus position, a 17-gauge Tuohy needle was inserted at the L4–5 interspace. The epidural space was confirmed with loss of resistance technique on the second attempt. A

19-gauge epidural catheter was inserted through the needle. On aspiration, there was no cerebrospinal fluid or blood. Then, an initial loading dose of 0.125% levobupivacaine (9 ml) and 50 micrograms of fentanyl was injected through the epidural catheter. The background infusion rate was 4 ml/h with 0.0625% levobupivacaine and self-administered 5 ml boluses at intervals of 10 min. Two hours later, she delivered a 2.38 kg female. The Apgar score of the infant at 1 min was 7 and at 5 min was 9.

Next morning, the patient complained of an occipital headache. The pain was worse when she sat down, but did not improve when she lay down. There were too many discrepancies to diagnose postdural puncture headache. There was no definite evidence of dural puncture and the symptoms were not specific. However, there was a possibility of an unrecognized dural puncture and symptoms of postdural puncture headache can vary from patient to patient. After consult with obstetrician and written informed consent by her husband, the epidural blood patch for diagnostic and therapeutic purpose with 10 ml autologous blood was performed. The patient said that symptoms were somewhat improved. At that time, she was diagnosed with postdural puncture headache.

That night, she had an episode of seizures. Endotracheal intubation was done to secure the airway. She was transferred to an intensive care unit. Magnetic resonance image (MRI) showed superior sagittal sinus thrombosis with acute infarct and mild subarachnoid haemorrhage (Fig. 1). For CVT treatment, low molecular weight heparin (enoxaparin sodium, Cnoxane, 60 mg) was injected subcutaneously two times during one day and for intracranial pressure control, an osmotic diuretics (Cerol) was injected. Despite these medical treatments, intracranial pressure continued to rise. The next day, her mental state changed to stupor. Brain CT showed diffuse brain swelling and aggravating venous infarct. An emergency decompressive craniectomy was performed. During the surgery, severe brain oedema and venous thrombosis were noted. (Fig. 2). After surgery, low molecular weight heparin was continuously administered with previous method during 10 days and monitoring aPTT according to neurologist consultation. Her

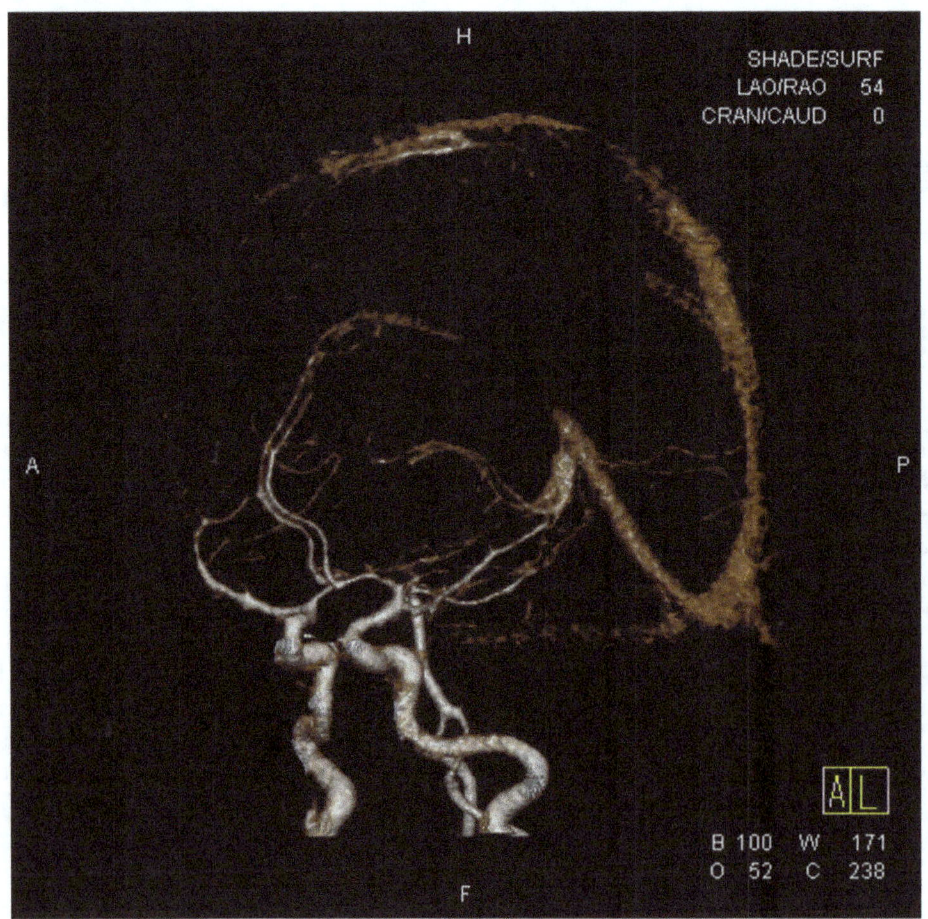

Fig. 1 MRI image showed superior sagittal sinus thrombosis with acute infarct and mild subarachnoid haemorrhage

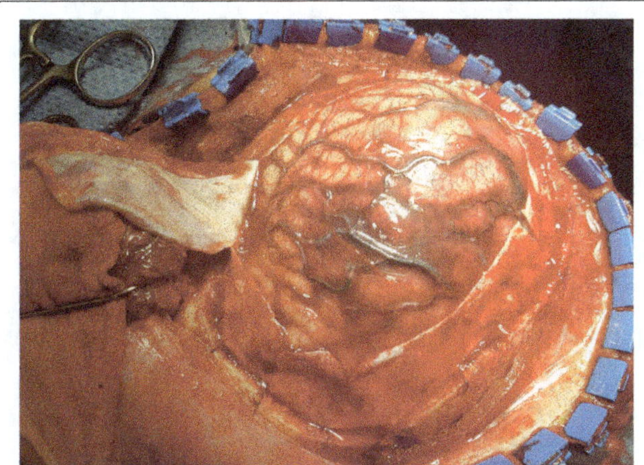

Fig. 2 Photograph of operation field. There were severe cerebral edema and venous thrombosis

mental state improved rapidly after the operation. A week later, she was transferred to a general ward. After that, apart from some neurological sequelae and right-side motor weakness, her health recovered and she was discharged.

Discussion and conclusions

Cerebral venous thrombosis can be a fatal complication of the postpartum period. The incidence of venous thrombosis during pregnancy or in the puerperium has been reported to vary from 0.018 to 0.2% depending on the study [1–3]. Because 13.4% of CVT patients are known to be at an increased risk of an unfavourable outcome [4], it is important to diagnose and treat the condition correctly.

During pregnancy, coagulation factors I, II, VII, VII, IX and XII increase [5]. In addition, physiologically, oestrogen contributes to vein expansion and congestion. Venous stasis results in a coagulation enhanced state in which thrombosis is likely to occur. Virchow's three signs (hypercoagulation, venous congestion, and tissue damage) reduce the risk of bleeding during labour, but they increase the risk of thromboembolism in the puerperium. Other risk factors for thrombosis include postpartum haemorrhage, varicose veins, caesarean section, obesity, and history of thromboembolic disease at previous pregnancy, preeclampsia, associated malignancy, a genetic defect of coagulation inhibitor, anaemia (< 9.9 g/dL) and placental abruption [4, 6, 7]. A large population-based cohort study [6] reported that risk of venous thromboembolism was peak during the first 3 week postpartum and women in their third trimester have 6 fold risk than their time outside trimester. Preeclampsia, hypertensive disorders of pregnancy, can progress to eclampsia, which is characterized by seizure activity. Preeclampsia associated with posterior reversible encephalopathy syndrome may be differentially diagnosed with CVT [8]. In this case, CVT appeared without any other risk factors except pregnancy.

Diagnosis of CVT is difficult. In particular, the differential diagnosis between CVT and postdural puncture headache can be very difficult. In the USA, about 61% of patients who undergo normal spontaneous vaginal delivery use epidural analgesia [9]. The incidence of postdural puncture headache is estimated to be between 30 and 50% following diagnostic or therapeutic lumbar puncture, 0–5% following spinal anaesthesia and up to 81% following accidental dural puncture during epidural insertion in the pregnant woman. Symptoms of CVT include papilledema, seizures, focal sensory or motor signs, aphasia, psychiatric disturbances, and cranial nerve palsies, but headache is common as an early symptom [10]. The incidence of CVT is much lower than postdural puncture headache. Therefore, patients who complain of postpartum headache are more likely to be diagnosed with postdural puncture headache even if they have CVT, such as in this case. Because the timing of the diagnosis is important in the prognosis of CVT, this delay can be fatal. Therefore, it is necessary to closely observe symptoms in patients who complain of postpartum headache. Then, if CVT is suspected, it is important to perform image studies, such as contrast-enhanced MRI and CT, without delay [11].

On the other hand, CVT is known to be associated with dural puncture [12, 13]. Dural puncture can result in low CSF pressure, which can affect the brain blood vessels and sinuses if the brain shifts down. This can lead to venous wall deformation which can induce thrombosis. As we mentioned above, it is difficult to distinguish between a headache due to postdural puncture and that due to CVT. In general, a dural puncture headache improves when the patient lies down and is completely resolved by an epidural blood patch. However, if it is accompanied by CVT, headaches may recur or more serious symptoms may occur later. Therefore, in patients who have had a dural puncture, if the symptoms are ambiguous or if the headache continues after the blood patch, CVT should be considered.

The treatment of CVT can be divided into anticoagulant therapy and symptomatic treatment including control of seizure and elevated intracranial pressure [13]. Anticoagulant therapy can avoid thrombus extension. Subcutaneous LMWH, intravenous heparin or oral anticoagulation are all known to be useful. Systemic or local thrombolytic therapy is not recommended. Approximately 40–50% of CVT patients also have intracranial cerebral haemorrhage, and these anticoagulant therapies may worsen that [4]. However, it is recommended that anticoagulant treatment is continued in patients with CVT even in the presence of intracranial cerebral haemorrhage [13]. Also, patient with CVT should be treated either dose-adjusted intravenous heparin or with body-weight –adjusted subcutaneous LMWH with monitoring activated partial thromboplastin time (at least double time) and INR (goal of 2–2.5) [13].

Cerebral venous thrombosis is one of the rare complications of the postpartum period. Because CVT is known to be related to an unfavourable outcome, it is very important to diagnose and treat it correctly. However, it is difficult to diagnose because the symptoms of CVT are not specific. If the patient has many risk factors associated with the CVT and shows symptoms, it is important to use appropriate diagnostic methods, such as contrast-enhanced CT or MRI.

In conclusion, we experienced postpartum cerebral venous thrombosis misdiagnosed as postdural puncture headache. We hope that this case report would be helpful in situation which a postpartum young woman complains severe headache in spite of management for headache including autologous epidural blood patch.

Abbreviations

CVT: Cerebral venous thrombosis; MRI: Magnetic resonance image

Acknowledgements

The authors thank the Hanyang University E-world center for considerable help during the preparation of the manuscript.

Authors' contributions

All authors including MKO, JHR, WJJ, CWL and SYC participated in the care of the patient and revise this manuscript, have read and approved final manuscript.

Author details

[1]Department of Anesthesiology and Pain Medicine, Hanyang University Guri Hospital, Guri-si, Gyeonggi-do, Republic of Korea. [2]Department of Anesthesiology and Pain Medicine, Hanyang University Guri Hospital, Guri-si, Gyeonggi-do, Republic of Korea. [3]Department of Anesthesiology and Pain Medicine, Hanyang University Guri Hospital, Guri-si, Gyeonggi-do, Republic of Korea. [4]Department of Anesthesiology and Pain Medicine, Hanyang University Guri Hospital, Guri-siGyeonggi-doRepublic of Korea. [5]Department of Anesthesiology and Pain Medicine, Hanyang University Guri Hospital, 249-1, Gyomun-dong, Guri-si, Gyeonggi-do 471-701, Republic of Korea.

References

1. Kontogiorgi M, Kalodimou V, Kollias S, Exarchos D, Nanas S, Ghiatas A, Routs C. Postpartum fatal cerebral vein thrombosis: a case report and review. Open J Clin Diagnostics. 2012;2:1–3..
2. Heit JA, Kobbervig CE, James AH, Petterson TM, Bailey KR, Melton LJ 3rd. Trends in the incidence of venous thromboembolism during pregnancy or postpartum: a 30-year population-based study. Ann Intern Med. 2005; 143(10):697–706.
3. Ferro JM, Canhão P, Stam J, Bousser MG. Barinagarrementeria F; ISCVT investigators. Prognosis of cerebral vein and dural sinus thrombosis: results of the international study on cerebral vein and Dural sinus thrombosis (ISCVT). Stroke. 2004;35(3):664–70.
4. Lanska DJ, Kryscio RJ. Risk factors for peripartum and postpartum stroke and intracranial venous thrombosis. Stroke. 2000;31(6):1274–82.
5. Bremme KA. Haemostatic changes in pregnancy. Best Pract Res Clin Haematol. 2003;16(2):153–68.
6. Sultan AA, West J, Tata LJ, Fleming KM, Nelson-Piercy C, Grainge MJ. Risk of first venous thromboembolism in and around pregnancy: a population-based cohort study. Br J Haematol. 2012;156(3):366–73.
7. Osterman MJ, Martin JA. Epidural and spinal anesthesia use during labor: 27-state reporting area, 2008. Natl Vital Stat Rep. 2011;59(5):1–13 16.
8. McDermott M, Miler EC, Rundek T, Hurn PD, Bushnell CD. Preeclampsia association with posterior encephalopathy syndrome and stroke. Stroke. 2018;49:524–30.
9. Crassard I, Bousser MG. Cerebral venous thrombosis. J Neuroophthalmol. 2004;24:156–63.
10. Saposnik G, Barinagarrementeria F, Brown RD Jr, Bushnell CD, Cucchiara B, Cushman M, de Veber G, Ferro JM, Tsai FY. Diagnosis and management of cerebral venous thrombosis: a statement for healthcare professionals from the American Heart Association/American Stroke Association. Stroke. 2011; 42:1158–92.
11. Stam J. Thrombosis of the cerebral veins and sinuses. N Engl J Med. 2005; 352(17):1791–8.
12. Borum SE, Naul LG, McLeskey CH. Postpartum dural venous sinus thrombosis after postdural puncture headache and epidural blood patch. Anesthesiology. 1997;86(2):487–90.
13. Einhäupl K, Stam J, Bousser MG, De Bruijn SF, Ferro JM, Martinelli I, Masuhr F, European Federation of Neurological Societies. EFNS guideline on the treatment of cerebral venous and sinus thrombosis in adult patients. Eur J Neurol. 2010;17(10):1229–35.

10

GPR30 receptor promotes preoperative anxiety-induced postoperative hyperalgesia by up-regulating $GABA_A$-α4β1δ subunits in periaqueductal gray in female rats

Ming Jiang[1†], Yu'e Sun[1†], Yishan Lei[1], Fan Hu[2], Zhengrong Xia[2], Yue Liu[1], Zhengliang Ma[1] and Xiaoping Gu[1*]

Abstract

Background: G-protein coupled estrogen receptor 30 (GPR30) was proved the specific estrogen receptor relating to mechanical hyperalgesia. Studies have shown that the $GABA_A$ receptor subunits α4, β1, and δ in the periaqueductal gray (PAG) neurons promote the descending facilitation system. This study inquired into whether and how GPR30 and $GABA_A$-α4β1δ in the PAG promote preoperative anxiety-induced postoperative hyperalgesia in female rats.

Methods: All the female rats were subjected to the single prolonged stress (SPS) to stimulate preoperative anxiety. Subsequently, mechanical allodynia was evaluated before and after the incision, based on the paw withdrawal mechanical threshold (PWMT). The selective GPR30 agonist G1 and antagonist G15 were locally microinjected into the PAG. The expression of GPR30, protein kinase A (PKA), and $GABA_A$ receptor subunits α4, β1, and δ in the PAG neurons were detected using western blotting and immunofluorescence.

Results: Behavioral testing revealed that Group S and Group I decreased the nociceptive threshold levels of PWMT in female rats. PWMT in Group S + I decreased more than that of Group S and Group I. Further, results of western blotting showed the expression of GPR30, PKA, and $GABA_A$ α4, β1, and δ subunits significantly up-regulated in Group S + I, and immunofluorescence indicated that the neurons of PAG in Group S + I appeared simultaneously immunopositive for GPR30 and $GABA_A$ α4, β1, and δ receptors. After microinjection of G1 into the PAG, female rats with plantar incision continued to exhibit significant hyperalgesia until postoperative 48 h. On the other hand, microinjection of G15 with SPS and plantar incision procedure relieved postoperative hyperalgesia in female rats. Western blotting demonstrated that intra-PAG injection of G15 markedly decreased the GPR30, PKA, and $GABA_A$ α4, β1, and δ levels in Group G15 + I.

Conclusions: Our results indicate that the GPR30-PKA-$GABA_A$α4β1δ pathway in the PAG promotes preoperative anxiety-induced postoperative hyperalgesia in female rats. This mechanism might be a potential novel therapeutic target for hyperalgesia in females.

Keywords: GPR30 receptor, $GABA_A$-α4β1δ subunits, Preoperative anxiety, Postoperative hyperalgesia, Female rat

* Correspondence: doctorgxp@163.com
†Ming Jiang and Yu'e Sun contributed equally to this work.
[1]Department of Anesthesiology, Affiliated Drum Tower Hospital of Nanjing University Medical School, Nanjing 210008, Jiangsu Province, China

Background

Preoperative anxiety is a clinically significant problem, with an incidence rate of 60 to 92%, for surgical patients [1]. Previous studies have demonstrated the positive correlativity between preoperative anxiety and postoperative pain [2]. Further, preoperative anxiety is often related to a slower and more algesic postoperative recovery of patients undergoing surgery [3]. Enhanced nociception and pain sensitivity due to exposure to physical or psychological stressors is described as stress-induced hyperalgesia (SIH) [4]. Although experimental studies have been conducted to investigate this phenomenon in male animals [5], the potential underlying mechanism has not been fully elucidated in female animals.

The G-protein coupled receptor 30 (GPR30), a specific estrogen receptor localized in the cell membrane, mediates the fast, non-genomic effects of estrogen [6]. It has been shown that estrogen-induced mechanical hyperalgesia is produced by selective agonists of the GPR30 receptor, and is inhibited by knockdown of the GPR30 receptor [7]. Required for complex functions, the periaqueductal gray (PAG) is associated with anxiety, fear, pain and analgesia [8]. A recent study shows that, via the p38 MAPK signaling pathway, descending facilitation of neuropathic pain is stimulated by glial activation in the PAG [9]. Further role of the GPR30 are demonstrated by studies showing GPR30 expression in the amygdala and PAG [10]. Given that PAG plays a vital part in the descending pain pathway and emotion response, it is of great importance to explore how this structure mediates anxiety-induced allodynia in females.

Accumulating evidence has indicated that $GABA_A$-mediated activation of neurons facilitates hypersensitivity in the central nervous system (CNS) [11]. Study has shown the up-regulation of $GABA_A\alpha4$ subunit is associated with anxiety disorders in the female rat [12]. It has been demonstrated that the increase in GPR30 levels under stress significantly reverses the attenuation of $GABA_A$ receptor, and causes its up-regulation in the amygdala of female mice [13]. Moreover, the up-regulation of $GABA_A$ subunits $\alpha4\beta1\delta$ in the PAG promotes the endogenous descending facilitation system [14]. However, whether GPR30 and $GABA_A$ subunits in the PAG contribute to preoperative anxiety-induced postoperative hyperalgesia in females remains unknown.

This study aims to test the hypothesis that preoperative anxiety-induced elevated GPR30 in the PAG evoked the up-regulation of extrasynaptic $\alpha4$, $\beta1$, and δ $GABA_A$ receptor subunits through protein kinase A (PKA), and thus exacerbated postoperative pain in female rats. We conducted the experiment in a model of preoperative anxiety-induced postoperative hyperalgesia [15], with single prolonged stress (SPS) procedure and plantar incision.

Methods

Laboratory animals and estrogen replacement

Laboratory Animal Centre of Drum Tower Hospital (Nanjing, China) supplied adult female Sprague-Dawley rats, weighing 250 to 300 g. In total, 6 rats were housed in one cage under a 12 h light/dark cycle at 20 °C, with a relative humidity of 55% and with free access to water and food. The experimental procedures were agreed by the Laboratory Animal Ethics Committee of the Affiliated Drum-Tower Hospital of Medical College of Nanjing University [16] (Approval number 20150603), and efforts were put forth to reduce the quantity of rats and relieve the suffering.

All the female rats received bilateral ovariectomy (OVX). According to the study by Xu [17], the OVX rats were subcutaneously injected with 17β-estradiol-3-benzoate (E2) ($0.1\ mg{\cdot}kg^{-1}{\cdot}day^{-1}$) for 10 days. This replacement therapy has been demonstrated to maintain an average concentration of plasma E2 between the nadir and peak levels of normal estrous cycle in the OVX rats [18].

Drugs and experimental grouping

Drugs were prepared and administered referring to previous studies. We used 17β-estradiol-3-benzoate (E2, Sigma, St. Louis, MO) for E2 replacement therapy. G1, (GPR30 agonist) and G15 (GPR30 antagonist) were administered for the local PAG microinjection (Cayman Chemical, Ann Arbor, MI, USA). The dosages of E2 and G1/G15 were adopted according to previous studies [18], and our preliminary experiments. The E2 was diluted in sesame seed oil, and other drugs were administered with dimethyl sulfoxide (DMSO) as the vehicle.

The rats were randomly divided into the 10 groups ($n = 6$ rats per group): All the female rats received bilateral ovariectomy on day 1, and subcutaneously received estrogen replacement for 10 days. Group C was a control for sham SPS and sham incision surgery experiments; Group S underwent SPS procedure on day 7; Group I was subjected to surgical incision on day 8 only; Group S + I underwent the SPS experimentation on day 7, and received incision surgery on day 8 after estrogen replacement. To investigate the effect of GPR30 in PAG, the PAG of Group G1 (10 μmol/L, 0.5 μL) and Group Vehicle1 (0.5 μL) were microinjected once per day, from day 6 to 8 without SPS and surgical incision; Group G1 + I and Group Vehicle1 + I were microinjected with the same conditions, from day 6 to 8, without SPS (30 min before surgical incision on day 8); Group G15 + I (20 μmol/L, 0.5 μL) and Group Vehicle2 + I (0.5 μL) were treated with PAG microinjection from day 6 to 8 (30 min before SPS on day 7, and 30 min before surgical incision on day 8). The procedures and treatments in 10 groups in this study are shown in Table 1, and the

Table 1 Procedures and treatments in 10 groups in this study

Group	Procedures and treatments
Group C	sham SPS and sham incision surgery
Group S	SPS procedure
Group I	incision surgery
Group S + I	SPS procedure and incision surgery
Group G1	PAG microinjection of G1
Group Vehicle1	PAG microinjection of Vehicle1
Group G1 + I	PAG microinjection of G1 and incision surgery
Group Vehicle1 + I	PAG microinjection of Vehicle1 and incision surgery
Group G15 + I	PAG microinjection of G15, SPS procedure, and incision surgery
Group Vehicle2 + I	PAG microinjection of Vehicle2, SPS procedure, and incision surgery

schematic representation of the experimental design and time schedule of the protocol are shown in Fig. 1.

SPS procedure and surgical incision

The SPS procedure was carried out according to the previous studies [19]. On day 7 after the estrogen replacement, female rats were confined in animal holders for 2 h, after which they were immediately forced to swim for 20 min individually in a clear acrylic cylinder (with a diameter of 30 cm and a height of 60 cm) filled with water (24 to 26 °C) to two-thirds of its height. After that, the female rats took a rest for 15 min and then exposed to the anesthetic ether until their consciousness vanished. After the animals were fully anesthetized following the administration of ether, we observed that righting reflex and corneal reflex of the rats disappeared. Control rats, untreated, were observed in another room.

The model of postoperative pain was operated on as described by Brennan [20] on day 8 after estrogen replacement. After sterilization of the right hind paw with 10% povidone-iodine, a 1 cm incision was operated on the skin and fascia. In this step, the muscle was remained intact. The skin was stitched up with 5–0 silk thread, after carefully maintaining hemostasis with pressure. Finally, the wound was covered with erythromycin ointment. The control group received sham surgery, consisting of sterilization of the hind paw, and application of erythromycin ointment on the plantar surface, without plantar incision.

Pain-related behavioral test

To assess the pain-related behaviors in the female rats, the paw withdrawal mechanical threshold (PWMT) was measured on day 6 (24 h prior to SPS, baseline), 8, 9, and 10 (2, 6, 24, and 48 h after the incision surgery). The PWMT was evaluated by the "up-and-down" method, using a set of von Frey filaments. The OVX female rats were kept in mesh-bottomed plastic cases (20 × 20 × 15 cm) with an approximately 30 min habituation. Each von Frey filament was positioned beneath the right hind paw, and was adjacent to the wound for 6 to 8 s. Positive responses were considered as paw lifting or licking of the paw following stimulation. We repeated the stimulation 3 times, with intervals of 5 min, recorded the data,

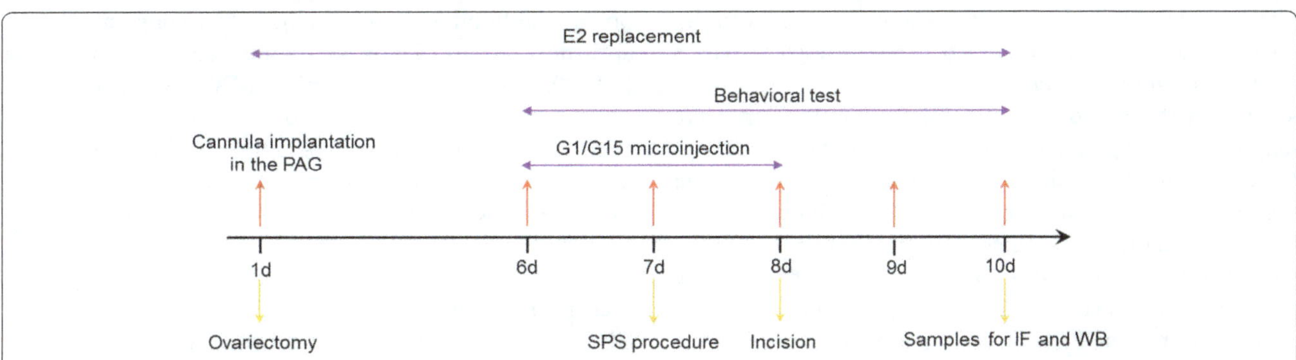

Fig. 1 The schematic representation of the experimental design and time schedule of the protocol. All the female rats were subjected to bilateral ovariectomy and cannula implantation in the periaqueductal gray on day 1, and received estrogen replacement for 10 days. The single prolonged stress was administered on day 7, and G1/G15 microinjection was once per day from day 6 to 8 after the estrogen replacement. Behavioral tests were conducted on day 6 prior to the incision surgery, and on day 8, 9, and 10 after the surgical incision. Samples were collected for immunofluorescence and western blotting analysis on day 10 after behavioral tests

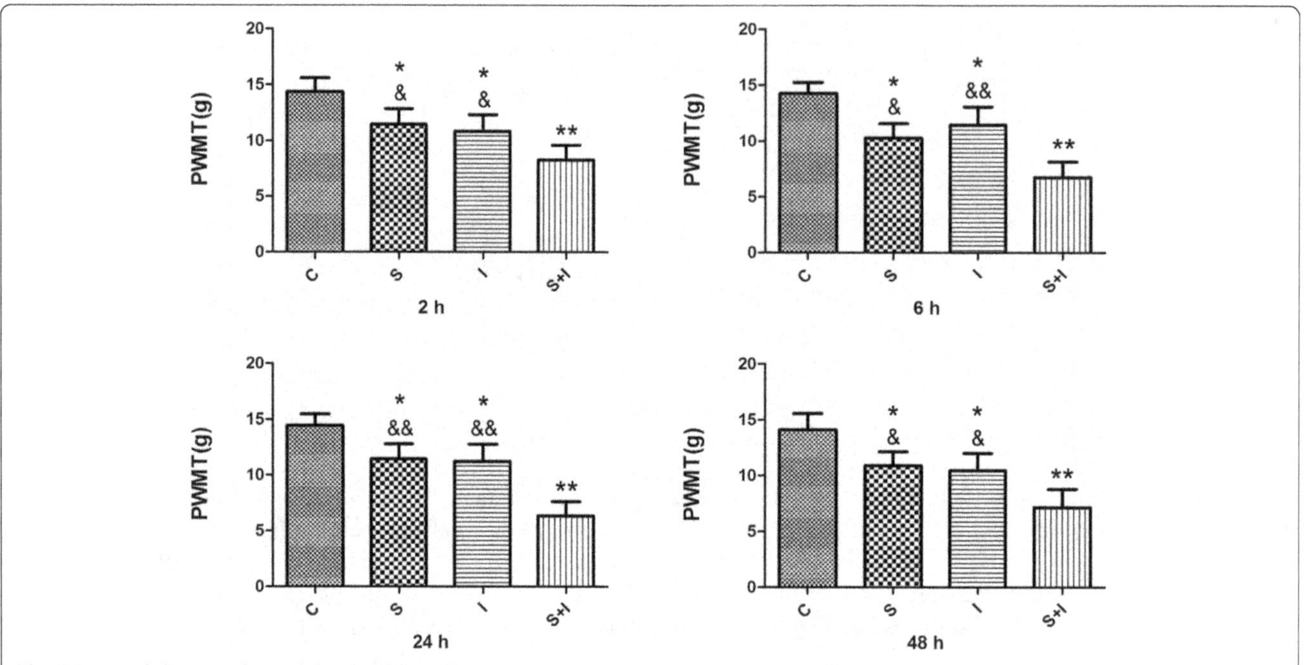

Fig. 2 Paw withdraw mechanical threshold (PWMT) was examined at 2 h, 6 h, 24 h and 48 h after the plantar incision ($n = 6$/each group). Decrease PWMT in Group S, Group I and Group S + I were observed at each time-point after the incision. $^{*}P < 0.05$, $^{**}P < 0.01$ compared with Group C; $^{\&}P < 0.05$, $^{\&\&}P < 0.01$ compared with Group S + I

and analyzed the data using the method described by Chaplan [21].

Intra-PAG microinjection

Rats were anesthetized with sevoflurane by a nose mask (induction, 3%; surgery, 1%; Heng Rui Co., Shanghai, China) and placed in a stereotaxic frame. After locating the bregma by exposing the skull of the rat, a small hole was drilled for cannula implantation in the PAG (bregma, − 7.8 mm, 0.6 mm laterally, and − 4.5 mm ventrally from the skull surface). The microinjection cannula was immobilized with dental cement. In the preliminary experiment, we used the stereotaxic instrument to perform multiple injections of Evans blue in the PAG of female rats to determine the correct injection site. Rats were given 5 days to recover after implantation, and body weights were measured. On the day of intra-PAG injection, the rats were left without being disturbed for 1 h before the microinjection. In this study, drugs were injected over a 2-min period, and the volume of drug administered into the PAG was 0.5 μL. To examine the active role of GPR30 in the PAG in SPS-enhanced postoperative hyperalgesia, the selective GPR30 agonist G1 and antagonist G15 were administered into the PAG by local microinjection.

Immunofluorescence

Immunofluorescence was used to further study the female rats. The animals were anesthetized deeply with 5% sevoflurane and sacrificed by cervical dislocation. Rats were then perfused with 4% paraformaldehyde in 0.1 M phosphate buffer (pH = 7.4) on day 10 after behavioral tests. Next, the brain was removed, post-fixed in the same fixative, and transferred to 30% sucrose. The PAG tissues were cut into 25 μm-thick sections, and they were incubated overnight with the primary antibodies: rabbit polyclonal to GPR30 (Abcam, Cambridge, UK; 1:200), goat polyclonal antibody against the $GABA_A\alpha4$ receptor (N-19; Santa Cruz Biotechnology, TX, USA; 1:250), mouse monoclonal to $GABA_A$ β1 receptor (S96–55; Abcam; 1:200), or goat polyclonal antibody against the $GABA_A\delta$ receptor (R-20; Santa Cruz Biotechnology; 1:250). After washing, sections were incubated with secondary antibodies: Alexa Fluor 555-conjugated goat anti-mouse, Alexa Fluor 488-conjugated goat anti-rabbit (1:1000, ThermoFisher Scientific, MA, USA) and NorthernLights 557-conjugated donkey anti-goat (1:1500, R&D Systems, MN, USA) for 1 h at room temperature. The stained sections were mounted on glass slides, and examined under a LSM710 (Carl Zeiss, Germany) confocal microscope.

Western blotting

The segments of PAG were removed rapidly from deeply anesthetized rats, and stored at − 80 °C. The collected tissue samples were homogenized in lysis buffer and centrifuged (4 °C) at 13,000 rpm for 10 min. Protein samples were separated using sodium dodecyl sulfate polyacrylamide gel electrophoresis (SDS-PAGE, 10%), and

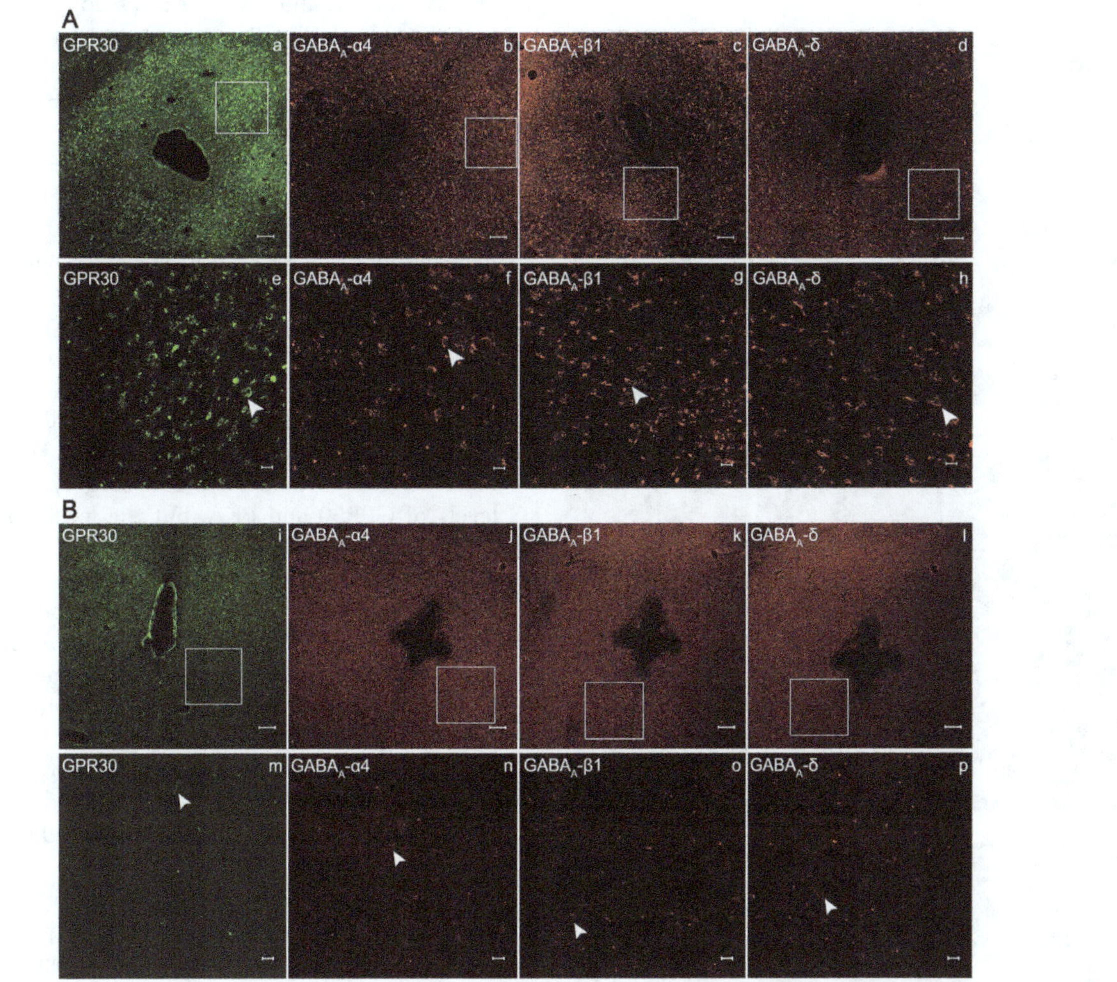

Fig. 3 Confocal fluorescence micrographs of the periaqueductal gray (PAG) neurons with the immunolabeled GPR30 (a, e, i, m), GABA$_A$α4 (b, f, j, n), GABA$_A$β1 (c, g, k, o), and GABA$_A$δ (d, h, l, p) receptors. **a** Representative images of Group S + I. **b** Representative images of Group I. Scale bar is 100 μm in a–d and i–l, and 20 μm in e–h and m–p

transferred onto a nitrocellulose membrane. The membranes were incubated overnight at 4 °C with primary antibodies against GPR30 (1:500, Abcam), PKA (1:500, R&D Systems), GABA$_A$α4 (1:1000, Santa Cruz Biotechnology), GABA$_A$β1 (1:1000, Abcam), and GABA$_A$δ (1: 1000, Santa Cruz Biotechnology). The membranes were washed and incubated with secondary antibody for 1 h at room temperature. β-actin was used as a loading control. The immune complexes were detected using enhanced chemiluminescence. Density of specific bands was analyzed using Image-Pro Plus software.

Statistical analysis

All data were expressed as mean ± standard deviation (S.D.). Two-way repeated measures analysis of variance (ANOVA) was performed to analyze differences in pain-related behaviours. Bonferroni post-hoc tests were conducted to determine the source(s) of differences when significant main effects were observed. Kruskal-Wallis test was used for comparisons of the non-parametric data regarding western blot. All statistical analyses were performed using SPSS 17.0 software (SPSS Inc., Chicago, IL, USA), and $P \leq 0.05$ was set as the level of statistical significance.

Results

Preoperative SPS-induced postoperative hyperalgesia in female rats

The baseline PWMT was not significantly different of PWMT across groups on day 6 before incision surgery. PWMT in Group S, Group I and Group S + I were observed significantly lower than Group C at each time-point from day 8 to 10 (Fig. 2). SPS and surgical incision in Group S + I significantly enhanced mechanical allodynia compared to the Group S. Meanwhile, the PWMT in

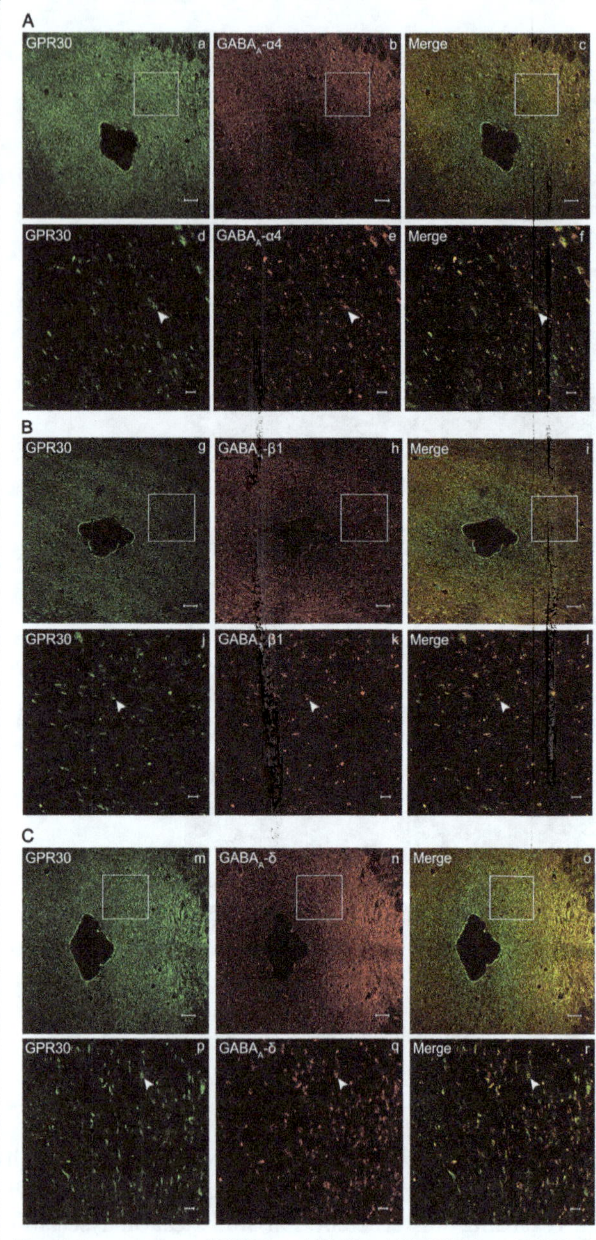

Fig. 4 Co-expression of GPR30 and GABA$_A$α4 (**a**), GPR30 and GABA$_A$β1 (**b**), as well as GPR30 and GABA$_A$δ (**c**) in periaqueductal gray (PAG) after incision surgery. Double immunofluorescence staining for confocal laser scanning microscopy showing a transverse section of PAG. In Group S + I, GPR30/GABA$_A$α4 (c, f), GPR30/GABA$_A$β1 (i, l), and GPR30/GABA$_A$δ (o, r), simultaneously immunopositive in neurons in PAG were co-localized, as indicated by yellow overlay. Scale bar is 100 μm in a–c, g–i, and m–o, and 20 μm in d–f, j–l, and p–r

Group S + I significantly decreased compared to the Group I from day 8 to 10.

Up-regulation of GPR30 and GABA$_A$α4β1δ in the PAG of female rats

The neuronal receptors of PAG were observed under the confocal microscope. The receptors GPR30 and GABA$_A$ α4, β1, and δ were expressed in the PAG of rats in Group S + I (Fig. 3a) and Group I (Fig. 3b). Double immunofluorescence staining for co-expression of GPR30 and GABA$_A$α4, GPR30 and GABA$_A$β1, as well as GPR30 and GABA$_A$δ were observed in Group S + I (Fig. 4a–c). The results showed that GPR30/GABA$_A$α4 (Fig. 4a), GPR30/GABA$_A$β1 (Fig. 4b), and GPR30/GABA$_A$δ (Fig. 4c), simultaneously immunopositive in neurons in PAG were co-localized, as indicated by yellow overlay.

Western blotting demonstrated that the expression of GPR30, PKA, and GABA$_A$ α4, β1, and δ of Group S + I rats were significantly higher than that of other groups (Fig. 5a-f). The expression level of GPR30 and PKA in Group S was higher than in Group C. Female rats that received SPS without incision surgery showed higher levels of GPR30 and PKA, but the levels of GABA$_A$ receptors were not different from those of Group C. Moreover, there were no significant changes in the levels of GPR30, PKA, and GABA$_A$ receptors between Group I and Group C. Furthermore, we compare the female rats only exposed to the anesthetic ether according to the SPS procedure with the control rats without the ether, and no significant changes were found in the levels of GABA$_A$-α4β1δ subunits between the two groups.

Effects of GPR30 in PAG for SPS-enhanced postoperative allodynia in female rats

Our results showed no significant difference in PWMT between the sham and model groups prior to incision surgery. Decreases in PWMT were observed in Group G1, Group I, Group G1 + I, Group Veh1 + I, Group G15 + I and Group Veh2 + I at each time-point after the incision (Fig. 6). A decreased tolerance to nociceptive stimulus was observed in Group G1 compared with Group C from 2 h to 48 h. Furthermore, in Group G1 + I, intra-PAG microinjection of G1 significantly declined in nociceptive thresholds after the surgical procedure compared with Group I. No significant changes were found in PWMT between Group G15 + I and Group I, while the threshold levels of Group G15 + I were relatively higher than those of Group Veh2 + I. Moreover, there were no significant differences in the PWMT between the groups receiving vehicle and the groups undergoing the same procedure without DMSO (Fig. 6).

Results from the western blotting showed that microinjection of G1 in the PAG significantly up-regulated the expression of GPR30, PKA, and GABA$_A$ α4, β1, and δ after incision operation compared with the Group C, but no significant difference was found compared with Group S + I (Fig. 5). The expressions of GPR30 and PKA in Group G1 and Group S + I were significantly higher than in other groups (Fig. 7). Further, Group S + I showed higher intensity of the GPR30 and PKA than

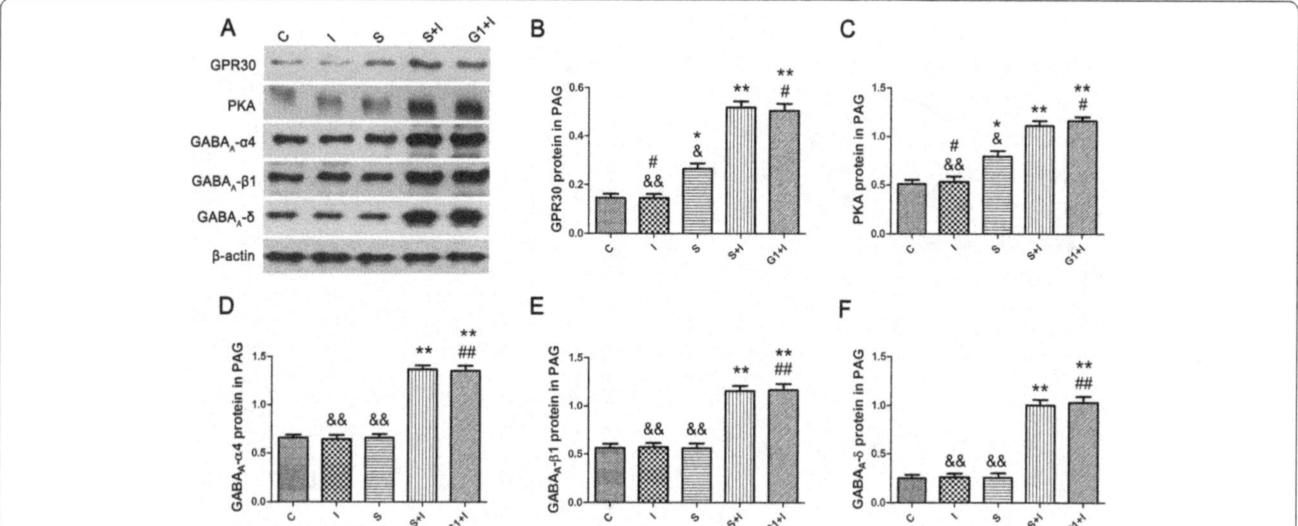

Fig. 5 Western blotting of GPR30, PKA, and GABA$_A$ α4, β1, and δ subunits in periaqueductal gray neurons of different groups ($n = 6$/each group). β-actin was used as a loading control. The expressions of GPR30 and PKA in Group S + I and Group G1 + I were significantly higher than in other groups (**a-f**). The expression level of GPR30 and PKA in Group S was higher than in Group C. $^{*}P < 0.05$, $^{**}P < 0.01$ compared with Group C; $^{\#}P < 0.05$, $^{\#\#}P < 0.01$ compared with Group S; $^{\&}P < 0.05$, $^{\&\&}P < 0.01$ compared with Group S + I

Group G1. In Group G1, the expression of GPR30 and PKA significantly increased, but no significant difference of GABA$_A$ α4, β1, and δ was found compared with Group C. In contrast, intra-PAG injection of G15 markedly decreased the GPR30, PKA, and GABA$_A$ α4, β1, and δ levels in the PAG compared with Group S + I (Fig. 7). Additionally, the staining expression of GPR30 and GABA$_A$ α4, β1, and δ in the PAG were observed in Group G1 + I, which was microinjected with G1, and underwent incision surgery (Fig. 8a). Double

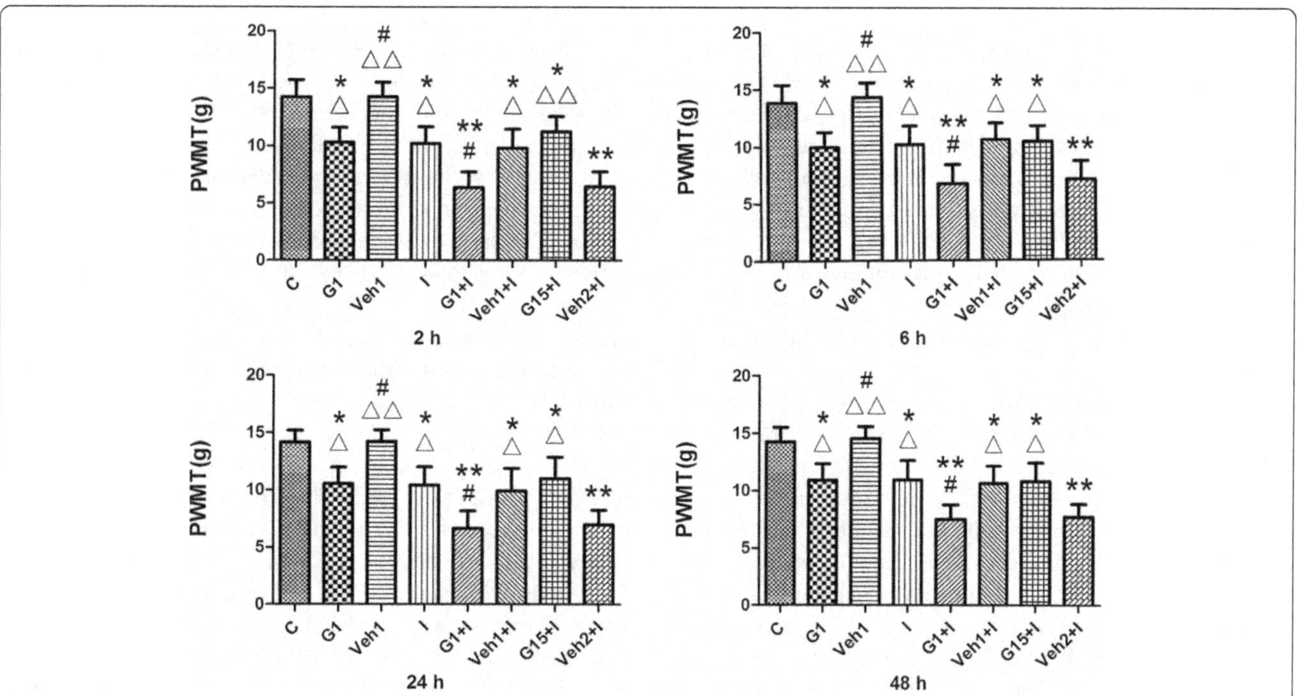

Fig. 6 Paw withdraw mechanical threshold (PWMT) was examined at 2 h, 6 h, 24 h and 48 h after the plantar incision (n = 6/each group). Decreases in PWMT were observed in Group G1, Group I, Group G1 + I, Group Veh1 + I, Group G15 + I and Group Veh2 + I at each time-point after the incision. $^{*}P < 0.05$, $^{**}P < 0.01$ compared with Group C; $^{\#}P < 0.05$ compared with Group I; $^{\triangle}P < 0.05$, $^{\triangle\triangle}P < 0.01$ compared with Group Veh2 + I

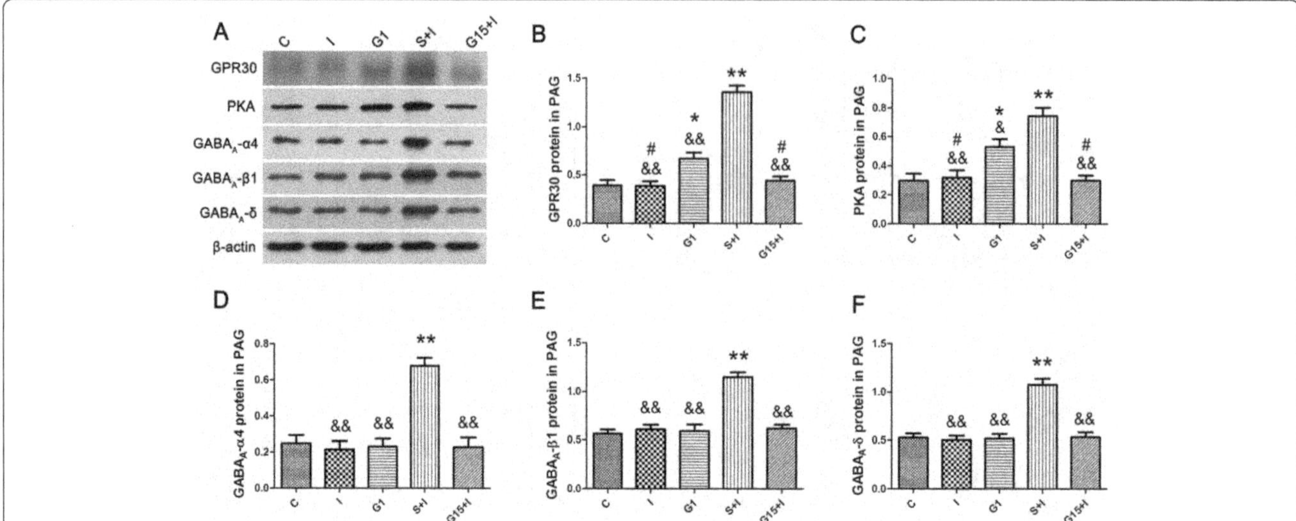

Fig. 7 Western blotting of GPR30, PKA, and $GABA_A$ α4, β1, and δ subunits in periaqueductal gray neurons of different groups (n = 6/each group). β-actin was used as a loading control. The expressions of GPR30 and PKA in Group G1 and Group S + I were significantly higher than in other groups (**a-f**). Further, Group S + I showed higher intensity of the GPR30 and PKA than Group G1. $^{*}P < 0.05$, $^{**}P < 0.01$ compared with Group C; $^{\#}P < 0.05$ compared with Group G1; $^{\&}P < 0.05$, $^{\&\&}P < 0.01$ compared with Group S + I

immunofluorescence images of the PAG showed the co-expression of GPR30 and $GABA_A$ α4, β1, and δ in the rats of Group G1 + I (Fig. 8b).

Discussion

In this study, we demonstrated (1) that preoperative SPS-induced postoperative hyperalgesia in female rats via up-regulation of GPR30, PKA and $GABA_A$α4β1δ in the PAG, (2) the previously unknown effects of GPR30 on SPS-induced postoperative allodynia in PAG of female rats with incisions, (3) microinjection of G1 in the PAG continued to exhibit significant hyperalgesia in female rats with plantar incision, and microinjection of G15 with SPS and plantar incision procedure relieved postoperative hyperalgesia in female rats. These findings support the hypothesis that upregulation of neuronal GPR30-PKA-$GABA_A$α4β1δ pathway in the PAG promotes preoperative anxiety-induced postoperative hyperalgesia in female rats.

Among patients undergoing surgery, preoperative anxiety has a very high incidence [1], which is related to acute postoperative pain, and even the chronic postoperative pain [22]. However, only a few studies have been conducted to investigate this phenomenon in females. The PAG, a core component of the descending pain-modulatory network, is a pre-eminent central trigger site for behavioral and pain transmission via the rostral ventromedial medulla (RVM), projecting to the spinal dorsal horn [23, 24]. The PAG has been demonstrated to be associated with vibration stress-induced reduction in tail flick latency [25], and spinal nerve ligation in mice exposed to SIH results in an increase in glial fibrillary acidic protein mRNA expression in the PAG [26]. In this study, the OVX female rats with E2 replacement using SPS, and incision surgery, exhibited postoperative hyperalgesia. Taken together, these data suggest that the GPR30 up-regulates extrasynaptic $GABA_A$ α4, β1, and δ subunits in the PAG neurons, and makes a difference in the progress of preoperative anxiety-induced postoperative hyperalgesia in female rats.

As a novel estrogen receptor, 7-transmembrane spanning G protein-coupled receptor, GPR30 is located in the plasma membrane, endoplasmic reticulum, Golgi complexes, and the physiological functions of GPR30 have been described in almost every organ [27]. Current evidences suggest GPR30 expression in multiple regions of the CNS in rodents (e.g. cortex, hypothalamus, hippocampus, amygdala, and PAG) [10, 28]. Further, 17β-estradiol produced GPR30-dependent primary hyperalgesia [29], which was restrained with antagonist or knockdown of GPR30. Estrogen binding with GPR30 causes the dissociation of heterotrimeric G proteins to activate intracellular signaling cascades. The Gα subunit of GPR30 initiates cyclic adenosine monophosphate (cAMP) production [30]. The Gα subunit cascades can activate the adenylyl cyclase (AC) enzymes which catalyze the conversion of adenosine triphosphate (ATP) to cAMP [31], and the Gα subunit also mobilizes calcium stores in a phospholipase C dependent manner. The rapid rise of the cAMP and Ca^{2+} concentration caused by GPR30 can ultimately lead to gene regulation and other related cellular responses [32]. We found that preoperative SPS induced the expression of GPR30 and PKA in the PAG of the female rats. Microinjection of

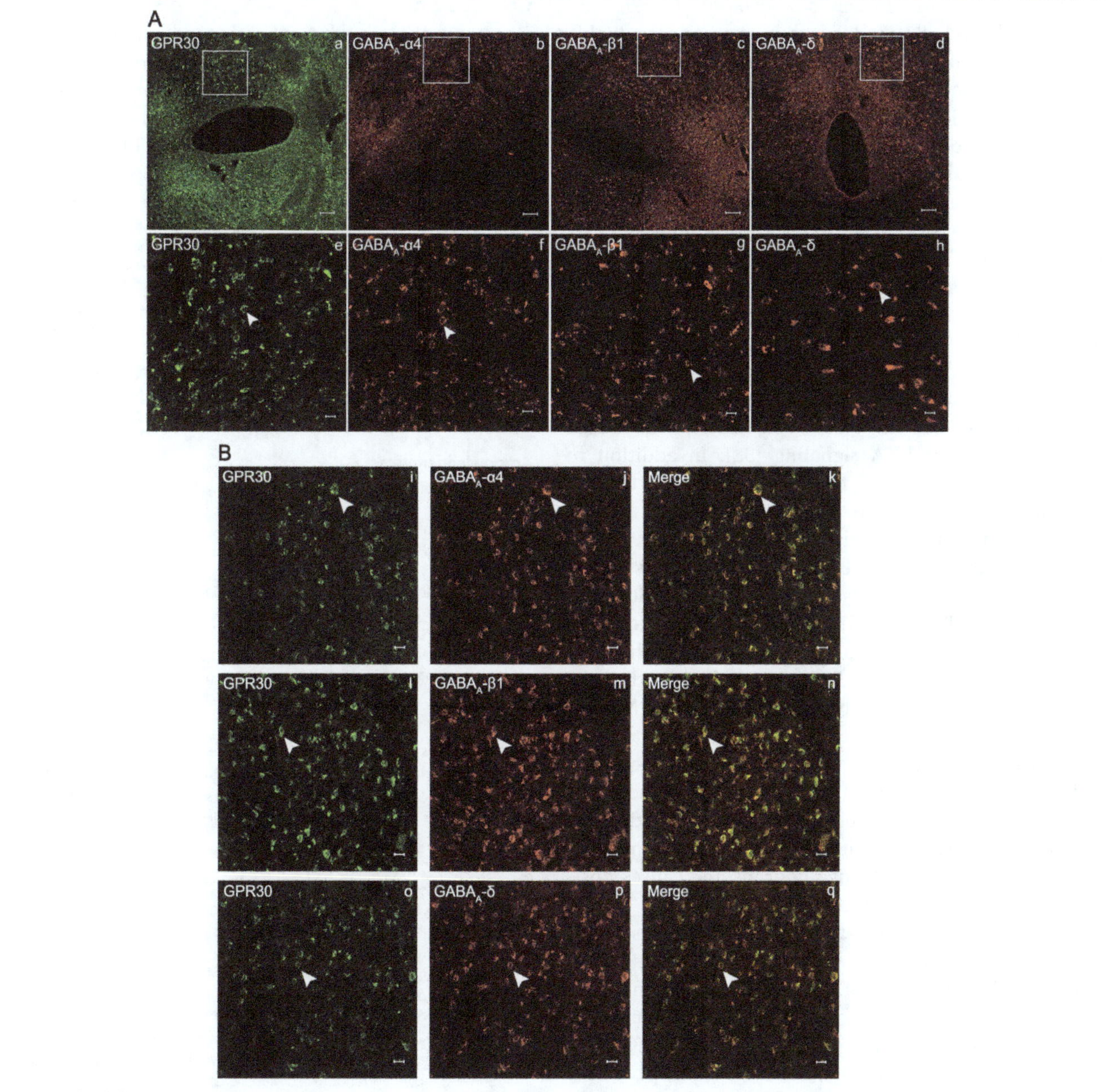

Fig. 8 Confocal fluorescent micrographs of the periaqueductal gray (PAG) neurons immunolabeled GPR30 and GABA$_A$ α4, β1, and δ subunits in Group G1 + I (**a**). GPR30/GABA$_A$α4, GPR30/GABA$_A$β1, and GPR30/GABA$_A$δ of neurons in PAG were co-localized, as indicated by yellow overlay (**b**). Scale bar is 100 μm in a–d and 20 μm in e–q

G1 into PAG significantly decreased the nociceptive threshold after the incision operation, and female rats treated with the antagonist G15 in the PAG alleviated hyperalgesia after incision surgery. Consistent with the behavioral tests, the expression of GPR30 and PKA were significantly increased in the process of postoperative hyperalgesia.

Generally, extrasynaptic GABA$_A$ receptors contain α4–6 subunits, together with either a γ2 or δ subunit, and mediate tonic inhibition [33]. It is acknowledged that the PAG is a source of descending facilitation and inhibitory pathways exerting paralleled but opposite influences on nociceptive transmission via the descending projections from the RVM to the dorsal horn [34]. The facilitation and inhibitory systems are both considered to be tonically active, and it has been indicated that a small net facilitation influence predominates under non-stressed conditions [35]. Studies have shown that the up-regulation of extrasynaptic GABA$_A$ receptors with the α4, β1, and δ subunits expressed on neurons in the PAG probably inhibit the endogenous descending inhibitory system, and promote the descending facilitation system function [14]. In this study, beside GPR30 and PKA, $GABA_A$ α4, β1, and δ subunits were also highly expressed in the PAG during preoperative anxiety-induced postoperative hyperalgesia. It has been shown that the expression of extrasynaptic $GABA_A$ α4 subunit in cultured cortical neurons can be enhanced by PKA activation, and simultaneous exposure to a PKA inhibitor can block this effect [36]. Moreover, ethanol modulation of extrasynaptic $GABA_A$ α4 and δ subunits is PKA-dependent, and PKA directly affects the expression and function of these receptors, which increase the tonic current in cortical neurons after exposure to a PKA activator, but PKC activation exerts no influence in the tonic current [37]. Aripiprazole increases the expression of $GABA_A$ (containing β-1 subunit) receptor in the nucleus accumbens of rats, which is significantly correlated with the enhanced PKA signaling [38]. In addition to hyperalgesia in behavioral tests, we found that the expression (based on western blotting) of $GABA_A$ α4, β1, and δ subunits significantly increased in the PAG of Group S + I and Group G1 + I, and the neurons of the PAG also appeared simultaneously immunopositive for GPR30 and $GABA_A$ α4, β1, and δ subunits. However, the levels of these receptors did not increase in the PAG of Group I and Group G15 + I. We speculate that the dissociation of Gα subunit of GPR30 through cAMP enhances PKA activation in female rats after SPS, and enhances the tonic currents caused by the extrasynaptic $GABA_A$ subunits α4, β1, and δ via PKA in the PAG, inhibiting the pain inhibitory system and activating the descending facilitation system, which decreases the excitation threshold of nociceptive neurons and causes postoperative hyperalgesia. Interestingly, although GPR30 and PKA expression increased in the female rats which only received the SPS, $GABA_A$ receptor subunits (α4, β1, δ) protein levels were not significantly different from Group C. The reason for this phenomenon might be that a certain degree of increase in GPR30 and PKA may not up-regulate the extrasynaptic $GABA_A$ α4, β1, and δ subunits without incision surgery. SPS without surgical incision were relatively lower in nociceptive thresholds than those of Group C might be through other downstream signaling pathways of GPR30-PKA system. Further in-depth studies are still needed to explore the detailed mechanisms. The limitation of our study is that not all groups were analyzed using immunofluorescence staining, and the changes in GPR30 and $GABA_A$ receptor subunits were only compared between different groups using western blotting. This limitation may affect the results in our study.

Overall, these findings might be relevant for understanding of the potential mechanisms involved, and for exploring the effective prevention and treatment for this clinical issue in females.

Conclusion

Together, the results further extend our understanding of the functional relevance of the GPR30-PKA-$GABA_A$α4β1δ pathway in the PAG promoting preoperative anxiety-induced postoperative hyperalgesia in female rats. The presence of GPR30 in the PAG is an important condition for the development of preoperative anxiety-induced postoperative allodynia.

Abbreviations

AC: Adenylyl cyclase; ANOVA: Analysis of variance; ATP: Adenosine triphosphate; cAMP: Cyclic adenosine monophosphate; CNS: Central nervous system; DMSO: Dimethyl sulfoxide; E2: 17β-estradiol-3-benzoate; ERα: Estrogen receptor-alpha; ERβ: Estrogen receptor- beta; GPR30: G-protein coupled estrogen receptor 30; OVX: Ovariectomy; PAG: Periaqueductal gray; PKA: Protein kinase A; PWMT: Paw withdrawal mechanical threshold; RVM: Rostral ventromedial medulla; SIH: Stress-induced hyperalgesia; SPS: Single prolonged stress

Acknowledgements

Not applicable.

Authors' contributions

All authors had full access to all the data in the study and take responsibility for the integrity of the data and the accuracy of the data analysis. Study concept and design: ZM. Analysis and interpretation of data: FH, YL1 and ZX. Drafting of the manuscript: MJ. Perform the experiments and contribute reagents: MJ, YL1 and YL2. Statistical analysis: ZM. Pain behavioral tests: YL2. Revise the manuscript: XG. All the authors approved the final manuscript and attest to the integrity of the original data and the analysis reported in this manuscript.

Author details

[1]Department of Anesthesiology, Affiliated Drum Tower Hospital of Nanjing University Medical School, Nanjing 210008, Jiangsu Province, China. [2]Analytical & Testing Center, Nanjing Medical University, Nanjing, Jiangsu Province, China.

References

1. Nigussie S, Belachew T, Wolancho W. Predictors of preoperative anxiety among surgical patients in Jimma University Specialized Teaching Hospital, South Western Ethiopia. BMC Surg. 2014;14:67.
2. Ip HY, Abrishami A, Peng PW, et al. Predictors of postoperative pain and analgesic consumption: a qualitative systematic review. Anesthesiology. 2009;111:657–77.
3. Clarke H, Kirkham KR, Orser BA, et al. Gabapentin reduces preoperative anxiety and pain catastrophizing in highly anxious patients prior to major surgery: a blinded randomized placebo-controlled trial. Can J Anaesth. 2013; 60:432–43.
4. Gibbons CH, Adler GK, Bonyhay I, et al. Experimental hypoglycemia is a human model of stress-induced hyperalgesia. Pain. 2012;153:2204–9.
5. Sun R, Zhao Z, Feng J, et al. Glucocorticoid-potentiated spinal microglia activation contributes to preoperative anxiety-induced postoperative Hyperalgesia. Mol Neurobiol. 2017;54:4316–28.
6. Prossnitz ER, Barton M. Estrogen biology: new insights into GPER function and clinical opportunities. Mol Cell Endocrinol. 2014;389:71–83.
7. Alvarez P, Bogen O, Levine JD. Role of nociceptor estrogen receptor GPR30 in a rat model of endometriosis pain. Pain. 2014;155:2680–6.
8. Mobbs D, Petrovic P, Marchant JL, et al. When fear is near: threat imminence elicits prefrontal-periaqueductal gray shifts in humans. Science. 2007;317:1079–83.
9. Ni HD, Yao M, Huang B, et al. Glial activation in the periaqueductal gray promotes descending facilitation of neuropathic pain through the p38 MAPK signaling pathway. J Neurosci Res. 2016;94:50–61.
10. Spary EJ, Chapman SE, Sinfield JK, et al. Novel G protein-coupled oestrogen receptor GPR30 shows changes in mRNA expression in the rat brain over the oestrous cycle. Neurosignals. 2013;21:14–27.

11. Kaushal R, Taylor BK, Jamal AB, et al. GABA-A receptor activity in the noradrenergic locus coeruleus drives trigeminal neuropathic pain in the rat; contribution of NAα1 receptors in the medial prefrontal cortex. Neuroscience. 2016;334:148–59.
12. Gulinello M, Gong QH, Li X, et al. Short-term exposure to a neuroactive steroid increases alpha4 GABA(a) receptor subunit levels in association with increased anxiety in the female rat. Brain Res. 2001;910:55–66.
13. Tian Z, Wang Y, Zhang N, et al. Estrogen receptor GPR30 exerts anxiolytic effects by maintaining the balance between GABAergic and glutamatergic transmission in the basolateral amygdala of ovariectomized mice after stress. Psychoneuroendocrinology. 2013;38:2218–33.
14. Devall AJ, Lovick TA. Differential activation of the periaqueductal gray by mild anxiogenic stress at different stages of the estrous cycle in female rats. Neuropsychopharmacology. 2010;35:1174–85.
15. Liu Y, Hou B, Zhang W, et al. The activation of spinal astrocytes contributes to preoperative anxiety-induced persistent post-operative pain in a rat model of incisional pain. Eur J Pain. 2015;19:733–40.
16. Zimmermann M. Ethical guidelines for investigations of experimental pain in conscious animals. Pain. 1983;16:109–10.
17. Xu HL, Vetri F, Lee HK, et al. Estrogen replacement therapy in diabetic ovariectomized female rats potentiates postischemic leukocyte adhesion in cerebral venules via a RAGE-related process. Am J Physiol Heart Circ Physiol. 2009;297:H2059–67.
18. Xu HL, Baughman VL, Pelligrino DA. Estrogen replacement treatment in diabetic ovariectomized female rats potentiates postischemic leukocyte adhesion in cerebral venules. Stroke. 2004;35:1974–8.
19. Liberzon I, Krstov M, Young EA. Stress-restress: effects on ACTH and fast feedback. Psychoneuroendocrinology. 1997;22:443–53.
20. Brennan TJ, Vandermeulen EP, Gebhart GF. Characterization of a rat model of incisional pain. Pain. 1996;64:493–501.
21. Chaplan SR, Bach FW, Pogrel JW, et al. Quantitative assessment of tactile allodynia in the rat paw. J Neurosci Methods. 1994;53:55–63.
22. Harden RN, Bruehl S, Stanos S, et al. Prospective examination of pain-related and psychological predictors of CRPS-like phenomena following total knee arthroplasty: a preliminary study. Pain. 2003;106:393–400.
23. Behbehani MM. Functional characteristics of the midbrain periaqueductal gray. Prog Neurobiol. 1995;46:575–605.
24. Floyd NS, Price JL, Ferry AT, et al. Orbitomedial prefrontal cortical projections to distinct longitudinal columns of the periaqueductal gray in the rat. J Comp Neurol. 2000;422:556–78.
25. Devall AJ, Santos JM, Lovick TA. Estrous cycle stage influences on neuronal responsiveness to repeated anxiogenic stress in female rats. Behav Brain Res. 2011;225:334–40.
26. Norman GJ, Karelina K, Zhang N, et al. Stress and IL-1beta contribute to the development of depressive-like behavior following peripheral nerve injury. Mol Psychiatry. 2010;15:404–14.
27. Prossnitz ER, Oprea TI, Sklar LA, et al. The ins and outs of GPR30: a transmembrane estrogen receptor. J Steroid Biochem Mol Biol. 2008;109: 350–3.
28. Hazell GG, Yao ST, Roper JA, et al. Localisation of GPR30, a novel G protein-coupled oestrogen receptor, suggests multiple functions in rodent brain and peripheral tissues. J Endocrinol. 2009;20:223–36.
29. Kuhn J, Dina OA, Goswami C, et al. GPR30 estrogen receptor agonists induce mechanical hyperalgesia in the rat. Eur J Neurosci. 2008;27:1700–9.
30. Filardo EJ, Thomas P. Minireview: G protein-coupled estrogen receptor-1, GPER-1: its mechanism of action and role in female reproductive cancer, renal and vascular physiology. Endocrinology. 2012;153:2953–62.
31. Filardo EJ, Quinn JA, Frackelton AR, et al. Estrogen action via the G protein-coupled receptor, GPR30: stimulation of adenylyl cyclase and cAMP-mediated attenuation of the epidermal growth factor receptor-to-MAPK signaling axis. Mol Endocrinol. 2002;16:70–84.
32. Thomas P, Dong J. Binding and activation of the seven-transmembrane estrogen receptor GPR30 by environmental estrogens: a potential novel mechanism of endocrine disruption. J Steroid Biochem Mol Biol. 2006;102: 175–9.
33. Farrant M, Nusser Z. Variations on an inhibitory theme: phasic and tonic activation of GABA(a) receptors. Nat Rev Neurosci. 2005;6:215–29.
34. Morgan MM, Whittier KL, Hegarty DM, et al. Periaqueductal gray neurons project to spinally projecting GABAergic neurons in the rostral ventromedial medulla. Pain. 2008;140:376–86.
35. Bee LA, Dickenson AH. Descending facilitation from the brainstem determines behavioural and neuronal hypersensitivity following nerve injury and efficacy of pregabalin. Pain. 2008;140:209–23.
36. Bohnsack JP, Carlson SL, Morrow AL. Differential regulation of synaptic and extrasynaptic α4 GABA(a) receptor populations by protein kinase a and protein kinase C in cultured cortical neurons. Neuropharmacology. 2016;105: 124–32.
37. Carlson SL, Bohnsack JP, Patel V, et al. Regulation of Extrasynaptic GABAA α4 receptors by ethanol-induced protein kinase a, but not protein kinase C activation in cultured rat cerebral cortical neurons. J Pharmacol Exp Ther. 2016;356:148–56.
38. Pan B, Lian J, Huang XF, et al. Aripiprazole increases the PKA Signalling and expression of the GABAA receptor and CREB1 in the nucleus Accumbens of rats. J Mol Neurosci. 2016;59:36–47.

11

Dexmedetomidine versus midazolam on cough and recovery quality after partial and total laryngectomy

Rui Xu[1†], Yun Zhu[2†], Yi Lu[1], Wenxian Li[1*] and Jie Jia[1*]

Abstract

Background: During emergence from anesthesia after partial and total laryngectomy, excessive airway reflex and systemic hypertension may lead to subcutaneous emphysema, hemorrhage or pneumothorax.

Methods: American Society of Anesthesiologist physical status III and IV male adults undergoing elective laryngectomy were recruited and randomly allocated to receive either dexmedetomidine (group D) or midazolam (group M). The primary outcome was incidence and severity of cough. Pulse oximetry results (SpO_2), heart rate (HR), systolic blood pressure (SBP), and diastolic blood pressure (DBP) were also recorded. The visual analog scale and the Ramsay sedation scale were recorded at the points of wakefulness and departure from the post-anesthesia care unit (PACU). Rescue analgesia consumption, the time of spontaneous breath recovery, duration of the PACU stay, and the incidence of adverse effects were also recorded.

Results: The prevalence of no coughing was significantly higher in group D than in group M at the points of wakefulness and departure. HR, SBP, and DBP were significantly lower in group D compared with group M, and SpO_2 was significantly higher in group D than in group M at the moment of laryngectomy. Pain scores were lower in group D than in group M. The Ramsay score at the point of wakefulness was higher in group D than in group M. There was no difference in time to spontaneous breathing recovery, duration of the PACU stay, and incidence of adverse effects.

Conclusions: Compared with midazolam, dexmedetomidine is an effective alternative to attenuate coughing and hemodynamic changes with a low incidence of adverse events during emergence from anesthesia after partial and total laryngectomy.

Keywords: Dexmedetomidine, Midazolam, Recovery quality, Laryngectomy

* Correspondence: liwenxian@eentanesthesia.com; jiajie@eentanesthesia.com
†Rui Xu and Yun Zhu contributed equally to this study and share first authorship.
[1]Department of Anesthesiology, The Eye, Ear, Nose and Throat Hospital of Fudan University, Shanghai Medical College of Fudan University, Fenyang Road #83, Shanghai 200031, People's Republic of China

Background

Laryngeal carcinoma is one of the most common malignant tumors worldwide and usually requires head and neck surgery [1, 2]. A study by the International Agency for Research on Cancer reported 177,422 new laryngeal cancer cases and 74,771 cancer-related deaths in 2018 [3]. The treatment of laryngeal carcinoma has largely improved in recent years [4]. Partial and total laryngectomy is considered to be the most effective method, except for early-stage laryngeal carcinoma.

After surgery, air no longer passes through the upper respiratory tract, and without warming, humidifying, and filtering, air directly causes irritation of the trachea-bronchial mucosa. A tracheostomy tube is also a strong stimulus to the tracheal mucosa. Coughing can lead to subcutaneous emphysema, pneumothorax, surgical bleeding, and lung intercostal hernia [5]. Therefore, minimal coughing and smooth emergence should be achieved.

Dexmedetomidine is a highly selective α_2 adrenoceptor agonist. Several studies have reported that dexmedetomidine may improve sympathetic tone, sedation, and analgesia without respiratory inhibition [6, 7]. To the best of our knowledge, there has been no study comparing recovery profiles between dexmedetomidine and midazolam after partial and total laryngectomy. Although the main drugs studied in our research are not commonly utilized during anesthesia for head and neck procedures, patients with tracheotomy after laryngeal carcinoma operation were chosen because of the strong discomfort and restlessness caused by the tracheotomy cannula, which is, however, guaranteed to keep the airway completely open. The aim of our study was to compare the effects of dexmedetomidine and midazolam on hemodynamics and recovery after partial and total laryngectomy.

Methods

Study design

This study was approved by the Ethics Committee of the Eye, Ear, Nose, and Throat Hospital of Fudan University, Shanghai, China (2013005). Written informed consent was obtained from all subjects participating in the trial. This prospective, randomized, double-blind, single-center clinical trial was registered prior to patient enrollment at clinicaltrials.gov (NCT03918889, principal investigator: Rui Xu, date of registration: March 28, 2019) and performed at the Department of Anesthesiology in the Eye, Ear, Nose, and Throat Hospital of Fudan University. All procedures adhered to the applicable CONSORT guidelines (Fig. 1).

Patients were randomly allocated to either the dexmedetomidine group (group D) ($n = 43$) or the midazolam group (group M) ($n = 43$). Randomized group allocation was performed using a computerized randomization table created by one staff member who was not involved in the patients' anesthesia or recovery care. The randomization result was kept sealed in an envelope; only the nurse who prepared the anesthetics could open the envelope in order to prepare the allocated drug. A total of 83 medical records were analyzed, 43 from group D and 40 from group M. The patients, the nurse in the post-anesthesia care unit (PACU), and attending anesthesiologists were blinded to the medicine administration.

Inclusion criteria

We enrolled 86 adult male patients with American Society of Anesthesiologist physical status III or IV, aged 25–70 years, scheduled for partial or total laryngectomy.

Exclusion criteria

Patients with cardiac disease, neuropsychiatric diseases, pharyngeal paraganglioma, or uncontrolled hypertension (i.e., systolic blood pressure > 160 mmHg or diastolic blood pressure > 90 mmHg), taking β-adrenoreceptor blockers, with long-term (> 6 months) abuse of alcohol, taking opioids or sedative-hypnotic drugs, with dexmedetomidine or midazolam allergies, undergoing awake fiberoptic intubation, with operation times shorter than 1 h or longer than 4 h, or with a tracheotomy history were excluded.

Anesthesia

Drugs, including sedative, analgesic, anti-emetic, and anti-itching drugs, were not given before an operation. After arrival at the operation room, the electrocardiogram, SpO_2 levels, blood pressure, the bispectral index, end-tidal carbon dioxide levels, and temperature were continuously monitored and recorded. General anesthesia was induced with sufentanil (0.2 µg/kg) and propofol (2.5 mg/kg), and after confirmation of adequate muscle relaxation with the administration of cisatracurium (0.2 mg/kg) iv, an endotracheal tube with an internal diameter of 7 mm was inserted into the trachea. Endotracheal tube cuff pressure was maintained at 25 cmH_2O measured using a calibrated handheld Portex Cuff Inflator Pressure Gauge (Portex Limited, Hythe, Kent, UK). Prior to the start of surgery, sufentanil (0.1 µg/kg) was given. Either dexmedetomidine (Precedex; Henrui Pharmaceutical, China) (group D, $n = 43$) infusion (0.5 µg/kg 10 min before tracheotomy, then adjusted to 0.3 µg/kg/h) or midazolam (Midazuolun injection; Enhua Pharmaceutical, China) (group M, $n = 43$) infusion (0.05 mg/kg 10 min before tracheotomy, then adjusted to 0.02 mg/kg′h) was administered in a blind mode. Anesthesia was maintained with a minimum alveolar end-tidal concentration of sevoflurane of 1–1.3 in

30% oxygen/air mixture to keep the bispectral index between 45 and 55. The maintenance infusion rate of cisatracurium was 1–1.5 μg/kg/min and the maintenance infusion rate of sufentanil was 0.002 μg/kg/min according to clinical needs. Granisetron (6 mg) was administered at the end of surgery to prevent post-operative nausea and vomiting (PONV). Endotracheal secretions were removed before tracheostomy tube insertion. Topical tetracaine hydrochloride gel was applied to the tracheostomy tube to enhance toleration.

After surgical procedures were finished, sevoflurane administration was discontinued, 100% oxygen was administered at 6 l/min, and patients were transferred to the PACU. Neostigmine (0.04 mg/kg) and atropine (0.02 mg/kg) were given to reverse residual neuromuscular block. After spontaneous ventilation returned, patients were considered to have fully recovered from muscle relaxation, and after patients opened their eyes, they were weaned from mechanical ventilation. Nurses who assessed subjects were blinded to the medicine intervention. If there was any adverse event, an attending anesthesiologist managed it. In the case of bradycardia (heart rate [HR] < 45 beats/min), 0.5 mg atropine was administered, and if systolic blood pressure (SBP) decreased to less than 90 mmHg, ephedrine (6 mg) was used.

Cough grading was based on a modified 4-point Minogue scale: grade 1, no cough; grade 2 (mild), coughing once or twice; grade 3 (moderate), fewer than 4 non-sustained coughs lasting 1–2 s each or overall coughing lasting less than 5 s; grade 4 (severe), at least 4 coughs lasting at least 2 s, or overall coughing duration more than 5 s [8]. Patients with grades 3 and 4 were categorized as "moderate to severe." The patients' levels of sedation were assessed by the Ramsay sedation scale (RSS): 1, the patient is anxious and restless or agitated, or both; 2, the patient is cooperative, tranquil, and oriented; 3, the patient responds to commands only; 4, the patient exhibits a brisk response to loud auditory stimuli or a light glabellar tap; 5, the patient exhibits a sluggish response to a loud auditory stimulus or a light glabellar tap; 6, the patient exhibits no response [9]. In addition, the nurse also assessed the post-operative pain score by a visual analog scale (VAS) (on a scale from 0 to 10, where 0 is no pain, and 10 is very much pain). If the pain score was above 5, sufentanil (0.1 μg/kg) was given to patients immediately as rescue analgesic; consumption of analgesics was recorded.

HR, SBP, diastolic blood pressure (DBP), and pulse oximetry results (SpO_2) were recorded before induction (T_1), after drug administration (T_2), after intubation (T_3), after medicine intervention (T_4), at the moment of laryngectomy (T_5), after completion of surgery (T_6), at the point of awareness (T_7), at departure from the PACU (T_8), 2 h after surgery (T_9), 24 h after surgery (T_{10}), and 48 h after surgery (T_{11}). Duration of surgery, respiratory recovery time, and duration of PACU stay were also recorded. The incidence of adverse events, including bradycardia, hypotension (< 30% decrease from baseline), hypertension (> 30% increase from baseline), vomiting, pale lips, delirium, subcutaneous emphysema, and hematoma, was noted by a nurse who was blinded to medicine intervention. The incidence of pneumonia 72 h after surgery was also recorded.

Statistical analysis

The primary endpoint was incidence and severity of cough. The secondary outcome measures were hemodynamic responses, post-operative pain scores, sedation scores, respiratory recovery time, duration of PACU stay, and incidence of adverse events.

PASS15 was used to calculate the sample size. On the basis of a preliminary study, the incidence of no cough in group M was about 65%, and in group D it was about 25% higher than in group M. The proportion in group D was assumed to be 0.65 under the null hypothesis and 0.90 under the alternative hypothesis. The proportion in group M was taken as 0.65. The test statistic used is the one-sided Z-test with unpooled variance. The significance level of the test is 0.025. Group sample sizes of 40 in group D and 40 in group M achieve 80% power to detect a difference between the group proportions of 0.25. Assuming a dropout rate of 8%, the final sample size was determined to be 43 patients per group, with a power of 80% and an alpha level of 0.05.

Student's t test was used for between-group comparisons of HR, SBP, DBP, and SpO_2. Repeated-measures ANOVA was used for within-group comparisons. The χ^2 test or the Fisher exact test was used to analyze coughing severity, sedation, pain scores, and adverse events. A P-value of 0.05 or less was considered statistically significant.

Results

Baseline characteristics

The incidence and severity of coughing

The prevalence of no coughing was significantly higher in group D than in group M, while patients were at the points of wakefulness (88% [38] vs. 65% [26], $P = 0.018$) and departure (100% [40] vs. 65% [28], $P = 0.009$) (Table 1). No patient in group D and 3 patients in group M experienced severe coughing. The incidence of mild cough was significantly lower in group D than in group M (14% [6] vs. 40% [16] of patients, $P = 0.015$). The incidence of "moderate to severe" cough was significantly higher in group M than in group D (5% [2] vs. 40% [16] of patients, $P = 0.012$).

Table 1 The incidence and severity of coughing in PACU

	No Cough		Mild Cough		Moderate Cough		Severe Cough	
	Awake	Departure	Awake	Departure	Awake	Departure	Awake	Departure
Group D	38*	40**	3	3	2&	0	0	0
Group M	26	28	7	9	5	2	2	1

*$p = 0.018$ vs Group M (awake)
**$p = 0.009$ vs Group M (departure)
Moderate+Severe, &$p = 0.012$ vs Group M

Perioperative hemodynamic changes

In group M, HR at T_3, T_4, T_5, T_6, and T_7 was significantly higher/lower than in group D. HR in group M was significantly higher at the moment of intubation and at the moment of laryngectomy compared with values before anesthesia (Fig. 2a).

As shown in Fig. 2b and c, SBP (131.98 vs. 120.33, $P = 0.005$) and DBP (82.88 vs. 76.98, $P = 0.042$) were significantly higher in group M than in group D at the moment of laryngectomy. Compared with pre-anesthesia values, SBP was significantly lower at other moments ($P < 0.01$) in group D. In group M, compared with pre-induction values, SBP was significantly lower at T_2, T_3, T_4, T_5, and T_6 ($P < 0.01$), but was not significantly different at the points of wakefulness and departure from the PACU ($P > 0.05$).

SpO_2 was significantly higher in group D than in group M at the moment of laryngectomy (97.77 vs. 96.60, $P = 0.040$). However, at 2 h post-surgery, SpO_2 was significantly higher in group M than in group D (96.14 vs. 97.03, $P = 0.041$) (Fig. 2d). Desaturation ($SpO_2 < 92\%$) was observed in 5 patients in group M and no patient in group D at the point of laryngectomy ($P = 0.029$) (Supplemental Table 2). The overall incidence of desaturation was lower in group D than in group M (20 [47%] vs. 29 [72%], $P = 0.029$) (Supplemental Table 2).

There was no significant difference in time to respiratory recovery and duration of PACU stay between the two groups (Table 2). As shown in Table 3, RSS at wakefulness in the PACU was higher in group D than in group M (1.98 vs. 1.80, $P = 0.025$).

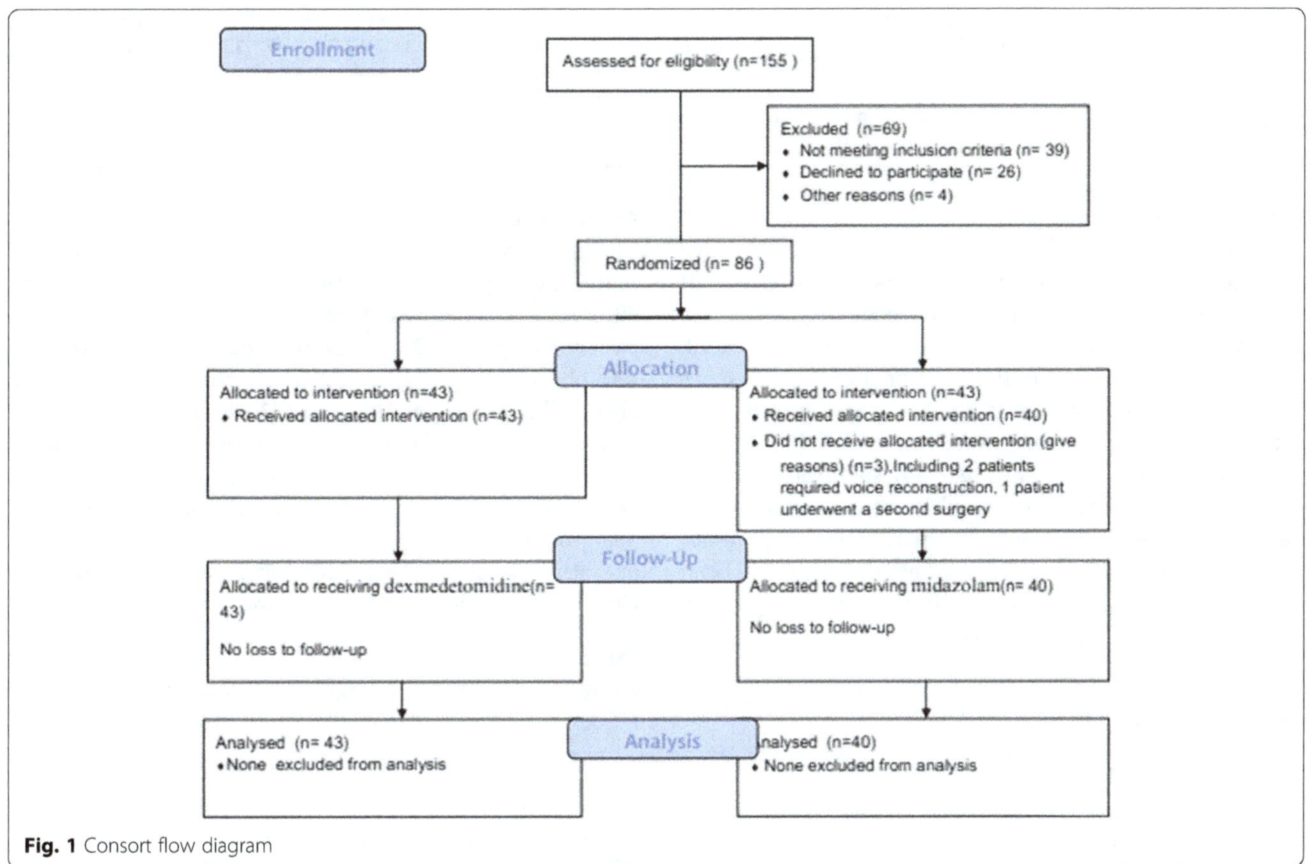

Fig. 1 Consort flow diagram

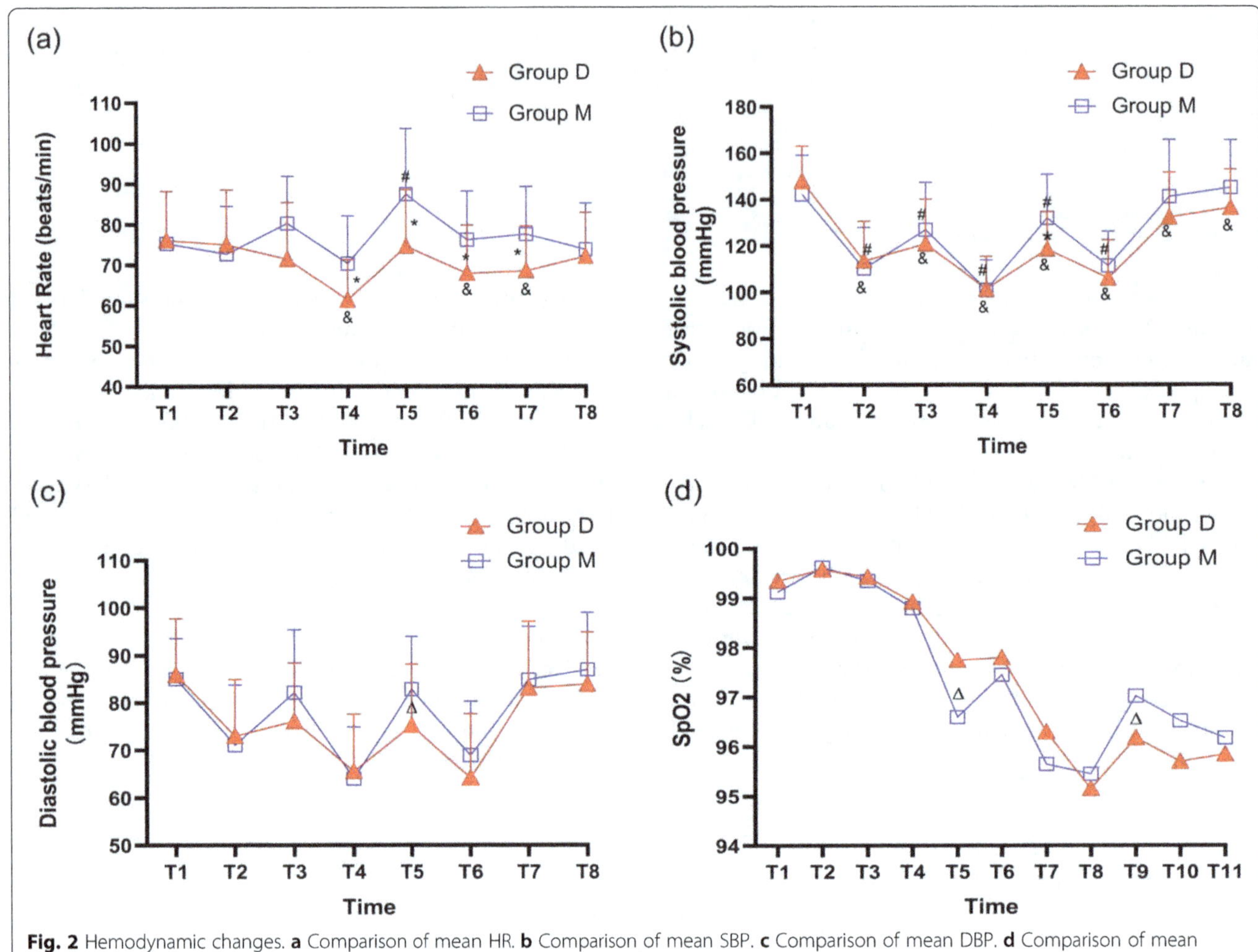

Fig. 2 Hemodynamic changes. **a** Comparison of mean HR. **b** Comparison of mean SBP. **c** Comparison of mean DBP. **d** Comparison of mean SpO_2. $^*P < 0.01$; $^{\&}P < 0.01$ group D versus T_1; $^{\#}P < 0.01$ group M versus T_1; $^{\Delta}P < 0.05$

Post-operative pain score

We observed no significant difference in post-operative pain scores between the two groups at the point of wakefulness. The requirement for rescue analgesics was significantly lower in group D than in group M (4 vs. 13, $P = 0.013$) (Table 4). But the post-operative pain score was significantly lower in group D than in group M at the moment of departure from the PACU (*1.2* vs *2.0*, $p < 0.05$), the difference is statistically significant but not clinically significant, patient who suffer postoperative pain in the PACU has been given rescue analgesics to relieve the pain, the number of patients who has been given rescue analgesics was significantly higher in group M than in group D (*13* vs *4*, $p < 0.05$).

Table 2 Recovery Profiles

Time	Group D($n = 43$)	Group M($n = 40$)	P
Recovery time (min)	26.6 ± 12.1	28.5 ± 12.3	0.475
Awake time (min)	46.5 ± 16.0	46.2 ± 14.7	0.938

Values are mean ± SD or number

Adverse events

The incidence of postoperative complications are presented in supplemental Table 3. There was no significant difference between two groups. Vomiting was noted in 7 patients in group D and 12 in group M. Hypertension was observed in 1 patient in each group. Pale lips was observed in 2 patients in group D, severe bradycardia in 1 patient in group D, delirium was reported in 2 patients in group M, subcutaneous emphysema in 1 patient in group M, while re-exploration of operation site for hematoma was observed in 1 patient in group M. Post-operative pneumonia was noted in 1 patient in group M. During the operation, vasopressor was used in 18

Table 3 Ramsay score

Ramsay score(1/2/3)	Group D($n = 43$)	Group M($n = 40$)	P
Awake	1/42/0	8/32/0	0.025
Departure	1/42/0	1/39/0	1.00
2 h after surgery	0/43/0	1/38/1	0.332

Grade of sedation, 1 = anxious and restless or agitated, 2 = cooperative, tranquil, and oriented, 3 = responds to commands only

Table 4 Pain scores and postoperative requirement for rescue analgesics at PACU

	Group D($n = 43$)	Group M($n = 40$)	P
VAS score (T_7)	1.6 ± 1.6	2.0 ± 2.0	0.261
VAS score (T_8)	1.2 ± 0.9	2.0 ± 2.0	0.024
Rescue analgesics(n)	4	13	0.013

Values are mean ± SD or number

patients in group D and 11 in group M, there was no significant difference in between two groups (*18* vs *11*, $p = 0.249$).

Discussion

This study showed dexmedetomidine provided adequate and satisfactory coughing suppression, stable hemodynamics, and good recovery for patients undergoing partial and total laryngectomy.

Coughing after laryngectomy is always related to airway secretions or the presence of a tracheostomy tube; we therefore used suction to remove oral and airway secretions before tube insertion. We used topical tetracaine hydrochloride gel for the tracheostomy tube to reduce tube stimulation of the peripheral nervous system. The prevalence of no coughing was significantly higher in group D than in group M. No patient in group D experienced severe coughing. This result is consistent with a previous study, which showed that dexmedetomidine is effective in attenuating the airway reflex to tracheal extubation [10]. Several pharmacological agents have been reported to decrease coughing, including lidocaine and opioids. Recently, a systematic review has been sponsored/carried out to investigate optimal pharmacological methods for reducing coughing after general anesthesia [11]. Opioids such as remifentanil and fentanyl are commonly used to prevent cough, but opioids can produce undesirable adverse events, such as respiratory depression, delayed awakening, and PONV. In the present study, we observed no significant differences in time to respiratory recovery and duration of PACU stay between the two groups, but the post-operative pain score was significantly lower in group D than in group M at the moment of departure from the PACU, fewer patients were given rescue analgesics to relieve the pain, and dexmedetomidine did not appear to induce respiratory depression.

Blunting the cardiovascular response can decrease the incidence of complications. Compared with group M, there was a significant decrease in HR, SBP, and DBP at the moment of laryngectomy. We did not combine dexmedetomidine and remifentanil due to the possibility of delayed awakening [12]. Dexmedetomidine can reduce the release of norepinephrine, resulting in decreased catecholamine release from nerve endings and a resultant central sympatholytic effect, leading to decreases in HR and blood pressure [13]. However, dexmedetomidine also has some disadvantages, including inducing bradycardia and hypotension in old patients. Severe bradycardia was observed in 1 patient in group D. A vasopressor was used in 18 patients in group D and 11 patients in group M. Hypotension and bradycardia occurred more often with the initial dose in group D. Previous studies have reported that midazolam had no significant effects on sympathetic tone but slightly decreased blood pressure for about 10 min due to decreased systemic vascular resistance and myocardial contractility [14, 15]. We speculated that a lower dose of dexmedetomidine may be more appropriate to elderly patients. SpO_2 levels were significantly higher in group D than in group M at the moment of laryngectomy. This may be attributed to decreased HR-induced lower oxygen consumption. Animal experiments have shown that dexmedetomidine preconditioning exerts cardioprotective effects against hypoxia injury and can improve peri-operative hypoxemia [16, 17].

Emergence agitation can result in cardiovascular instability, decreased venous return and increased intracranial pressure, decreased functional residual capacity, wound dehiscence, and hemorrhage [18]. Midazolam is an effective sedative anxiolytic that provides anterograde amnesia. But it has been reported that there is a high risk of drug accumulation and delirium when using midazolam in patients with liver dysfunction [19]. In our research, delirium was observed in 2 patients in group M, but this was relieved within 24 h. We found satisfactory sedation with dexmedetomidine. Dexmedetomidine exhibits a high specificity for α_2 vs. α_1 receptors [20], producing unique sedative effects similar to normal sleep. Dexmedetomidine has been reported to be used for long-term sedation during mechanical ventilation in critically ill patients at the intensive care unit and for decreasing patient agitation in the PACU [21]. Our results also confirmed that dexmedetomidine may be an effective agent for sedation in partial and total laryngectomy.

Partial and total laryngectomy is associated with a high level of pain [22]. Our results show that the postoperative pain scores and the requirement for rescue analgesics were significantly lower in group D than in group M. However, the analgesic efficacy of dexmedetomidine is still controversial [23], and the analgesic mechanism of dexmedetomidine remains to be further studied.

Although there were more adverse events in group M compared with group D, this difference was not statistically significant. Insertion of a stomach tube is also a risk factor of PONV, but all patients retained the stomach tube in our study. Patients who breathe via a tracheostomy tube cannot make use of their glottis [24].

Preservation of the cough reflex is mandatory to prevent pulmonary complications [25]. No patient developed pneumonia in group D. The finding that the prevalence of post-operative pneumonia did not differ between the two groups suggests that dexmedetomidine is not associated with post-operative pulmonary infections.

There were several limitations to the present study. The major limitation was that we investigated only one dose of dexmedetomidine. Second, the sample size was relatively small, so future multicenter studies comprising larger sample sizes are needed. Third, we did not include patients with bilateral cervical lymph node dissection, since the wounds are always larger, so our results are not generalizable to these patients. Fourth, we did not include patients older than 70, while in Europe and North America, approximately 30% of all head and neck cancer patients are aged over 70 years [26]. Finally, there were potential sources of heterogeneity, including the fitness of the patient's trachea and tracheostomy tube and the fact that surgery was performed by different surgeons.

Conclusions

In conclusion, intra-operative infusion of dexmedetomidine has advantages, including blunting the airway reflex, good sedation, stable hemodynamics, and a low risk of adverse events. Dexmedetomidine improved the outcome, alleviated patient discomfort caused by the tracheostomy tube, and allowed for a smooth emergence from anesthesia.

Supplementary information

Additional file 1: Table S1. Demographics and baseline variables of patients in the two groups.

Additional file 2: Table S2. Oxygen desaturation (SpO2 < 92%).

Additional file 3: Table S3. Incidence of drug-related adverse events.

Abbreviations

group D: Group dexmedetomidine; group M: Group midazolam; PACU: Postanesthesia care unit; SpO_2: Pulse oximetry; HR: Heart rate; SBP: Systolic blood pressure; DBP: Diastolic blood pressure; VAS: Visual Analogue Scale; RSS: Ramsay sedation scale; ASA: American Society of Anesthesiologist physical status; PONV: Postoperative nausea and vomiting

Acknowledgements

Not applicable.

Authors' contributions

RX helped to design the study, conduct the study, analyze the data, and write the manuscript. YZ helped to design the study, conduct the study, analyze the data. YL helped to design the study, conduct the study, analyze the data, and write the manuscript. LWX designed the study, analyzed the data, and wrote the manuscript. JJE designed the study, conducted the study, and analyzed the data. All authors have read and approved the manuscript.

Author details

[1]Department of Anesthesiology, The Eye, Ear, Nose and Throat Hospital of Fudan University, Shanghai Medical College of Fudan University, Fenyang Road #83, Shanghai 200031, People's Republic of China. [2]Department of Oro-maxillofacial Head and Neck Oncology, Shanghai Ninth People's Hospital, Shanghai Jiao Tong University School of Medicine, Shanghai Key Laboratory of Stomatology, Shanghai, China.

References

1. Vokes EE, Weichselbaum RR, Lippman SM, Hong WK. Head and neck cancer. N Engl J Med. 1993;328:184–94.
2. Zhi L, Wenli W, Pengfei G, Pengcheng C, Wenxian C, Jiasheng L, et al. Laryngotracheal reconstruction with autogenous rib cartilage graft for complex laryngotracheal stenosis and/or anterior neck defect. Eur Arch Otorhinolaryngol. 2014;271:317–22.
3. Bray F, Ferlay J, Soerjomataram I, Siegel RL, Torre LA, Jemal A. Global cancer statistics 2018: GLOBOCAN estimates of incidence and mortality worldwide for 36 cancers in 185 countries. CA Cancer J Clin. 2018;68:394–424.
4. Liu C, Liu H, Wen Y, Huang H, Hao J, Lv Y, et al. Aspernolide A Inhibits the Proliferation of Human Laryngeal Carcinoma Cells through the Mitochondrial Apoptotic and STAT3 Signaling Pathways. Molecules. 2019; 19(24):1074.
5. Kosałka J, Wawrzycka-Adamczyk K, Jurkiewicz P, Pawlik W, Milewski M, Musiał J. Cough-induced lung intercostal hernia. Pneumonol Alergol Pol. 2016;84:119–20.
6. Guler G, Akin A, Tosun Z, Ors S, Esmaoglu A, Boyaci A. Single-dose dexmedetomidine reduces agitation and provides smooth extubation after pediatric adenotonsillectomy. Paediatr Anaesth. 2005;15:762–6.
7. Kim H, Min KT, Lee JR, Ha SH, Lee WK, Seo JH, et al. Comparison of Dexmedetomidine and Remifentanil on airway reflex and hemodynamic changes during recovery after craniotomy. Yonsei Med J. 2016;57:980–6.
8. Reza M, Hasani V, Bagheri-aghdam A, Zamani MM, Pournajafian A, Rokhtabnak F, et al. Remifentanil infusion during emergence moderates hemodynamic and cough responses to the tracheal tube: a randomized controlled trial. J Clin Anesth. 2016;33:514–20.
9. Ramsay MA, Savege TM, Simpson BR, Goodwin R. Controlled sedation with alphaxalone-alphadolone. Br Med J. 1974;2:656–9.
10. Aksu R, Akin A, Biçer C, Esmaoğlu A, Tosun Z, Boyaci A. Comparison of the effects of dexmedetomidine versus fentanyl on airway reflexes and hemodynamic responses to tracheal extubation during rhinoplasty: a double-blind, randomized, controlled study. Curr Ther Res Clin Exp. 2009;70: 209–20.
11. Tung A, Fergusson NA, Ng N, Hu V, Dormuth C, Griesdale DGE. Pharmacological methods for reducing coughing on emergence from elective surgery after general anesthesia with endotracheal intubation: protocol for a systematic review of common medications and network meta-analysis. Syst Rev. 2019;8:32.
12. Lee JS, Choi SH, Kang YR, Kim Y, Shim YH. Efficacy of a single dose of dexmedetomidine for cough suppression during anesthetic emergence: a randomized controlled trial. Can J Anaesth. 2015;62:392–8.
13. Tobis JD. Dexmedetomidine: applications in pediatric critical care and pediatric anesthesiology. Pediatr Crit Care Med. 2007;8:111–31.
14. Liu X, Rabin PL, Yuan Y, Kumar A, Vasallo P, Wong J, et al. Effects of anesthetic and sedative agents on sympathetic nerve activity. Heart Rhythm. 2019;16:1875–82.
15. Watanabe Y, Higuchi H, Ishii-Maru M, Honda Y, Yabuki-Kawase A, Yamane-Hirano A, et al. Effect of a low dose of midazolam on high blood pressure in dental patients: a randomised, double-blind, placebo-controlled, two-center study. Br J Oral Maxillofac Surg. 2016;54:443–8.
16. Gao JM, Meng XW, Zhang J, Chen WR, Xia F, Peng K, et al. Dexmedetomidine protects Cardiomyocytes against hypoxia/Reoxygenation injury by suppressing TLR4-MyD88-NF-κB signaling. Biomed Res Int. 2017; 2017:1674613.
17. Chen Q, Wu W, Zhang GC, Cao H, Chen LW, Hu YN, et al. Dexmedetomidine attenuates hypoxemia during palliative reconstruction of the right ventricular outflow tract in pediatric patients. Medicine (Baltimore). 2014;93:e69.
18. Miller KA, Harkin CP, Bailey PL. Postoperative tracheal extubation. Anesth Analg. 1995;80:149–72.
19. Patel SB, Kress JP. Sedation and analgesia in the mechanically ventilated patient. Am J Respir Crit Care Med. 2012;185:486–97.

20. Tobias JD. Dexmedetomidine: applications in pediatric critical care and pediatric anesthesiology. Pediatr Crit Care Med. 2007;8:115–31.
21. Fraser GL, Devlin JW, Worby CP, Alhazzani W, Barr J, Dasta JF, et al. Benzodiazepine versus nonbenzodiazepine-based sedation for mechanically ventilated, critically ill adults: a systematic review and meta-analysis of randomized trials. Crit Care Med. 2013;41:S30–8.
22. Mom T, Bazin JE, Commun F, Dubray C, Eschalier A, Derbal C, et al. Assessment of postoperative pain after laryngeal surgery for cancer. Arch Otolaryngol Head Neck Surg. 1998;124:794–8.
23. Lee S. Dexmedetomidine: present and future directions. Korean J Anesthesiol. 2019;72:323–30.
24. Kowalski S, Macaulay K, Thorkelsson R, Girling L, Bshouty Z. Assessment of cough strength in patients with a tracheostomy. Can J Anaesth. 2017;64: 1284–5.
25. Di Santo D, Bondi S, Giordano L, Galli A, Tulli M, Ramella B, et al. Long-term swallowing function, pulmonary complications, and quality of life after Supracricoid Laryngectomy. Otolaryngol Head Neck Surg. 2019;12: 194599819835189.
26. Porceddu SV, Haddad RI. Management of elderly patients with locoregionally confined head and neck cancer. Lancet Oncol. 2017;18:e274–83.

12

Intranasal dexmedetomidine is an effective sedative agent for electroencephalography in children

Hang Chen, Fei Yang, Mao Ye, Hui Liu, Jing Zhang, Qin Tian, Ruiqi Liu, Qing Yu, Shangyingying Li and Shengfen Tu*

Abstract

Background: Intranasal dexmedetomidine (DEX), as a novel sedation method, has been used in many clinical examinations of infants and children. However, the safety and efficacy of this method for electroencephalography (EEG) in children is limited. In this study, we performed a large-scale clinical case analysis of patients who received this sedation method. The purpose of this study was to evaluate the safety and efficacy of intranasal DEX for sedation in children during EEG.

Methods: This was a retrospective study. The inclusion criteria were children who underwent EEG from October 2016 to October 2018 at the Children's Hospital affiliated with Chongqing Medical University. All the children received 2.5 $\mu g \cdot kg^{-1}$ of intranasal DEX for sedation during the procedure. We used the Modified Observer Assessment of Alertness/Sedation Scale (MOAA/S) and the Modified Aldrete score (MAS) to evaluate the effects of the treatment on sedation and resuscitation. The sex, age, weight, American Society of Anesthesiologists physical status (ASAPS), vital signs, sedation onset and recovery times, sedation success rate, and adverse patient events were recorded.

Results: A total of 3475 cases were collected and analysed in this study. The success rate of the initial dose was 87.0% (3024/3475 cases), and the success rate of intranasal sedation rescue was 60.8% (274/451 cases). The median sedation onset time was 19 mins (IQR: 17–22 min), and the sedation recovery time was 41 mins (IQR: 36–47 min). The total incidence of adverse events was 0.95% (33/3475 cases), and no serious adverse events occurred.

Conclusions: Intranasal DEX (2.5 $\mu g \cdot kg^{-1}$) can be safely and effectively used for EEG sedation in children.

Keywords: Children, Electroencephalography, Intranasal dexmedetomidine, Sedation

Background

Electroencephalography (EEG) is an important tool for the clinical diagnosis of epilepsy, mental disorders, intracranial tumours and other nervous system diseases. However, for children who have difficulty falling asleep due to a lack of cooperation or anxiety before the examination, a satisfactory form of sedation can make the examination process more efficient and comfortable [1].

Many sedative drugs have been used for paediatric sedation in the past, but the use of many sedative drugs for EEG is controversial. For example, ketamine, propofol and sevoflurane can affect brain waves, which may lead to an incorrect diagnosis based on an EEG. Midazolam and chloral hydrate have been used in the past but have some shortcomings with regard to safety and sedative efficacy, respectively [2].

* Correspondence: 595494227@qq.com
Department of Anesthesiology, Children's Hospital of Chongqing Medical University, No.136 Zhongshan 2nd Road, Yuzhong District, Chongqing, People's Republic of China

Dexmedetomidine (DEX) is a highly selective alpha-2 adrenergic receptor agonist that mainly acts on the alpha-2 receptor in the spinal cord and the nucleus of the locus coeruleus. DEX has little influence on haemodynamics or respiratory inhibition and has a short half-life [3, 4]. Previous studies have shown that DEX interferes little with the basic background waves of the brain; it slightly increases theta, alpha and beta activities but has no effect on the detection of an epileptic discharge [5, 6]. In addition, DEX produces a state similar to natural sleep, which can be reversed with conversation, enabling clinicians to assess a child's cognitive status after the completion of an EEG examination [7]. As animal studies have shown, drugs can be administered through the nasal cavity, which can effectively reduce first-pass elimination, and the drug can more efficiently enter the brain through the nervous olfactory system [8]. The overall bioavailability of DEX in children with intranasal administration was reported to be 84% [9]. The use of DEX alone in paediatric sedation provides adequate sedation [10, 11]. Thus, DEX is a sedative suitable for EEG, no comprehensive studies have been performed regarding the safety and effective dose of DEX. Evaluating the safety and efficacy of 2.5 $\mu g \cdot kg^{-1}$ intranasal DEX was the main objective of this study.

An increasing number of studies have reported the use of DEX in clinical practice. In children under deep sedation, failure to strictly meet the fasting requirement before anaesthesia did not lead to an increase in adverse events [12]. In contrast, prolonged fasting may cause anxiety in children, making them difficult to placate and leading to a reduction in sedation success rate [13].

The purpose of this study was to evaluate the safety and efficacy of intranasal DEX in paediatric EEG sedation and to provide a reference for clinical sedative use in paediatrics.

Methods

Patient population

This was a retrospective research study that was approved by the Ethics Committee of the Children's Hospital affiliated with Chongqing Medical University. Our study retrospectively analysed children who underwent EEG from October 2016 to October 2018 at our hospital. Patients were sedated with 2.5 $\mu g \cdot kg^{-1}$ intranasal DEX.

Sedation method

The inclusion criteria for this study were children who underwent EEG in our hospital who received 2.5 $\mu g \cdot kg^{-1}$ of intranasal DEX. Children were excluded when they met any of the following criteria: (1) A history of allergy to DEX, (2) difficult airway, (3) anatomical structural deformity of the nasal cavity, (4) severe liver or renal insufficiency and (5) severe bradycardia or atrioventricular block above II degree type 2.

Our standard sedation procedure was as follows. Children needed to fast for at least 1 h before sedation. An anaesthesiologist evaluated the patient's general condition, history of the present illness, previous medical history, surgical history, allergy history and sedative history. Then, the anaesthesiologist created an appropriate sedative plan, and an informed consent form was signed. The child was placed in a supine position and attended by a guardian, and a nurse administered a nasal drip of 2.5 $\mu g \cdot kg^{-1}$ DEX to the child. All the children remained lying flat for 1–2 min after the medicine was administered while we gently massaged the alae of the nose of the children to facilitate DEX absorption by the nasal mucosa. We used the Modified Observer Assessment of Alertness/Sedation Scale (MOAA/S) [14] (Table 1) to evaluate the children's sedation state. Successful sedation was defined as an MOAA/S score less than or equal to 3 within 30 mins after the first dose of DEX. If the MOAA/S score was greater than 3 within 30 min after the first dose of DEX, an additional 1 $\mu g \cdot kg^{-1}$ intranasal DEX was given as a "rescue" dose. If the EEG could still not be completed, inhaled sevoflurane were administered to allow the examination to be completed, which we defined as failed sedation. After drug administration, the anaesthesiologist not only assessed the child's sedation level but also recorded heart rate (HR), pulse oxygen saturation (SpO_2), and the occurrence of adverse events, which referred to postoperative nausea and vomiting (PONV), bradycardia, SpO_2 reduction, etc. The EEG was performed after successful sedation, while the attending physician used a portable monitor to track the patient's HR and SpO_2. We defined the onset time of sedation as the time from drug administration to successful sedation. Recovery time was defined as the time from successful sedation to recovery. After the examination, the children were sent back to the sedation recovery room for further observation. Patients were discharged upon attaining a Modified Aldrete score (MAS) [15] (Table 2)

Table 1 Modified Observer's Assessment of Alertness/Sedation Scale

Response	Score
Agitated	6
Responds readily to name spoken in normal tone	5
Lethargic response to name spoken in normal tone	4
Responds only after name is called loudly and repeatedly	3
Responds only after mild prodding or shaking	2
Does not respond to mild prodding or shaking	1
Does not respond to a deep stimulus	0

Table 2 Modified Aldrete score

Criterion	Score
Activity	
Move 4 extremities voluntarily or on command	2
Move 2 extremities voluntarily or on command	1
Unable to move extremities voluntarily or on command	0
Respiration	
Able to breathe deeply, cough, and/or cry	2
Dyspnoea or limited breathing	1
Apnoeic	0
Circulation	
Blood pressure ± 20 mmHg of preanaesthetic value	2
Blood pressure ± 21 to 49 mmHg of preanaesthetic value	1
Blood pressure ± 50 mmHg of preanaesthetic value	0
Consciousness	
Fully awake	2
Arousable on calling	1
Unresponsive	0
Oxygen saturation	
Able to maintain oxygen saturation > 92% on room air	2
Needs oxygen inhalation to maintain oxygen saturation > 90%	1
Oxygen saturation < 90% even with oxygen supplementation	0

of 9 or upon reaching the following states: (1) stable cardiovascular function and unobstructed respiratory tract; (2) awakened easily, with protective airway reflexes intact; (3) ability to communicate with others (age-appropriate assessment); (4) able to sit up unassisted (age-appropriate assessment); (5) for very small children or children with disabilities who were unable to exhibit the usual expected responses, a return to pre-sedation response levels or to as close to normal as possible; and (6) adequate hydration status.

Data collection

Sex, age, weight, American Society of Anesthesiologists physical status (ASAPS), vital signs, sedation onset and recovery times, success of sedation, adverse events, etc. were collected and recorded in Microsoft Excel 2010.

Adverse events and handling

Adverse events were classified as severe or minor, and the occurrences of adverse events was recorded. The serious adverse events were: (1) emergency airway intervention (the use of tracheal intubation or the placement of airway aids, such as oropharynx or larynx masks); (2) laryngospasm; (3) reflux aspiration; (4) severe arrhythmia; (5) respiratory and cardiac arrest. The minor adverse reaction events were as follows: (1) bradycardia, defined as a heart rate deceleration of greater than 20% of the normal age-adjusted rate during sedation and need drug intervention (treated with atropine intravenously); (2) a significant oxygen saturation decrease, defined as an SpO_2 of less than 90%; (3) upper respiratory tract obstruction (open airway; can be reversed with mask oxygen); (4) PONV (tilt the child's head to one side while removing vomit from the mouth); (5) recovery delay, defined as a sedation recovery time > 2 h; and (6) rash.

Statistical analysis

Quantitative data with a normal distribution are described with the mean ± standard deviation or median and interquartile ranges. Categorical variables are represented by a number, and the rate and 95% confidence interval (CI) were calculated. All clinical data were analysed using SPSS 17.0 for Windows (SPSS Inc., Chicago, IL, USA).

Results

Demographics and sedation characteristics

This study included 3475 cases of children who were examined by EEG from October 2016 to October 2018. There were 2229 (64.1%) males and 1246 (35.9%) females. The age of the children was 61.7 ± 38.9 months. The weight of the children was 19.5 ± 11.4 kg. In total, 1914 patients (55.1%) were assigned to ASAPS Class 1, 1523 patients (43.8%) were assigned to ASAPS Class 2 and 38 patients (1.1%) were assigned to ASAPS Class 3, as shown in Table 3.

Success rate of sedation

The success rate of the initial DEX dose was 87.0% (3024/3475 cases), and the success rate of intranasal sedation rescue was 60.8% (274/451 cases).

The time of sedation and examination

The median sedation onset time was 19 mins (IQR: 17–22 min), and the sedation recovery time was 41 mins (IQR: 36–47 min).

Table 3 Demographics and sedation characteristics

Characteristics	Value
N	3475
Sex (M/F)	2229 (64.1)/1246 (35.9)
Age (months)	61.7 ± 38.9
Weight (kg)	19.5 ± 11.4
ASAPS	
1	1914 (55.1)
2	1523 (43.8)
3	38 (1.1)
4	0 (0)

Age and weight are expressed as the mean ± standard deviation; the other data are expressed as numbers (%)

Adverse events

The total rate of adverse events in this study was 0.95% (33/3475 cases). Among the adverse events, no serious adverse events occurred. Among the minor adverse events, PONV was found in 20 cases (0.58, 95% CI: 0.3–0.8%); SpO_2 was reduced in 6 cases (0.17, 95% CI: 0–0.3%); upper respiratory tract obstruction was observed in 3 cases (0.09, 95% CI: 0–0. 2%); rash was observed in 2 cases (0.06, 95% CI: 0–0.1%); heart rate decreased by more than 20% of the normal age-adjustment and drug intervention was required in 1 case (0.03, 95% CI: 0–0.1%); and recovery delay occurred in 1 case (0.03, 95% CI: 0–0.1%), as shown in Table 4.

Discussion

In the past, many sedative drugs were used clinically for moderate and deep sedation during paediatric examinations, but EEG examination is unique. Many sedative drugs that act on the central nervous system interfere with brain waves. Some studies have shown that ketamine can selectively inhibit the thalamic neocortex system and activate the medulla oblongata and limbic system as well as indirectly excite the brain waves and increase the theta wave due to the "separation anaesthesia" effect of ketamine [16]. A small dose of propofol can increase beta waves, and a high dose of propofol increases the delta wave frequency due to the double action of propofol at different dosages [17]. Sevoflurane affects the number of slow delta and alpha waves [18]. The sedative drugs midazolam and chloral hydrate were used in the past; while they exhibited little interference with EEG, they had a long half-life, many side effects, high sedation failure rates and other undesirable characteristics [19, 20]. DEX has a good sedative effect when it is administered via intranasal administration or intravenous injection [21]. Additionally, DEX has been widely used for sedation before paediatric examinations [22]. Because DEX is a new sedative, its use in EEG procedures is limited. We summarized the experience of intranasal DEX in EEG, which can provide a reference for clinical practice.

In our study, the success rate of the initial dose of 2.5 $\mu g{\cdot}kg^{-1}$ DEX was 87.0% (3024/3475 cases). A recent study have found that 90% of the effective dose of intranasal DEX sedation was 3.28 $\mu g{\cdot}kg^{-1}$ in children [23]. Another study found that the 50% effective dose and the 95% effective dose of intranasal DEX increased with increasing age in patients under 3 years of age [24]. The success rate of sedation in our study was slightly lower than that in previous studies [11]. We believe the reason for this observation is that the age (61.7 ± 38.9 months) of the children in this study was higher than that in previous studies. Therefore, we speculate that when older children are sedated, the initial dose can be appropriately increased to improve the sedation success rate, but further research is needed to verify the safety and efficacy of this approach. Notably, Jenny Bua found DEX is an attractive and reliable sedative in preterm neonates undergoing MRI. We also hope to further study the safety of DEX in preterm neonates during EEG [25].

Table 4 Adverse events

Adverse events	N (%)	95% CI
PONV	20 (0.58)	0.30–0.80
Significant SpO_2 reduction	6 (0.17)	0–0.30
Upper airway obstruction	3 (0.09)	0–0.20
Rash	2 (0.06)	0–0.10
Bradycardia requiring drug intervention	1 (0.03)	0–0.10
Delayed awakening	1 (0.03)	0–0.10

In this study, no serious adverse events occurred in 3475 paediatric cases. In contrast to previous studies, there were no respiratory-related severe adverse events (such as laryngospasm and bronchospasm) while using intranasal DEX [26]. This result again confirms the safety of this sedation method.

The most common adverse event was PONV (0.58%), which resolves on its own after rest. Through the monitoring of vital signs after sedation, we found that DEX can slow the heart rate of children [27]. Therefore, we speculate that because of the specific physiology of children, the heart rate slowed down, and the symptoms of nausea and vomiting appeared. The incidence of PONV was higher in our study than in previous studies on the use of intranasal DEX for various paediatric examinations [26]. This observation may be due to the various nervous system diseases in patients who underwent EEG in our study.

There are still some limitations to our research. First, the subjects in this study were children aged from half a month to 204 months (61.7 ± 38.9 months), and there are differences in the physiological characteristics among different age groups. In addition, the anaesthetist evaluated the sedation depth of the children with external stimulation after nasal sedation, but this monitoring was not continuous, so there was a certain error while recording the onset time and recovery time of sedation; the recorded time was often longer than the actual time. Additionally, this was a retrospective study. Continuous blood pressure monitoring was not performed routinely as standard practice in hospital clinics, so we cannot report whether the children had hyper or hypotension as a possible side effect during the whole examination process, which also needs to be confirmed by prospective studies.

Conclusion

An intranasal DEX dose of 2.5 $\mu g{\cdot}kg^{-1}$ for paediatric EEG examinations has a high sedation success rate, quick recovery and low incidence of adverse reactions.

Abbreviations

ASAPS: American Society of Anesthesiologists physical status; DEX: Dexmedetomidine; EEG: Electroencephalography; HR: Heart rate; IQR: Interquartile ranges; kg: Kilogram; MAS: Modified Aldrete Score; mg: Milligram; min: Minute; ml: Millilitre; MOAA/S: Modified Observer's Assessment of Alertness and Sedation; PONV: Postoperative nausea and vomiting; SpO_2: Pulse oxygen saturation; μg: Microgram

Acknowledgements

Not applicable.

Authors' contributions

CH helped design and perform the study, and this author contributed significantly to the analysis and manuscript preparation. TSF participated in the design and draft the manuscript. YF performed the quality assessment, and helped to draft the manuscript. YM performed the quality assessment. LH and ZJ helped to perform statistical analyses and search strategy. TQ, LRQ, YQ, LSYY helped to perform the study. All authors have read and approved the manuscript.

References

1. Keidan I, Ben-Menachem E, Tzadok M, Ben-Zeev B, Berkenstadt H. Electroencephalography for children with autistic spectrum disorder: a sedation protocol. Paediatr Anaesth. 2015;25(2):200–5.
2. Zhang H, Fang B, Zhou W. The efficacy of dexmedetomidine-remifentanil versus dexmedetomidine-propofol in children undergoing flexible bronchoscopy: a retrospective trial. Medicine. 2017;96(1):e5815.
3. Berkenbosch JW. Options and considerations for procedural sedation in pediatric imaging. Paediatric drugs. 2015;17(5):385–99.
4. Tong Y, Ren H, Ding X, Jin S, Chen Z, Li Q. Analgesic effect and adverse events of dexmedetomidine as additive for pediatric caudal anesthesia: a meta-analysis. Paediatr Anaesth. 2014;24(12):1224–30.
5. Mason KP, O'Mahony E, Zurakowski D, Libenson MH. Effects of dexmedetomidine sedation on the EEG in children. Paediatr Anaesth. 2009; 19(12):1175–83.
6. Ray T, Tobias JD. Dexmedetomidine for sedation during electroencephalographic analysis in children with autism, pervasive developmental disorders, and seizure disorders. J Clin Anesth. 2008;20(5):364–8.
7. Mahmoud M, Mason KP. Dexmedetomidine: review, update, and future considerations of paediatric perioperative and periprocedural applications and limitations. Br J Anaesth. 2015;115(2):171–82.
8. Charlton ST, Whetstone J, Fayinka ST, Read KD, Illum L, Davis SS. Evaluation of direct transport pathways of glycine receptor antagonists and an angiotensin antagonist from the nasal cavity to the central nervous system in the rat model. Pharm Res. 2008;25(7):1531–43.
9. Miller JW, Balyan R, Dong M, Mahmoud M, Lam JE, Pratap JN, Paquin JR, Li BL, Spaeth JP, Vinks A, et al. Does intranasal dexmedetomidine provide adequate plasma concentrations for sedation in children: a pharmacokinetic study. Br J Anaesth. 2018;120(5):1056–65.
10. Yuen VM, Hui TW, Irwin MG, Yao TJ, Wong GL, Yuen MK. Optimal timing for the administration of intranasal dexmedetomidine for premedication in children. Anaesthesia. 2010;65(9):922–9.
11. Baier NM, Mendez SS, Kimm D, Velazquez AE, Schroeder AR. Intranasal dexmedetomidine: an effective sedative agent for electroencephalogram and auditory brain response testing. Paediatr Anaesth. 2016;26(3):280–5.
12. Clark M, Birisci E, Anderson JE, Anliker CM, Bryant MA, Downs C, Dalabih A. The risk of shorter fasting time for pediatric deep sedation. Anesth Essays Res. 2016;10(3):607–12.
13. Keidan I, Gozal D, Minuskin T, Weinberg M, Barkaly H, Augarten A. The effect of fasting practice on sedation with chloral hydrate. Pediatr Emerg Care. 2004;20(12):805–7.
14. Shetty SK, Aggarwal G. Efficacy of intranasal Dexmedetomidine for conscious sedation in patients undergoing surgical removal of impacted third molar: a double-blind Split mouth study. J Maxillofac Oral Surg. 2016; 15(4):512–6.
15. Mason KP, Robinson F, Fontaine P, Prescilla R. Dexmedetomidine offers an option for safe and effective sedation for nuclear medicine imaging in children. Radiology. 2013;267(3):911–7.
16. Ahnaou A, Huysmans H, Biermans R, Manyakov NV, Drinkenburg W. Ketamine: differential neurophysiological dynamics in functional networks in the rat brain. Transl Psychiatry. 2017;7(9):e1237.
17. Ke JD, Xu M, Wang PP, Wang M, Tian M, Chen ACN. Influence of propofol on the electroencephalogram default mode network in patients of advanced age. J Int Med Res. 2018;46(11):4660–8.
18. de Heer IJ, Bouman SJM, Weber F. Electroencephalographic (EEG) density spectral array monitoring in children during sevoflurane anaesthesia: a prospective observational study. Anaesthesia. 2019;74(1):45–50.
19. Sheta SA, Al-Sarheed MA, Abdelhalim AA. Intranasal dexmedetomidine vs midazolam for premedication in children undergoing complete dental rehabilitation: a double-blinded randomized controlled trial. Paediatr Anaesth. 2014;24(2):181–9.
20. Yuen VM, Li BL, Cheuk DK, Leung MKM, Hui TWC, Wong IC, Lam WW, Choi SW, Irwin MG. A randomised controlled trial of oral chloral hydrate vs. intranasal dexmedetomidine before computerised tomography in children. Anaesthesia. 2017;72(10):1191–5.
21. Mason KP, Lubisch NB, Robinson F, Roskos R. Intramuscular dexmedetomidine sedation for pediatric MRI and CT. AJR Am J Roentgenol. 2011;197(3):720–5.
22. Sulton C, McCracken C, Simon HK, Hebbar K, Reynolds J, Cravero J, Mallory M, Kamat P. Pediatric procedural sedation using Dexmedetomidine: a report from the pediatric sedation research consortium. Hospital pediatrics. 2016; 6(9):536–44.
23. Liu H, Sun M, Zhang J, Tian Q, Yu Q, Liu Y, Yang F, Li S, Tu S. Determination of the 90% effective dose of intranasal dexmedetomidine for sedation during electroencephalography in children. Acta Anaesthesiol Scand. 2019; 63(7):847–52.
24. Yu Q, Liu Y, Sun M, Zhang J, Zhao Y, Liu F, Li S, Tu S. Median effective dose of intranasal dexmedetomidine sedation for transthoracic echocardiography in pediatric patients with noncyanotic congenital heart disease: an up-and-down sequential allocation trial. Paediatr Anaesth. 2017;27(11):1108–14.
25. Bua J, Massaro M, Cossovel F, Monasta L, Brovedani P, Cozzi G, Barbi E, Demarini S, Travan L. Intranasal dexmedetomidine, as midazolam-sparing drug, for MRI in preterm neonates. Paediatr Anaesth. 2018;28(8):747–8.
26. Yang F, Liu Y, Yu Q, Li S, Zhang J, Sun M, Liu L, Lei Y, Tian Q, Liu H, et al. Analysis of 17 948 pediatric patients undergoing procedural sedation with a combination of intranasal dexmedetomidine and ketamine. Paediatr Anaesth. 2019;29(1):85–91.
27. Chrysostomou C, Komarlu R, Lichtenstein S, Shiderly D, Arora G, Orr R, Wearden PD, Morell VO, Munoz R, Jooste EH. Electrocardiographic effects of dexmedetomidine in patients with congenital heart disease. Intensive Care Med. 2010;36(5):836–42.

13

Comparison of ED95 of Butorphanol and sufentanil for gastrointestinal endoscopy sedation

Xiaona Zhu, Limei Chen, Shuang Zheng and Linmin Pan*

Abstract

Background: Butorphanol, a synthetic opioid partial agonist analgesic, has been widely used to control perioperative pain. However, the ideal dose and availability of butorphanol for gastrointestinal (GI) endoscopy are not well known. The aim of this study was to evaluated the 95% effective dose (ED_{95}) of butorphanol and sufentanil in GI endoscopy and compared their clinical efficacy, especially regarding the recovery time.

Methods: The study was divided into two parts. For the first part, voluntary patients who needed GI endoscopy anesthesia were recruited to measure the ED_{95} of butorphanol and sufentanil needed to achieve successful sedation before GI endoscopy using the sequential method (the Dixon up-and-down method). The second part was a double-blind, randomized study. Two hundred cases of painless GI endoscopy patients were randomly divided into two groups ($n = 100$), including group B (butorphanol at the ED_{95} dose) and group S (sufentanil at the ED_{95} dose). Propofol was infused intravenously as the sedative in both groups. The recovery time, visual analogue scale (VAS) score, hand grip strength, fatigue severity scores, incidence of nausea and vomiting, and incidence of dizziness were recorded.

Results: The ED_{95} of butorphanol for painless GI endoscopy was 9.07 μg/kg (95% confidence interval: 7.81–19.66 μg/kg). The ED_{95} of sufentanil was 0.1 μg/kg (95% CI, 0.079–0.422 μg/kg). Both butorphanol and sufentanil provided a good analgesic effect for GI endoscopy. However, the recovery time for butorphanol was significantly shorter than that for sufentanil ($P < 0.05$, group B vs. group S:21.26 ± 7.70 vs. 24.03 ± 7.80 min).

Conclusions: Butorphanol at 9.07 μg/kg was more effective than sufentanil for GI endoscopy sedation and notably reduced the recovery time.

Keywords: Butorphanol, Sufentanil, Gastrointestinal endoscopy, Sedation

Background

The morbidity from gastric and intestinal cancer is ranked second and fifth highest for cancers in China, respectively [1]. Gastrointestinal (GI) examination has been used as a standard method for the diagnosis of esophageal, gastroduodenal, and colorectal disease. However, unbearable abdominal pain can be caused by the distension and traction of viscera during GI endoscopy, eventually resulting in poor conditions for observation and severe arrhythmia [2]. Presently, sedative drugs combined with analgesics are typically used to alleviate pain and nervousness during GI endoscopy.

* Correspondence: panlinmina@163.com
Department of Anesthesiology, the First Affiliated Hospital, Wenzhou Medical University, Shangcai village, Nanbaixiang town, Ouhai District, Wenzhou City 325000, Zhejiang Province, China

Currently, opioid μ receptor agonists, such as sufentanil and fentanyl, are the most commonly used analgesics. The stomach and intestine are mainly innervated by the sympathetic and parasympathetic nervous systems [3] and the kappa receptor agonist is found at higher concentrations in the spinal cord thus is involved in relieving visceral pain [4]. Butorphanol is a kappa receptor agonist, which has the advantages of light respiratory depression, stable hemodynamics, a rapid onset, and a moderate effective duration [5], and it may be a more suitable intraoperative and postoperative analgesic for painless GI endoscopy.

Butorphanol is a more effective analgesic than morphine, while its respiratory depression is as low as 1/5 that of morphine [6]. At present, butorphanol can be safely applied as a maternal analgesic, especially for pregnant women with pre-eclampsia and chronic hypertension, it dose not cause severe fluctuations in blood pressure [7]. Butorphanol has also been used in outpatients undergoing laparoscopic tubal sterilization in the early stage [8], although the analgesic dose has not been standardized [9, 10]. It is imperative that the optimal butorphanol dose that produces analgesia and minimizes side effects during outpatient sedation is found.

The objective of this study was to detect the ED_{50}, ED_{95}, and 95% confidence intervals for butorphanol using the sequential method and to compared these to the ED_{95} dose of sufentanil to assess the feasibility and superiority of butorphanol in GI endoscopy.

Methods

This clinical study was approved by the Hospital Ethics Committee of the First Affiliated Hospital of Wenzhou Medical University and was registered in the Clinical Trial Registration Center of China (ChiCTR1900022780). Informed consent was obtained from all individual participants included in the study. This study adhered to CONSORT guidelines.

This study was based on the medical records of ASA I-II patients aged 18 to 65 who underwent an outpatient GI endoscopy (diagnostic esophagogastroduodenoscopy and colonoscopy, without therapeutic procedures), who required anesthesia and an operation of no more than 30 min in duration at the endoscopy center from May to July 2019. Patients were excluded from the study based on the following criteria: not willing or able to finish the whole study; acute upper respiratory tract infection; hepatitis and renal failure; habitual sedative or analgesic use; analgesic use for acute pain; chronic fatigue syndrome; low potassium; myasthenia gravis; psychiatric disease; and allergy to butorphanol, sufentanil, or propofol.

This study was divided into two parts: (1) determination of the ED_{95} of butorphanol and sufentanil; (2) comparison of the clinical efficacy of butorphanol with the efficacy of the equivalent sufentanil.

ED_{95} of butorphanol and sufentanil

All patients underwent routine GI preparation before endoscopy, fasting from solids for 8 h and liquids for 2 h before the operation. The anesthesia machine was inspected, and intravenous access was established. Before inducting anesthesia in the outpatient operating room, standard monitoring was applied, including for non-invasive blood pressure (BP), electrocardiogram (ECG), and oxygen saturation (SpO_2), and the patients were placed in the left lateral position. All the patients received 3 L per minute supplemental oxygen via nasal inhalation and were asked to hold the facial mask themselves.

Butorphanol (Batch number: 190411BP, Jiangsu Hengrui Pharmaceutical Co., Ltd.) or sufentanil (Batch number: 3018511505, Yichang Humanwell Pharmaceutical Co., Ltd.) was slowly injected intravenously. Given the 3 min onset time, propofol (Batch number: 1811236 Beijing Fresenius Kabi Pharmaceutical Co., Ltd.) was administrated intravenously at a constant speed until the patient lost consciousness and dropped the hand-held mask, followed by a continuous intravenous infusion at a rate of $50–150\,\mu g{\bullet}kg^{-1}{\bullet}min^{-1}$.The bispectral index (BIS) was monitored (BIS Complete Monitoring System, Covidien), and a controlled BIS value of between 50 and 60 was maintained by adjusting propofol speed. Then, the endoscopy was begun (operated by the same gastroenterologist). If the patient showed "failed sedation" (definition of failed sedation: occurrence of gag reflex [11], coughing, or body movement during esophagogastroduodenoscopy, or body movement during colonoscopy) during the GI endoscopy, an additional propofol dose of 0.5–1 mg/kg was administered. Once the SpO_2 fell to 90%, assisted ventilation with oxygen via a facial mask was applied. If the heart rate dropped below 45 beats per minute, atropine (0.5 mg) was applied. If the mean arterial pressure was less than 50 mmHg, ephedrine 5–10 mg was administered. After surgery, the patients were transported to the postanesthesia care unit (PACU) to rest and recover.

Dixon up-and-down method

The dose of butorphanol administered to each patient was determined by the Dixon up-and-down method [12]. According to geometric progression, the dose gradient was divided into six steps: 12.00, 10.00, 8.33, 6.94, 5.79, and 4.82 μg/kg. In a preliminary experiment, the ED_{95} of butorphanol for "successful sedation" (definition of successful sedation: without gag reflex, coughing, or body movement in esophagogastroduodenoscopy and body movement in colonoscopy) with propofol in outpatient GI endoscopy was 9.8 μg/kg. Therefore, the first patient was prescribed a dose of 10.00 μg/kg. The dose grade was increased or decreased using the up-down method based on the failure or success of the sedation in the previous patient. This process was repeated until there were nine cross-over pairs [13] (i.e., one successful sedation, followed by one failed sedation).

The dose of sufentanil given to each patient was also determined by the Dixon up-and-down method. According to geometric progression, the dose gradient was divided into six steps: 0.12, 0.1, 0.083, 0.069, 0.058, and 0.048 μg/kg. In the preliminary experiment, the ED_{95} of sufentanil for "successful sedation" with propofol in outpatient GI endoscopy was 0.085 μg/kg. Thus, the first patient was prescribed a dose of 0.083 μg/kg. The following process was similar to that used for testing the ED_{95} of butorphanol.

Comparison with sufentanil

Groups

Two hundred cases of painless GI endoscopy patients were recruited. The patients were randomly divided into two groups: the butorphanol group (group B, $n = 100$) and the sufentanil group (group S, n = 100).

Anesthesia methods

This part of the study was double-blind and randomized. The patients were grouped according to the envelope method. The dispensing nurse dispensed the drugs according to the directions of the anesthetist. The preoperative preparation and anesthesia methods were the same as in the first part of the study and were performed by the anesthetist. The ED_{95} dose of butorphanol (9.07 μg/kg) was administered to group B. The ED_{95} doses of sufentanil (0.1 μg/kg) was administered to group S. The ED_{95} doses of butorphanol and sufentanil were estimated in the first part of the study. Postoperative indications in the PACU were evaluated and recorded by another postoperative observer who was blinded to the group division.

Efficacy measurements and variables

The primary outcome in this study was the recovery time, which represented the time from completion of the examination and to the patient's departure from the PACU. The standards for hospital discharge were our outpatient operational standards [14] (including vital signs, pain, orientation, dizziness, and walking). The secondary outcomes included the demographic and medical data, i.e., the incidence of respiratory depression (respiratory rate < 10 beats/min or $SpO_2 < 90\%$ in nasal catheter oxygenation with 3 L/min), the incidence of circulatory inhibition (MAP < 50 mmHg or HR < 45 beats /min), dosage of propofol, the incidence of failed sedation, fatigue severity scores (assessed with an 11-point (0–10) scale [15] 15 min after awakening time), VAS score of abdominal pain (15 min after awakening time), value of hand grip strength before and 15 min after operation (assessed using an electronic hand dynamometer [EH101, Camry Co. Zhongshan, China]), the incidence of nausea and vomiting, and dizziness after awakening.

Statistical analysis

SPSS statistical software (IBM Corporation, version 19) was used for statistical analyses. The median effective dose (ED_{50}), ED_{95}, and the 95% confidence intervals (CI) of butorphanol and sufentanil were determined by binary regression (probit) [16].

The sample size in part two was evaluated by PASS 11.0. The primary indicator was recovery time. The pre-experimental measurements showed that the recovery time was 22.12 ± 7.9 min in the butorphanol group and 25.57 ± 8.1 min in the sufentanil group. A sample size of 93 in each group was determined to be required for a β value of 0.10 and an α value of 0.05. Considering the loss of data and the number of patients who could not be interviewed after endoscopy, 100 patients were selected in each group to ensure that the experiment had a large enough sample size.

Normally distributed data were analyzed with the mean ± standard deviation, and a two independent sample *t*-test was used to evaluate the differences between the two groups. The non-parametric data were analysed using the median (Q1, Q3) or ratio, and a non-parametric test was used to evaluate the differences between the two groups. The complication rates were compared using a four-square table Chi-squared test. A *P*-value < 0.05 was considered to be statistically significant.

Results

The data of 30 patients were screened in the first part of the study. One patient was excluded due to poor GI preparation, thus 29 cases remained. The individual responses to butorphanol assessed using Dixon's up-and-down method are shown in Fig. 1. The ED_{50} of butorphanol for inhibiting body movement during painless GI endoscopy was 6.58 μg/kg (95% CI, 5.57–7.49 μg/kg), and the ED_{95} of butorphanol was 9.07 μg/kg (95% CI, 7.81–19.66 μg/kg) for the same procedure. A total of 37 patients were included in the second part of the study. The individual responses to sufentanil assessed using Dixon's up-and-down method are shown in Fig. 2. The ED_{50} of sufentanil for inhibiting body movement during painless GI endoscopy was 0.060 μg/kg (95% CI, 0.048–0.073 μg/kg) and the ED_{95} of sufentanil was 0.100 μg/kg (95% CI, 0.079–0.422 μg/kg) for the same procedure. No significant

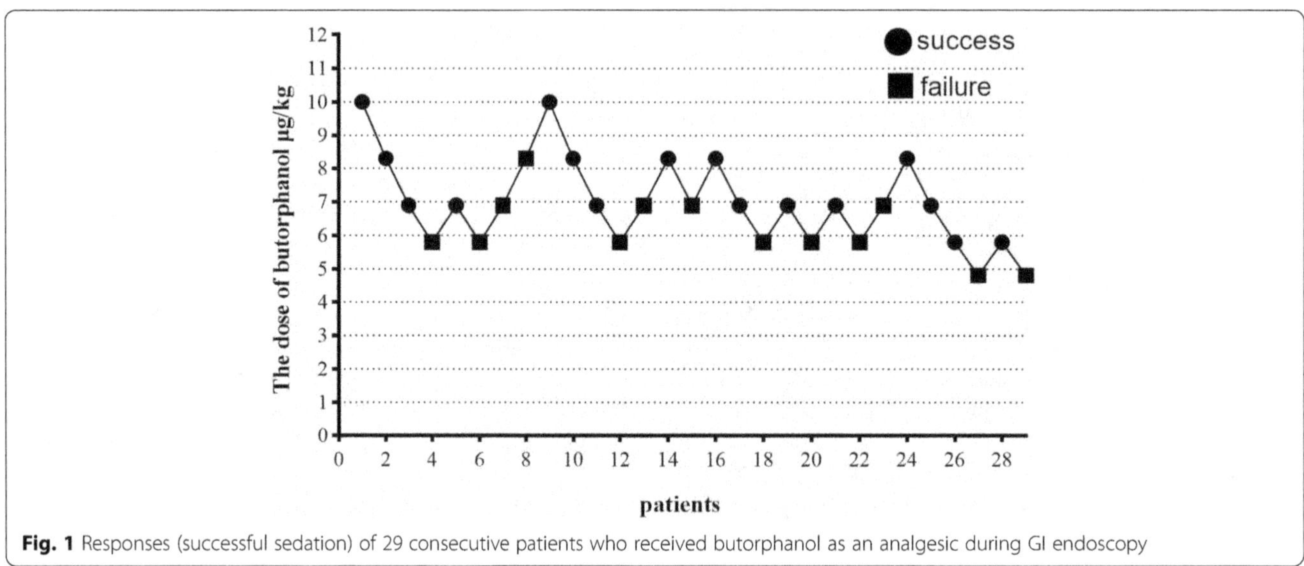

Fig. 1 Responses (successful sedation) of 29 consecutive patients who received butorphanol as an analgesic during GI endoscopy

circulatory or respiratory depression occurred during the operation.

A total of 200 patients were recruited to completed the second part of the study, and their data were analyzed to produce the final results ($n = 100$ per group). The characteristics of the enrolled subjects are shown in Table 1. There were no significant differences between the two groups regarding patient age-gender composition, SBP (Systolic Blood Pressure), heart rate, weight, height, BMI, GI endoscopy operation time, preoperative hand grip strength, and ASA (American Society of Anesthesiologists) grade composition ($P > 0.05$).

There were no statistically significant differences in the incidences of respiratory depression ($P = 0.469$), circulatory inhibition ($P = 0.489$), failed sedation ($P = 0.352$), dizziness ($P = 0.205$), and propofol dosage ($P = 0.171$). Compared to group S, group B showed lower fatigue severity scores ($P = 0.001$) and better postoperative hand grip strength ($P < 0.001$). Furthermore, the recovery time for group B was significantly shorter than for group S ($P = 0.012$). The incidence of nausea and vomiting for group B was significantly lower than for group S ($P = 0.014$), as shown in Table 2.

Discussion

In our study, the ED_{50} of butorphanol for inhibiting body movement in painless GI endoscopy was 6.58 μg/kg, (95%CI: 5.57–7.49 μg/kg) and the ED_{95} was 9.07 μg/kg (95%CI: 7.81–19.66 μg/kg). The ED_{50} for inhibiting body movement of sufentanil in painless GI endoscopy

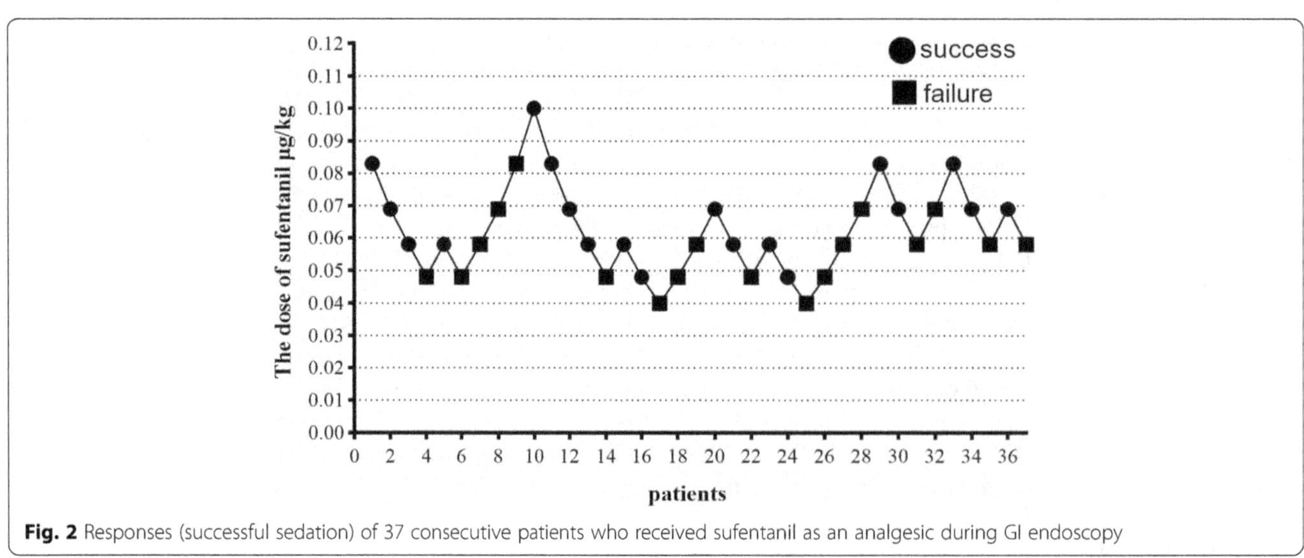

Fig. 2 Responses (successful sedation) of 37 consecutive patients who received sufentanil as an analgesic during GI endoscopy

Table 1 General comparison between group S and group B

	S group(n = 100)	B group(n = 100)
Weight, kg	63 ± 11	64 ± 10
Sex (male, female)	(60, 40)	(63, 37)
SBP, mmHg	128 ± 15	130 ± 21
Heat rate, beats/min	69 ± 17	77 ± 13
Height, cm	165 ± 8	166 ± 8
BMI, kg/m^2	23.3 ± 3.0	23.4 ± 2.8
Operation time, min	14.4 ± 4.9	14.6 ± 4.9
Preoperative hand grip strength, kg	42.9 ± 9.5	44.4 ± 8.9
ASA classification, I/II	60/40	66/34

ASA American Society of Anesthesiologists ASA physical status classification. Normally distributed statistics dates were mean ± SD, and a two independent sample t-test was used to evaluate the differences between the two groups. Sex and ASA classification were ratio and were compared by χ2 test. There were no significant differences between the two groups ($P > 0.05$)

was 0.060 μg/kg (95% CI, 0.048–0.073 μg/kg) and the ED_{95} was 0.100 μg/kg (95% CI, 0.079–0.422 μg/kg). In the second part of our study, the primary indicator (recovery time) in group B was significantly shorter than that in group S. Compared to group S, the VAS score, fatigue severity score, incidence of postoperative nausea and vomiting were lower in group B.

A sequential method was used to accurately select the optimal doses of butorphanol and sufentanil for GI endoscopy. An advantage of this method is that it can be used to evaluate the efficacy of drugs using fewer cases over a short time. The ED_{95} values of butorphanol and sufentanil were 9.07 μg/kg and 0.1 μg/kg, respectively, which were close to the doses used in the first patients in whom we administered the drugs (10 and 0.83 μg/kg, respectively). In our study, we confirmed that there was no difference in the incidences of successful sedation using the ED_{95} of butorphanol and sufentanil during GI endoscopy.

With a published in vitro affinity for opioid receptors of 1:4:25 (mu: delta: kappa), butorphanol has been known to act on kappa-opioid receptors of the upper spinal cord to inhibit nociceptive stimulus conduction [5]. Ozaki et al. demonstrated that kappa-, but not mu- or delta-, opioid receptor agonists modulate visceral sensations conveyed by the vagal afferent fibers innervating the stomach [17]. Soichiro et al. reported that butorphanol-induced visceral chemical antinociception was entirely blocked by pretreatment with a kappa-opioid receptor antagonist [18]. Kappa receptor shows absent related to respiratory depression, nausea, and vomiting. The mu receptor has strong effects on respiratory depression and is associated with nausea and vomiting [19]. Our experimental results are consistent with previous findings; they also confirm that butorphanol is less likely to cause nausea and vomiting and show that butorphanol resulted in a lower postoperative VAS score than the pure mu-opioid receptor agonist sufentanil at the ED_{95} dose. The most likely reason for this is the difference between the kappa and mu receptors. In addition, the doses of butorphanol and sufentanil used in our study were low, thus led to a low incidence of respiratory depression and did not result in a significant difference between them. The duration of the analgesic effect of butorphanol is about 4 h. Although the average examination time of painless GI endoscopy is not that long, the patient still needs excellent analgesia after waking up. PremyslFalt et al. reported that, with an intravenous injection of 2 mg midazolam after routine air-inflated GI endoscopy, 1% of patients still reported abdominal pain and 2% of patients had flatulence during the 3 h and 30 min after the procedure had finished [20]. It is essential to have excellent analgesia during this period, and butorphanol is a suitable choice.

Postoperative fatigue influences the emotional and mental state of the patients after surgery and affects

Table 2 Comparison of the indicators between group S and group B

	S group(n = 100)	B group(n = 100)	P value
Incidence of respiratory depression	11%	8%	0.469
Incidence of circulatory inhibition	12%	9%	0.489
Dosage of propofol, mg	222.6 ± 38.4	215.0 ± 39.7	0.171
Incidence of failed sedation	7%	4%	0.352
VAS score	2 (1,3)	2 (1,2)	0.001*
Fatigue severity scores	2.18 ± 1.30	1.66 ± 0.87	0.001*
Postoperative grip strength, kg	31.8 ± 6.8	35.5 ± 7.7	0.000*
Incidence of nausea and vomiting	7%	0	0.014*
Incidence of dizzness	6%	11%	0.205
Recovery time, min	24.03 ± 7.80	21.26 ± 7.70	0.012*

The VAS scores are the median (Q1, Q3). The Mann-Whitney U-test was used to evaluate the differences. Normally distributed statistics dates were mean ± SD, and a two independent sample t-test was used to evaluate the differences. Ratios were compared by χ2 test.* $P < 0.05$

their recovery [21]. Sufentanil is the classic analgesic drug used for painless GI endoscopy. However, during its clinical in our study, several patients experienced fatigue phenomenon lasting more than 1 h. In C^{11}- labeled positron emission tomography, it was found that exercise can evoke and be related to changes in μ receptors in most of the limbic system, and deactivation of the μ receptor is the main reason for fatigue [22]. There was a strong correlation between grip strength and fatigue, after adjustment for age and height, that was independent of physical activity levels [23, 24]. Butorphanol resulted in less fatigue than sufentanil according to both subjective and objective indicators. We speculated that butorphanol can reduce visceral pain in GI endoscopy, as it targets the kappa receptor and decreases deactivation of the μ receptor, thereby reducing postoperative fatigue.

Compared with sufentanil, we believe that butorphanol, reduces postoperative nausea and vomiting, improves postoperative analgesia, and reduces postoperative fatigue, thus reducing the time at PACU after GI endoscopy.

This study had several limitations: (1) Fatigue is a multi-factor subjective experience. We only evaluated one objective indicator of fatigue, grip strength, and used a simplified scale. (2) Clinical examinations of outpatients were usually incomplete. The existence of hidden diseases and different sensitivities to drugs in individuals may have affected the results of the trial.

Conclusion

In summary, the ED_{95} for butorphanol in inhibiting body movement during painless GI endoscopy was 9.07 μg/kg. Butorphanol combined with propofol as anesthesia for GI endoscopy reduced the recovery time, and, therefore, presents an excellent sedation strategy.

Abbreviations

ED95: Effective dose; CI: Confidence intervals; GI: Gastrointestinal; ASA: American Society of Anesthesiologists; BP: Blood pressure; ECG: Electrocardiogram; SpO2: Oxygen saturation; BIS: Bispectral index; PACU: Postanesthesia care unit

Acknowledgments

We thank all the patients, doctors, and nurses who participated in this study.

Authors' contributions

XZ Contribution: Design and conduct the study, analyze the data, and write the manuscript. LC Contribution: Write the manuscript and critical manuscript review. SZ Contribution: Design and conduct the study. LP: Design the study, analyze the data, and write the manuscript. All authors read and approved the final manuscript.

References

1. Chen W, Zheng R, Baade PD, Zhang S, Zeng H, Bray F, Jemal A, Yu XQ, He J. Cancer statistics in China, 2015. CA Cancer J Clin. 2016;66(2):115–32.
2. Abraham NS, Fallone CA, Mayrand S, Huang J, Wieczorek P, Barkun AN. Sedation versus no sedation in the performance of diagnostic upper gastrointestinal endoscopy: a Canadian randomized controlled cost-outcome study. Am J Gastroenterol. 2004;99(9):1692–9.
3. Altschuler SM, Escardo J, Lynn RB, Miselis RR. The central organization of the vagus nerve innervating the colon of the rat. Gastroenterology. 1993;104(2): 502–9.
4. Kivell B, Prisinzano TE. Kappa opioids and the modulation of pain. Psychopharmacology. 2010;210(2):109–19.
5. Commiskey S, Fan LW, Ho IK, Rockhold RW. Butorphanol: effects of a prototypical agonist-antagonist analgesic on kappa-opioid receptors. J Pharmacol Sci. 2005;98(2):109–16.
6. Horan PJ, Ho IK. Comparative pharmacological and biochemical studies between butorphanol and morphine. Pharmacol Biochem Behav. 1989;34(4): 847–54.
7. Garrity K, Jang A, Wagner S. Butorphanol use in laboring patients with preeclampsia or chronic hypertension. Pregnancy Hypertension. 2016;6(4): 288–90.
8. Wetchler BV, Alexander CD, Shariff MS, Gaudzels GM. A comparison of recovery in outpatients receiving fentanyl versus those receiving butorphanol. J Clin Anesth. 1989;1(5):339–43.
9. Zhang L, Shu R, Zhao Q, Li Y, Yu Y, Wang G. Preoperative butorphanol and flurbiprofen axetil therapy attenuates remifentanil-induced hyperalgesia after laparoscopic gynaecological surgery: a randomized double-blind controlled trial. Br J Anaesth. 2016;117(4):504–11.
10. Kong M, Yang L, Li J, Zhong Z, Cheng Y, Wu Z, Guo R. Low-dose butorphanol alleviates remifetanil-induced hyperalgesia in patients undergoing laparoscopic cholecystectomy. J Clin Anesth. 2016;34:41–5.
11. Borrat X, Valencia JF, Magrans R, Gimenez-Mila M, Mellado R, Sendino O, Perez M, Nunez M, Jospin M, Jensen EW, et al. Sedation-analgesia with propofol and remifentanil: concentrations required to avoid gag reflex in upper gastrointestinal endoscopy. Anesth Analg. 2015;121(1):90–6.
12. Dixon WJ. Staircase bioassay: the up-and-down method. Neurosci Biobehav Rev. 1991;15(1):47–50.
13. Hui MT, Subash S, Wang CY. The 50 and 95% effective doses of desflurane for removal of the classic laryngeal mask airway in spontaneously breathing anaesthetised adults. Anaesthesia. 2011;66(4):274–7.
14. Chen L, Zhou Y, Cai Y, Bao N, Xu X, Shi B. The ED95 of Nalbuphine in outpatient-induced abortion compared to equivalent Sufentanil. Basic Clin Pharmacol Toxicol. 2018;123(2):202–6.
15. Terkawi AS, Durieux ME, Gottschalk A, Brenin D, Tiouririne M. Effect of intravenous lidocaine on postoperative recovery of patients undergoing mastectomy: a double-blind, placebo-controlled randomized trial. Reg Anesth Pain Med. 2014;39(6):472–7.
16. Gorges M, Zhou G, Brant R, Ansermino JM. Sequential allocation trial design in anesthesia: an introduction to methods, modeling, and clinical applications. Paediatr Anaesth. 2017;27(3):240–7.
17. Ozaki N, Sengupta JN, Gebhart GF. Differential effects of mu-, delta-, and kappa-opioid receptor agonists on mechanosensitive gastric vagal afferent fibers in the rat. J Neurophysiol. 2000;83(4):2209–16.
18. Ide S, Minami M, Ishihara K, Uhl GR, Satoh M, Sora I, Ikeda K. Abolished thermal and mechanical antinociception but retained visceral chemical antinociception induced by butorphanol in mu-opioid receptor knockout mice. Neuropharmacology. 2008;54(8):1182–8.
19. Gunther T, Dasgupta P, Mann A, Miess E, Kliewer A, Fritzwanker S, Steinborn R, Schulz S. Targeting multiple opioid receptors - improved analgesics with reduced side effects? Br J Pharmacol. 2018;175(14):2857–68.
20. Falt P, Liberda M, Smajstrla V, Kliment M, Bartkova A, Tvrdik J, Fojtik P, Urban O. Combination of water immersion and carbon dioxide insufflation for minimal sedation colonoscopy: a prospective, randomized, single-center trial. Eur J Gastroenterol Hepatol. 2012;24(8):971–7..
21. Salmon P, Hall GM. A theory of postoperative fatigue: an interaction of biological, psychological, and social processes. Pharmacol Biochem Behav. 1997;56(4):623–8.
22. Hiura M, Sakata M, Ishii K, Toyohara J, Oda K, Nariai T, Ishiwata K. Central mu-Opioidergic system activation evoked by heavy and severe-intensity cycling exercise in humans: a pilot study using positron emission tomography with 11C-Carfentanil. Int J Sports Med. 2017;38(1):19–26.
23. Strandkvist V, Andersson M, Backman H, Larsson A, Stridsman C, Lindberg A. Hand grip strength is associated with fatigue among men with COPD: epidemiological data from northern Sweden. Physiother Theory Pract. 2020; 36(3):408–16.
24. Goldblatt J, James OF, Jones DE. Grip strength and subjective fatigue in patients with primary biliary cirrhosis. Jama. 2001;285(17):2196–7.

14

Quadratus lumborum block versus transversus abdominis plane block for postoperative analgesia in patients undergoing abdominal surgeries

Xiancun Liu[1], Tingting Song[1], Xuejiao Chen[2], Jingjing Zhang[1], Conghui Shan[1], Liangying Chang[1] and Haiyang Xu[1*]

Abstract

Background: Abdominal surgery is common and is associated with severe postoperative pain. The transverse abdominal plane (TAP) block is considered an effective means for pain control in such cases. The quadratus lumborum (QL) block is another option for the management of postoperative pain. The aim of this study was to conduct a meta-analysis and thereby evaluate the efficacy and safety of QL blocks and TAP blocks for pain management after abdominal surgery.

Methods: We comprehensively searched PubMed, EMBASE, EBSCO, the Cochrane Library, Web of Science and CNKI for randomized controlled trials (RCTs) that compared QL blocks and TAP blocks for pain management in patients undergoing abdominal surgery. All of the data were screened and evaluated by two researchers. RevMan5.3 was adopted for the meta-analysis.

Results: A total of 8 RCTs involving 564 patients were included. The meta-analysis showed statistically significant differences between the two groups with respect to postoperative pain scores at 2 h (standardized mean difference [Std.MD] = − 1.76; 95% confidence interval [CI] = − 2.63 to − 0.89; $p < .001$), 4 h (Std.MD = -0.77; 95% CI = -1.36 to − 0.18; $p = .01$),6 h (Std.MD = -1.24; 95% CI = -2.31 to − 0.17; $p = .02$),12 h (Std.MD = -0.70; 95% CI = -1.27 to − 0.13; p = .02) and 24 h (Std.MD = -0.65; 95% CI = -1.29 to − 0.02; $p = .04$); postoperative morphine consumption at 24 h (Std.MD = -1.39; 95% CI = -1.83 to − 0.95; $p < .001$); and duration of postoperative analgesia (Std.MD = 2.30; 95% CI = 1.85 to 2.75; p < .001). There was no statistically significant difference between the two groups with regard to the incidence of postoperative nausea and vomiting (PONV) (RR = 0.55;95% CI = 0.27 to 1.14;$p = 0.11$).

(Continued on next page)

* Correspondence: haiyang1975@163.com
[1]Department of Anesthesiology, The First Hospital of Jilin University, No.71 Xinmin street, Changchun, Jilin 130021, China

(Continued from previous page)

Conclusion: The QL block provides better pain management with less opioid consumption than the TAP block after abdominal surgery. In addition, there are no differences between the TAP block and QL block with respect to PONV.

Keywords: Pain scores, Abdominal surgery, Quadratus lumborum (QL) block, Transversus abdominis plane (TAP) block, Meta-analysis

Background

There are many kinds of abdominal surgeries, including but not limited to colorectal resection, appendectomy, cesarean section, hysterectomy, and laparoscopic cholecystectomy [1]. Postoperative pain is severe in patients undergoing abdominal surgery, and severe pain not only affects the rate of recovery of patients but also induces a series of pathophysiological reactions [1]. Therefore, it is very important for perioperative patients to have a safe and effective pain management model. Although classic postoperative analgesia methods can provide effective pain relief after surgery, their administration has a well-defined risk of side effects [2–4]. Recently, with the rise in enhanced recovery after surgery, nerve blocks have become the key link in multimodal analgesic regimes [5].

As effective constituents of multimode analgesia, quadratus lumborum (QL) block and transversus abdominis plane (TAP) block are mainly used for postoperative analgesia in abdominal surgery. At present, there have been meta-analyses [6–9] comparing a QL block to a placebo, a TAP block to a placebo, and QL and TAP blocks to other types of analgesia, and the results have shown that TAP blocks and QL blocks can reduce postoperative pain scores, the amount of opioids consumed and opioid-related side effects. Despite the reliability, widespread application and effectiveness of TAP blocks, there are several limitations and complications [10].TAP blocks should not be administered to patients with active infections at the injection site. Other limitations involve the need for a bilateral block for midline incisions and the lack of effectiveness for visceral pain [10].

Compared with TAP blocks, the QL block, which is a regional variation of the TAP block, has been suggested to be a more reliable approach for pain after abdominal surgery. QL blocks result in more extensive sensory blocks than TAP blocks (T10-L3vs.T10-T12, [11]).

Some studies [12–14] have shown that compared with TAP blocks, QL blocks are more effective at postoperative analgesia and can prolong the analgesic time of patients. However, some scholars [15] have confirmed that the analgesic effects of the two treatments are the same in the postoperative period, and there is no difference in the incidence of postoperative adverse reactions. Whether QL blocks offer superior analgesia and faster postoperative recovery than TAP blocks after abdominal surgery remains controversial.

Therefore, the purpose of this study was to evaluate, in the form of a meta-analysis, whether QL blocks or TAP blocks are superior for postoperative pain management and reduce the incidence of adverse reactions after abdominal surgery.

Methods

The study was a meta-analysis, and ethics approval was not needed. This review and meta-analysis was reported on the basis of the Preferred Reporting Items for Systematic Reviews and Meta-Analyses (PRISMA).

Search strategy

We searched the following databases (the time limit was from the establishment of the database to September 2019): PubMed, EMBASE, EBSCO, the Cochrane Library, Web of Science and CNKI. We identified randomized controlled trials (RCTs) comparing the use of QL blocks and TAP blocks for analgesia after abdominal surgery. The reference lists within these publications were also investigated to identify other qualified trials not found in the initial database search. No limitations were set with regard to the language of publication. The search terms included “quadratus lumborum block”, “QL block”, “transversus abdominis plane block”, “TAP block”, “abdominal surgery”, “abdominal wall”, “abdominal muscles”, “pain management”, “postoperative pain control”, and “postoperative pain management”.

Inclusion criteria and study selection

The inclusion criteria were as follow: (1) population: patients undergoing abdominal surgery; (2) study design: RCTs; (3) intervention: QL block; (4) comparison: TAP block; (5) primary outcomes: postoperative pain scores; and (6) secondary outcomes: postoperative opioid consumption, PONV incidence and postoperative analgesia duration. Two reviewers searched for and selected studies according to the abovementioned strategy. The specific process was as follows: (1) retrieved references were deduplicated using Endnote software; (2) screening was initially performed by reading the titles and abstracts; (3) the full texts of the initially identified articles were read, eligible studies were selected and the risk of bias was assessed for each included article; (4) the third researcher made the final decision in any cases of disagreement with respect to the inclusion of studies.

Data extraction

Two investigators extracted the data from each included study, including basic information (author name, number of cases, sex, age, type of surgery, published year), primary outcomes (pain scores) and secondary outcomes (opioid consumption, postoperative analgesia duration and PONV incidence). All opioids were converted into equianalgesic doses of IV morphine for analysis (IV morphine 10 mg = IVfentanyl 100 μg = IVsufentanil 10 μg) [5]. Pain scores reported as visual, verbal, or numeric rating scale scores were converted to a standardized 0 to 10 analog scale for the quantitative evaluations.

Assessment of methodological quality

The methodological quality of each RCT was evaluated by two investigators, who used the Cochrane Handbook, and the third researcher made the final decision in any case of disagreement. The following aspects were assessed: random sequence generation, allocation scheme concealment, blinding, accuracy of data results, freedom from selective reporting and other biases. The quality of the outcomes in the meta-analysis was evaluated by the Grading of Recommendations Assessment, Development and Evaluation (GRADE) (Table 1).

Statistical analysis

The statistical analysis was conducted using RevMan 5.3. We performed a heterogeneity test on the included studies and calculated the statistics. When I^2 was < 0.5 or p was > 0.1, the level of heterogeneity was low, and a fixed-effects model was applied. Otherwise, a random-effects model was used to analyze the sources of heterogeneity. Continuous outcomes are represented as the standardized mean difference (Std.MD) with the associated 95% confidence interval (CI). Dichotomous outcomes are represented as the relative risk (RR) with the associated 95% CI. Due to the limited number (< 10) of included studies, publication bias was not evaluated.

Results

Literature search and study characteristics

A total of 135 relevant studies were initially identified, and 8 studies [13–20] were eventually included, with 564 patients. The literature screening process and results are shown in Fig. 1. The basic features of the 8 RCTs included in the meta-analysis are summarized in Table 2.

Risk of bias

The Cochrane Handbook for Systematic Reviews of Interventions was used to evaluate the risk of bias of the RCTs. Five studies [13, 15, 17–19] employed random number tables, two studies [16, 20] adopted computer generated random numbers, and one study [14] used sealed envelopes. All studies described the allocation concealment. One study [19] did not mention the method used to blind the subjects. The researchers were blinded as well. Three studies [16, 18, 20] made use of blinding for outcome measurements, and five studies did not. In addition, all studies reported the completion of the trial without withdrawals. Only one study [20] reported high levels of other biases. (See Fig. 2 and Fig. 3.)

Table 1 The GRADE evidence quality for main outcomes

Quality assessment							No of patients			
No of Studies	Design	Risk of bias	Inconsistency	Indirectness	Imprecision	Other considerations	QL block groups	TAP block groups	Effect	Quality
Postoperative pain scores at 2 h										
3	RCT	No serious risk of bias	serious	No serious indirectness	No serious imprecision	None	90	90	SMD = −1.76 95%CI: (−2.63 to −0.89)	Moderate
Postoperative pain scores at 4 h										
6	RCT	No serious risk of bias	serious	No serious indirectness	No serious imprecision	None	199	198	SMD = −0.74 95%CI: (−1.34 to − 0.14)	Moderate
Postoperative pain scores at 6 h										
4	RCT	No serious risk of bias	serious	No serious indirectness	No serious imprecision	None	144	143	SMD = −1.24 95%CI: (−2.31 to −0.17)	Moderate
Postoperative pain scores at 12 h										
7	RCT	No serious risk of bias	serious	No serious indirectness	No serious imprecision	None	253	251	SMD = −0.70 95%CI: (−1.27 to − 0.13)	Moderate
Postoperative pain scores at 24 h										
7	RCT	No serious risk of bias	serious	No serious indirectness	No serious imprecision	None	253	251	SMD = −0.60 95%CI: (−1.21 to 0)	Moderate

GRADE Grading of Recommendations Assessment, Development, and Evaluation, *RCT* randomized controlled trial, *SMD* standard mean difference, *QL* quadratus lumborum,*TAP* transversus abdominis plane

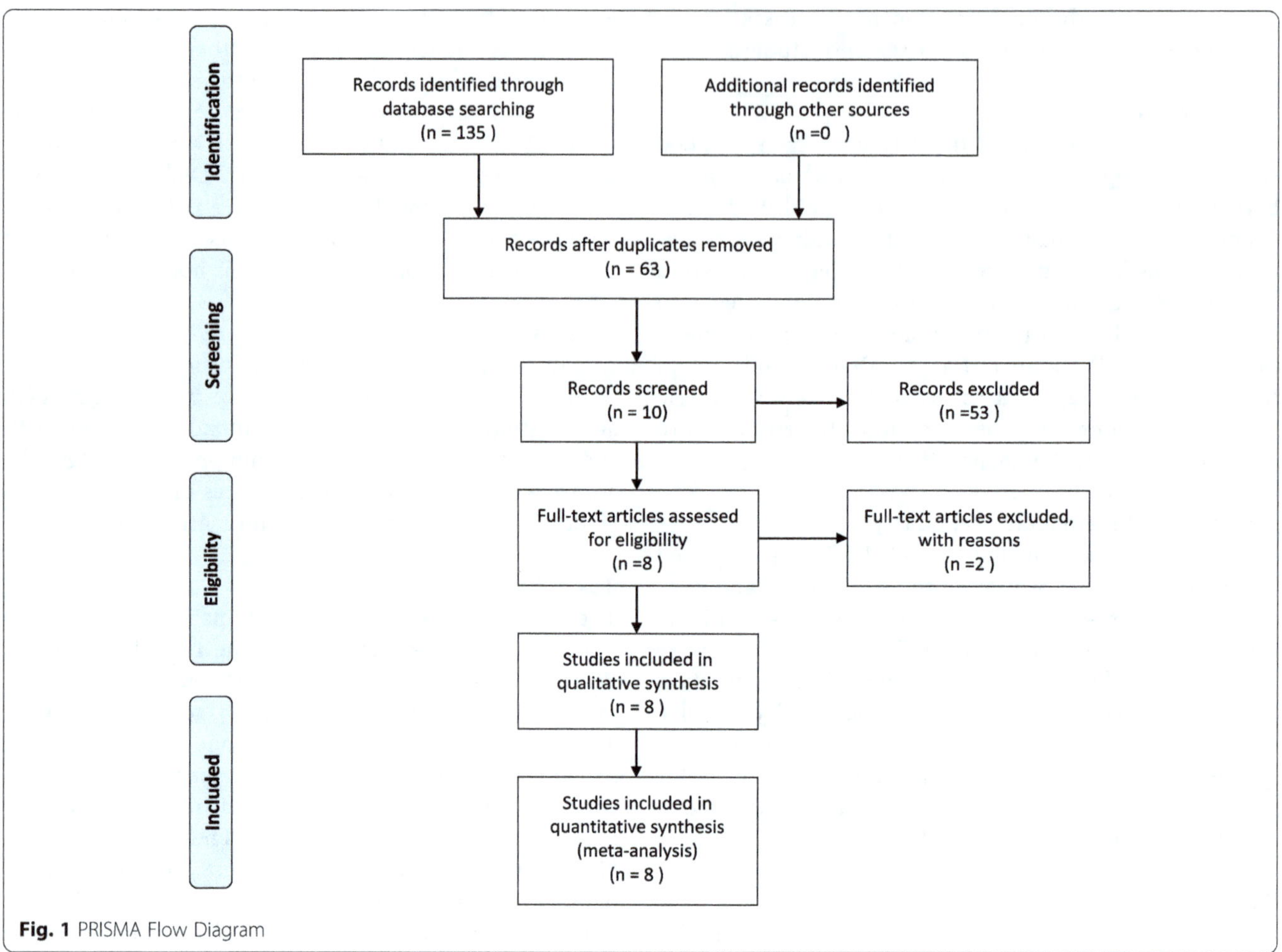

Fig. 1 PRISMA Flow Diagram

Table 2 Trails characteristics

Author	Research type	Location	Numbers (E/C)	Mean age (E/C)	QL block group	TAP block group	Surgery type	Follow-up
Blanco et al	RCT	UAE	38/38	30.2/31.3	0.125%bupivacaine (0.2 ml/kg)	0.125%bupivacaine (0.2 ml/kg)	Cesarean delivery	4 months
Oksuz et al	RCT	Turkey	25/25	3.13/3.02	0.2% bupivacaine (0.5 ml/kg)	0.2% bupivacaine (0.5 ml/kg)	Low abdominal surgery	5 months
Han et al	RCT	China	39/38	26.3/27.8	20 ml of ropivacaine (concentration of 0.25%)	20 ml of ropivacaine (concentrationof0.25%)	Appendectomy	2 months
Yousef et al	RCT	India	30/30	56.5/50.7	20 ml ofbupivacaine (concentration of 0.25%)	20 ml ofbupivacaine (concentration of 0.25%)	Total abdominal hysterectomy	3 months
Kumar et al	RCT	Egypt	35/35	39.2/38.4	20 ml of ropivacaine (concentration of 0.25%)	20 ml of ropivacaine (concentration of 0.25%)	Low abdominal surgery	2 months
Li et al	RCT	China	40 /40	30/31	20 ml of ropivacaine (concentration of0.375%)	20 ml of ropivacaine (concentration of0.375%)	Cesarean delivery	4 months
Zhu et al	RCT	China	30/30	51/52	20 ml of ropivacaine (concentration of 0.25%)	20 ml of ropivacaine (concentration of 0.25%)	Total abdominal hysterectomy	2 months
Baytar et al	RCT	Turkey	54/53	46.4/48.1	20 ml ofbupivacaine (concentration of 0.25%)	20 ml ofbupivacaine (concentration of 0.25%)	Laparoscopic cholecystectomy	3 months

E experimental groups, *C* controlled groups, *RCT* randomized controlled trials, *QL* quadratus lumborum, *TAP* transversus abdominis plane

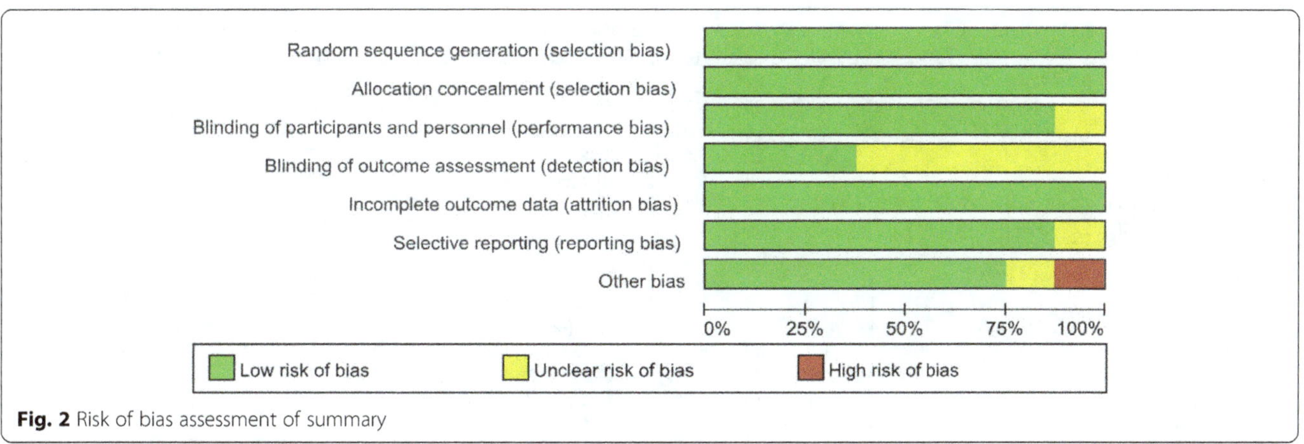

Fig. 2 Risk of bias assessment of summary

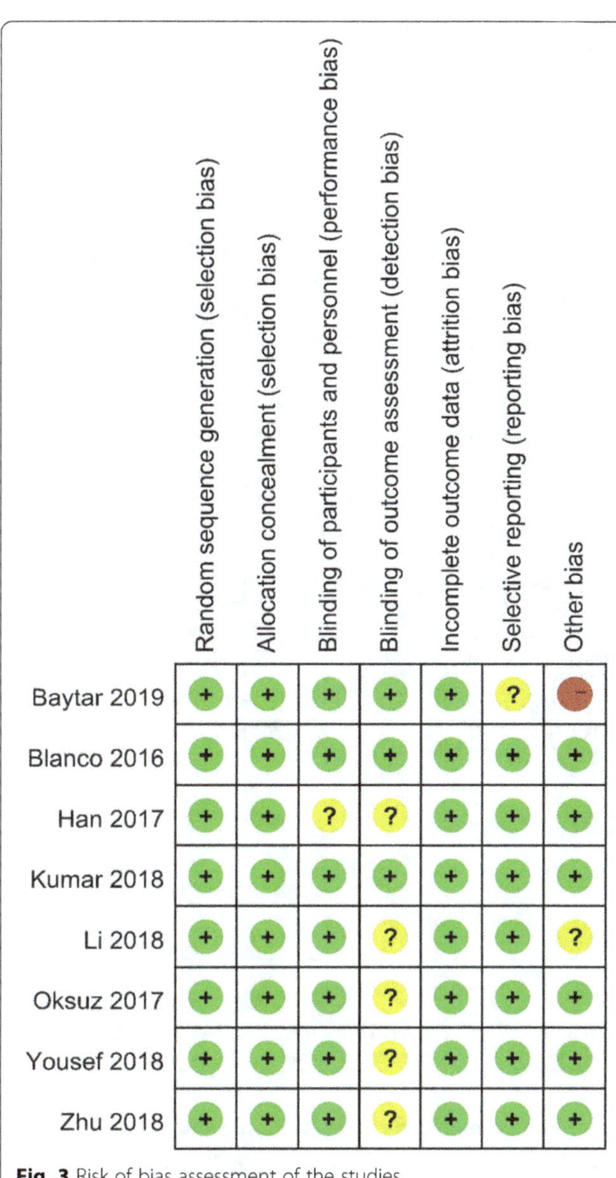

Fig. 3 Risk of bias assessment of the studies

Outcomes of the meta-analysis

Postoperative pain scores at 2 h

Three studies [13, 14, 18] with 180 patients reported pain scores 2 h after abdominal surgery. A random-effects model was used because significant heterogeneity was found among the studies (I^2 = 0.83, $p < .10$). There was a significant difference in postoperative pain scores at 2 postoperative hours between the 2 groups (Std.MD = -1.76; 95% CI = -2.63 to-0.89; $p < .001$; Fig. 4).

Postoperative pain scores at 4 h

Six studies [13–15, 17–19] with 397 patients reported pain scores 4 h after abdominal surgery. A random-effects model was applied because significant heterogeneity was found among the studies (I^2 = 0.87, $p < .10$). There was a significant difference in postoperative pain scores at 4 postoperative hours between the 2 groups (Std.MD = -0.77; 95% CI = -1.36 to – 0.18; $p = .01$;Fig. 4).

Postoperative pain scores at 6 h

Four studies [13, 14, 18, 20] with 287 patients reported pain scores 6 h after abdominal surgery. A random-effects model was applied because significant heterogeneity was found among the studies (I^2 = 0.94, $p < .10$). There was no significant difference in postoperative pain scores at 6postoperative hours between the 2 groups (Std.MD = -1.24; 95% CI = -2.31 to – 0.17; $p = .02$;Fig. 4).

Postoperative pain scores at 12 h

Seven studies [13–15, 17–20] with504 patients reported pain scores 12 h after abdominal surgery. A random-effects model was used because significant heterogeneity was found among the studies (I^2 = 0.89, $p < .10$). There was a significant difference in postoperative pain scores at 12 postoperative hours between the 2 groups (Std.MD = -0.70; 95% CI = -1.27 to – 0.13; p = .02;Fig. 4).

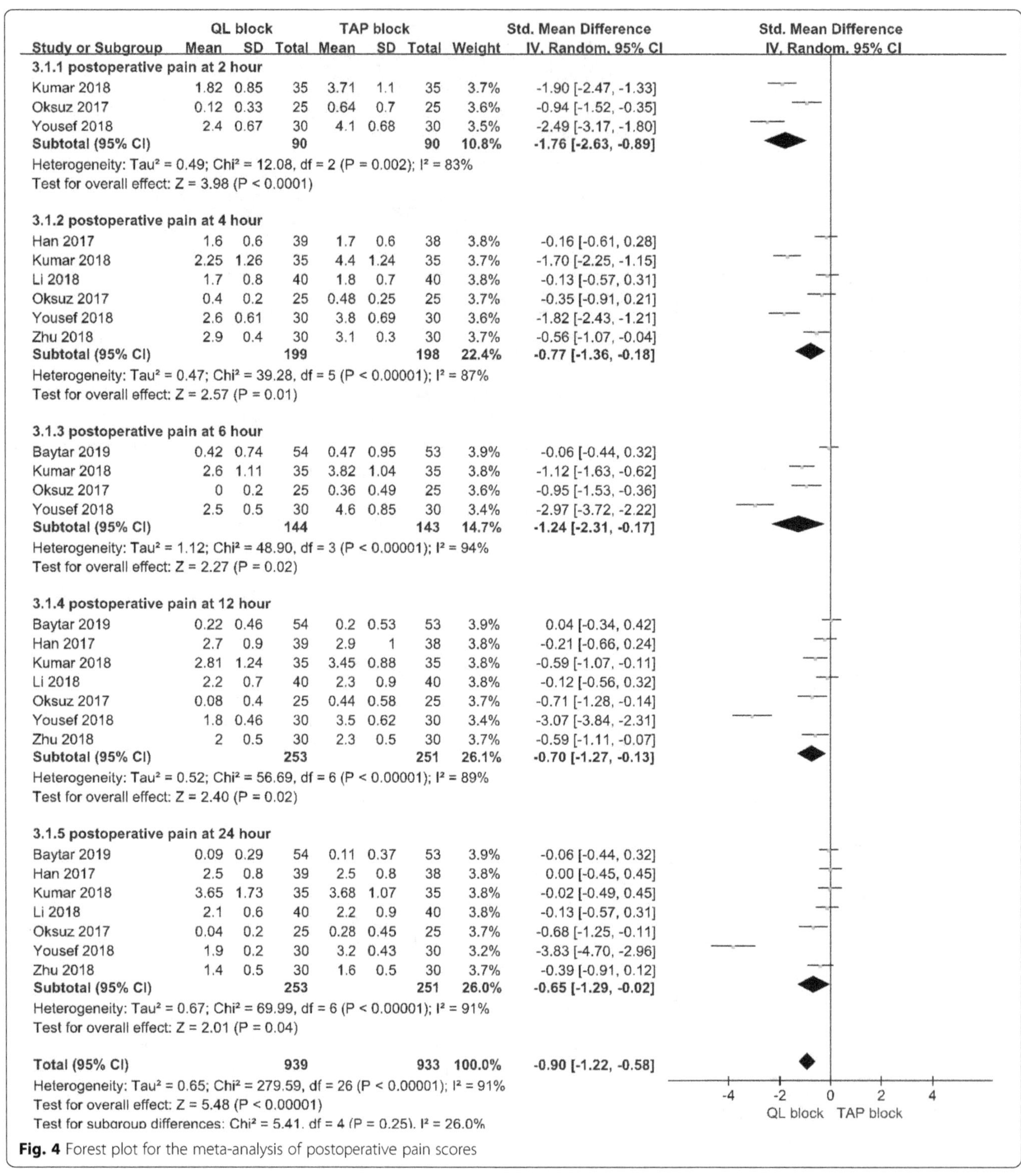

Study or Subgroup	QL block Mean	SD	Total	TAP block Mean	SD	Total	Weight	Std. Mean Difference IV, Random, 95% CI
3.1.1 postoperative pain at 2 hour								
Kumar 2018	1.82	0.85	35	3.71	1.1	35	3.7%	-1.90 [-2.47, -1.33]
Oksuz 2017	0.12	0.33	25	0.64	0.7	25	3.6%	-0.94 [-1.52, -0.35]
Yousef 2018	2.4	0.67	30	4.1	0.68	30	3.5%	-2.49 [-3.17, -1.80]
Subtotal (95% CI)			**90**			**90**	**10.8%**	**-1.76 [-2.63, -0.89]**
Heterogeneity: Tau² = 0.49; Chi² = 12.08, df = 2 (P = 0.002); I² = 83%								
Test for overall effect: Z = 3.98 (P < 0.0001)								
3.1.2 postoperative pain at 4 hour								
Han 2017	1.6	0.6	39	1.7	0.6	38	3.8%	-0.16 [-0.61, 0.28]
Kumar 2018	2.25	1.26	35	4.4	1.24	35	3.7%	-1.70 [-2.25, -1.15]
Li 2018	1.7	0.8	40	1.8	0.7	40	3.8%	-0.13 [-0.57, 0.31]
Oksuz 2017	0.4	0.2	25	0.48	0.25	25	3.7%	-0.35 [-0.91, 0.21]
Yousef 2018	2.6	0.61	30	3.8	0.69	30	3.6%	-1.82 [-2.43, -1.21]
Zhu 2018	2.9	0.4	30	3.1	0.3	30	3.7%	-0.56 [-1.07, -0.04]
Subtotal (95% CI)			**199**			**198**	**22.4%**	**-0.77 [-1.36, -0.18]**
Heterogeneity: Tau² = 0.47; Chi² = 39.28, df = 5 (P < 0.00001); I² = 87%								
Test for overall effect: Z = 2.57 (P = 0.01)								
3.1.3 postoperative pain at 6 hour								
Baytar 2019	0.42	0.74	54	0.47	0.95	53	3.9%	-0.06 [-0.44, 0.32]
Kumar 2018	2.6	1.11	35	3.82	1.04	35	3.8%	-1.12 [-1.63, -0.62]
Oksuz 2017	0	0.2	25	0.36	0.49	25	3.6%	-0.95 [-1.53, -0.36]
Yousef 2018	2.5	0.5	30	4.6	0.85	30	3.4%	-2.97 [-3.72, -2.22]
Subtotal (95% CI)			**144**			**143**	**14.7%**	**-1.24 [-2.31, -0.17]**
Heterogeneity: Tau² = 1.12; Chi² = 48.90, df = 3 (P < 0.00001); I² = 94%								
Test for overall effect: Z = 2.27 (P = 0.02)								
3.1.4 postoperative pain at 12 hour								
Baytar 2019	0.22	0.46	54	0.2	0.53	53	3.9%	0.04 [-0.34, 0.42]
Han 2017	2.7	0.9	39	2.9	1	38	3.8%	-0.21 [-0.66, 0.24]
Kumar 2018	2.81	1.24	35	3.45	0.88	35	3.8%	-0.59 [-1.07, -0.11]
Li 2018	2.2	0.7	40	2.3	0.9	40	3.8%	-0.12 [-0.56, 0.32]
Oksuz 2017	0.08	0.4	25	0.44	0.58	25	3.7%	-0.71 [-1.28, -0.14]
Yousef 2018	1.8	0.46	30	3.5	0.62	30	3.4%	-3.07 [-3.84, -2.31]
Zhu 2018	2	0.5	30	2.3	0.5	30	3.7%	-0.59 [-1.11, -0.07]
Subtotal (95% CI)			**253**			**251**	**26.1%**	**-0.70 [-1.27, -0.13]**
Heterogeneity: Tau² = 0.52; Chi² = 56.69, df = 6 (P < 0.00001); I² = 89%								
Test for overall effect: Z = 2.40 (P = 0.02)								
3.1.5 postoperative pain at 24 hour								
Baytar 2019	0.09	0.29	54	0.11	0.37	53	3.9%	-0.06 [-0.44, 0.32]
Han 2017	2.5	0.8	39	2.5	0.8	38	3.8%	0.00 [-0.45, 0.45]
Kumar 2018	3.65	1.73	35	3.68	1.07	35	3.8%	-0.02 [-0.49, 0.45]
Li 2018	2.1	0.6	40	2.2	0.9	40	3.8%	-0.13 [-0.57, 0.31]
Oksuz 2017	0.04	0.2	25	0.28	0.45	25	3.7%	-0.68 [-1.25, -0.11]
Yousef 2018	1.9	0.2	30	3.2	0.43	30	3.2%	-3.83 [-4.70, -2.96]
Zhu 2018	1.4	0.5	30	1.6	0.5	30	3.7%	-0.39 [-0.91, 0.12]
Subtotal (95% CI)			**253**			**251**	**26.0%**	**-0.65 [-1.29, -0.02]**
Heterogeneity: Tau² = 0.67; Chi² = 69.99, df = 6 (P < 0.00001); I² = 91%								
Test for overall effect: Z = 2.01 (P = 0.04)								
Total (95% CI)			**939**			**933**	**100.0%**	**-0.90 [-1.22, -0.58]**
Heterogeneity: Tau² = 0.65; Chi² = 279.59, df = 26 (P < 0.00001); I² = 91%								
Test for overall effect: Z = 5.48 (P < 0.00001)								
Test for subgroup differences: Chi² = 5.41, df = 4 (P = 0.25), I² = 26.0%								

Fig. 4 Forest plot for the meta-analysis of postoperative pain scores

Postoperative pain scores at 24 h

Seven studies [13–15, 17–20] with 504 patients reported pain scores 24 h after abdominal surgery. A random-effects model was adopted because significant heterogeneity was found among the studies ($I^2 = 0.91$, $p < .10$). There was a significant difference in postoperative pain scores at 24 postoperative hours between the 2 groups (Std.MD = -0.65; 95% CI = -1.29 to − 0.02; $p = .04$;Fig. 4).

Postoperative morphine consumption at 24 h

Five studies [13, 15, 16, 18, 19] with 363 patients reported morphine consumption 24 h after abdominal

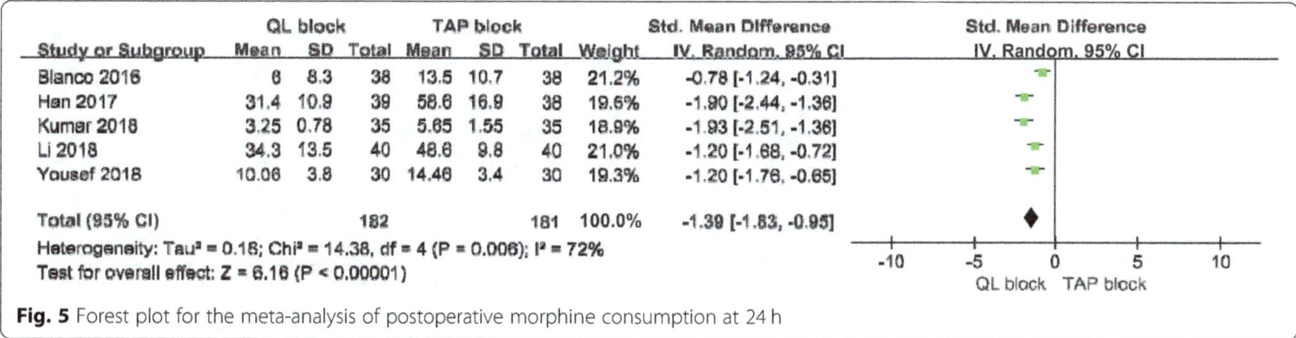

Fig. 5 Forest plot for the meta-analysis of postoperative morphine consumption at 24 h

surgery. A random-effects model was used because significant heterogeneity was found among the studies ($I^2 = 0.72$, $p < .10$). There was a significant difference in morphine consumption at 24 postoperative hours between the 2 groups (Std.MD = -1.39;95% CI = -1.83 to -0.95; $p < .001$; Fig. 5).

Duration of postoperative analgesia

Two studies [13, 18] with 130 patients reported the analgesia duration after abdominal surgery. A fixed-effects model was adopted because significant heterogeneity was not found among the studies ($I^2 = 0$, $p > .10$). There was a significant difference in postoperative analgesia duration between the 2 groups (Std.MD = 2.30; 95% CI 95% CI = 1.85 to 2.75; $p < .001$; Fig. 6).

Postoperative nausea and vomiting

Four studies [16, 17, 19, 20] with304 patients showed the incidence of PONV. A fixed-effects model was used because significant heterogeneity was not found among the studies ($I^2 = 0$, $p > .10$). There was no significant difference in PONV between the 2 groups (RR = 0.55; 95% CI = 0.27 to 1.14; $p = 0.11$;Fig. 7).

Discussion

The meta-analysis of 8RCTs showed that the pain scores at 2, 4, 6, 12 and 24 postoperative hours were significantly lower in the QL group than in the TAP group. The amount of postoperative morphine consumption was lower in the QL group than in the TAP group. The duration of postoperative analgesia was longer in the QL group than in the TAP group. In addition, there were no differences in PONV.

In the UK, approximately 700,000 people undergo abdominal surgery every year [21]. Patients experience severe pain, which leads to a series of complications. Due to pain and discomfort, patients do not cough and cannot carry out their normal activities, resulting in respiratory complications that may lead to pulmonary infections [4, 22]. If the symptoms are severe, patients may have postoperative delirium, myocardial ischemia and other serious complications. If the pain cannot be controlled in a timely fashion, acute pain can transform into chronic pain, which distresses the patient, affects wound healing, reduces the quality of life of the patient, and prolongs his or her length of hospital stay [23, 24]. Therefore, adequate postoperative analgesia has important clinical significance. In recent years, regional blocks, as a key link in multimodal analgesia, have been increasingly widely used for postoperative analgesia after abdominal surgery. TAP blocks and QL blocks belong to this treatment category [5, 25]. Thus, the potential for effective analgesia after abdominal surgery is becoming increasingly promising.

TAP blocks were first described by Rafi in 2001 [26]. TAP blocks involve the Petit triangle (that is, the lower lumbar triangle: the outer boundary is the posterior edge of the abdominal external oblique muscle, the inner boundary is the leading edge of the latissimus dorsi muscle, and the lower boundary is the iliac crest). The TAP is a nanatomical space between the transverse abdominal muscle and the medial oblique muscle [27]. The thoracolumbar nerve originates from the T6 to L1

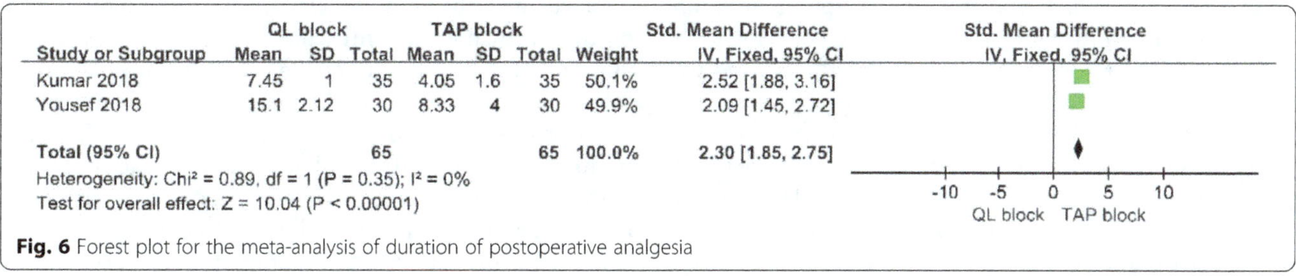

Fig. 6 Forest plot for the meta-analysis of duration of postoperative analgesia

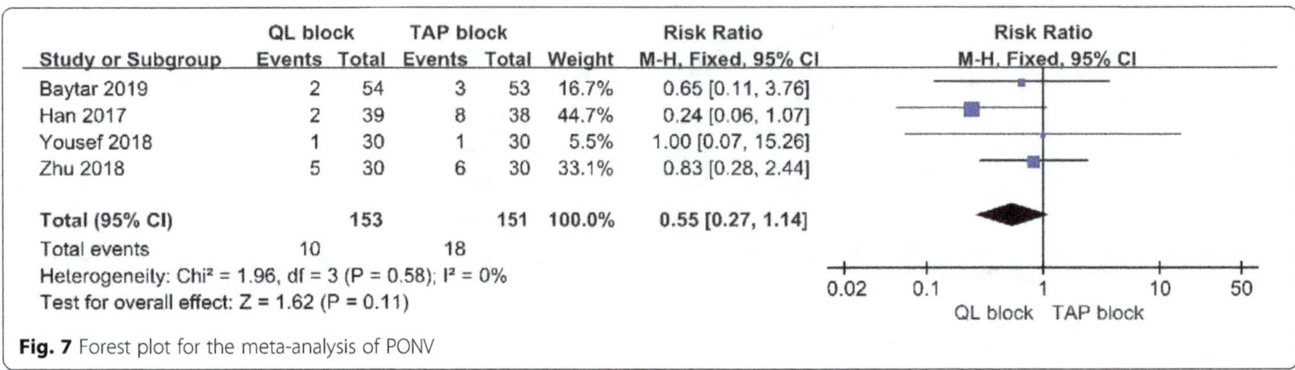

Fig. 7 Forest plot for the meta-analysis of PONV

segment of the spinal nerve root and innervates the abdominal wall, providing anterolateral sensation. The injection of local anesthetics into this space can block nerve afferents and provide adequate analgesia for the anterolateral abdominal wall [28]. However, due to the narrow range of abdominal transverse muscle plane blocks, they are often limited to use as postoperative analgesia for lower abdominal surgery, and the application of these blocks as postoperative analgesia for upper abdominal surgery is limited. As a new technique for abdominal trunk block, QL blocks were first proposed by Blanco in 2007; anesthetic is injected adjacent to the anterolateral aspect of the QL muscle and its fascia, blocking the posterior abdominal wall [16]. The block level is high (T7-L1), which can provide postoperative analgesia for both upper and lower abdominal surgery. The key to the analgesic effect of a QL block is the thoracolumbar fascia (TLF). The TLF is a complex tubular structure formed by connective tissue. Local anesthetics can spread through the TLF to the paravertebral space to generate an indirect paraspinal block [29, 30]. Therefore, it has an effect on visceral pain and abdominal incision pain. Additional studies [7, 12, 31] have shown that two different trunk blocks have adequate analgesic effects for the management of pain after abdominal surgery. FuscoP [32] et al. confirmed the analgesic effect of TAP blocks after cesarean section. Blanco [16] et al. conducted a RCT of 76 patients after cesarean section to compare the effects of pain management via QL block and TAP block. The results showed that TAP blocks were better able to reduce postoperative morphine requirements. However, there was no significant difference in postoperative pain scores between the two groups. In addition to clinical trials, other meta-analyses have confirmed the feasibility of the use of TAP blocks and QL blocks as analgesia after abdominal surgery.

Previous studies have reported the effectiveness and safety of QL blocks and TAP blocks for postoperative pain management after abdominal surgery. However, it is not yet clear which option is better. Zhu [17] et al. found no significant difference in VAS scores between patients receiving QL blocks and those receiving TAP blocks 4 h and 8 h after surgery, while the resting and motor scores 12 h and 24 h after surgery were lower in the QL block group than in the TAP block group. However, Oksuz [14] et al. reported that QL blocks provided superior analgesic relief. They compared the numbers of patients who needed analgesia in the first 24 h and the pain scores at 30 min and 1, 2, 4, 6, 12, and 24 h(s), and they found that the QL block was significantly superior to the TAP block. At the same time, Kumar's study [18] demonstrated that the pain scores of the patients in the QL block group were lower than those of the patients in the TAP block group 2, 4, 8, 12 and 24 h after lower abdominal surgeries.

In contrast to the above studies, we systematically evaluated the analgesic effects and adverse reactions of QL blocks and TAP blocks to determine which is the better regional blocking technique for pain management after abdominal surgery. The results of our meta-analysis, which included 8 RCTs, indicated that the QL block is superior to the TAP block with respect to the analgesic effect at 2, 4, 6, 12 and 24 h after surgery. Overall, the present study suggests that the effect of the QL block is better than that of the TAP block for the early management of pain after abdominal surgery. We found that the QL block is superior to the TAP block with regard to reducing postoperative opioid requirements and that pain control lasts longer after the QL block, which is consistent with the findings of Blanco et al. The reason may be that the TLF is formed by the arrangement of the anterior, middle and posterior layers. After the posterior layer and the middle layer meet at the lateral edge of the vertical spinal muscle, they converge with the anterior layer at the lateral edge of the lumbar quadratus muscle to form the aponeuros is starting point of the transverse abdomen muscle. When QL block is performed, the local anesthetics can spread not only within the TLF but also to the abdominal transverse muscle plane and paraspinal space, creating an effect similar to the effect of a paravertebral nerve block

[33]. The TLF has receptors that can regulate autonomic nerve function and pain mechanisms. Local anesthetics applied to the QL block some sympathetic nerves and thereby achieve a better effect. There was no significant difference in the incidence of PONV between the two groups. The reasons may be related to the different methods of anesthesia but may also stem from the sample size; therefore, a large number of consistent clinical trials are still needed.

Regarding the sensitivity analysis, there was still significant heterogeneity when performing the analysis by omitting one study in turn and when performing subgroup analyses. The main reasons for heterogeneity include the following: (1) Five RCTs originated in Asia, and the patient sample of one of the RCTs was limited to children. There may be relevant differences in the analytical results of the integrated data.(2) The types of surgery varied, including cesarean sections, total abdominal hysterectomies and appendectomies. The degree of postoperative pain varies among patients undergoing different abdominal surgeries. (3) The anesthetic drugs and concentrations used in the RCTs were different. Bupivacaine was used in 4 RCTs at concentrations of 0.125, 0.2 and 0.25%. The concentrations of ropivacaine used in the other 4 RCTs were 0.25 and 0.375%. (4) Three RCTs used subarachnoid anesthesia, and five RCTs employed general anesthesia.

The limitations of this meta-analysis are as follows: in the data extraction, some observation indexes in the literature were only reported as the mean and median or in the form of graphics and text; thus, these results could not be included in the analysis, which may have excluded some high-quality studies. Furthermore, there was no explicit mention of the optimal drug type and concentration for the two trunk plane blocks, which need to be further studied to arrive at a satisfactory approach. During the data collection process, the original data from requested from the author by e-mail, but no response was received. Finally, although our meta-analysis has shown that there is a statistically significant difference in postoperative pain scores between patients receiving QL blocks and TAP blocks, a difference in pain scores that is less than 2 points has limited clinical relevance. Further studies are needed to clarify the more subtle clinical differences in pain after receiving a QL block compared with a TAP block after abdominal surgery.

Conclusions

Compared with the TAP block, the QL block provides better pain management with less opioid consumption after abdominal surgery. However, further large RCTs are needed to confirm these findings.

Abbreviations

CI: Confidence interval, St.; MD: Standard mean difference; PONV: Postoperative nausea and vomiting; RCT: Randomized controlled trial; RR: Relative risk; VAS: visual analogue scale

Acknowledgments

Not applicable.

Author contributions

HX,JZ and LC designed and conceived of the study, performed the statistical analysis.and drafted the manuscript. XC and CS participated in theinterpretation of data and drafting of the manuscript. XL and TSparticipated in the study design and helped draft the manuscript. All authors read and approved the final manuscript.

Author details

[1]Department of Anesthesiology, The First Hospital of Jilin University, No.71 Xinmin street, Changchun, Jilin 130021, China. [2]Department of Anesthesiology, China-Japan Friendship Hospital, Beijing 100029, China.

References

1. Borglum J, Gogenur I, Bendtsen TF. Abdominal wall blocks in adults. Curr Opin Anaesthesiol. 2016;29(5):638–43.
2. Wu CL, Cohen SR, Richman JM, Rowlingson AJ, Courpas GE, Cheung K, Lin EE, Liu SS. Efficacy of postoperative patient-controlled and continuous infusion epidural analgesia versus intravenous patient-controlled analgesia with opioids: a meta-analysis. Anesthesiology. 2005;103(5):1079–88 quiz 1109-1010.
3. Cho JS, Kim HI, Lee KY, Son T, Bai SJ, Choi H, Yoo YC. Comparison of the effects of patient-controlled epidural and intravenous analgesia on postoperative bowel function after laparoscopic gastrectomy: a prospective randomized study. Surg Endosc. 2017;31(11):4688–96.
4. Salicath JH, Yeoh EC, Bennett MH. Epidural analgesia versus patient-controlled intravenous analgesia for pain following intra-abdominal surgery in adults. The Cochrane database of systematic reviews. 2018;8:Cd010434.
5. Wick EC, Grant MC, Wu CL. Postoperative multimodal analgesia pain management with nonopioid analgesics and techniques: a review. JAMA surgery. 2017;152(7):691–7.
6. Liu L, Xie YH, Zhang W, Chai XQ. Effect of Transversus Abdominis plane block on postoperative pain after colorectal surgery: a meta-analysis of randomized controlled trials. Med Princ Pract. 2018;27(2):158–65.
7. De Oliveira GS Jr, Castro-Alves LJ, Nader A, Kendall MC, RJ MC. Transversus abdominis plane block to ameliorate postoperative pain outcomes after laparoscopic surgery: a meta-analysis of randomized controlled trials. Anesth Analg. 2014;118(2):454–63.
8. Yu N, Long X, Lujan-Hernandez JR, Succar J, Xin X, Wang X. Transversus abdominis-plane block versus local anesthetic wound infiltration in lower abdominal surgery: a systematic review and meta-analysis of randomized controlled trials. BMC Anesthesiol. 2014;14:121.
9. Brogi E, Kazan R, Cyr S, Giunta F, Hemmerling TM. Transversus abdominal plane block for postoperative analgesia: a systematic review and meta-analysis of randomized-controlled trials. Can J Anaesth. 2016;63(10):1184–96.
10. Taylor R Jr, Pergolizzi JV, Sinclair A, Raffa RB, Aldington D, Plavin S, Apfel CC. Transversus abdominis block: clinical uses, side effects, and future perspectives. Pain Pract. 2013;13(4):332–44.
11. Urits I, Ostling PS, Novitch MB, Burns JC, Charipova K, Gress KL, Kaye RJ, Eng MR, Cornett EM, Kaye AD. Truncal regional nerve blocks in clinical anesthesia practice. Best Pract Res Clin Anaesthesiol. 2019; 33(4):559–71.
12. McCrum CL, Ben-David B, Shin JJ, Wright VJ. Quadratus lumborum block provides improved immediate postoperative analgesia and decreased opioid use compared with a multimodal pain regimen following hip arthroscopy. J Hip Preserv Surg. 2018;5(3):233–9.
13. Yousef NK. Quadratus Lumborum block versus Transversus Abdominis plane block in patients undergoing Total abdominal hysterectomy: a randomized prospective controlled trial. Anesth Essays Res. 2018;12(3):742–7.
14. Oksuz G, Bilal B, Gurkan Y, Urfalioglu A, Arslan M, Gisi G, Oksuz H. Quadratus Lumborum block versus Transversus Abdominis plane block in children undergoing low abdominal surgery: a randomized controlled trial. Reg Anesth Pain Med. 2017;42(5):674–9.

15. Li G, Gai DX. Postoperative analgesia efficacy of quadratus lumborum block versus transversus abdominis plane block in patients undergoing caesarean section. Int J Anesthesiol Resuscitation. 2018;39(4):338–340,345.
16. Blanco R, Ansari T, Riad W, Shetty N. Quadratus Lumborum block versus Transversus Abdominis plane block for postoperative pain after cesarean delivery: a randomized controlled trial. Reg Anesth Pain Med. 2016;41(6): 757–62.
17. Zhu MH, Tang Y, Xu Q, Qin Q, Chen Y. Quadratys lumborum block versus transversus abdominis plane block for analgesia after total abdominal hysterectomy. Int J Anesthesiol Resuscitation. 2018;39(8):741–5.
18. Kumar GD, Gnanasekar N, Kurhekar P, Prasad TK. A comparative study of Transversus Abdominis plane block versus Quadratus Lumborum block for postoperative analgesia following lower abdominal surgeries: a prospective double-blinded study. Anesth Essays Res. 2018;12(4):919–23.
19. Han B, Wang WT, He AH. Comparison of ultrasound-guided quadratus lumborum block and transversus abdominis plane block combined with patient controlled intravenous analgesia with sufentani on post-operation analgesia after pendectomy. J Clin Anesthesiol. 2017;33(10):984–6.
20. Baytar C, Yilmaz C, Karasu D, Topal S. Comparison of ultrasound-guided subcostal Transversus Abdominis plane block and Quadratus Lumborum block in laparoscopic cholecystectomy: a prospective, randomized, Controlled Clinical Study. Pain Res Manag. 2019;2019:2815301.
21. Brennan F, Carr DB, Cousins M. Pain management: a fundamental human right. Anesth Analg. 2007;105(1):205–21.
22. Ueshima H, Hiroshi O. Intermittent bilateral anterior sub-costal quadratus lumborum block for effective analgesia in lower abdominal surgery. J Clin Anesth. 2017;43:65.
23. Simpson JC, Bao X, Agarwala A. Pain Management in Enhanced Recovery after surgery (ERAS) protocols. Clin Colon Rectal Surg. 2019; 32(2):121–8.
24. Kehlet H, Dahl JB. Anaesthesia, surgery, and challenges in postoperative recovery. Lancet (London, England). 2003;362(9399):1921–8.
25. Gelman D, Gelmanas A, Urbanaite D, Tamosiunas R, Sadauskas S, Bilskiene D, Naudziunas A, Sirvinskas E, Benetis R, Macas A. Role of Multimodal Analgesia in the Evolving Enhanced Recovery after Surgery Pathways. Medicina (Kaunas, Lithuania). 2018;54(2). https://doi.org/10.3390/medicina54020020.
26. Rafi AN. Abdominal field block: a new approach via the lumbar triangle. Anaesthesia. 2001;56(10):1024–6.
27. McDonnell JG, O'Donnell BD, Farrell T, Gough N, Tuite D, Power C, Laffey JG. Transversus abdominis plane block: a cadaveric and radiological evaluation. Reg Anesth Pain Med. 2007;32(5):399–404.
28. Hebbard P, Fujiwara Y, Shibata Y, Royse C. Ultrasound-guided transversus abdominis plane (TAP) block. Anaesth Intensive Care. 2007;35(4):616–7.
29. Sa M, Cardoso JM, Reis H, Esteves M, Sampaio J, Gouveia I, Carballada P, Pinheiro C, Machado D. Quadratus lumborum block: are we aware of its side effects? A report of 2 cases. Rev Bras Anestesiol. 2018;68(4): 396–9.
30. Dhanjal S, Tonder S. In: StatPearls, editor. Quadratus Lumborum block. Treasure Island: StatPearls Publishing StatPearls Publishing LLC; 2019.
31. Blanco R. The 'pecs block': a novel technique for providing analgesia after breast surgery. Anaesthesia. 2011;66(9):847–8.
32. Fusco P, Scimia P, Petrucci E, Di Carlo S, Paladini G, Marinangeli F. Transversus Abdominis plane block as analgesic technique for postoperative pain management after cesarean section: no more? Reg Anesth Pain Med. 2017;42(4):541.
33. Willard FH, Vleeming A, Schuenke MD, Danneels L, Schleip R. The thoracolumbar fascia: anatomy, function and clinical considerations. J Anat. 2012;221(6):507–36.

15

The relationship between the level of μ-opioid receptor (μORs) and postoperative analgesic use in patients undergoing septoplasty

Muzaffer Gencer[1*†] and Ayşe Yeşim Göçmen[2†]

Abstract

Background: In this study, the μ-Opioid receptor activity was assessed pre-operatively for its association with postoperative pain level and second analgesic requirement in patients undergoing septoplasty.

Methods: In our prospective study, 120 adult patients underwent septoplasty from June 2015 to January 2019 were randomly divided into 2 pre-operative groups. The first group ($n = 60$) was patients given tramadol (1–2 mg/kg) for post-operative analgesia, and the second group (control group) ($n = 60$) was initially prescribed only fentanyl (1 μg/kg-i.v.) in the induction. Acetaminophen with codeine analgesic 325/30 mg (p.o.) was used as an rescue painkiller in the post-operative period. The μ-Opioid receptor activity was investigated in pre-operative blood samples and compared to post-operative pain level and time required for second round of analgesic administration. The visual analogue score (VAS) was used to evaluate the post-operative pain degree (0 no pain; 10 worst pain). The patients' post-operative VAS scores were evaluated upon arrival to recovery room, and at the 1st, 3rd, 7th, 10th, and 24th hour post-operative period.

Results: Demographic data and peri-operative variables were similar in both study group ($p < 0.05$).There was no significant difference between the receptor levels in both groups and the mean receptor level was 200.94 ± 15.34 pg/mL (max:489.92 ± 22.36 pg/mL, min: 94.56 ± 11.23 pg/mL).In patients who used tramadol as the levels of μ-Opioid receptors increased, VAS scores of patients and second analgesic use decreased in post-operative period.The VAS scores in patients with higher receptor levels were lower in the recovery room ($p < 0.05$), 1st ($p < 0.05$) and 3rd hours ($p < 0.05$).The VAS scores were lower in the tramadol group compared to the control group ($p < 0.05$).Number of secondary analgesic requirement was significantly lower in patients of the tramadol group with higher receptor levels compared to the ones with lower receptor ($p < 0.05$) for arrival at the recovery room and 1st hour. Patients in the tramadol group needed a second pain killer much later than patients in the control group.

(Continued on next page)

* Correspondence: dr.m.gencer07@gmail.com
†Muzaffer Gencer and Ayşe Yeşim Göçmen contributed equally to this work.
[1]Department of Anesthesia, Istinye University Medical Faculty, Istanbul, Turkey

(Continued from previous page)
Conclusions: Our study demonstrates that patients with higher μOR levels have a higher efficacy of opioid analgesic agents and an lesser need for additional analgesic agents.

Keywords: Analgesic agent, μ-Opioid receptor (μORs), Septoplasty, Tramadol

Background

Nasal septal surgery is one of the most common operations in otorhinolaryngology; alone or in combination with other procedures, such as inferior turbinoplasty, endoscopic sinus surgery, and rhinoplasty. Nasal septal surgery performed by an otolaryngologists may cause severe pain post-operatively. In the post-surgery term, patients usually suffer from severe pain for several days and the pain slowly decreases over the following 4 days [1]. *Non-steroidal* anti-inflammatory *drugs* (NSAIDs), acetaminophen, and opioid analgesics can be used as medications for post-surgical pain control. Different methods and techniques have been used to reduce pain, including improved intraoperative anesthetic pain regimens, adjustment of surgical technique, and intra-operative local anesthesia infiltration. Presently, the drugs used in the field of post-operative analgesia are mainly opioids. Opioid analgesics provide significant benefits for relief of moderate-to-severe pain. A number of opioids are available for clinical use such as fentanyl, remifentanil, and tramadol. Tramadol is commonly used as an opioid analgesic for post-operative analgesia. Tramadol has important advantages compared to the other opioids including a long duration of action, rapid recovery, and limited hemodynamic and respiratory depressant effects. Tramadol and the metabolite O-desmethyl-tramadol (M1) are agonists of the mu (μ) opioid receptor [2]. Tramadol, a centrally acting analgesic, also stimulates pre-synaptic release of serotonin and inhibits serotonin reuptake. Therefore, tramadol increases inhibitory effects on pain transmission both by opioid and monoaminergic mechanisms [3, 4]. Due to its pharmacological properties, tramadol is a safe drug that has a low risk of drug abuse and dependence, respiratory depression, and cardiovascular side effects unlike other opioids [5].

Opioid receptors are classified as the mu-opioid receptors (MOP-R), kappa-opioid receptors (KOP-R) and delta-opioid receptors (DOP-R) and can be heterogeneous upon multimerization [6].

The pharmacological effects of opioid analgesics are derived from their complex interactions with three opioid receptor types (mu, delta, and kappa). The mu opioid receptor gene (*OPRM1*) (opioid receptor, mu 1) produces a receptor (the MOP-r) that is a site of action for commonly used opioid analgesics [7]. μ-Opioid receptors (μORs) are the major receptors that mediate the analgesic effects of opioids. (μ)-Opioid receptor agonists such as fentanyl, remifentanil, and morphine are the gold standard treatment for severe pain. However, opioid analgesic agents are prone to abuse due to their highly addictive effect and their use may cause undesirable side-effects including respiratory distress, sedation, locomotor activity, constipation, narcotic addiction, and tolerance. The use of these agents in post-operative analgesia is limited due to mechanisms such as respiratory depression, sedation, tolerance and dependence [8]. μ-Opioid receptors bind to G proteins, and their activity in periaqueductal gray matter and brainstem is associated with analgesic effects [9].

In a recent study, the researchers revealed that polymorphism in the μ-Opioid receptor gene may cause a change in the patient's pain threshold and susceptibility to opioid drugs [10]. When the current literature is reviewed, there is limited number of studies related to the relationship between opioid agents and the μ-Opioid receptor level.

In our study, we aimed to investigate the relationship between the μ-Opioid receptor activities with post-operative pain level and second analgesic administration requirement in nasal septal surgery patients.

Methods

This study was a randomized, double-blind, and prospective trial. Between June 2015 and January 2019, 120 adult patients underwent septoplasty at Otorhinolaryngology Clinic of Bozok University Research Hospital were included to the study. The approval of the Ethics Committee was obtained (date: May 25, 2015, number: 25/12). This trial was registered retrospectively (The ACTRN: ACTRN12619001652167, registration date: 26/11/2019).

The informed consents were obtained from all patients and followed the guidelines of Helsinki. In the operation room, all patients were randomly classified into two groups by using a computer-generated randomization table with an allocation ratio of 1:1. The randomization table was obtained from the website http://www.randomization.com. The randomization was performed by an anesthesiologist who was not involved in the anesthetic management. Intraoperative and post-operative data was collected by an anesthesiologist and *anesthetic nurses* who did not participate in the study. For post-operative analgesia, the first group ($n = 60$) used tramadol and the second group ($n = 60$) were given fentanyl in the induction initially. In both groups, fentanyl (1 μg/ kg-i.v.), propofol (2–3 mg/ kg), and muscle relaxant (rocuronium bromide 0.6 mg/ kg) were administered to all patients for induction. After endotracheal intubation, the rest of the anesthesia procedure was maintained with 2–3% sevoflurane. Sixty percent NO_2 in 40% O_2 was delivered to the patients in both groups. Although at the end of the surgery to first group patients was given tramadol (1–2 mg/ kg) for post-operative analgesia, no agent was given to the control group for post-operative analgesia. The patients in control group received same amount of placebo instead of tramadol *100 mg* vial (50 mg/ml, 2 mL). The medications given intravenously to each group before awakening were performed by the *Anesthesia* Care *Team.* Acetaminophen with codeine analgesic 325/30 mg (p.o.) was used as an additional analgesic agent in the post-operative period.

The inclusion criteria for the study consisted of patients between the age of 18–45 years, who were categorized as I and II according to the American Society of Anesthesiology physical status classification and scheduled for elective surgery for septoplasty operation under general anesthesia. The exclusion criteria consisted of the patients who had electrocardiogram (ECG) changes, receiving opioids for chronic pain, additional nasal pathologies and thus receiving additional surgical intervention, and history of allergies to local anesthetics, pregnancy, renal insufficiency, cognitive dysfunction and refusal of participation to the study.

All patients were operated by the same surgical team with similar techniques under general anesthesia by using the classic septoplasty operation technique including the correction of a deviated septum, classic submucosal resection, traditional septoplasty, and open techniques [11]. Since the genetic analysis of the samples was not available in our institute, venous blood samples were obtained from patients for research to determine the μ-Opioid receptors activities in the pre-operative period. The sera were transferred into unused cover tubes. The tubes were stored at − 20 °C in the deep-freezer and analyzed for μ-Opioid receptors levels using an Olympus AU 600 auto-analyzer (Olympus Optical Co., Japan) using Randox kits.

All the patients' vital signs were monitored during the operation. In all patients, the changes of mean arterial pressure, heart rate and Ramsay Sedation Scales (RASS) were measured at predetermined time points as arrival to the recovery room, and at the 1st, 3rd, 7th, 10th, and 24th hours in post-operative period.

To determine the level of post-operative pain, a continuous 10 cm visual analog scale (VAS), was used. On the scale, 0 indicated 'no pain', and 10 indicated 'severe pain'. The patients were asked to mark their pain at different times on the scale, and the results were recorded. First measurements were made on arrival to the recovery room in postoperative period, and they were repeated at the 1st, 3rd, 7th, 10th, and 24th hours. When VAS pain scale was evaluated at postoperative 1st hour (in addition to the patient's level of consciousness), clinical signs and vital signs were also evaluated. At the times when the pain was severe (VAS ≥ 4), the patients were given upon arrival to the recovery room: Acetaminophen 1 g (10 mg/mL, 100 mL) intravenously due to difficult peroral intake, at other time points: Acetaminophen with codeine analgesic 325/30 mg perorally as rescue analgesic, and both timing and amount of analgesics used were recorded. The relations between μ-Opioid receptors level and VAS pain scale and second analgesic need was investigated in patients. The primary outcome was the postoperative pain level difference in relation with pre-operative μORs level. The secondary outcomes were the needed rescue analgesic agent (Acetaminophen with codeine analgesic 325/30 mg. peroral) timing and amount, the changes of mean arterial pressure, heart rate, the degree of sedation of the patients, incidence of postoperative nause and vomiting in post-operative period.

Statistical analysis

Sample size calculation were performed with a power analysis based on data from a previous study [12]. In this study, which included a total of 96 patients, the relationship between Human mu opioid receptor gene A118G polymorphism and efficacy of a combination of tramadol and acetaminophen was investigated in painful neuropathy. In the study, the researchers revealed that Human mu opioid receptor gene A118G polymorphism decreased analgesic efficacy of opioid agents in pain control. Power estimation analysis suggested that 53 patients per group with a power of 80% (1-β error = 0.80), considering a type I error of 0.05 (α error = 0.05). To compensate for unexpected losses, recruitment was increased by 20%. The data were analyzed using the SPSS 21.0 software package. The number, mean and standard deviations of the demographic variables were tabulated, and student t test was used to compare the groups. ANOVA test (two ways classification with repeated measures) was used for statistical analysis of VAS values. A *p*-value of less than 0.05 was accepted as statistically significant.

Results

One hundred twenty adult patients underwent septoplasty were randomly selected for two groups. There were 52 female and 68 male patients (ranged from 18 to 45 years of age). One hundred twenty-six patients were enrolled randomly and 120 were included in the analysis. Six patients were excluded the study because they did not agree to participate. A consort flow diagram of the study is shown in Fig. 1.

The two groups were comparable with respect to age, gender, American Society of Anesthesiologists Scale (ASA), body mass index (BMI), surgical time, and anesthesia time. There was no statistically significant difference between the two groups in terms of demographic data and perioperative variables (Table 1).

In tramadol group, compared to patients with a μORs level of 200.94 ± 15.34 pg/mL-489.92 ± 22.36 pg/mL and patients with a μORs level of 94.56 ± 11.23 pg/mL-200.94 ± 15.34 pg/mL, patients with a higher receptor level were less painful and the VAS scores were lower at the recovery room, ($p < 0.001$), 1st hour ($p < 0.001$), 3rd hour ($p < 0.05$), 7th hour ($p < 0.05$), 10th hour ($p < 0.05$) in post-operative period. In the control group, while the VAS scores in patients with higher receptor levels (range: 200.94 ± 15.34–489.92 ± 22.36 pg/mL) were lower in the recovery room, ($p < 0.05$), 1st ($p < 0.05$) and 3rd hours ($p < 0.05$), there was no significant difference in other time points. Additionally, compared to the control group, the VAS scores were significantly lower in the tramadol group with both receptor levels 200.94 ± 15.34–489.92 ± 22.36 pg/mL (p values were < 0.001 for arrival at the recovery room and 1st hour, p values were < 0.05 for 3rd, 7th and 10th hours, not significant for 24th hour) and receptor levels 94.56 ± 11.23–200.94 ± 15.34 pg/mL (p values were < 0.01 for arrival at the recovery room and 1st hour, p values were < 0.05 for 3rd and 7th hour, not significant for 10th and 24th hours). We commented these data as follow: the severity of pain of post septoplasty in study group patients was less observed in the tramadol group than the control group at post-operative arrival, 1st, 3rd, 7th, and, 10th hours. Moreover, the effect of time (post-operative hours) on VAS values was significant in both the tramadol group and the control group (Table 2). The second analgesic agent requirement was significantly different between tramadol group and control group. The patients in the tramadol group required a second painkiller at a later hours and less amount than the control group who only received fentanyl in induction.

Compared to patients with μORs level: 200.94 ± 15.34–489.92 ± 22.36 pg/mL and patients with μORs level: 94.56 ± 11.23–200.94 ± 15.34 pg/mL; number of secondary analgesic requirement was significantly lower

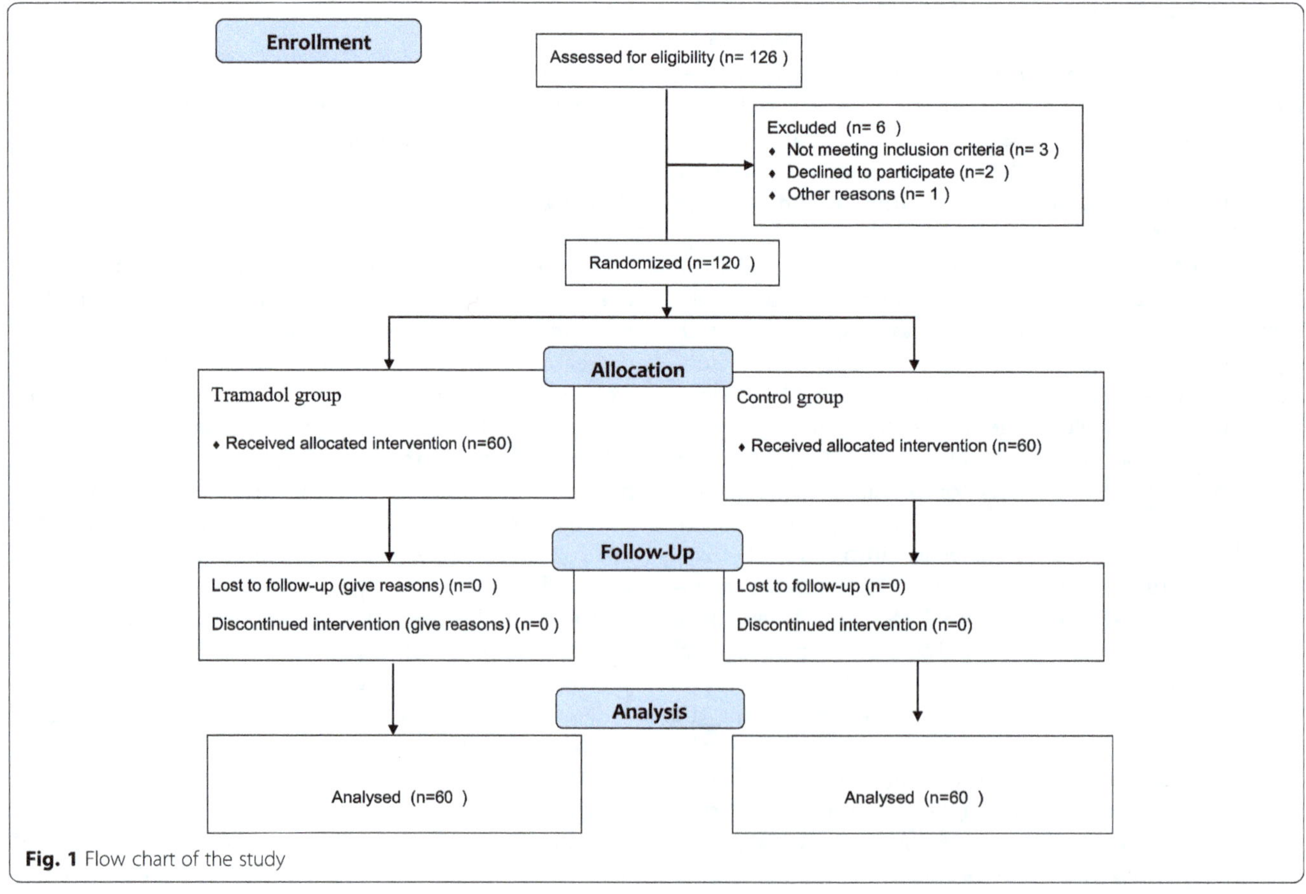

Fig. 1 Flow chart of the study

Table 1 Demographic data and perioperative variables

	Tramadol ($n = 60$)	Control ($n = 60$)	*P value
Age (yr)	28.4 ± 10.02	32.26 ± 11.78	0.352
Sex (F/M)	24/36	28/32	0.466
ASA Score I/II	21/39	31/29	0.231
BMI (kg/m^2)	23.4 ± 3.0	25.3 ± 5.0	0.285
Duration of surgery (min)	74.44 ± 23.81	80.48 ± 25.14	0.406
Duration of anesthesia (min)	82.91 ± 25.75	85.38 ± 29.31	0.763

Data are expressed as number of patients and mean ± SD. *ASA* American society of Anesthesiologists, *BMI* Body Mass Index, *F* Female, *M* Male.* Student t test, $p > 0.05$

in patients of the tramadol group with higher receptor levels compared to the ones with lower receptor (p values were < 0.05 for arrival at the recovery room and 1st hour whereas not significant for the other time points). In the control group, when the patients whose μORs level were above the average (200.94 ± 15.34 pg/mL) and those below the mean were compared, number of secondary analgesic use was higher in patients with μORs level: 94.56 ± 11.23–200.94 ± 15.34 pg/mL (p values were < 0.05 for arrival at the recovery room and 1st hour whereas not significant for the other time points) (Table 2). These results suggest opioids effect patients more with high receptor levels and therefore; patients felt lower pain in the postoperative period. *VAS* and a second analgesic need in both the tramadol group and the control group are shown in Table 2.

Mean arterial pressure was significantly lower in the 1st and 3rd hours in post-operative period in the tramadol group compared to the control group. Similarly, the heart rate of patients was higher in the control group than in the tramadol group at the time of arrival in the recovery room and post-operative 1st and 3rd hours (Table 3).

Ramsay Sedation Scale (RASS) scores were similar in both groups. However, patients in the control group were observed to be more agitated at the post-operative 3rd and 7th hour time points, but it did not reach to level of clinical significance. RASS of the patients in both study groups are shown in Table 4.

Comparison of the incidence of vomiting between the groups did not show any significant difference during post-operative period. Five patients in the tramadol group and three patients in the control group had nausea and vomiting in the recovery room during the post-operative period ($p = 0.464$). Three patients developed respiratory distress in the tramadol group, and two patients were *reintubated* due to decrease in peripheral oxygen saturation (SpO_2) in the control group. Only 3 patients had bleeding as postoperative complications.

Table 2 Visual analogue *scale* (*VAS*) and second analgesic use between the groups

	Arriva	1st h	3rd h	7th h	10th h	24th h
μORs level: **200.94–489.92 pg/mL**						
Group T ($n = 32$) VAS score	1	1	2	1	1	1
	(0–2)[b]	(0–2)	(1–3)	(0–2)	(0–1)	(0–1)
R. Analgesic[a]	0	0	1	0	0	0
Group C ($n = 31$) VAS score	5	4	3	2	2	1
	(3–8)[b]	(3–5)	(2–5)	(1–3)	(1–2)	(0–2)
R.Analgesic	2	0	0	0	1	0
μORs level: **94.56–200.94 pg/mL**						
Group T ($n = 28$) VAS score	3	3	3	2	2	1
	(2–5)[b]	(1–5)	(1–5)	(1–3)	(1–2)	(0–1)
R. Analgesic	1	1	1	1	1	0
Group C ($n = 29$) VAS score	6	5	4	3	2	1
	(4–8)[b]	(3–7)	(3–5)	(1–3)	(1–2)	(0–2)
R. Analgesic	2	2	1	1	1	0

[a]R. Analgesic: Rescue analgesic use

[b]Min-Max values. Group T: Tramadol group; Group C: Control Group. VAS scores were expressed in median. Acetaminophen 1 g (10 mg/ml,100 ml) intravenously was given at arrival to the recovery room as a rescue analgesic, Acetaminophen with codeine analgesic 325/ 30 mg (p.o) was given at other time points as a rescue analgesic; 0: analgesic was not given; 1: one dose was given; 2: two doses were given

Table 3 The changes of mean arterial pressure and heart rate at different time points

	Tramadol group (***n*** = 60)	Control group (***n*** = 60)	***p***-value
Arterial pressure (Mean ± SD)			
Arrival	116.54 ± 15.92	124.91 ± 11.06	0.354
1st h	98.54 ± 15.88	106.88 ± 11.66	0.048**
3rd h	91.78 ± 3.36	93.62 ± 2.12	0.030**
7th h	83.34 ± 10.06	84.20 ± 10.96	0.846
10th h	78.20 ± 7.62	77.00 ± 6.82	0.636
24th h	71.54 ± 3.34	72.76 ± 2.46	0.172
Heart rate (Mean ± SD)			
Arrival	88.03 ± 5.22	104.14 ± 5.82	0.001*
1st h	86.51 ± 5.15	102.73 ± 5.78	0.001*
3rd h	85.93 ± 5.02	100.86 ± 5.86	0.001*
7th h	79.12 ± 3.20	92.14 ± 2.60	0.192
10th h	78.50 ± 2.32	86.58 ± 1.82	0.146
24th h	72.84 ± 4.93	94.34 ± 5.74	0.318

SD Standard deviation, *h* hour. Student t test * $p < 0.01$, ** $p < 0.05$

Discussion

This is the first prospective study investigating the relationship between μ-opioid receptor level and post-operative pain and analgesic use. As the level of the μ-Opioid receptors increased, the effect of opioid analgesics such as the tramadol increased in study group.

After elective rhinologic surgery, pain is prominent in the first 3 days, but rapidly decreases in the days that follow [13]. Patients who undergo septoplasty operations will experience the most pain within the first 24 h, and patients often need additional analgesics during this period. The pain that occurs in the post-operative period is mostly associated with surgical trauma and the release of pain mediators into the circulation [1]. Controlling pain during the post-operative period reduces pain-related anxiety in the patient and thus, prevents the development of a cascade that may have negative consequences for the patient [14]. Low pain level of the patient will speed up recovery, provide a comfortable process, and minimize the cost [15]. It is beneficial for the patient to apply a local anesthetic agent to the surgical area during the surgery as it causes decreased post-operative pain scores and additional analgesic requirements [16]. In a recent study, the addition of a local anesthetic agent to the nasal packs after septal surgery has been shown to have positive effects in reducing post-operative pain within the first 12 h [17].

In our study, we investigated the relationship between μ-Opioid receptor level and opioid analgesics and evaluated with post-operative pain and analgesic use. However, the current studies revealed that the μ-Opioid receptors are not only associated with pain, but are also closely related to some tumor cells. Recently μ-opioid receptors have been shown to be in many cancer cell lines including non-small cell lung cancer, breast cancer, adenocarcinoma, and gastric carcinoma [18, 19]. The current studies have revealed that MOR expression correlated with, tumor aggressiveness, progression-free survival, and survival [20]. Levins KJ and colleagues [21] reported that there are the relationship between some tumor cells in the body and the anesthetic technique and μ-Opioid receptors. In their study, they emphasized that tumor MOR expression is a key difference and that this difference has prognostic importance in most types of cancer. It is possible that difference in μ-Opioid receptors may be caused by the interaction between opioid analgesic use (morphine) and the OPRM1 gene causing an increase in MOR expression. They reported a relationship between MOR expression and anesthetic technique and suggested that the use of regional anesthetic techniques and total intravenous anesthesia could be more appropriate anesthesia methods in oncoanesthesia.

Steroids such as methylprednisolone are used due to anti-inflammatory and immunosuppressive effects in addition to opioid analgesics for post-operative pain [22]. Their effects take place by altering the gene expression with specific intracellular receptor action; this leads to the blockage of the formation of certain substances, and the acceleration of the production of others. As a result, there is reduced edema and fibrosis during healing [23]. Dexamethasone may reduce inflammation at the surgery site by reducing release of inflammatory mediators into the circulation [24]. Dexamethasone significantly reduced the μ-opioid receptor binding in the adrenal cortex and affects differently opioid receptor binding in the hypothalamus and pituitary gland [25].

In addition to opioid analgesics and steroids, some drugs may also be used in post-operative pain. Kim et al. [26] revealed that oral administration of 150 mg of pregabalin twice in the early postoperative period is an effective and safe option in early postoperative pain relief in patients undergoing septoplasty. Non-opioid analgesics and NSAIs are commonly used drugs to reduce pain and inflammation after surgery. However, the use of these drugs by clinicians is limited, as excessive use of

Table 4 The comparison of Ramsay sedation scores of the tramadol and the control groups

Time points	Tramadol (*n* = 60)	Control (*n* = 60)	*p* values
Arrival	3 (2–3)	3 (1–3)	0.452
1th hour	2 (2–2)	2 (1–2)	0.406
3th hour	2 (2–2)	1 (1–2)	0.132
7th hour	2 (2–2)	1 (1–1)	0.095
10th hour	2 (2–2)	2 (1–2)	0.314
24th hour	2 (2–2))	2 (1–2)	0.324

Data are expressed as median

these agents can lead to gastrointestinal damage, which can be serious enough to cause bleeding.

Although opioid analgesics have side effects, they are commonly used agents for post-operative analgesia. Tramadol has been used frequently in recent decades and opioid drugs show their analgesic effects by affecting μ-Opioid receptors. One of the ways under the analgesic effect of tramadol is the affinity to μ-opioid receptors. It binds stronger to μ-Opioid receptors than the δ-Opioid or κ-Opioid receptors [2]. Another factor contributing to the analgesic effect of tramadol is the inhibition of the reuptake of monoamines such as norepinephrin and 5-Hydrositriptamin, which play a role in the transmission of pain in the central nervous system (CNS) [15]. Agents such as carbamazepine and cimetidine, which induce hepatic enzyme decreases the effect of tramadol. It has been shown in studies that the dose of tramadol should be increased when used with such drugs [27]. Tramadol's analgesic effect lasts 2–3 times longer than fentanyl and provides analgesia for about 7–8 h [2]. Fentanyl is a synthetic, lipophilic phenylpiperidine opioid agonist, and produces its potent analgesic effects for the treatment of moderate to severe pain via activation of the μORs with low affinity for delta and kappa opioid receptors. Unlike tramadol, which is a centrally acting weak μ opioid agonist, fentanyl is a highly efficacious agonist at the μORs, and it has a faster onset, much shorter duration of analgesic action, and higher analgesic potency compared to tramadol [28]. Undesirable side effects associated with opioid analgesic use can be seen, and opioid misuse, abuse, dependence, addiction, and overdose deaths are a major cause of concern for clinicians [8]. Since tramadol is a weak μ-opioid agonist that affects the centrally, its tolerability is higher compared to fentanyl, and adverse side effects such as respiratory depression, constipation, abuse, dependence and abuse potential are lower than other opioids [29]. Acetaminophen used as rescue analgesic in the study is a centrally acting analgesic that appears to relieve pain through both spinal and supraspinal levels. The combination of tramadol and acetaminophen may provide pain relief with synergistic effect in a 1: 8 ratio through analgesic effect in multiple pathways [30]. Granados-Soto and colleagues showed that tramadol combined with gabapentin showed a synergistic effect in both systemic and spinal administration [31]. Tramadol can cause serotonin syndrome when with serotonin reuptake inhibitors (SSRIs) and tricyclic antidepressant (TCA). A case of serotonin syndrome has been reported in the literature related to sertraline [32].

Endogenous opioids acting by binding to μ-Opioid receptors are likely to interact with hormones released from the hypothalamic-pituitary-adrenal axis in physiological and pathophysiological conditions [33].

There are a few limitations in the study. First, we used the weak μ-Opioid receptor agonist, tramadol in our study to investigate the relationship between the μ-Opioid receptor activities with post-operative pain level and second analgesic administration requirement. In similar studies, more efficient results may be obtained when using other opioid analgesics, which are more potent, highly efficacious agonists at the μORs. Second, genetic analysis of spinal or supraspinal tissue samples could be used for the measurement of mu opioid receptors. However, genetic analysis of samples is not available in our institute, patients' venous blood samples were used for research to determine the μ-Opioid receptors activities in the pre-operative period. Finally, we included 120 adult patients in the study. Similar studies may be carried out with more participants.

Conclusions

In this study, we found that the efficacy of opioid analgesic agents was higher and the need for additional analgesics was lower in patients with higher μ-Opioid receptor levels. As the level of the μ-Opioid receptor increased in the study groups, the duration of the second analgesic requirement increased. Patients with a high level of μORs in both study group experienced less analgesic need in the post-operative period. Additionally, Tramadol is a safe and effective opioid analgesic agent that reduces the postoperative pain and it may be effective analgesic agent of choice in septoplasty operations. We recommend the use of opioids such as tramadol in patients with higher opioid receptor levels for more comfortable post-operative periods.

Abbreviations

μORs: Mu-opioid receptor; KORs: Kappa-opioid receptors (KOP-R); DOP-R: Delta-opioid receptors (DOP-R); VAS: Visual analog scale; RASS: The ramsay sedation scale; NE: *Norepinephrine*; 5-HT: *5-Hidroksitriptofan*; SSRIs: Serotonin reuptake inhibitors

Acknowledgements

Each of the authors has contributed to, read and approved this manuscript. The authors thank all the patients who participated in this study and Bozok University Scientific Research Projects Unit for their support.

Authors' contributions

MG conceived the study. AYG collected the data and drafted the manuscript. MG and AYG revised the manuscript and language. AYG conducted the data analysis. All authors have read and approved the manuscript.

Author details

[1]Department of Anesthesia, Istinye University Medical Faculty, Istanbul, Turkey. [2]Department of Biochemistry, Bozok University Medical Faculty, Yozgat, Turkey.

References

1. Moumoulidis I, Draper MR, Patel H. A prospective randomized controlled trial comparing Merocel and rapid rhino nasal tampons in the treatment of epistaxis. Eur Arch Otorhinolaryngol. 2006;263:719–22.
2. Gillen C, Haurand M, Kobelt DJ, Wnendt S. Affinity, potency and efficacy of

tramadol and its metabolites at the cloned human mu-opioid receptor. Naunyn Schmiedeberg's Arch Pharmacol. 2000;362:116–21.
3. Tsai YC, Won SJ. Effects of tramadol on T lymphocyte proliferation and natural killer cell activity in rats with sciatic constriction injury. Pain. 2001;92: 63–9.
4. Minami K, Uezono Y, Ueta Y. Pharmacological aspects of the effects of tramadol on Gprotein coupled receptors. J Pharmacol Sci. 2007;103:253–60.
5. Raffa RB, Friderichs E. Profile of tramadol and tramadol analog. In: Bountra C, Munglani R, Schmidt K, editors. Pain-current understanding, emerging therapies, and novel approaches to drug discovery. New York: Marcel Dekker; 2003. p. 731–42.
6. Wolf ME, O'Brien CP. in Basic Neurochemistry (Eighth Edition); 2012.
7. Vecchiola A, Collyer P, Figueroa R, Labarca R, Bustos G, Magendzo K. Differential regulation of mu-opioid receptor mRNA in the nucleus accumbens shell and core accompanying amphetamine behavioral sensitization. Brain Res Mol Brain Res. 1999 May 21;69(1):1–9.
8. Gendron L, Cahill CM, von Zastrow M, Schiller PW, Piñeyro G. Molecular pharmacology of δ-opioid receptors. Pharmacol Rev. 2016;68(3):631–700.
9. Latapy C, Jean Martin Beaulieu JM. In Progress in Molecular Biology and Translational Science; 2013.
10. Hayashida M, Nagashima M, Satoh Y, et al. Analgesic requirements after major abdominal surgery are associated with OPRM1 gene polymorphism genotype and haplotype. Pharmacogenomics. 2008;9:1605–16.
11. Fettman N, Sanford T, Sindwani R. Surgical Management of the Deviated Septum: techniques in Septoplasty; 2009. p. 241–52.
12. Liu YC, Wang WS. Human mu opioid receptor gene A118G polymorphism predicts the efficacy of tramadol/ acetaminophen combination tablets (ultracet) in oxaliplatin-induced painful neuropathy. Cancer. 2012;118(6): 1718–25.
13. Riley CA, Kim M, Sclafani AP, Kallush A, Kjaer K, Kacker AS, et al. Opioid analgesic use and patient-reported pain outcomes after rhinologic surgery. Int Forum Allergy Rhinol. 2018. https://doi.org/10.1002/alr.22260.
14. Driessen B, Reimann W. Interaction of the central analgesic, tramadol, with the uptake and release of 5-hydroxytryptamin in the rat brain in vitro. Br J Pharmacol. 1992;105:147–51.
15. Sagata K, Minami K, Yanagihara N, Shiraishi M, Toyohira Y, Ueno S, et al. Tramadol inhibits norepinephrine transporter function at desipramine-binding sites in cultured bovine adrenal medullary cells. Anesth Analg. 2002; 94:901–6.
16. Nguyen BK, Yuhan BT, Folbe E, Eloy JA, Zuliani GF, Hsueh WD, et al. Perioperative analgesia for patients undergoing Septoplasty and Rhinoplasty: an evidence-based review. Laryngoscope. 2018. https://doi.org/10.1002/lary.27616.
17. Fujiwara T, Kuriyama A, Kato Y, Fukuoka T, Ota E. Perioperative local anaesthesia for reducing pain following septal surgery. Cochrane Database Syst Rev. 2018;8:CD012047. https://doi.org/10.1002/14651858.CD012047.
18. Lennon FE, Mirzapoiazova T, Mambetsariev B, Salgia R, Moss J, Singleton PA. Overexpression of the μ-opioid receptor in human non-small cell lung cancer promotes Akt and mTOR activation, tumor growth, and metastasis. Anesthesiology. 2012;116:857–67.
19. Zylla D, Gourley BL, Vang D, Jackson S, Boatman S, Lindgren B, et al. Opioid requirement, opioid receptor expression, and clinical outcomes in patients with advanced prostate cancer. Cancer. 2013;119:4103–10.
20. Singleton PA, Mirzapoiazova T, Hasina R, Salgia R, Moss J. Increased μ-opioid receptor expression in metastatic lung cancer Br. J Anaesth. 2014;113(suppl 1):i103–8.
21. Levins KJ, Prendeville S, Conlon S, Buggy DJ. The effect of anesthetic technique on μ-opioid receptor expression and immune cell infiltration in breast cancer. J Anesth. 2018;32(6):792–6.
22. Kaygusuz I, Susaman N. The effects of dexamethasone, bupivacain and topical lidocain spray on pain after tonsillectomy. Int J Pediatr Ontolaryngol. 2003;67:737–42.
23. Tewary AK, Cable HR, Barr GS. Steroids and control of post tonsillectomy pain. J Laryngol Otol. 1993;107:605–6.
24. Elhakim M, Ali NM, Rashed I, Riad MK, Refat M. Dexamethasone reduces postoperative vomiting and pain after pediatric tonsillectomy. Can J Anesth. 2003;50:392–7.
25. Pierzchała-Koziec K, Dziedzicka-Wasylewska M, Oeltgen P, Zubel-Łojek J, Latacz A, Ocłon E. The effect of CRH, dexamethasone and naltrexone on the mu, Delta and kappa opioid receptor agonist binding in lamb hypothalamic-pituitary-adrenal Axis. Folia Biol (Krakow). 2015;63(3):187–93.
26. Kim JH, Seo MY, Hong SD, Lee J, Chung SK, Kim HY, et al. The efficacy of preemptive analgesia with pregabalin in septoplasty. Clin Exp Otorhinolaryngol. 2014;7(2):102–5.
27. Lee CR, McTavish D, Sorkin EM. Tramadol: a priliminary review of its pharmacodynamic and pharmacokinetic properties, and therapeutic potential in acute and chronic pain states. Drugs. 1993;46:313–40.
28. Comer SD, Cahill CM. Fentanyl: receptor pharmacology, abuse potential, and implications for treatment. Neurosci Biobehav Rev. 2019;106:49–57.
29. Wolfe AM, Kennedy LH, Na JJ, Nemzek-Hamlin JA. Efficacy of tramadol as a sole analgesic for postoperative pain in male and female mice. J Am Assoc Lab Anim Sci. 2015;54(4):411–9.
30. Tallarida RJ, Raffa RB. Testing for synergism over a range of fixed ratio drug combinations: replacing the isobologram. Life Sci. 1996;58:PL23–8.
31. Granados-Soto V, Argüelles CF. Synergic Antinociceptive interaction between tramadol and gabapentin after local, spinal and systemic administration. Pharmacology. 2005;74:200–8.
32. Mason BJ, Blackburn KH. Possible serotonin syndrome associted with tramadol and sertralin coadministration. Ann Pharmacother. 1997;31:175–7.
33. O'Rourke TK Jr, Wosnitzer MS. Opioid-induced androgen deficiency (OPIAD): diagnosis, management, and literature review. Currrent Urol Rep. 2016; 17(10):76.

16

Effects of transversus abdominis plane block versus quadratus lumborum block on postoperative analgesia

Yanqing Wang[1†], Xiaojia Wang[2†] and Kexian Zhang[1*]

Abstract

Background: Trunk block technique has been used in postoperative analgesia for patients undergoing surgery, specifically, transversus abdominis plane block (TAPB) and quadratus lumborum block (QLB) have been proved effective. The purpose of this meta-analysis is to evaluate the effects of TAPB and QLB in postoperative analgesia.

Methods: Online databases, including MEDLINE, EMBASE, Cochrane Library (&Trail), Web of Science, CNKI, Wanfang and QVIP were applied to collect the randomized controlled trials (RCTs) from inception to Dec. 9th, 2019. Twenty-two studies were finally included containing 777 patients in the TAPB group and 783 cases in QLB group. RCTs comparing TAPB and QLB in postoperative analgesia were included in this meta-analysis. The indicators including total analgesia consumption postoperatively, operative time, duration of anesthesia, visual analogue scale (VAS) score at 24 h postoperatively, duration of postoperative analgesia, the number of patients requiring analgesia postoperatively and adverse reactions were analyzed.

Results: our findings showed that morphine consumption (mg) (WMD = 3.893, 95%CI: 2.053 to 5.733, $P < 0.001$), fentanyl consumption (μg) (WMD = 23.815, 95%CI: 15.521 to 32.109, $P < 0.001$), VAS score at 24 h postoperatively (WMD = 0.459, 95%CI: 0.118 to 0.801, $P = 0.008$), the number of patients requiring analgesia postoperatively (WMD = 3.893, 95%CI: 2.053 to 5.733, $P < 0.001$), and the incidence of dizziness (WMD = 2.691, 95%CI: 1.653 to 4.382, $P < 0.001$) in TAPB group were higher than in QLB group.

Conclusions: QLB is superior to TAPB in reducing morphine consumption, fentanyl consumption, VAS score at 24 h postoperatively, the number of patients requiring analgesia postoperatively, and the incidence of dizziness.

Keywords: Transversus abdominis plane block, Quadratus lumborum block, Postoperative analgesia, Outcomes

* Correspondence: kxzhangdoctor@hotmail.com
†Yanqing Wang and Xiaojia Wang contributed equally to this work.
[1]Department of Anesthesiology, Sichuan Cancer Hospital & Institute, Sichuan Cancer Center, School of Medicine, University of Electronic Science and Technology of China, No.55, Section 4, South Renmin Road, Chengdu 610041, People's Republic of China

Background

Postoperative pain, including acute postoperative pain and persistent chronic postoperative pain, remains a main clinical problem. Without timely and effective treatment, acute postoperative pain can turn into persistent chronic postoperative pain [1]. Previous studies showed that 10–50% of patients undergoing surgery suffered from postoperative pain lasting more than 1 month, and 2–10% of these patients continued to experience moderate to severe chronic pain. Furthermore, inadequate postoperative analgesia continues to occur despite advances in analgesia techniques [2, 3]. Inadequate management of postoperative pain can lead to serious consequences, such as poor immediate postoperative effect, prolonged stay and/or hospital readmission, poor patient satisfaction, increased burden on patients and health systems [3, 4]. Therefore, effective prevention and control of postoperative pain is of great significance.

Multimodal analgesia technique has been widely applied in postoperative analgesia [3, 5]. Truncal block, including transversus abdominis plane block (TAPB), quadratus lumborum block (QLB), rectus sheath block and hernia block, plays important roles in multimodal analgesia [6, 7]. TAPB involves injecting local anesthetic into the plane between the transverse abdominis and the internal oblique, it can block the sensory nerve supply to the anterior abdominal wall by deposition of local anesthetics and has shown promising in managing postoperative pain [8–10]. QLB, similar to TAPB, was first introduced as a different form of TAPB in 2007 [11]. It is also known as an interfascial plane block because it involves injecting local anesthetics into the thoracolumbar fascia which is different from TAPB. QLB can result in a widespread sensory suppression via a wide distribution of local anesthetics, and has been increasingly used for postoperative analgesia [11–14].

In recent years, many randomized controlled trials (RCTs) have been conducted to compare the effects of TAPB and QLB in postoperative analgesia [6, 15–18]. However, the results of outcomes of postoperative analgesia were inconsistent. In the current study, we aimed to compare the efficacy of TAPB versus QLB in postoperative analgesia based on RCT articles with a meta-analysis. The indicators for this meta-analysis included total analgesia consumption postoperatively, operative time, duration of anesthesia, visual analogue scale (VAS) score at 24 h postoperatively, duration of postoperative analgesia, the number of patients requiring analgesia postoperatively and adverse reactions.

Methods

Search strategy

The literatures were retrieved from MEDLINE, EMBASE, Cochrane Library (&Trail), Web of Science, CNKI, Wanfang and QVIP the deadline for searching documents was Dec. 9th, 2019. The index words for searching literatures as follows: 'transversus abdominis' OR 'transversus abdominis plane block' OR 'transverse abdominis' OR 'transverse abdominis plane block' OR 'TAP' OR 'TAP block' OR 'TAPB' AND 'quadratus lumborum' OR 'quadratus lumborum block' OR 'quadrate lumborum' OR 'quadrate lumborum block' OR 'QL' OR 'QL block' OR 'QLB'.

Inclusion and exclusion criteria

Inclusion criteria: (1) RCTs; (2) comparison of TAPB and QLB in postoperative analgesia; (3) English and Chinese literatures; (4) outcome indicators: total analgesia consumption postoperatively, operative time, duration of anesthesia, VAS score at 24 h postoperatively, duration of postoperative analgesia, the number of patients requiring analgesia postoperatively and adverse reactions.

Exclusion criteria: (1) reviews, meta-analyses, conference articles and letters; (2) animal experiments; (3) repetitive studies; (4) articles that cannot extract the valid data.

Methodological quality appraisal

The studies were screened independently by two researchers Y Wang and X Wang. In the event of disagreements, a third party (K Zhang) would participate in the discussion. The modified Jadad scale (Table 1) was applied to evaluate the quality of literatures. The scale was

Table 1 The modified Jaded Scale

Classification	Score	Description
Randomization		
Inappropriate	0	Semi-randomized or quasi-randomized trials
Unclear	1	Randomized trials without describing methods for generating random sequences
Appropriate	2	Random sequences produced by a computer or a random number table
Allocation concealment		
Inappropriate	0	Regular grouping
Unclear	1	Only use of a random number table or other random assignment scheme
Appropriate	2	A method for assigning sequences without prediction
Blinding		
Inappropriate	0	Use of double blindness without an appropriate method
Unclear	1	Only mention of double blindness
Appropriate	2	A description of the specific and appropriate method of double blindness
Withdrawals or dropouts		
No	0	No description of withdrawal or dropouts
Yes	1	A description of withdrawal or dropouts

Table 2 Characteristics of studies included in meta-analysis

Author	Year	Country	Score	Treatment	TAPB_n (M/F)	TAPB_age# (years)	QLB_n (M/F)	QLB_age# (years)	Quality	Outcomes
Baytar	2019	Turkey	4	TAPB vs QLB	53 (11/42)	48.12 ± 12.42	54 (15/39)	46.42 ± 16.57	HQ	b f g
Yousef	2018	Egypt	5	TAPB vs QLB	30 (0/30)	50.70 ± 6.8	30 (0/30)	56.5 ± 6.97	HQ	a b c d e f
Kumar	2018	India	4	TAPB vs QLB	35 (15/20)	38.34 ± 11.59	35 (15/19)	39.20 ± 11.64	HQ	a b d f
Öksüz	2017	Turkey	3	TAPB vs QLB	25 (21/4)	3.02 ± 1.82	25 (21/4)	3.13 ± 0.20	LQ	e f
Blanco	2016	Arab	3	TAPB vs QLB	38 (0/38)	NA	38 (0/38)	NA	LQ	a
Verma	2019	India	6	TAPB vs QLB	30 (0/30)	28 ± 3	30 (0/30)	30 ± 3	HQ	b d f
Ipek	2019	Turkey	3	TAPB vs QLB	29 (19/10)	4.16 ± 2.55	35 (28/7)	3.89 ± 3.26	LQ	e f g
Shan	2019	China	3	TAPB vs QLB	30 (0/30)	30 ± 3	30 (0/30)	29 ± 6	LQ	c f
Deng	2019	China	6	TAPB vs QLB	34 (12/22)	53.5 ± 10.6	34 (14/20)	51.1 ± 13.8	HQ	b c f
Fu	2019	China	4	TAPB vs QLB	30 (NA)	71.8 ± 5.8	30 (NA)	72.2 ± 6.9	HQ	b f
Han	2017	China	4	TAPB vs QLB	38 (24/14)	27.8 ± 3.9	39 (20/19)	26.3 ± 3.2	HQ	b c f
He	2018	China	2	TAPB vs QLB	36 (20/16)	67.3 ± 2.3	36 (19/17)	67.7 ± 2.1	LQ	e f
Li G	2018	China	5	TAPB vs QLB	40 (0/40)	31 ± 4	40 (0/40)	30 ± 5	HQ	b c f
Li N	2019	China	3	TAPB vs QLB	30 (0/30)	42.10 ± 5.26	30 (0/30)	41.07 ± 4.75	LQ	b e f
Ma	2019	China	3	TAPB vs QLB	30 (17/13)	55. 2 ± 4. 4	30 (16/14)	53.1 ± 4.6	LQ	e
Ren	2018	China	3	TAPB vs QLB	82 (44/38)	45.7 ± 15.2	78 (40/38)	46.3 ± 15.1	LQ	b c
Xia	2018	China	4	TAPB vs QLB	30 (15/15)	48 ± 8	30 (12/18)	46 ± 11	HQ	f
Yang	2019	China	3	TAPB vs QLB	30 (0/30)	NA	30 (0/30)	NA	LQ	a b
Yang	2019	China	5	TAPB vs QLB	30 (0/30)	38.5 ± 14.8	30 (0/30)	43.9 ± 15.04	HQ	b c e f
Ye	2019	China	4	TAPB vs QLB	28 (12/16)	48.9 ± 2.1	30 (14/16)	50.3 ± 2.8	HQ	c f
Zhu	2019	China	3	TAPB vs QLB	39 (20/19)	68.8 ± 3.4	39 (18/21)	69.1 ± 3.2	LQ	e f
Zhu	2018	China	3	TAPB vs QLB	30 (0/30)	52 ± 6	30 (0/30)	51 ± 7	LQ	b e f

#: mean ± standard deviation
TAPB transversus abdominis plane block, *QLB* quadratus lumborum block, *VAS* visual analog scale, *HQ* high-quality, *LQ* low-quality, *NA* unavailable
a: morphine consumption; b: VAS score at 24 h postoperatively; c: fentanyl consumption; d: duration of postoperative analgesia; e: the number of patients requiring analgesia postoperatively; f: operative time; g: duration of anesthesia

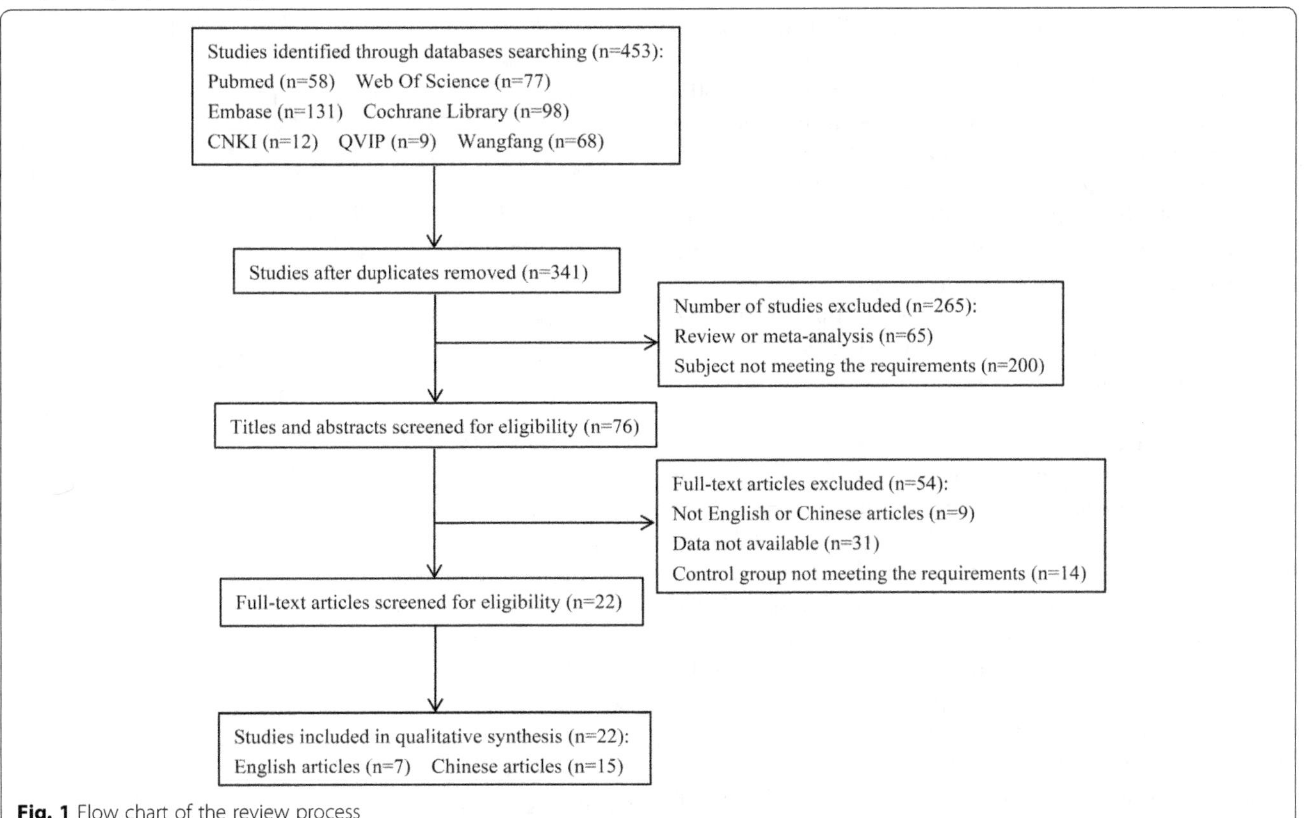

Fig. 1 Flow chart of the review process

divided into 7 points, 1–3 were defined as low quality, and 4–7 were defined as high quality.

Statistical analysis

Heterogeneity test was conducted for each indicator and measured by statistics of I^2, with $I^2 > 50\%$ indicating significant heterogeneity. If $I^2 > 50\%$, a random effects model was used; if $I^2 < 50\%$, the fixed effects model was applied, and the heterogeneity was assessed. The software Stata 15.0 (Stata Corporation, College Station, TX, USA) was used for statistical analysis, effect index relative risk (RR) was used for enumeration data and weighted mean difference (WMD) for measurement data. $P < 0.05$ was considered statistically significant.

Results

Included studies

According to the search strategy, literature searches via the databases identified 453 articles. Following removing duplicates, screening titles or abstracts, and after assessing the full texts of relevant studies, 22 articles [6, 15–35] were finally included containing 777 patients in the TAPB group and 783 cases in QLB group (Table 2 and Fig. 1).

Overall meta-analysis

As shown in Table 3, our findings showed that morphine consumption (mg) (WMD = 3.893, 95%CI: 2.053 to 5.733, $P < 0.001$), fentanyl consumption (μg) (WMD = 23.815, 95%CI: 15.521 to 32.109, $P < 0.001$), VAS score at 24 h postoperatively (WMD = 0.459, 95%CI: 0.118 to 0.801, $P = 0.008$), the number of patients requiring analgesia postoperatively (WMD = 3.893, 95%CI: 2.053 to 5.733, $P < 0.001$), and the incidence of dizziness (RR = 2.691, 95%CI: 1.653 to 4.382, $P < 0.001$) in TAPB group were higher than in QLB group. No significant differences were observed between the two groups regarding the operative time (min) ($P = 0.573$), duration of anesthesia (min) ($P = 0.733$), duration of postoperative analgesia (h) ($P = 0.258$), and nausea and vomiting ($P = 0.141$).

Total analgesia consumption postoperatively

Total analgesia consumption postoperatively (mg) as an outcome was reported containing 4 studies ($n = 266$) on morphine consumption (mg) and 8 articles ($n = 623$) on fentanyl consumption (μg). Patients in TAPB group consumed more morphine than QLB group (WMD = 3.893, 95%CI: 2.053 to 5.733; $P < 0.001$) (Table 3 and Fig. 2a). Heterogeneity among the included studies was statistically significant ($I^2 = 72.7\%$). Subgroup analysis was performed to identify sources of heterogeneity. According to operation types and literature quality, there were significant differences in abdominal surgery (WMD = 2.400, 95%CI: 1.825 to 2.975, $P < 0.001$), pelvic surgery (WMD: 4.731,

Table 3 Overall results of the meta-analysis

Outcomes	WMD/RR (95%CI)	*P*	I^2
Morphine consumption (mg)			
Overall	3.893 (2.053, 5.733)	< 0.001	72.7
Operation types			
Abdominal surgery	2.400 (1.825, 2.975)	< 0.001	NA
Pelvic surgery	4.731 (2.634, 6.829)	< 0.001	44.5
Quality			
High-quality	3.205 (1.283, 5.127)	0.001	76.2
Low-quality	6.443 (0.098, 12.788)	0.047	72.2
Fentanyl consumption (μg)			
Overall	23.815 (15.521, 32.109)	< 0.001	96.0
Operation types			
Abdominal surgery	14.077 (7.412, 20.742)	< 0.001	92.3
Pelvic surgery	34.808 (14.079, 55.537)	0.001	96.5
Quality			
High-quality	26.576 (13.594, 39.558)	< 0.001	96.9
Low-quality	16.264 (7.527, 25.000)	< 0.001	73.3
Operative time			
Overall	0.324 (−0.805, 1.454)	0.573	0.0
Duration of anesthesia (min)			
Overall	-2.139 (−14.423, 10.146)	0.733	80.8
VAS score at 24 h postoperatively			
Overall	0.459 (0.118, 0.801)	0.008	94.8
Operation types			
Abdominal surgery	0.224 (−0.033, 0.480)	0.088	80.1
Pelvic surgery	0.671 (0.103, 1.240)	0.021	95.4
Quality			
High-quality	0.576 (0.048, 1.104)	0.032	96.3
Low-quality	0.218 (−0.019, 0.455)	0.071	66.1
Duration of postoperative analgesia			
Overall	-21.882 (−59.774, 16.010)	0.258	100.0
Operation types			
Abdominal surgery	-3.400 (−4.038, −2.762)	< 0.001	NA
Pelvic surgery	−31.125 (−78.851, 16.600)	0.201	100.0
Number of patients requiring analgesia postoperatively			
Overall	2.618 (2.040, 3.361)	< 0.001	13.2
Adverse reactions			
Dizziness			
Overall	2.691 (1.653, 4.382)	< 0.001	0.0
Nausea and vomiting			
Overall	1.918 (0.805, 4.571)	0.141	50.9
Quality			
High-quality	4.100 (1.932, 8.699)	< 0.001	0.0
Low-quality	0.417 (0.054, 3.239)	0.403	70.9

CI confidence interval, *RR*, risk ratio, *WMD* weighted mean difference, *VAS* visual analog scal, *NA* unavailable

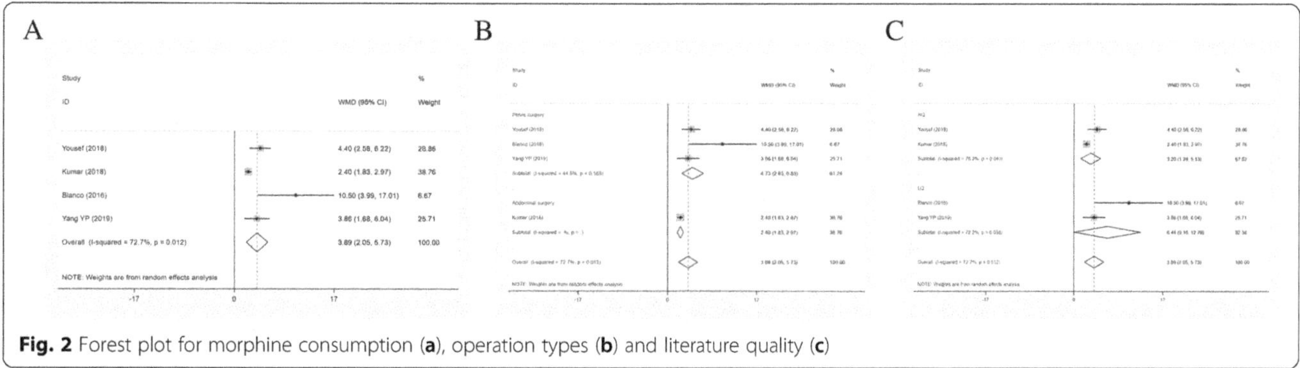

Fig. 2 Forest plot for morphine consumption (**a**), operation types (**b**) and literature quality (**c**)

95%CI: 2.634 to 6.829, $P < 0.001$), high-quality (WMD = 3.205, 95%CI: 1.283 to 5.127, $P = 0.001$) and low-quality (WMD = 6.443, 95%CI: 0.098 to 12.788, $P = 0.047$) between the two groups (Fig. 2b and c). The fentanyl consumption in TAPB group was higher than that in QLB group (WMD = 23.815, 95%CI: 15.521 to 32.109, $P < 0.001$) (Table 3 and Fig. 3a). We also found statistical differences in abdominal surgery (WMD = 14.077, 95%CI: 7.412 to 20.742, $P < 0.001$), pelvic surgery (WMD: 34.808, 95%CI: 14.079 to 55.537, $P < 0.001$), high-quality (WMD = 26.576, 95%CI: 13.594 to 39.558, $P < 0.001$) and low-quality (WMD = 16.264, 95%CI: 7.527 to 25.000, $P < 0.001$) between the two groups (Fig. 3b and c).

Operative time

Eighteen articles ($n = 1204$) on operative time (min) were included containing 597 patients in TAPB group and 607 patients in QLB group. The operative time in TAPB group was similar to QLB group, with no significant differences (WMD = 0.324, 95%CI: – 0.805 to 1.454, $P = 0.573$).

Duration of anesthesia

The data of duration of anesthesia (min) as a clinical outcome was extracted from 2 articles including 171 cases. Duration of anesthesia in TAPB group was near to QLB group, with no significant differences (WMD = - 2.139, 95%CI: – 14.423 to10.146, $P = 0.733$).

VAS score at 24 h postoperatively

Thirteen studies, including 982 patients, reported VAS score at 24 h postoperatively for pain as an outcome (I^2 = 94.8%). The VAS score at 24 h postoperatively in TAPB group was higher than that in QLB group (WMD = 0.459, 95% CI: 0.118 to 0.801; $P = 0.008$) (Fig. 4a). The results of subgroup analysis showed statistical differences in pelvic surgery (WMD = 0.671, 95% CI: 0.103 to 1.240, $P = 0.021$) and high-quality (WMD = 0.576, 95% CI: 13.594 to 39.558, $P < 0.001$) (Fig. 4b and c).

Duration of postoperative analgesia

The duration of postoperative analgesia (h) was reported as an outcome in 3 studies ($n = 190$) (I^2 = 100.00%). Duration of postoperative analgesia in TAPB group was shorter than QLB group (WMD = -21.882, 95% CI: – 59.774 to 16.010, $P = 0.258$) (Fig. 5a). The findings also showed differences in abdominal surgery (WMD = - 3.400, 95% CI: – 4.038 to – 2.762, $P < 0.001$) (Fig. 5b).

The number of patients requiring analgesia postoperatively

Nine studies (564 patients) on the number of patients requiring analgesia postoperatively were analyzed (I^2 = 13.2%). The results founded that the number of patients requiring analgesia after surgery in TAPB group were higher than QLB group (RR = 2.618, 95% CI: 2.040 to 3.361, $P < 0.001$).

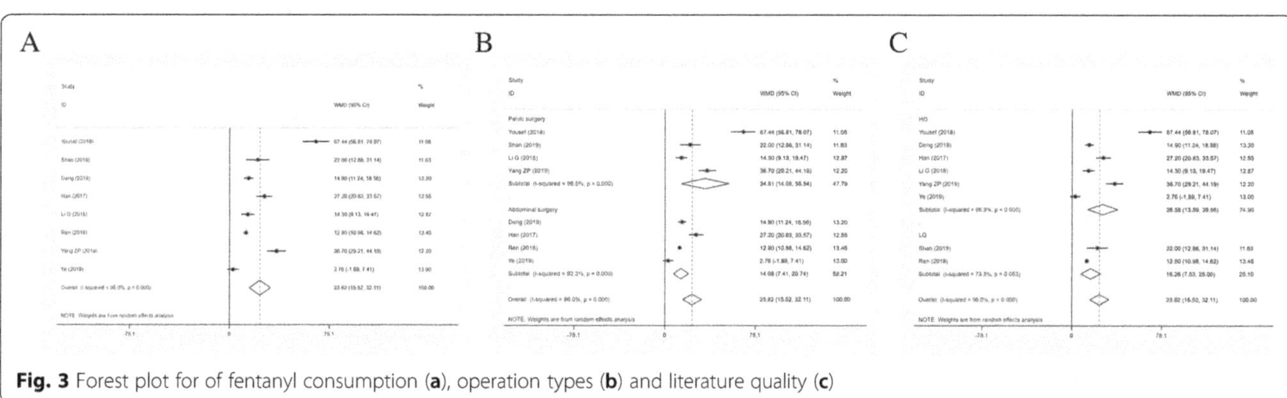

Fig. 3 Forest plot for of fentanyl consumption (**a**), operation types (**b**) and literature quality (**c**)

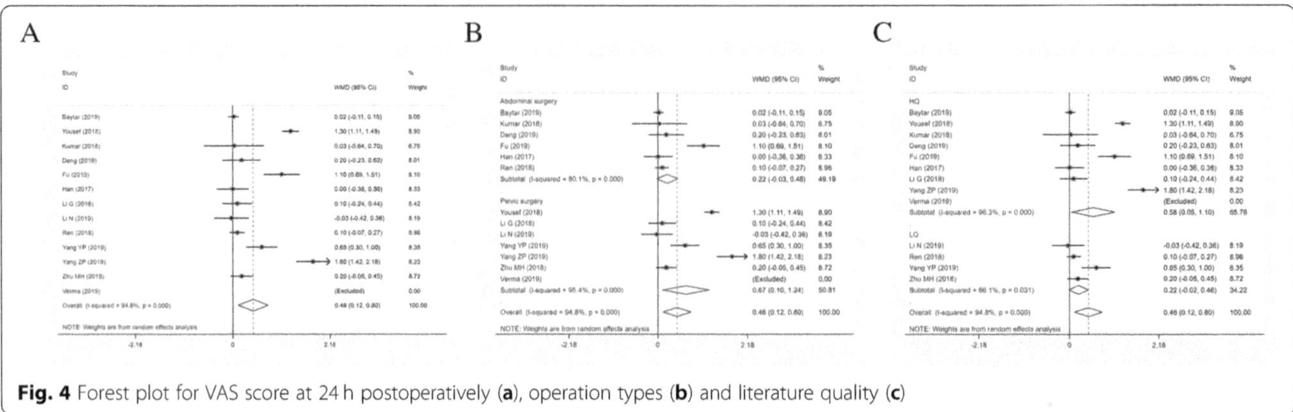

Fig. 4 Forest plot for VAS score at 24 h postoperatively (**a**), operation types (**b**) and literature quality (**c**)

Adverse reactions

The incidence of dizziness in TAPB group from 5 articles was ($n = 361$) higher than that in QLB group ($I^2 = 0.0\%$, RR = 2.691, 95% CI: 1.653 to 4.382, $P < 0.001$) (Fig. 6). 8 studies ($n = 535$) on the incidence of nausea and vomiting were no differences between the two groups ($I^2 = 50.9\%$, RR = 1.918, 95% CI: 0.805 to 4.571, $P = 0.141$).

Publication bias

Publication bias was performed using Begg' test. There were no distinct publication bias in morphine consumption (Z = 1.36, $P = 0.174$), operative time (Z = 1.17, $P = 0.240$), duration of anesthesia (Z = 1.00, $P = 0.317$), VAS score at 24 h postoperatively (Z = 1.10, $P = 0.273$), duration of postoperative analgesia (Z = -1.00, $P = 0.317$), the number of patients requiring analgesia postoperatively (Z = -0.42, $P =$ 0.677), the incidence of dizziness (Z = 0.49, $P = 0.624$), and nausea and vomiting (Z = -0.12, $P = 1.000$), except fentanyl consumption (Z = 2.23, $P = 0.026$).

Discussion

Twenty-two studies [6, 15–20] on effects of TAPB vs. QLB in postoperative analgesia were included in this meta-analysis. Overall results showed that QLB showed more effective analgesia than TAPB in regards to morphine consumption, fentanyl consumption, VAS score at 24 h postoperatively, the number of patients requiring analgesia postoperatively, and the incidence of dizziness.

Pain was regarded as the fifth vital sign by the joint commission on accreditation of medical institutions (JCAHO) in 2000, ignoring pain management equals disrespecting human rights [36]. Postoperative pain is a major concern for patients and clinicians. Inadequate management of postoperative pain remains a common clinical problem worldwide [3, 4, 37]. TAPB has been described as a successful adjunct procedure for postoperative analgesia, however with some complications: failure of block, abdominal organ injury, nerve injury, vascular injury and so on [38–40]. Fortunately, the application of ultrasound can display injection point, the tap plane and the needle. With the guidance of ultrasound, the accuracy of puncture is improved, and the related complications are reduced [13, 41]. However, TAPB only blocks the anterolateral skin, muscles and parietal peritoneal sensory nerve fibers of the abdominal wall, and has no inhibitory effect on visceral pain [42]. QLB, as an

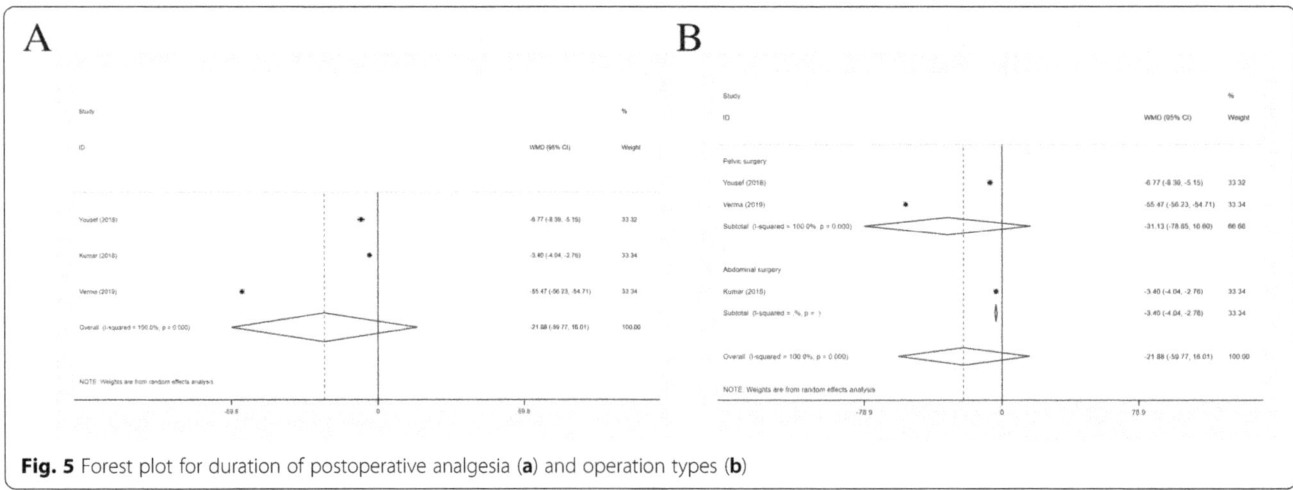

Fig. 5 Forest plot for duration of postoperative analgesia (**a**) and operation types (**b**)

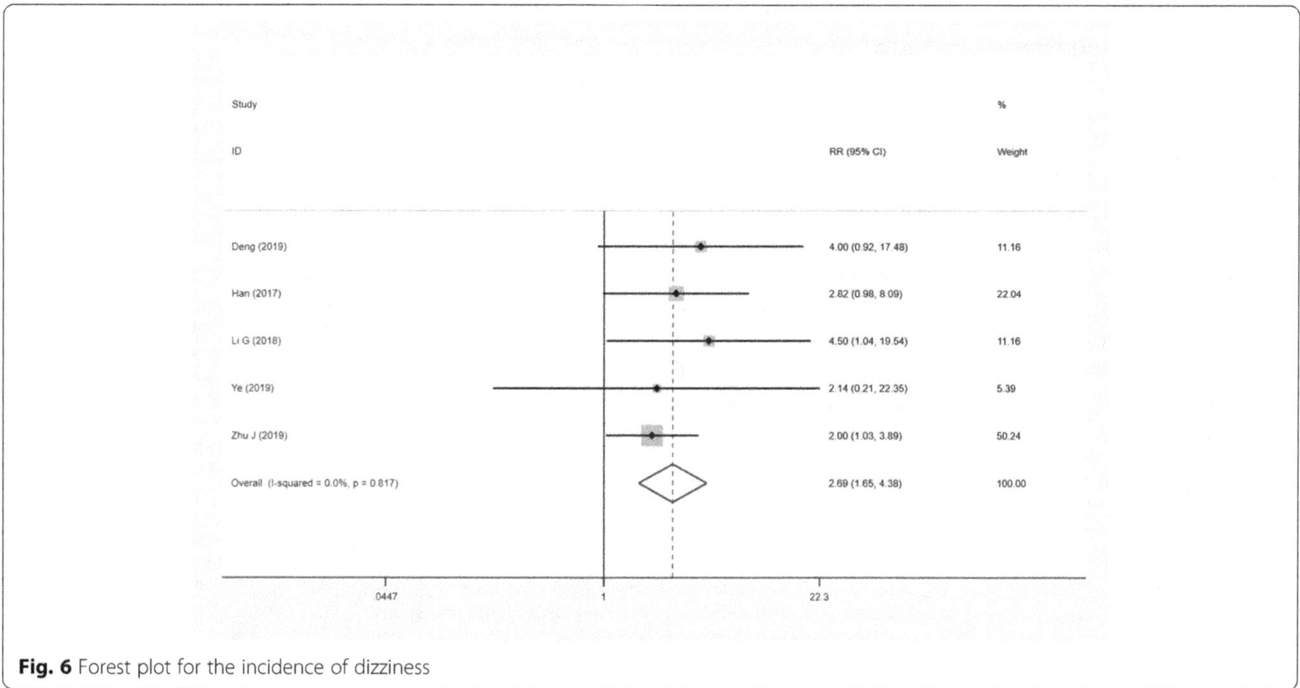

Fig. 6 Forest plot for the incidence of dizziness

effective and reliable option for relieving postoperative pain, is performed exclusively under the guidance of ultrasound, and the passage of the needle and the site of the local anesthetic application are far from the abdominal organs, great vessels and peritoneal cavity [43–47]. QLB can block the sympathetic nerves distributed between the thoracolumbar fascias. Some scholars suggested that QLB may alleviate the visceral pain to a certain extent [48]. Compared with TAPB, the drug diffusion range of QLB drugs was relatively wide, even reaching the paravertebral space of chests [49].

In this meta-analysis, VAS score at 24 h postoperatively of TAPB group was higher than that of QLB group, which may cause high consumption of analgesics. We also found that morphine and fentanyl consumption postoperatively in TAPB group were higher than QLB group. Similarly, a previous study showed that QLB type 1 significantly reduced morphine consumption up to postoperative 48 h [50]. Salama et al. found that QLB performed after cesarean section provided an ideal effect in reducing total postoperative morphine consumption [44]. The reason why the patients in TAPB group consumed more morphine than QLB group may be that TAPB only provides effective somatic analgesia, however poor effect in visceral analgesia [47]. Yousef reported that patients undergoing hysterectomy bilateral QLB provided more effective intraoperative and postoperative analgesia with less intraoperative fentanyl consumption and less postoperative morphine consumption compared with bilateral TAPB [18]. As we all know, morphine and fentanyl are common analgesic drugs for pain, and excessive use may cause several adverse reactions. Herein, it is significant for postoperative analgesia to explore an adjunct procedure that can reduce analgesia consumption.

The number of patients requiring analgesia postoperatively in QLB group was less than TAPB group. Zhu et al. [51] have studied the rate at patients who receive QLB requested analgesia postoperatively. They performed ultrasound-guided subcostal approach to QLB in an ipsilateral parasagittal oblique plane at the L1-L2 level on patients who underwent laparoscopic nephrectomy, and they reported that QLB was related with reducing rate of patients requiring rescue analgesia postoperatively. There were no significant differences in the operative time, duration of anesthesia, duration of postoperative analgesia, and nausea and vomiting between the two groups. The reasons may be less number of articles and small sample size included in this study. More high-quality studies with large samples are needed to further verify these results.

Because of representing the high level of evidences, the meta-analysis of RCTs can help patients, doctors and policy-makers to make decisions [52]. This meta-analysis was conducted to compare the effect of TAPB and QLB on postoperative analgesia based on RCT studies. However, several limitations of this study should be noted. First, heterogeneity existed in some measurements, and subgroup analyses failed to change the heterogeneity. Furthermore, there was a publication bias in fentanyl consumption, which may be attributed to the fact that the positive results were easy to publish, and only one English article and 2 low-quality studies were included in this meta-analysis. These factors mentioned above may affect our results. Therefore, the current results should be interpreted with caution.

Conclusions

In summary, compared with TAPB, QLB provided effective intraoperative and postoperative analgesia with less morphine consumption, less fentanyl consumption, lower VAS score at 24 h postoperatively, decreased number of patients requiring analgesia postoperatively, and reduced incidence of dizziness. In addition, QLB is comparable with TAPB as regards to operative time, duration of anesthesia, and the incidence of nausea and vomiting. More researches with well-designed and adequate sample size are required to confirm these findings.

Abbreviations

TAPB: Transversus abdominis plane block; QLB: Quadratus lumborum block; RCTs: Randomized controlled trials; VAS: Visual analogue scale; RR: Relative risk; WMD: Weighted mean difference; JCAHO: Joint commission on accreditation of medical institutions

Acknowledgements

Not applicable.

Authors' contributions

All authors conceived and designed the study. YQW and XJW participated in manuscript writing, data collection and data analysis. KYZ critically reviewed and edited the manuscript. All authors read and approved the final manuscript.

Author details

[1]Department of Anesthesiology, Sichuan Cancer Hospital & Institute, Sichuan Cancer Center, School of Medicine, University of Electronic Science and Technology of China, No.55, Section 4, South Renmin Road, Chengdu 610041, People's Republic of China. [2]Department of Pain management, West China Hospital, Sichuan University, Chengdu 610041, People's Republic of China.

References

1. Lovich-Sapola J, Smith CE, Brandt CP. Postoperative pain control. Surg Clin N Am. 2015;95(2):301–18.
2. Grosu I, de Kock M. New concepts in acute pain management: strategies to prevent chronic postsurgical pain, opioid-induced hyperalgesia, and outcome measures. Anesthesiol Clin. 2011;29(2):311–27.
3. Rawal N. Current issues in postoperative pain management. Eur J Anaesthesiol. 2016;33(3):160–71.
4. Wu MS, Chen KH, Chen IF, Huang SK, Tzeng PC, Yeh ML, Lee FP, Lin JG, Chen C. The efficacy of acupuncture in post-operative pain management: a aystematic review and meta-analysis. PLoS One. 2016;11(3):e0150367.
5. Chandon M, Bonnet A, Burg Y, Barnichon C, DesMesnards-Smaja V, Sitbon B, Foiret C, Dreyfus JF, Rahmani J, Laloe PA, et al. Ultrasound-guided transversus abdominis plane block versus continuous wound infusion for post-caesarean analgesia: a randomized trial. PLoS One. 2014;9(8):e103971.
6. Oksuz G, Bilal B, Gurkan Y, Urfalioglu A, Arslan M, Gisi G, Oksuz H. Quadratus lumborum block versus transversus abdominis plane block in children undergoing low abdominal surgery: a randomized controlled trial. Reg Anesth Pain Med. 2017;42(5):674–9.
7. Chakraborty A, Khemka R, Datta T. Ultrasound-guided truncal blocks: a new frontier in regional anaesthesia. Indian J anaesth. 2016;60(10):703–11.
8. Dal Moro F, Aiello L, Pavarin P, Zattoni F. Ultrasound-guided transversus abdominis plane block (US-TAPb) for robot-assisted radical prostatectomy: a novel '4-point' technique-results of a prospective, randomized study. J Robot Surg. 2019;13(1):147–51.
9. Sun N, Wang S, Ma P, Liu S, Shao A, Xiong L. Postoperative analgesia by a transversus abdominis plane block using different concentrations of ropivacaine for abdominal surgery: a meta-analysis. Clin J Pain. 2017;33(9): 853–63.
10. Ghisi D, Fanelli A, Vianello F, Gardini M, Mensi G, La Colla L, Danelli G. Transversus abdominis plane block for postoperative analgesia in patients undergoing total laparoscopic hysterectomy: a randomized, controlled, observer-blinded trial. Anesth Analg. 2016;123(2):488–92.
11. Yuan Q, Cui X, Fei Y, Xu Z, Huang Y. Transmuscular quadratus lumborum block versus thoracic paravertebral block for acute pain and quality of recovery after laparoscopic renal surgery: study protocol for a randomized controlled trial. Trials. 2019;20(1):276.
12. Bjelland TW, Yates TGR, Fagerland MW, Froyen JK, Lysebraten KR, Spreng UJ. Quadratus lumborum block for postoperative analgesia after full abdominoplasty: a randomized controlled trial. Scand J Pain. 2019; 19(4):671–8.
13. Bak H, Bang S, Yoo S, Kim S, Lee SY. Continuous quadratus lumborum block as part of multimodal analgesia after total hip arthroplasty: a case report. Korean J Anesthesiol. 2020;73(2):158–62.
14. Dhanjal S, Tonder S. Quadratus Lumborum block. In: StatPearls. Edn. Treasure Island (FL): StatPearls Publishing StatPearls Publishing LLC; 2019.
15. Kumar GD, Gnanasekar N, Kurhekar P, Prasad TK. A comparative study of transversus abdominis plane block versus quadratus lumborum block for postoperative analgesia following lower abdominal surgeries: a prospective double-blinded study. Anesth Essays Res. 2018;12(4):919–23.
16. Baytar C, Yilmaz C, Karasu D, Topal S. Comparison of ultrasound-guided subcostal transversus abdominis plane block and quadratus lumborum block in laparoscopic cholecystectomy: a prospective, randomized, controlled clinical ptudy. Pain Res Manag. 2019;2019:2815301.
17. Blanco R, Ansari T, Riad W, Shetty N. Quadratus lumborum block versus transversus abdominis plane block for postoperative pain after cesarean delivery: a randomized controlled trial. Reg Anesth Pain Med. 2016;41(6): 757–62.
18. Yousef NK. Quadratus lumborum block versus transversus abdominis plane block in patients undergoing total abdominal hysterectomy: a randomized prospective controlled trial. Anesth Essays Res. 2018;12(3):742–7.
19. Verma K, Malawat A, Jethava D, Jethava DD. Comparison of transversus abdominis plane block and quadratus lumborum block for post-caesarean section analgesia: a randomised clinical trial. Indian J Anaesth. 2019;63(10): 820–6.
20. Ipek CB, Kara D, Yilmaz S, Yesiltas S, Esen A, Dooply S, Karaaslan K, Turkoz A. Comparison of ultrasound-guided transversus abdominis plane block, quadratus lumborum block, and caudal epidural block for perioperative analgesia in pediatric lower abdominal surgery. Turk J Med Sci. 2019;49(5): 1395–402.
21. Shan T, Bao HG. Efficiency of ultrasound-guided quadratus lumborum block for postoperative analgesia in puerperants underwent cesarean section. Jiangsu Med J. 2019;45(7):704–6.
22. Zheng W: Application of quaratus lumborum block versus transversus abdominis plane block on enhanced recovery after laparoscopic radical resection of colorectal cancer. Master. Nanchang University; 2019.
23. Ma CZ, Chen QY, Lin ZX, Zhang CC, Zhang Z. Effect of ultrasound-guided quadratus lumborum block for peritoneal dialysis catheter placement. J Clin Anesthesiol. 2019;35(10):961–4.
24. Fu K, Wei JY, Zhou FF, Hu QH. Comparison for the analgesic effect after inguinal herniorrhaphy in the elderly. Jiangxi Med J. 2019;54(5):551–3.
25. Han B, Wang B, He AP. Comparison of ultrasound-guided quadratus lumborum block and transversus abdominis plane block combined with patient controlled intravenous analgesia with sufentanil on post-operation analgesia after appendectomy. J Clin Anesthesiol. 2017;33(10):984–6.
26. Ye P, Lin YL, Liu YJ, Yu ZG. Comparison of analgesia effects between ultrasound-guided quadratus lumborum block and transversus abdominis plane block with assistance of patient controlled intravenous analgesia after laparoscopic cholecystectomy. J Trauma Emerg. 2019;7(2):93–7.
27. Yang ZP, Zhao WB. Effects of ultrasound-guided quadrate lumbar block and transverse abdominal block on postoperative analgesia of gynecological tumors. Sichuan Med J. 2019;40(6):566–70.
28. Zhu J, Ma JL, Gao YP. Effect of low back quadratus block and transverse abdominis block on postoperative analgesia in elderly patients undergoing radical gastrectomy. Guizhou Med J. 2019;43(9):1368–71.
29. Li N, Yue XQ. Analgesia effect study of ultrasound-guided lumbar quadratus block after laparoscopic myomectomy. Smart Healthcare. 2019;5(9):102–5.

30. Yang YP, Sun ZP, Xu JJ. Comparison of analgesic effect of dexmedetomidine combined with different nerve block pathways after cesarean section. Zhejiang Med J. 2019;21(9):1275–6.
31. Xia ZY, Bu HL, Wang ZF, Wang ZY, Zhang W. Efficiency of ultrasound-guided quadratus lumborum block for analgesia after laparoscopic cholecystectomy. Clin J Anesthesiol. 2018;38(8):950–2.
32. Ren BL, Feng AM, Qiao YS, Wang JW, Lu XH. Comparison of the analegesic effect between quadratus lumborum block and transversus abdominis plane block in laparoscopic operation. J Xinxiang Med Univ. 2018;35(8):719–21.
33. Zhu MH, Tang Y, Xu Q, Qin Q. Chen Y: quadratus lumborum block versus transversus abdominis plane block for analgesia after total abdominal hysterectomy. Int J Anesth Resus. 2018;39(8):741–5.
34. He WQ, Li YS, Zhang XH, Yi B, Lu KZ. Comparison of quadratus lumborum block and transversus abdominis plane block for postoperative analgesia in elderly patients undergoing abdominal surgery. Clin J Anesthesiol. 2018; 38(1):40–3.
35. Li G, Mamat R, Gai DX. Postoperative analgesia efficacy of quadratus lumborum block versus transversus abdominis plane block in patients undergoing caesarean section. Int J Anesth Resus. 2018;39(4):338–40.
36. White PF, Kehlet H. Improving pain management: are we jumping from the frying pan into the fire? Anesth Analg. 2007;105(1):10–2.
37. Mahama F, Ninnoni JPK. Assessment and management of postoperative pain among nurses at a resource-constraint teaching hospital in Ghana. Nurs Res Pract. 2019;2019:9091467.
38. Baeriswyl M, Zeiter F, Piubellini D, Kirkham KR, Albrecht E. The analgesic efficacy of transverse abdominis plane block versus epidural analgesia: a systematic review with meta-analysis. Medicine. 2018;97(26):e11261.
39. Soltani Mohammadi S, Dabir A, Shoeibi G: Efficacy of transversus abdominis plane block for acute postoperative pain relief in kidney recipients: a double-blinded clinical trial. Pain Med (Malden, Mass) 2014, 15(3):460–464.
40. Baker BW, Villadiego LG, Lake YN, Amin Y, Timmins AE, Swaim LS, Ashton DW. Transversus abdominis plane block with liposomal bupivacaine for pain control after cesarean delivery: a retrospective chart review. J Pain Res. 2018; 11:3109–16.
41. Jin Y, Li Y, Zhu S, Zhu G, Yu M. Comparison of ultrasound-guided iliohypogastric/ilioinguinal nerve block and transversus abdominis plane block for analgesia after cesarean section: a retrospective propensity match study. Exp Ther Med. 2019;18(1):289–95.
42. Kargar R, Minas V, Gorgin-Karaji A, Shadjoo K, Padmehr R, Mohazzab A, Enzevaei A, Samimi-Sadeh S, Kamali K, Khazali S. Transversus abdominis plane block under laparoscopic guide versus port-site local anaesthetic infiltration in laparoscopic excision of endometriosis: a double-blind randomised placebo-controlled trial. BJOG. 2019;126(5):647–54.
43. Murouchi T, Iwasaki S, Yamakage M. Quadratus lumborum block: analgesic effects and chronological ropivacaine concentrations after laparoscopic surgery. Reg Anesth Pain Med. 2016;41(2):146–50.
44. Salama ER. Ultrasound-guided bilateral quadratus lumborum block vs. intrathecal morphine for postoperative analgesia after cesarean section: a randomised controlled trial. Korean J Anesthesiol. 2020;73(2):121–8.
45. Zhu Q, Li L, Yang Z, Shen J, Zhu R, Wen Y, Cai W, Liu L. Ultrasound guided continuous Quadratus Lumborum block hastened recovery in patients undergoing open liver resection: a randomized controlled, open-label trial. BMC Anesthesiol. 2019;19(1):23.
46. Ueshima H, Hiroshi O. Intermittent bilateral anterior sub-costal quadratus lumborum block for effective analgesia in lower abdominal surgery. J Clin Anesth. 2017;43:65.
47. Akerman M, Pejcic N, Velickovic I. A review of the quadratus lumborum block and ERAS. Front Med (Lausanne). 2018;5:44.
48. Putzu M, Gambaretti E, Rizzo F, Latronico N. Postoperative analgesia for laparotomic surgery provided by bilateral single-shot quadratus lumborum block. Minerva Anestesiol. 2018;84(10):1231–2.
49. Hussein MM. Ultrasound-guided quadratus lumborum block in pediatrics: trans-muscular versus intra-muscular approach. J Anesth. 2018;32(6):850–5.
50. Mieszkowski MM, Mayzner-Zawadzka E, Tuyakov B, Mieszkowska M, Zukowski M, Wasniewski T, Onichimowski D. Evaluation of the effectiveness of the quadratus lumborum block type I using ropivacaine in postoperative analgesia after a cesarean section - a controlled clinical study. Ginekol Pol. 2018;89(2):89–96.
51. Zhu M, Qi Y, He H, Lou J, Pei Q, Mei Y. Analgesic effect of the ultrasound-guided subcostal approach to transmuscular quadratus lumborum block in patients undergoing laparoscopic nephrectomy: a randomized controlled trial. BMC Anesthesiol. 2019;19(1):154.
52. Young D. Policymakers, experts review evidence-based medicine. Am J Health Syst Pharm. 2005;62(4):342–3.

17

Effectiveness of wound infusion of 0.2% ropivacaine by patient control analgesia pump after minithoracotomy aortic valve replacement

Gordan Mijovski[1*], Matej Podbregar[1], Juš Kšela[2], Matej Jenko[1] and Maja Šoštarič[1]

Abstract

Background: Local anesthetic wound infusion has become an invaluable technique in multimodal analgesia. The effectiveness of wound infusion of 0.2% ropivacaine delivered by patient controlled analgesia (PCA) pump has not been evaluated in minimally invasive cardiac surgery. We tested the hypothesis that 0.2% ropivacaine wound infusion by PCA pump reduces the cumulative dose of opioid needed in the first 48 h after minithoracothomy aortic valve replacement (AVR).

Methods: In this prospective, randomized, double-blind, placebo-controlled study, 70 adult patients (31 female and 39 male) were analyzed. Patients were randomized to receive 0.2% ropivacaine or 0.9% saline wound infusion by PCA pump for 48 h postoperatively. PCA pump was programmed at 5 ml h^{-1} continuously and 5 ml of bolus with 60 min lockout. Pain levels were assessed and recorded hourly by Numeric Rating Scale (NRS). If NRS score was higher than three the patient was administered 3 mg of opioid piritramide repeated and titrated as needed until pain relief was achieved. The primary outcome was the cumulative dose of the opioid piritramide in the first 48 h after surgery. Secondary outcomes were frequency of NRS scores higher than three, patient's satisfaction with pain relief, hospital length of stay, side effects related to the local anesthetic and complications related to the wound catheter.

Results: The cumulative dose of the opioid piritramide in the first 48 h after minithoracotomy AVR was significantly lower ($p < 0.001$) in the ropivacaine (R) group median 3 mg (IQR 6 mg) vs. 9 mg (IQR 9 mg). The number of episodes of pain where NRS score was greater than three median 2 (IQR 2), vs 3 (IQR 3), ($p = 0.002$) in the first 48 h after surgery were significantly lower in the ropivacaine group, compared to control. Patient satisfaction with pain relief in our study was high. There were no wound infections and no side-effects from the local anesthetic.

(Continued on next page)

* Correspondence: gord@healthgrouper.com
[1]Department of Anaesthesiology and Surgical Intensive Therapy, University Medical Centre Ljubljana, Faculty of Medicine, University of Ljubljana, Zaloška cesta 2, 1000 Ljubljana, Slovenia

(Continued from previous page)

Conclusions: Wound infusion of local anesthetic by PCA pump significantly reduced opioid dose needed and improves pain control postoperatively. We have also shown that it is a feasible method of analgesia and it should be considered in the multimodal pain control strategy following minimally invasive cardiac surgery.

Keywords: Wound catheter, PCA, AVR, Minithoracotomy, Multimodal analgesia

Background

Multimodality in pain management, during and after surgery, has long been established and well accepted [1]. Since, it has become a central part of most enhanced recovery protocols and its use has received high evidence level and strong recommendation [2, 3]. Despite the wide acceptance of the concept and the ever greater focus on postoperative pain relief and fast tracking of patients there are numerous reports of suboptimal pain management [4, 5]. While wound infusion catheter is becoming more and more popular way of pain relief management after surgery [6], opioids are still a mainstream medication for pain relief after cardiac surgery. The concept of multimodal analgesia implies combining medications with different mechanisms of action to achieve effective postoperative pain relief while avoiding their adverse effects, mainly those of opioids [7]. The most frequent side effects of opioid analgesics being respiratory depression, nausea, constipation and pruritus [8–11]. To avoid these side effects of opioid medications postoperatively, they are often combined with NSAIDs in cardiac surgery [12–14]. Still, opioids have remained the main analgesia of choice following cardiac surgery in the early postoperative period and serve as a reference point to which most analgesic protocols are compared to.

Delivering local anesthetic through a wound catheter was proven to be a successful way of postoperative pain relief throughout most surgical fields [15–17]. In cardiac surgery however, it has produced mixed results when used after full sternotomy [18–21]. The increasing use of minimally invasive surgical techniques in heart surgery offers more opportunities for successfully implementing multimodality by administering local anesthetic through a wound catheter. The effectiveness of wound infusion of 0.2% ropivacaine delivered by patient controlled analgesia (PCA) pump has not been evaluated in minimally invasive cardiac surgery.

We designed a prospective, randomized, double-blind, placebo-controlled trial, to analyze the effectiveness of wound infusion of 0.2% ropivacaine delivered by patient control analgesia (PCA) pump for pain relief after minimally invasive right anterior minithoracotomy aortic valve replacement (AVR).

Methods

This study was approved by the National Medical Ethics Committee of Republic of Slovenia (No. MZ 0120–145/2016–3, 10.06.2016) and registered at ClinicalTrials.gov (NCT03079830). The study was conducted in a tertiary level university hospital from March 2017 to January 2018. With this prospective, randomized, double-blind, placebo-controlled study we analyzed the effectiveness of wound infusion of local anesthtetic 0,2% ropivacaine after minimally invasive - right anterior minithoracotomy AVR. The study adheres to the CONSORT guidelines for reporting research.

All patients were preoperatively given a detailed description of the study by an anesthetist. After obtaining written consent, the patients were familiarized with the numeric rating scale (NRS) for pain evaluation where "0" represents no pain and "10" represents worst possible pain.

The protocol we describe was a result of a small pilot study we carried out before the main study. Inclusion criteria were all adult patients scheduled to have an elective right anterior minithoracotomy AVR who consented to be included in the study. Preoperative exclusion criteria were patients not consenting to the study, emergency surgery, patients allergic to local anesthetic and patients with chronic pain syndromes. Postoperative exclusion criteria were reoperation in the first 48 h after surgery and prolonged need for intubation postoperatively. In total 76 adult patients scheduled to have an elective right anterior minithoracotomy AVR were randomly allocated into two groups. All patients were operated by the same surgical team and all patients received the same sutureless aortic valve (Perceval - LivaNova PLC, London, UK).

All patients were premedicated one hour before the surgery with 5 mg diazepam orally. Fentanyl 5–10 μg kg^{-1}, ethomidate 0.2 mg kg^{-1} were used as induction agents and rocuronium 0.6 mg kg^{-1} was used as neuromuscular blocking drug. Intubation was performed with a single lumen tube. Total intravenous anesthesia was maintained with 0.3 μg kg^{-1} min^{-1} remifentanyl and 5 mg kg^{-1} h^{-1} propofol. Standard haemodynamic monitoring for cardiac surgery was used during the procedure. Our standard monitoring includes direct arterial blood pressure, central venous pressure, transoesophageal echocardiography, body temperature, urinary catheter and cerebral oximeter.

At the end of the operation after wound closure, the surgeon inserted a 7.5 cm long wound catheter (PAINfusor - Plan 1 Health Srl, Amaro UD, Italy) by using an introducer needle. The catheter was placed above the ribs in the deep subcutaneous tissue followed by a bolus of 10 ml of 0.75% ropivacaine through the catheter (Fig. 1). We administered a bolus of 0.75% ropivacaine to patients of both groups at the end of the operation, regardless of the group they were randomized to as we were using an ultra short-acting opioid for maintaining analgesia perioperatively. A PCA pump (Mini Rythmic Evolution, Micrel Medical Devices SA - Athens, Greece) was connected to the catheter and started in theatre at 5 ml h^{-1}. Before stopping the remifentanil infusion at the end of the operation all patients were administered 2.5 g i.v. metamizole, a non-opioid analgesic. After the operation patients were admitted to the ICU. Once patients met the standard extubation protocol requirements they were extubated (Tab1). The feasibility of intervention was evaluated in a pilot study of 20 patients, as part of protocol development of the RCT.

The patients were randomized into two groups: Study group - R (ropivacaine) - 38 patients and Control group - C (0.9% saline) - 38 patients. A dedicated nurse that was not part of the performing anesthetic team was in charge of the randomization process. Randomization was done by covariate adaptive randomization using an on-line program for randomization at www.graphpad.com. The dedicated nurse who was the only person to know which group the patient was randomized to, prepared the mixtures. The bags containing both mixtures were of same shape, taped and covered with aluminum foil.

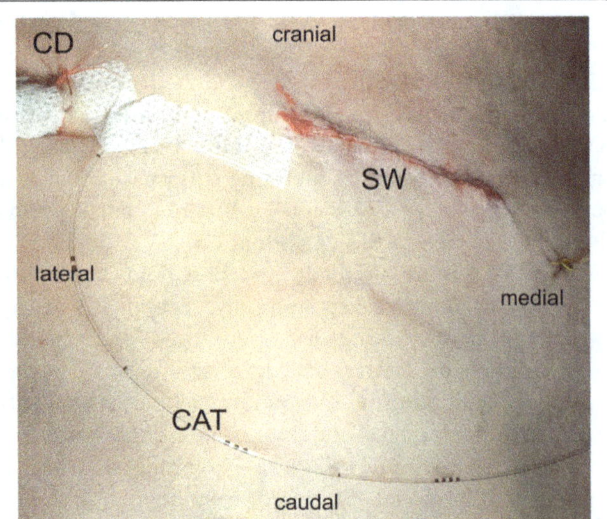

Fig. 1 Wound catheter position. CAT-wound catheter, CD-chest drain, SW-surgical wound

The anesthetist in the operating theatre, the intensivists and the nurses in the ICU and HDU were all blinded to which group a patient was randomized to. The PCA pump was programmed the same way for both groups, to continuously administer the mixture at 5 ml h^{-1} and a bolus of 5 ml if needed with a lock out time of 60 min.

1. Patients in the ropivacaine group were administered 5 ml h^{-1} of 0.2% ropivacaine continuously per PCA pump through the wound catheter and a single 5 ml bolus if needed with 60 min of lock-out time.
2. Patients in the 0,9% saline group were administered 5 ml h^{-1} of 0.9% saline continuously per PCA pump through the wound catheter and a single 5 ml bolus if needed with 60 min of lock-out time.

Postoperatively in the ICU, patients in both groups regularly received metamizole 2,5 g/12 h i.v. Once the patient was awake, extubated and able to communicate, the ICU nurse hourly assessed and recorded the pain level by NRS score, except when patients were asleep. If the pain level was higher than three, the patient at first administered a bolus of 5 ml of the mixture delivered by the PCA pump through the wound catheter. If the NRS pain score remained higher than three, 15 min after the PCA bolus, the patient was administered i.v. bolus of 3 mg piritramide - an opioid 0.75 times as potent as morphine [22], by a nurse or physician, repeated and titrated as needed until pain relief was achieved. The wound infusion was administered during the first 48 h after surgery when the catheter was removed. The patients were continuously clinically assessed for side effects related to local anesthetic - neurotoxicity and cardiotoxicity, and complications related to the wound catheter - wound infection or delayed healing.

The dedicated nurse using Stratified Randomization randomly selected 20 patients to have total plasma ropivacaine concentration measured (ten from each group). Also 20 patients (ten from each group) were randomly selected, using the same method, to have the tips of wound catheters' sent for microbiology analysis after removal. Venous blood samples for total plasma ropivacaine concentration were taken at 1 h, 24 h and 48 h after surgery. The blood samples were centrifuged immediately at 3000 rpm for 5 min and plasma was aspirated and pipetted into a separate tube. The tubes with the plasma samples were then frozen at $-60°$ and analyzed after all the samples from all 20 patients were taken.

The primary outcome of our study was the cumulative dose of the opioid piritramide required in the 48 h after surgery, compared between the two groups. Our secondary outcomes were the frequency of NRS scores higher

Table 1 Extubation criteria in the ICU

Parameter	Values
Consciousness	Alert, obeys simple commands
Ventilation	Spontaneous, respiratory rate 10–18/min, TV ≥ 6 ml/kg, SaO2 ≥ 94% on FiO2 ≤ 0.35
Haemodynamics	MAP 60–80 mmHg, heart rate 50–90 beats/min, no signs of myocardial ischemia nor vasoplegia
Bleeding	≤ 2 ml/kg/h in first two hours
Body temperature	Between 37 °C–36 °C

MAP - mean arterial pressurre; TV - tidal volume

than three, patients' satisfaction with the pain relief, the time to recovery and discharge from hospital, side effects related to local anesthetic and complications related to the wound catheter. Patients' satisfaction with the pain relief was assessed on the third postoperative day by anesthetist trainees, that were blinded of the treatment allocation, on a patient satisfaction scale with the possible answers ranging from 1.completely satisfied, 2.satisfied, 3.neither satisfied nor dissatisfied, 4.dissatisfied, to 5.completely dissatisfied.

Statistical analysis

Before carrying out the main study, we performed a small pilot study with 20 patients, to assess the feasibility of the method and for sample size calculations. Results are based on the primary outcome, piritramide consumption in the first 48 h after surgery. To achieve 85% of statistical power at least 35 patients per group had to be included into the study. Effect size for our calculaction was 1.09. Groups of patients were compared by Mann-Whitney U test or $\chi 2$ test where appropriate. P -value below 0.05 was used for statistical significance. Statistical analysis was performed using the R project, a language and environment for statistical computing - R Foundation for Statistical Computing, Vienna, Austria.

Results

Overall, 76 eligible patients consented to participate in the study. Postoperatively 3 patients from the ropivacaine group and 2 patients from the 0.9% saline group were excluded due to occlusion of the wound catheter. Also, one patient from the 0.9% saline group was excluded due to prolonged need for intubation postoperatively, not related to the wound catheter. Thirty-five patients in each group completed the study and their results were analyzed (Fig. 2). Patients in both groups had similar baseline demographic (Tab. 2) and clinical characteristics (Tab. 3).

The primary outcome of the cumulative dose of the opioid piritramide in the first 48 h after minithoracotomy AVR was significantly lower ($p < 0.001$, Mann-Whitney U test) in the ropivacaine group. The median cumulative dose of piritramide in 48 h in the ropivacaine group was 3 mg (IQR 6 mg). The median dose of piritramide in the 0.9% saline group was 9 mg (IQR 9 mg). We found that the difference between the two groups was statistically significant ($p < 0.001$), (Fig. 3).

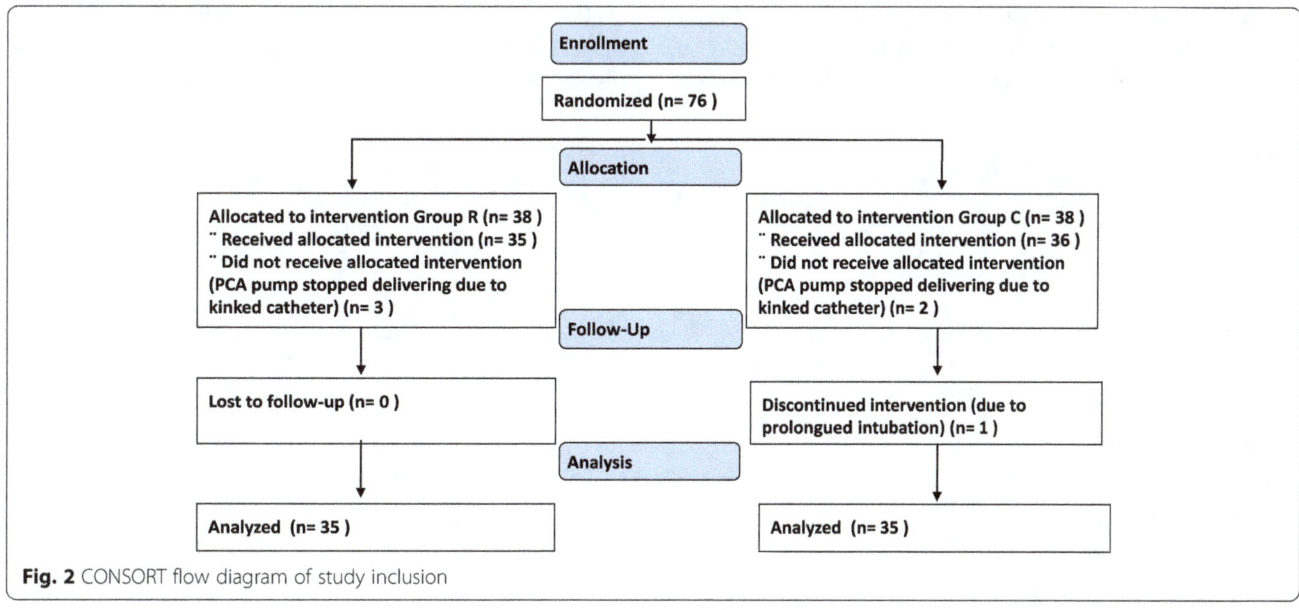

Fig. 2 CONSORT flow diagram of study inclusion

Table 2 Demographic data for both groups

Demographic data	Ropivacaine group	0,9% saline group	*P* value
No. of patients studied	35	35	
Age, median (25th–75th percentilles) in years	76 (69–78)	76 (72–81)	0.083[1]
Female	15	16	0.810[2]
Male	20	19	
No. of patients smoking	7	6	0.758[2]

1 – Mann-Whitney U test 2 – χ^2 test

Among the secondary outcomes, only the frequency of NRS scores higher than three in the first 48 h postoperatively reached statistical significance ($p = 0.002$). The median number of episodes of pain where NRS score was greater than three in the ropivacaine group was 2 (IQR2). The median in the 0.9% saline group was 3 (IQR 3) (Fig. 4).

The median patient satisfaction with the pain relief measured by patient satisfaction scale ranging from 1-best to 5-worst, in the ropivacaine group was 1 (IQR 1). The median patient satisfaction with the pain relief in the 0.9% saline group was 2 (IQR 1). There was no significant difference between the two groups regarding pain relief satisfaction, Mann-Whitney U test, $p = 0.130$ (Fig. 5).

The median length of hospital stay in the ropivacaine group was 8 days (IQR 4 days). The median length of hospital stay in the 0.9% saline group was 8 days (IQR 2 days). There was no significant difference between the two groups in length of hospital stay, Mann-Whitney U test, $p = 0.652$ (Fig. 6).

There were no clinical signs of local anesthetic neurotoxicity nor cardiotoxicity in any one of the patients studied. No sample reached the maximum tolerated total plasma level of ropivacaine of 2.2 mg l^{-1} as suggested by an earlier study on volunteers [23]. There were no clinical signs of wound infection nor delayed wound healing in any of the patients studied. All twenty tips of the wound catheters, (ten from each group) that were sent for microbiology analysis returned sterile.

Discussion

The results of our study have shown that by administering a local anesthetic using a PCA pump there was a significant reduction of the opioid dose needed postoperatively. We also found significantly lower frequency of NRS scores higher than three in the ropivacaine group.

In recent decade, minimally invasive cardiac surgery has gained momentum in everday clincal practice mainly due to continuously growing medical technological innovations, progress in surgical techniques and advancement in anesthesiological experitse, involving modified patient monitoring, innovations in anesthesia drug delivery pathways, and utilization of short-acting anesthetics and multimodality in pain management.

Effective postoperative pain relief through multimodal approach is the goal every perioperative team aims to achieve. Improving postoperative analgesia leads to faster mobilizing, higher patient satisfaction and better surgical results [24, 25]. Even though the multimodal pain relief is central to most enhanced recovery protocols, it has been widely accepted that the treatment

Table 3 Clinical data for both groups

Clinical data median (25th–75th percentilles)	Ropivacaine group	0,9% saline group	P value
Euroscore II	1.35 (0.99–2.01)	1.56 (1.17–2.15)	0.173[1]
CPB time in minutes	60 (54–69)	66 (58–77)	***0.047***[1,3]
Cross clamp time in minutes	33 (30–37)	36 (32–45)	0.057[1]
Time of surgery in minutes	136 (122–145)	144 (132–154)	0.101[1]
Time to extubation in minutes	120 (120–180)	120 (120–180)	0.703[1]
PCA boluses attempted	2 (1–4)	4 (2–6)	***0.022***[1,3]
PCA boluses given	2 (1–4)	3 (2–5)	***0.021***[1,3]
No. of patients with PONV	7	8	0.778[2]

1 – Mann-Whitney U test, 2 – χ^2 test
3-statistically significant difference

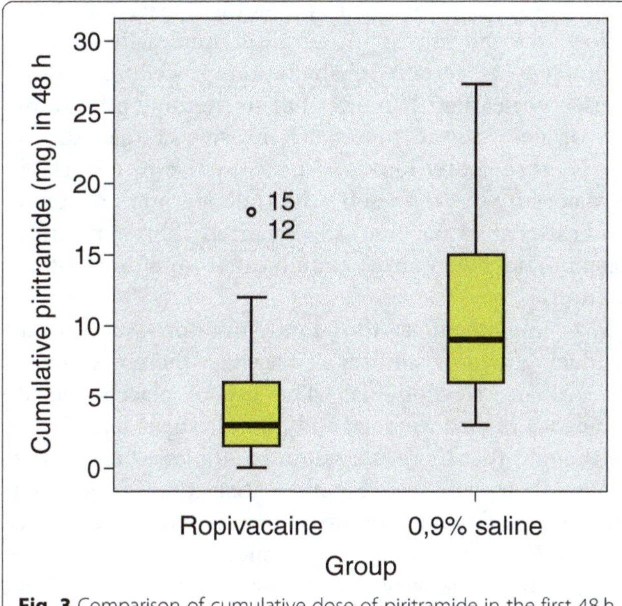

Fig. 3 Comparison of cumulative dose of piritramide in the first 48 h postoperatively between the ropivacaine group and the 0.9% saline group

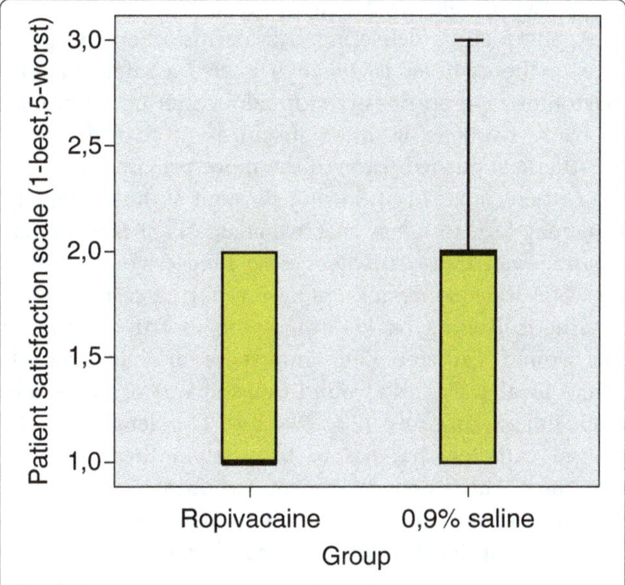

Fig. 5 Comparison of patient satisfaction between the ropivacaine group and the 0,9% saline group

improvements need to be achieved at every step of the recovery process [2, 3], while at the same time also emphasizing the importance of adapting the protocols for each patient individually [26]. Using a PCA pump for delivering a local anesthetic in the surgical wound is a step closer to personalizing the multimodal analgesia to every patient. So far, most of the reports that studied wound infusion of local anesthetics have used an elastomeric pump as a delivery system [18, 27, 28]. To our knowledge, this is the first study that evaluates the effectiveness of PCA delivered local anesthetic at a mini-thoracotomy wound for AVR. Administering local anesthetic by PCA pump has certain advantages over an elastomeric pump. However, this concept assumes that the setting allows for an intensive care nurse or a physician to be available during the 48 h postoperatively to

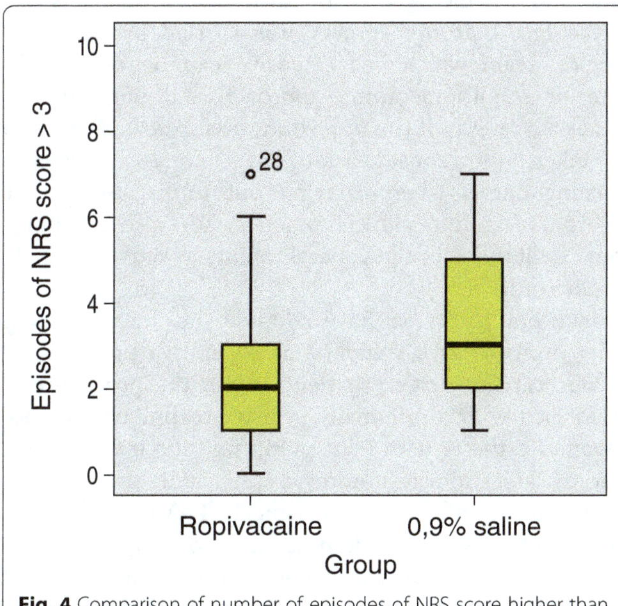

Fig. 4 Comparison of number of episodes of NRS score higher than three in the first 48 h postoperatively between the ropivacaine group and the 0,9% saline group

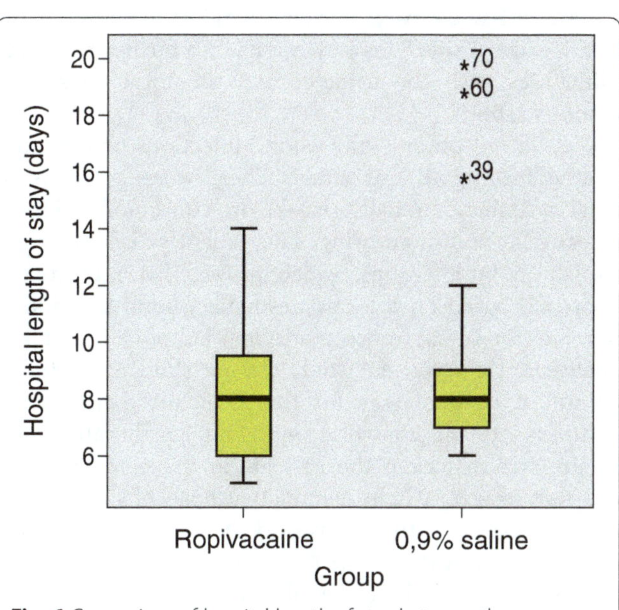

Fig. 6 Comparison of hospital length of stay between the ropivacaine group and the 0,9% saline group

administer opioid i.v. when needed. The fact that the PCA pump stops delivering and alarms when the pressure in the catheter is too high is also a safety system. Elastomeric pump doesn't stop administering, and what probably happens in these instances is that the local anesthetic is pushed through the more proximal holes of the catheter instead of flowing through all holes equally. This may lead to a less effective analgesia at the surgical wound, even more so when using longer wound catheters. Not least, some authors have reported cases of local anesthetic leaking back through the insertion point of the wound catheter [29], and there are also reports where local anesthetic wound infusion was of no benefit after full sternotomy [20, 29, 30]. The length of the wound catheter that has to be used in these patients combined with a delivery system without pressure alarm, may play a role. On the other hand using a PCA pump for delivering local anesthetic also allows the patient to administer a bolus, if needed. We had also encountered and had to overcome some technical difficulties as there is also a learning curve with correctly placing the catheter. During the pilot study we tested two ways of placing the wound catheter, one before wound closure and the other after the wound was closed. Placing the catheter before wound closure resulted in too many catheter occlusions probably due to the subcutaneous or the intradermal sutures causing the wound catheter to kink. We then realized that most patients undergoing AVR procedure, had only a thin muscle tissue if any, above the ribs II and III to serve as a cushion between the skin and the ribs which makes the catheter more likely to kink. Therefore inserting the wound catheter into the deep subcutaneous tissue and importantly after the wound was closed prevents kinking of the catheter at this sugical site. This way, we had no further technical difficulties with the catheter and the local anesthetic administration.

We did not observe any wound infections or impaired wound healing in this study. There were no signs of local anesthetic toxicity, based on continuous clinical assessment and monitoring. The patient satisfaction was similar in both groups, which proves that multimodal approach based on a local anesthetic wound infusion is not inferior to the more traditional i.v. opioid centered analgesia. However, our study did not show a shortened length of hospital stay for the local anesthetic group compared to the control group. This can be attributed to the fact that even the patients in the control group did not receive a large cumulative dose of opioid. We acknowledge that there was also the effect of the bolus of 0.75% ropivacaine that we administered to both groups at the end of the operation. It was done for ethical reasons as we were using an ultra short-acting opioid during the surgery. It is also important for the whole postoperative team (physiotherapists, nurses) to follow the advances in surgical minimally invasive techniques as certain rehabilitation procedures can be carried out earlier than after full sternotomy procedures. We argue that the minimally invasive cardiac surgery needs a separate recovery pathway from the classic cardiac surgery approach with full sternotomy. Other medical centers have already reported shorter length of hospital stay than in our study after minithoracotomy AVR [31].

We implemented the randomisaiton successfully, producing groups similary at baseline, thereby reducing the risk of selection bias. The use of placebo ensure avoidance of performance and measurement bias. It may be thought that there is a potential of bias when patients report their pain scores and satisfaction subjectively. However as this is randomized placebo-controlled study, the subjectivity probably influences patients in both groups the same way due to practitioner and patient blinding, thereby avoid the risk of bias arising in the main findings. Another limitation of our study is that patients in both groups received a bolus of 0.75% ropivacaine at the end of the operation in line with the ethical requirements for this study. Furthermore the multimodal protocol also included metamizole a non-opioid analgesic administered to patients in both groups regularly. Therefore, we may be critisized that baseline analgesic requirement and pain were relatively low, such that a prominent effect of continuous wound infiltration is hard to demonstrate. However, as we did show a significant difference this concern did not materialize in our study. Thus we are confident that our findings are valid and reliable. An additional limitation of our study is the fact that the surgery was carried by the same surgical team which has extensive experience in right anterior minithoracotomy approach. Although this is rather a strength of the procedure performed, it needs to be taken into consideration as it creates a steeper learning curve, when carrying out future analysis or incorporation into clinical practice. We also recognize some limitations in the generalisability as ours is a single center study.

Since our study, we have adopted the described pain relief protocol as a standard postoperative protocol for all our cardiac surgery patients when the procedure is performed with a minimally invasive technique. We use a wound catheter with PCA pump for all our minithoracotomy and ministernotomy AVRs, and also for our minithoracotomies for transapical TAVI procedures. The protocol is also made possible by our organisational structure which provides continuous monitoring of cardiac patients at least for the first 48 h, from ICU to HDU, where a nurse can check for pain levels hourly and administer an opioid bolus if needed.

Conclusion

We found that wound infusion of local anesthetic by PCA pump significantly reduced opioid dose needed postoperatively. We have also shown that it is a feasible multimodal method of analgesia and it is in our opinion better suited to minimally invasive surgical techniques. Patient satisfaction with pain relief in our study was high. Therefore, we conclude that infusion of local anesthetic by PCA pump should be included in the multimodal pain control method following minimally invasive surgery.

Abbreviations

AVR: Aortic valve replacement; HDU: High dependency unit; ICU: Intensive care unit; NSAIDs: Nonsteroidal anti-inflammatory drugs; PCA: Patient controlled analgesia; RCT: Randomized controlled trial; NRS: Numeric rating scale

Acknowledgements

Not applicable.

Authors' contributions

GM designed the study, recruited patients, collected data, analysed data, wrote the first draft. MP helped with the study design, contributed to writing the manuscript. JK was part of the surgical team, helped with the correct placement of catheter and reviewed the manuscript. MJ helped with the statistics, analysed data, interpreted the results. MŠ designed the study, recruted patients, treated patients in ICU, contributed to writing the manuscript. All authors have read and approved the manuscript.

Author details

[1]Department of Anaesthesiology and Surgical Intensive Therapy, University Medical Centre Ljubljana, Faculty of Medicine, University of Ljubljana, Zaloška cesta 2, 1000 Ljubljana, Slovenia. [2]Department of Cardiovascular Surgery, University Medical Centre Ljubljana, Faculty of Medicine, University of Ljubljana, Ljubljana, Slovenia.

References

1. Kehlet H, Dahl JB. The value of "multimodal" or "balanced analgesia" in postoperative pain treatment. Anesth Analg. 1993;77(5):1048–56.
2. Batchelor TJP, Rasburn NJ, Abdelnour-Berchtold E, Brunelli A, Cerfolio RJ, Gonzalez M, Ljungqvist O, Petersen RH, Popescu WM, Slinger PD, et al. Guidelines for enhanced recovery after lung surgery: recommendations of the enhanced recovery after surgery (ERAS(R)) society and the European Society of Thoracic Surgeons (ESTS). Eur J Cardiothorac Surg. 2019;55(1):91–115.
3. Gustafsson UO, Scott MJ, Hubner M, Nygren J, Demartines N, Francis N, Rockall TA, Young-Fadok TM, Hill AG, Soop M, et al. Guidelines for perioperative Care in Elective Colorectal Surgery: enhanced recovery after surgery (ERAS((R))) society recommendations: 2018. World J Surg. 2019;43(3): 659–95.
4. Sommer M, de Rijke JM, van Kleef M, Kessels AG, Peters ML, Geurts JW, Gramke HF, Marcus MA. The prevalence of postoperative pain in a sample of 1490 surgical inpatients. Eur J Anaesthesiol. 2008;25(4):267–74.
5. Apfelbaum JL, Chen C, Mehta SS, Gan TJ: Postoperative pain experience: results from a national survey suggest postoperative pain continues to be undermanaged. Anesth Analg 2003, 97(2):534–540, table of contents.
6. Thompson C, French DG, Costache I. Pain management within an enhanced recovery program after thoracic surgery. J Thorac Dis. 2018; 10(Suppl 32):S3773–s3780.
7. Buvanendran A, Kroin JS. Multimodal analgesia for controlling acute postoperative pain. Curr Opin Anaesthesiol. 2009;22(5):588–93.
8. Cashman JN, Dolin SJ. Respiratory and haemodynamic effects of acute postoperative pain management: evidence from published data. Br J Anaesth. 2004;93(2):212–23.
9. Pattinson KT. Opioids and the control of respiration. Br J Anaesth. 2008; 100(6):747–58.
10. Babul N, Provencher L, Laberge F, Harsanyi Z, Moulin D. Comparative efficacy and safety of controlled-release morphine suppositories and tablets in cancer pain. J Clin Pharmacol. 1998;38(1):74–81.
11. Ahmedzai S, Brooks D. Transdermal fentanyl versus sustained-release oral morphine in cancer pain: preference, efficacy, and quality of life. The TTS-fentanyl comparative trial group. J Pain Symptom Manag. 1997;13(5):254–61.
12. Fayaz MK, Abel RJ, Pugh SC, Hall JE, Djaiani G, Mecklenburgh JS. Opioid-sparing effects of diclofenac and paracetamol lead to improved outcomes after cardiac surgery. J Cardiothorac Vasc Anesth. 2004;18(6):742–7.
13. Maddali MM, Kurian E, Fahr J. Extubation time, hemodynamic stability, and postoperative pain control in patients undergoing coronary artery bypass surgery: an evaluation of fentanyl, remifentanil, and nonsteroidal antiinflammatory drugs with propofol for perioperative and postoperative management. J Clin Anesth. 2006;18(8):605–10.
14. Rafiq S, Steinbruchel DA, Wanscher MJ, Andersen LW, Navne A, Lilleoer NB, Olsen PS. Multimodal analgesia versus traditional opiate based analgesia after cardiac surgery, a randomized controlled trial. J Cardiothorac Surg. 2014;9:52.
15. Forastiere E, Sofra M, Giannarelli D, Fabrizi L, Simone G. Effectiveness of continuous wound infusion of 0.5% ropivacaine by on-Q pain relief system for postoperative pain management after open nephrectomy. Br J Anaesth. 2008;101(6):841–7.
16. Aguirre J, Baulig B, Dora C, Ekatodramis G, Votta-Velis G, Ruland P, Borgeat A. Continuous epicapsular ropivacaine 0.3% infusion after minimally invasive hip arthroplasty: a prospective, randomized, double-blinded, placebo-controlled study comparing continuous wound infusion with morphine patient-controlled analgesia. Anesth Analg. 2012;114(2):456–61.
17. Chan SK, Lai PB, Li PT, Wong J, Karmakar MK, Lee KF, Gin T. The analgesic efficacy of continuous wound instillation with ropivacaine after open hepatic surgery. Anaesthesia. 2010;65(12):1180–6.
18. Dowling R, Thielmeier K, Ghaly A, Barber D, Boice T, Dine A. Improved pain control after cardiac surgery: results of a randomized, double-blind, clinical trial. J Thorac Cardiovasc Surg. 2003;126(5):1271–8.
19. White PF, Rawal S, Latham P, Markowitz S, Issioui T, Chi L, Dellaria S, Shi C, Morse L, Ing C. Use of a continuous local anesthetic infusion for pain management after median sternotomy. Anesthesiology. 2003;99(4):918–23.
20. Magnano D, Montalbano R, Lamarra M, Ferri F, Lorini L, Clarizia S, Rescigno G. Ineffectiveness of local wound anesthesia to reduce postoperative pain after median sternotomy. J Card Surg. 2005;20(4):314–8.
21. Amour J, Cholley B, Ouattara A, Longrois D, Leprince P, Fellahi JL, Riou B, Hariri S, Latremouille C, Remy A, et al. The effect of local anesthetic continuous wound infusion for the prevention of postoperative pneumonia after on-pump cardiac surgery with sternotomy: the STER NOCAT randomized clinical trial. Intensive Care Med. 2019;45(1):33–43.
22. Hinrichs M, Weyland A. Bantel C: [Piritramide : A critical review]. Schmerz. 2017;31(4):345–52.
23. Knudsen K, Beckman Suurkula M, Blomberg S, Sjovall J, Edvardsson N. Central nervous and cardiovascular effects of i.v. infusions of ropivacaine, bupivacaine and placebo in volunteers. Br J Anaesth. 1997;78(5):507–14.
24. Peters ML, Sommer M, de Rijke JM, Kessels F, Heineman E, Patijn J, Marcus MA, Vlaeyen JW, van Kleef M. Somatic and psychologic predictors of long-term unfavorable outcome after surgical intervention. Ann Surg. 2007; 245(3):487–94.
25. Beaussier M, El'Ayoubi H, Schiffer E, Rollin M, Parc Y, Mazoit JX, Azizi L, Gervaz P, Rohr S, Biermann C, et al. Continuous preperitoneal infusion of ropivacaine provides effective analgesia and accelerates recovery after colorectal surgery: a randomized, double-blind, placebo-controlled study. Anesthesiology. 2007;107(3):461–8.
26. Shepherd SJ, Klein AA, Martinez G. Enhanced recovery for thoracic surgery in the elderly. Curr Opin Anaesthesiol. 2018;31(1):30–8.
27. Hoenecke HR Jr, Pulido PA, Morris BA, Fronek J. The efficacy of continuous bupivacaine infiltration following anterior cruciate ligament reconstruction. Arthroscopy. 2002;18(8):854–8.
28. Kushner DM, LaGalbo R, Connor JP, Chappell R, Stewart SL, Hartenbach EM. Use of a bupivacaine continuous wound infusion system in gynecologic oncology: a randomized trial. Obstet Gynecol. 2005;106(2):227–33.
29. Florkiewicz P, Musialowicz T, Hippelainen M, Lahtinen P. Continuous Ropivacaine infusion offers no benefit in treating postoperative pain after cardiac surgery. J Cardiothorac Vasc Anesth. 2019;33(2):378–84.

30. Eljezi V, Imhoff E, Bourdeaux D, Pereira B, Farhat M, Schoeffler P, Azarnoush K, Duale C. Bilateral sternal infusion of ropivacaine and length of stay in ICU after cardiac surgery with increased respiratory risk: a randomised controlled trial. Eur J Anaesthesiol. 2017;34(2):56–65.
31. Glauber M, Gilmanov D, Farneti PA, Kallushi E, Miceli A, Chiaramonti F, Murzi M, Solinas M: Right anterior minithoracotomy for aortic valve replacement: 10-year experience of a single center. J Thorac Cardiovasc Surg 2015, 150(3): 548–556.e542.

18

Interscalene brachial plexus block for surgical repair of clavicle fracture

Magnus Olofsson[1*], Patrick Taffé[2], Kyle Robert Kirkham[3], Frédéric Vauclair[4], Bénédict Morin[1] and Eric Albrecht[1]

Abstract

Background: Innervation of the clavicle is complex and debated, with scarce data on the analgesic and clinical impact of regional anaesthesia after surgical repair of clavicle fracture.

Methods: In order to assess the analgesic efficiency of an interscalene brachial plexus block (ISB) for surgical repair of clavicle fracture, 50 consecutive patients scheduled for surgical fixation of middle/lateral clavicle fracture under general anaesthesia with ISB were prospectively enrolled. This cohort was compared to a historical control of 76 retrospective patients without regional block. The primary outcome was total intravenous morphine equivalent consumption at 2 postoperative hours. To assess the ISB impact, both an overall cohort analysis and a case-matched analysis with each ISB-treated patient matched to a Non-ISB-treated patient was performed. Matching employed a 1-to-1, nearest-neighbour approach using the Mahalanobis metric.

Results: In the overall cohort, patients with ISB had significantly lower i.v. morphine equivalent consumption at 2 postoperative hours (0.7 mg (95% CI 0.1 to 1.2) versus controls 8.8 mg (95% CI 7.1 to 10.4); $P < 0.0001$). These results persisted after case-matching the cohorts (mean difference for the primary outcome: 8.3 mg (95% CI 6.5 to 10.0); $P < 0.001$).

Conclusions: ISB provides effective analgesia after surgical fixation of middle and lateral clavicle fracture. These results should help physicians in establishing an analgesic strategy for this type of surgery. Further research is needed to identify the optimal regional technique for medial third clavicle fractures and the clinically relevant contributions of the cervical and brachial plexus.

Keywords: Clavicle, Locoregional anaesthesia, Pain, Surgery, Postoperative, Ultrasound, Brachial plexus

Background

Surgical fixation of clavicular fractures may result in moderate to severe postoperative pain that does not always respond well to opioid therapy. If effective, a regional technique may therefore represent an analgesic improvement with the potential to reduce postoperative opioid consumption [1–3]. However, innervation of the clavicle remains a source of much debate. A recent report illustrated the state of current anatomic knowledge on this topic suggesting that contributions might come from: the cervical plexus through the supraclavicular nerve or from the brachial plexus with contributions from the subclavian nerve, the long thoracic nerve or the suprascapular nerve [4]. This anatomic uncertainty means anaesthetists struggle to determine the optimal analgesic strategy [4–6]. Furthermore, to date there has been no study that evaluates the analgesic efficacy of an interscalene brachial plexus block in patients with

* Correspondence: ms.olofsson@gmail.com
[1]Department of Anaesthesia, Lausanne University Hospital, Rue du Bugnon 46, BH 05.311, 1011 Lausanne, Switzerland

clavicular fractures. With the goal to resolve this clinical dilemma, we undertook a matched case-control cohort study assessing the analgesic impact of ultrasound-guided interscalene brachial plexus block (US-ISB) for patients scheduled for open reduction and internal fixation (ORIF) of middle or lateral clavicle fracture.

Methods

We followed the recommended process described in the Strengthening the Reporting of Observational Studies in Epidemiology (STROBE) statement [7].

Recruitment

After approval by the Lausanne University Hospital Ethics Committee (Commission d'Ethique Romande, protocol number CHUV 317/15, Chairperson Prof. André Pannatier) on 26th October 2015, this study was prospectively registered on clinicaltrials.gov (NCT02565342). All patients aged 18 to 70 years, American Society of Anesthesiologists score (ASA) I-II, scheduled for middle or lateral clavicle fracture ORIF at the Lausanne University Hospital were eligible to participate in this study. Exclusion criteria included existing neurological deficit in the upper limb, history of neck surgery or radiotherapy, moderate to severe pulmonary disease, contraindications to peripheral nerve block (e.g., allergy to local anaesthetics, coagulopathy, infection in the area), pre-existing opioid treatment, any distracting pain (i.e. polytraumatized patients), pregnancy and cognitive or psychiatric condition that might affect patient assessment. All surgeries were performed electively. Written informed consent was obtained prior to the day of surgery.

Ultrasound-guided interscalene brachial plexus block

All US-ISB were performed prior to surgery in a dedicated block procedure room, following an extrafascial approach without nerve stimulation [8–10]. These blocks were administered or directly supervised by one of the authors (EA) who had no further involvement in the study protocol. Patients were positioned supine with the head turned 45 degrees to the non-operative side. Electrocardiogram, pulse oximetry, and blood pressure monitors were routinely applied, and supplemental oxygen was provided. Peripheral intravenous (i.v.) access was established and midazolam 1 to 4 mg i.v. was administered for anxiolysis and sedation as needed. The needle insertion site was sterilized with a solution of chlorhexidine 2% in isopropyl alcohol 70%. Under sterile conditions, a high-frequency linear array transducer (18–6 MHz, HF Linear Array 8870, BK Ultrasound, Peabody, Massachusetts) was placed over the interscalene region to visualize the carotid artery and brachial plexus in the short axis view. The C5, C6, and C7 roots were identified as described by Martinoli and colleagues [11]. After skin infiltration with 1 to 3 mL of lidocaine 1%, a 22-gauge 50-mm insulated block needle (SonoPlex Stim cannula, Pajunk®, Geisingen, Germany) was inserted in-plane with the US beam on the lateral side of the transducer. The needle was then advanced under direct US guidance through the middle scalene muscle and toward the lateral border of the brachial plexus sheath. The brachial plexus sheath was identified as the linear hyperechoic layer surrounding the roots of the brachial plexus. The final needle tip was positioned extrafascially, about 3 to 5 mm laterally to the brachial plexus sheath, at a depth equidistant between C5 and C6 roots. All patients received 20 mL of bupivacaine 0.5% with epinephrine 1: 200,000 through the block needle without repositioning, except in cases of reported paraesthesia.

Intraoperative and postoperative procedure

After application of routine monitors in the operating theatre, patients received a standard general anaesthetic. Anaesthesia was induced using Sufentanil 0.1 to 0.2 $\mu g\,kg^{-1}$ i.v. and Propofol 2 to 4 $mg\,kg^{-1}$ i.v. with endotracheal intubation facilitated by rocuronium 0.6 $mg\,kg^{-1}$ i.v. Maintenance of anaesthesia was via inhaled sevoflurane 1.6 to 2.4% in a 40:60 mixture of oxygen and air. Positive pressure ventilation was initiated with tidal volume and rate adjusted to maintain an end-tidal PCO_2 of 35 to 40 mmHg. Sufentanil 2.5–5.0 μg i.v. was administered as needed to treat increases in blood pressure or heart rate of more than 15% above pre-induction baseline values. Muscle relaxation was antagonized with neostigmine 50 $\mu g\,kg^{-1}$ and glycopyrrolate 5 to 10 $\mu g\,kg^{-1}$ at the end of surgery. In the Post-Anesthesia Care Unit (PACU), pain (numeric rating scale [NRS] ≥ 4 or patient request for analgesia) was treated with i.v. morphine 1–2 mg every 10 min as needed for 2 h following our institutional procedure. Once oral intake was initiated, patients received oral acetaminophen 1000 mg every 6 h and oxycodone 5 mg every 4 h as needed. Antiemetic medications on the ward included ondansetron 4 mg i.v. and metoclopramide 10 mg i.v. as needed.

Block assessment and definition of successful block

Assessment of sensory and motor blocks was performed by a research assistant every 5 min after local anaesthetic injection, for a total duration of 30 min. Sensory block was tested in the C5 and C6 dermatomes using a blunt tip needle pinprick test (0, no perception; 1, decreased sensation; 2, normal sensation). Motor block was tested using arm abduction (C5), and forearm flexion (C6) (inability to overcome gravity, 0; reduced force compared to contralateral arm, 1; no loss of force, 2). A successful block was defined as complete sensory (score, 0) and motor (score, 0) block in the distribution of the C5 and C6 nerve roots within 30 min of performing the US-ISB block.

Outcomes

The primary outcome was total i.v. morphine consumption at 2 postoperative hours upon departure from the PACU. Secondary outcomes were intraoperative Sufentanil administration; i.v. morphine equivalent consumption at 24 postoperative hours; pain scores at rest (NRS 0–10) at 2 and 24 postoperative hours; and rate of postoperative nausea and vomiting (PONV) within 24 postoperative hours. Opioids were converted into equianalgesic doses of i.v. morphine for analysis (i.v. morphine 10 mg = oral oxycodone 20 mg) [3, 12].

Control cohort selection

All patients aged 18 to 70 years old, ASA score I-II, who had undergone middle or lateral clavicle fracture ORIF under general anaesthesia only, between September 2012 and August 2015 at the same institution as this study was conducted, were included in the historical control cohort. Exclusion criteria included pre-existing opioid tolerance, any distracting pain (i.e. polytraumatized patients), pregnancy and cognitive or psychiatric condition that might affect patient pain assessment. All surgeries were performed electively. The data was collected using the surgical calendar software in use at our institution.

Statistical analysis and matching procedure

Categorical variables are presented as frequencies and continuous variables are summarized as mean values with 95% confidence intervals (95% CI). In the preliminary analysis, ISB-treated and Non-ISB-treated patients were compared using the Student's t test or Mann–Whitney U test for continuous variables, and the Fisher's exact test or Pearson Chi-square test for categorical variables, as appropriate. To assess the impact of the US-ISB procedure on the outcomes, we matched each ISB-treated patient with a Non-ISB-treated patient and computed the difference in means. The matching procedure was 1-to-1 nearest-neighbour matching using the Mahalanobis metric [13]. Therefore, for each exposed (ISB) individual, one unexposed (Non-ISB) individual, having the smallest possible Mahalanobis distance between the two vectors of covariates, (patients' and intervention characteristics), was selected, and reversely for each non-exposed individual. Patients characteristics considered for the matching procedure were the gender, the age, the body mass index, the ASA score, the fracture location, the total dose of Propofol at induction and the duration of surgery. The standardized mean differences were computed for each variable before and after matching to assess the performance of the matching procedure (i.e. balance checking). We also used a logistic regression approach to assess whether some variables (gender, age, body mass index, ASA score, fracture location) were associated with the allocation of US-ISB. Significance was considered at $P < 0.05$ based on a two-tailed probability. Statistical analyses were performed using the Stata 15 statistical package (Stata Corporation, College Station, Texas, U.S.A.).

Results

Fifty patients with an US-ISB were prospectively included and compared with 76 patients who did not receive an interscalene brachial plexus block. All US-ISBs attempted were successful. Table 1 presents patients' characteristics.

Primary outcome

Before matching, patients who received the US-ISB had a significantly lower i.v. morphine equivalent consumption at 2 postoperative hours (0.7 mg (CI 95% 0.1 to 1.2)) compared to control patients (8.8 mg (CI 95% 7.1 to 10.4); $P < 0.0001$; Fig. 1). After matching, the mean difference was 8.3 mg (95% CI 6.5 to 10.0), which remained significant ($P < 0.001$). The logistic regression analysis results indicated that none of the patients' characteristics were associated with US-ISB group allocation, suggesting equivalent cohort selection for both the control and intervention groups (Additional file 1).

Secondary outcomes

Tables 2 and 3 shows the secondary outcomes before and after the matching procedure respectively. All secondary

Table 1 Patient characteristics and clinical data presented as means (95% confidence interval) or percentages as appropriate

	Control group ($n = 76$)	US-ISB group ($n = 50$)	p value
Gender (male / female)	82% / 18%	84% / 16%	0.73
Age (years)	35 (32–38)	36 (32–41)	0.66
Height (cm)	177 (175–179)	177 (174–180)	0.94
Weight (kg)	74 (71–76)	75 (71–78)	0.67
Body Mass Index (kg.m^{-2})	23.4 (22.7–24.1)	23.6 (22.8–24.4)	0.67
ASA (I / II)	53% / 47%	50% / 50%	0.77
Fracture location (middle / distal)	78% / 22%	72% / 28%	0.47
Total dose of Propofol at induction (mg)	249 (231–267)	265 (242–287)	0.29
Duration of surgery (minutes)	96 (89–104)	101 (94–108)	0.35

ASA American Society of Anaesthesiologists

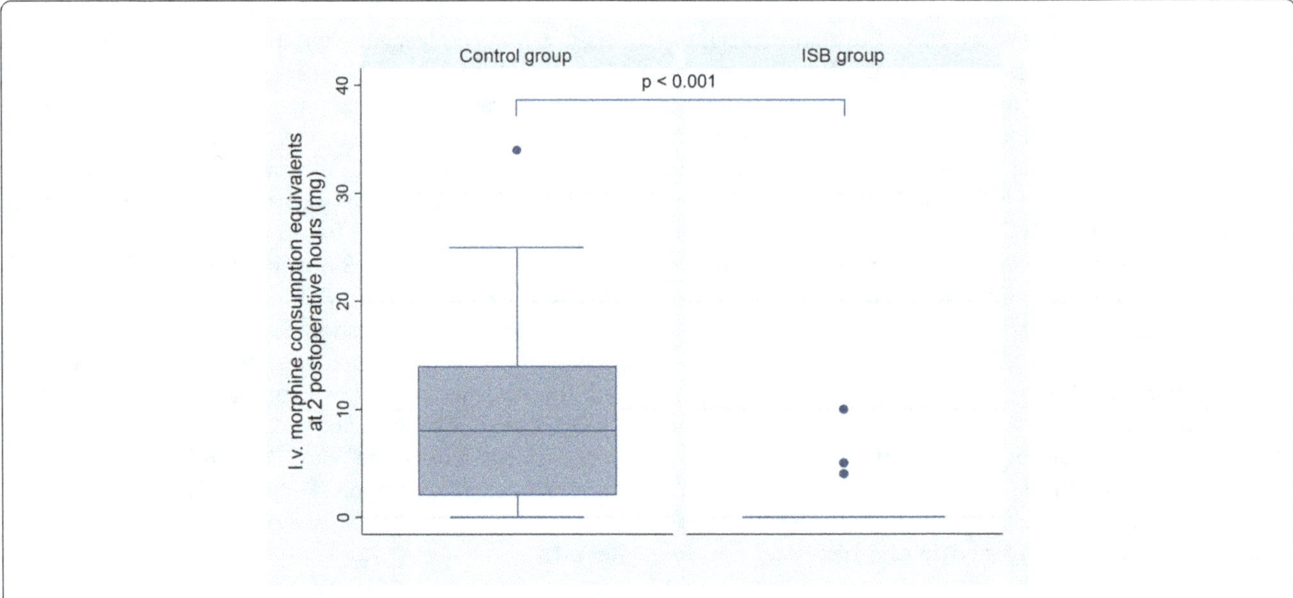

Fig. 1 I.v. morphine consumption equivalents at 2 postoperative hours (mg). Data are expressed as the median with 25th and 75th percentiles (box), along with upper adjacent and lower adjacent values (whiskers)

outcomes were significantly lower in the US-ISB group, before and after the matching procedure, except resting pain scores and rate of PONV at 24 postoperative hours. Patients who received the US-ISB consumed significantly less Sufentanil intraoperatively with a mean difference of 28 µg (24-33 µg, $P < 0.001$). This also translated into lower pain scores for the US-ISB group in the PACU with a mean difference of 1.7 (0.8–2.5, $P < 0.001$) and lower morphine equivalent consumption at 24 h. Although the rate of PONV at 24 h did not retain a significant difference after the matching procedure, it is noteworthy to mention that 17% of patients who did not receive the US-ISB reported an episode of PONV at 24 h compared to 4% of patients who received the US-ISB. Balance checking results are provided in the Additional file 2.

Discussion

This matched case-control cohort study investigated the analgesic efficacy of US-ISB for patients undergoing middle or lateral clavicle fracture ORIF. Our analyses showed that, when compared with patients who did not receive the regional procedure, patients with US-ISB received less intraoperative Sufentanil, consumed less opioid in i.v. morphine equivalents at 2 and 24 postoperative hours, and reported lower resting pain scores at 2 postoperative hours.

As summarized by Tran and colleagues, the clavicle may be innervated either by the supraclavicular nerve with its origin from the cervical plexus, or by the long thoracic nerve, the suprascapular nerve or even the subclavian nerve derived from the brachial plexus; a combined innervation from both plexuses is also possible [4]. We believe that our study brings clinically relevant evidence to this anatomic dilemma and, given the analgesic impact of US-ISB on postoperative analgesia after clavicle fracture ORIF, points towards a clavicle innervated at least in part by branches from the brachial plexus. The contribution of the cervical plexus remains unclear and further studies comparing analgesia provided with an ISB or a superficial cervical plexus block, or a detailed cadaveric study, may help to clarify remaining anatomic uncertainty.

Table 2 Secondary outcomes before matching. Data are presented as means and 95% confidence intervals

	Control group ($n = 76$)	US-ISB group ($n = 50$)	p value
Perioperative Sufentanil administration (µg)	45 (42–49)	17 (15–18)	< 0.001
Pain scores at rest at 2 postoperative hours (NRS, 0–10)	2.2 (1.8–2.6)	0.6 (0.2–1.1)	< 0.001
I.v. morphine equivalent consumption at 24 postoperative hours (mg)	16.7 (14.6–18.7)	6.9 (5.1–8.8)	< 0.001
Pain scores at rest at 24 postoperative hours (NRS, 0–10)	2.0 (1.5–2.4)	2.5 (1.9–3.1)	0.12
Rate of PONV within 24 postoperative hours	17%	4%	0.02

NRS numeric rating scale, *PONV* postoperative nausea and vomiting

Table 3 Secondary outcomes after matching. Data are presented as means with 95% confidence intervals

	Difference in means	*p* value
Perioperative Sufentanil administration (μg)	28 (24–33)	< 0.001 < 0.0001
Resting pain scores at 2 postoperative hours (NRS, 0–10)	1.7 (0.8–2.5)	< 0.001
I.v. morphine equivalent consumption at 24 postoperative hours (mg)	9.9 (6.7–13.0)	< 0.001
Resting pain scores at 24 postoperative hours (NRS, 0–10)	− 0.5 (− 0.4–1.3)	0.21
Rate of PONV within 24 postoperative hours	7% (− 3–17%)	0.23

PONV postoperative nausea and vomiting

Limitations

Our study contains several limitations. First, this matched case-control cohort study suffers from the inherent weaknesses and potential biases of non-randomized interventions. Despite the inclusion of a detailed matching procedure, there may remain unknown confounding factors that might contribute to overestimation of the US-ISB's analgesic efficacy during surgical fixation of middle or lateral clavicle fractures. We believe the likelihood of this is minimal given that our logistic regression analysis suggested equivalent allocation of patients across the two cohorts. Second, it could be argued that local anaesthetic may have spread from the interscalene groove towards the superficial cervical plexus, thereby limiting interpretation of our results. However, the US-ISB technique we adopted with an extrafascial needle tip location minimizes or eliminates the risk of spread towards the superficial cervical block, as recently demonstrated [8–10]. Finally, further exploration of the medial clavicle is needed given the middle/lateral distribution of fracture in this cohort.

Conclusions

In conclusion, patients who received an US-ISB benefited from better analgesia after middle or lateral clavicle fracture ORIF, when compared with patients without US-ISB, and these results should help physicians establish an adequate analgesic strategy for managing this type of surgery. Further research is needed to identify the optimal regional technique for medial third clavicle fractures and the clinically relevant contributions of the cervical and brachial plexus.

Supplementary information

Additional file 1: Appendix 1. Logistic regression analysis. Data are presented as log odds ratios with 95% confidence interval.

Additional file 2: Appendix 2. Balance checking: standardized difference in means.

Abbreviations

ASA: American society of Anesthesiologists score; ISB: Interscalene brachial plexus block; US-ISB: Ultrasound-guided interscalene brachial plexus block; ORIF: Open reduction and internal fixation; STROBE: Strengthening the Reporting of Observational Studies in Epidemiology; PACU: Post-Anesthesia Care Unit; NRS: Numeric rating scale; PONV: Postoperative nausea and vomiting; CI: Confidence intervals

Acknowledgements

The abstract has been presented as a poster at the annual meeting of the Swiss Society of Anaesthesiology and Resuscitation SGAR/SSAR on November 9th 2018 in Interlaken, Switzerland, and at the European Society of Regional Anaesthesia and Pain Therapy ESRA congress on September 14th 2018 in Dublin, Ireland.

Authors' contributions

MO: Methodology, Investigation, Datas Curation, Writing – Original Draft, Writing – Review & Editing, Visualisation. PT: Formal Analysis. KK: Conceptualization, Validation. FV: Conceptualization, Investigation, Resources. BM: Investigation, Resources, Dats Curation. EA: Conceptulization, Methodology, Validation, Resources, Investigation, Writing – Review & Editing, Project Administration, Supervision. All authors read and approved the final manuscript.

Author details

[1]Department of Anaesthesia, Lausanne University Hospital, Rue du Bugnon 46, BH 05.311, 1011 Lausanne, Switzerland. [2]Institute of Social and Preventive Medicine (IUMSP), Lausanne University Hospital, Lausanne, Switzerland. [3]Department of Anaesthesia, Toronto Western Hospital, University of Toronto, Toronto, Canada. [4]Department of Orthopaedic, Lausanne University Hospital, Lausanne, Switzerland.

References

1. Herring AA, Stone MB, Frenkel O, Chipman A, Nagdev AD. The ultrasound-guided superficial cervical plexus block for anesthesia and analgesia in emergency care settings. Am J Emerg Med. 2012;30:1263–7.
2. Albrecht E, Morfey D, Chan V, et al. Single-injection or continuous femoral nerve block for total knee arthroplasty? Clin Orthop Relat Res. 2014;472: 1384–93.
3. Baeriswyl M, Kirkham KR, Kern C, Albrecht E. The analgesic efficacy of ultrasound-guided transversus abdominis plane block in adult patients: a meta-analysis. Anesth Analg. 2015;121:1640–54.
4. Tran DQ, Tiyaprasertkul W, González AP. Analgesia for clavicular fracture and surgery: a call for evidence. Reg Anesth Pain Med. 2013;38:539–43.
5. Tran DQ, Finlayson RJ. Reply to Drs Valdés-Vilches and Sánchez-del Águila. Reg Anesth Pain Med. 2014;39:259–60.
6. Valdés-Vilches LF, Sánchez-del Águila MJ. Anesthesia for clavicular fracture: selective supraclavicular nerve block is the key. Reg Anesth Pain Med. 2014; 39:258–9.
7. von Elm E, Altman DG, Egger M, et al. The strengthening the reporting of observational studies in epidemiology (STROBE) statement: guidelines for reporting observational studies. Lancet. 2007;370:1453–7.
8. Palhais N, Brull R, Kern C, et al. Extrafascial injection for interscalene brachial plexus block reduces respiratory complications compared with a conventional intrafascial injection: a randomized, controlled, double-blind trial. Br J Anaesth. 2016;116:531–7.
9. Albrecht E, Kirkham KR, Taffe P, et al. The maximum effective needle-to-nerve distance for ultrasound-guided interscalene block: an exploratory study. Reg Anesth Pain Med. 2014;39:56–60.
10. Albrecht E, Bathory I, Fournier N, Jacot-Guillarmod A, Farron A, Brull R.

Reduced hemidiaphragmatic paresis with extrafascial compared with conventional intrafascial tip placement for continuous interscalene brachial plexus block: a randomized, controlled, double-blind trial. Br J Anaesth. 2017;118:586–92.

11. Martinoli C, Bianchi S, Santacroce E, Pugliese F, Graif M, Derchi LE. Brachial plexus sonography: a technique for assessing the root level. Am J Roentgenol. 2002;179:699–702.
12. Baeriswyl M, Kirkham KR, Jacot-Guillarmod A, Albrecht E. Efficacy of perineural vs systemic dexamethasone to prolong analgesia after peripheral nerve block: a systematic review and meta-analysis. Br J Anaesth. 2017;119: 183–91.
13. Stuart EA. Matching methods for causal inference: a review and a look forward. Stat Sci. 2010;25:1–21.

19

Sufentanil postoperative analgesia reduce the increase of T helper *17* (Th*17*) cells and FoxP*3*⁺ regulatory T (Treg) cells in rat hepatocellular carcinoma surgical model

Yanhua Peng[1], Jinfeng Yang[1*], Duo Guo[1], Chumei Zheng[1], Huiping Sun[1], Qinya Zhang[1], Shuangfa Zou[1], Yanping Zhang[2], Ke Luo[1] and Keith A. Candiotti[2]

Abstract

Background: Surgery-related pain and opioids might exacerbate immune defenses in immunocompromised cancer patients which might affect postoperativd overall survival. Sufentanil is a good postoperative pain control drug,the present study aimed to figure out whether it effect T cell immunity in rat hepatocellular carcinoma surgical model.

Methods: A rat hepatocellular carcinoma (HCC) models was established by N-nitrosodiethylamine. Forty-eight of them were randomly divided into 3 equal groups: surgery without postoperative analgesia (Group C), surgery with morphine postoperative analgesia (Group M), surgery with sufentanil postoperative analgesia (Group S). Each animal underwent a standard left hepatolobectomy, and intraperitoneally implanted with osmotic minipumps filled with sufentanil, morphine or normal saline according to the different group. The food and water consumptions, body weight changes, locomotor activity and mechanical pain threshold (MPT) were observed. The ratio of $CD4^+/CD8^+$, proportions of Th1, Th2, Th17 and Treg cells in blood were detected using flow cytometry. The liver function and the rats' survival situation of each group were observed.

Results: The food and water consumption, locomotor activity and MPT of group C declined than those of group S and M on d1, d2, d3 ($P < 0.05$). The $CD4^+/CD8^+$ ratio and the proportion of Th1 cells were significantly higher while the proportion of Th2, Th17 and Treg cells were significantly lower in group S and group M compared with group C. The rats of group S have higher $CD4^+/CD8^+$ ratio on d3, while lower proportion of Treg cells on d7 compared with group M. The plasma ALT and AST values in group C were significantly higher than that of group S and group M on both d3 and d7. There were not significant differences in mortality rate between 3 groups.

(Continued on next page)

* Correspondence: yangjinfeng@hnca.org.cn
[1]Department of Anesthesiology, Hunan Cancer Hospital, The Affiliated Cancer Hospital of Xiangya School of Medicine, Central South University, Changsha 410013, Hunan, China

(Continued from previous page)

Conclusions: Sufentanil and morphine postoperative analgesia in HCC rats accepted hepatectomy could relieve postoperative pain, promote the recovery of liver function after surgery, alleviate the immunosuppressive effect of pain. Furthermore, Compared to morphine, sufentanil might have a slighter effect on CD4+/CD8+ ratio and Treg frequencies. Therefore, sufentanil postoperative analgesia is better than morphine in HCC hepatectomy rats.

Keywords: Sufentanil, Postoperative analgesia, Th17, Treg

Background

Hepatocellular carcinoma (HCC) is one of the most common malignant tumors, characteristic of relatively poor overall survival and increasing morbidity and mortality, which is reportedly the third cancer-related mortality worldwide [1, 2]. Surgery-related pain and opioid analgesics are factors known to adversely affect the anti-tumor immune defenses which may promote tumor growth and metastasis [3]. In view of the growing interest in the immune system in control of neoplasia, further efforts toward the discovery of a good analgesia agent for postoperative pain treatment with a reduced impaction on immunity are urgently needed.

The helper T cells were mainly divided into T helper 1(Th1), Th2, Th9, Th17, Th21, T follicular helper (Thf) and regulatory T (Treg) cells according to the function and phenotype [4, 5]. Among them, Th1, Th2, Th17 and Treg cells are more concerned in tumor immunity. Th17 cells could increase tumor progression by activating angiogenesis and immunosuppressive activities [6, 7]. Treg cells might inhibit the tumor-specific T cell-mediated immune response and have been observed increased quantity in tumor tissues or peripheral blood of patients or animal models with gastric cancer [8], ovarian cancer [9], breast cancer [10] and hepatocellular carcinoma [11].

Immune cells express appropriate receptors such as the μ receptor and toll-like receptor. Opioids modulate the immune system by binding to the μ receptor [12]. Sufentanil has a higher affinity to μ1-opioid receptor which has the closest relationship with analgesia than morphine, but the selectivity for binding to μ2 receptor is opposite which is related to adverse effects such as nausea, vomiting, respiratory depression, urinary retention, and itching, so sufentanil has stronger analgesic effect than morphine, and adverse effects are weaker than morphine [13].

The results of opioid-induced immunomodulation are conflicting in experimental and human studies. Previous studies manifested that morphine could decrease the expressions of peripheral T lymphocytes (CD3+, CD4+, CD8+) and natural killer cells (CD3+, CD56+) in vivo [14] and could increase the ratio of CD4+/CD8+ T cells and Treg populations in vitro [15]. The Epidural postoperative analgesia with ropivacaine plus sufentanil significantly decreased Blymphocytes, T-helper cells and Natural killer cells compared with patient-controlled IV analgesia (PCIA) with morphine in patients after major spine surgery [16]. However, little or nothing is known concerning the effect of sufentanil postoperative analgesia on Th17 and Treg cells. The primary purpose of this study was to observe the effects of sufentanil and morphine postoperative analgesia on immunity through analysis of CD4+/CD8+ ratio, proportion of Th1, Th2, Th17 and Treg cells using flow cytometry, and the secondary target was liver function changes and mortality in HCC rats undergoing left hepatolobectomy.

Methods

Ethics

All animal procedures were approved (Permit Number: 2015001) by the Institutional Animal Care and Use Committees of Hunan Cancer Hospital, Changsha, China on 27 March 2015, and were performed in strict accordance with recommendations of the Guide to the Care and Use of Laboratory Animals of the National Institutes of Health.

Animals

Eighty male Sprague-Dawley rats (100 ± 20 g; Center of Experimental Animals of Hunan Cancer Hospital, Hunan, China) were used in this experiment. Rats were housed under controlled conditions with a temperature of 25 ± 2 °C, relative humidity of 60 ± 10%, room air changes of 12–18 times/h and a 12 h light/dark cycle and were acclimated for 7 days before experiments. They were allowed free access to food and water.

Experimental protocol

Eighty Sprague-Dawley rats were intraperitoneal administrated with 0.19% N-nitrosodiethylamine (DENA, Sigma Aldrich, USA)(50 $mgkg^{-1}$) every 3 days for a total of 16 weeks to make HCC models [17]. After 16 weeks, 58 of these rats were successfully modeled, 48 HCC rats were randomly selected and stochasticly assigned to 3 groups by digital random method(n = 16): surgery without postoperative analgesia (Control, Group C), surgery with morphine postoperative analgesia (Group M), surgery with sufentanil postoperative analgesia (Group S). All animals underwent a standard left hepatolobectomy under 2–3% isoflurane anesthesia. Rats' abdominal region was shaved and thoroughly cleaned with complex iodine. A 2 cm midline incision was made in the abdomen. After reaching the abdomen cavity, the left lateral leaf of the liver was exposed, and the left leaves were ligated from the root and excised. A implanted osmotic minipumps (volume 2 ml, pump speed $10\mu lh^{-1}$ for 72 h, Alzet, USA) for postoperative analgesia was placed in the abdominal cavity, which is filled with morphine of 0.25 $mgKg^{-1}h^{-1}$ for 72 h in Group M [18], sufentanil of 0.25$ugKg^{-1}h^{-1}$ for 72 h in Group S (the dose of sufentanil was calculated in accordance with its analgesic potency in comparison to morphine), or 0.9% saline 10ul h^{-1} for 72 h in Group C. Finally, the muscle and skin were closed with sterile sutures. During surgery, the rats' temperatures were maintained using a thermal insulation blanket.

We measured the following parameters in each operated rat on 1 day before surgery (d0), the first, second and third day after surgery(d1, d2, d3): Food and water consumption, body weight changes. The locomotor activity was surveyed using open field test [19]. Mechanical pain threshold (MPT) comprehensively evaluated using standard von Frey monofilaments [20]. We randomly sacrificed four rats per group on 1 day before surgery (d0), six rats on the third day after surgery (d3), and all of the remaining rats on the seventh day after surgery (d7) to collect blood samples by cardiac puncturing method, and all the rats were euthanized by the method of cercical vertebra decoupling under anesthesia after collecting blood samples. The level of cluster of $CD4^+$, $CD8^+$, Th1, Th2, Th17 and Treg cells in blood were detected to assess immune function using flow cytometry on d0, d3 and d7. The serum alanine aminotransferase (ALT) and aspartate transaminase (AST) were measured to assess liver function at the same time point. The rats' survival situation of each group left after 7 days of surgery were observed.

Locomotor activity—open field test

Rats were individually exposed to the same open field (100 cm × 100 cm) for 5 min trials with an interval of 30 min between each trial. The open field behavior was videotaped using a camera that was placed above the arena. The videos were subsequently analyzed digitally using EthoVisionXT (Noldus, The Netherlands). Parameters measured were the total distance traveled throughout the arena.

Mechanical pain threshold (MPT)

Rats were placed in test cages prior to the experiment and allowed to fully acclimate to the environment for 3 h. A 0.1 to 12 g single fiber test needle was used to stimulate the position of the rat's abdominal incision about 0.5 cm perpendicular to the skin surface until the filament was slightly curved in an S shape for 5–6 s. The MPT for this region was measured using the Chaplan up-down method [21]. If the rat appears to be licking or scratching the stimulated area during the stimulation time or removing the von Frey filament, or a sudden withdrawal or jump occurs, it is recorded as a positive behavioral response.

Assessment of liver function

Blood samples were collected and sera were obtained by centrifugation in low temperature on d0, d3, d7. Serum AST and ALT were measured using the modified Jaffe rate reaction in the clinical laboratory of The Hunan Cancer Hospital, Changsha, China.

Flow cytometry

Fresh heparinized blood samples of rats were collected on d0, d3, d7. Then Peripheral Blood Mononuclear Cells (PBMCs) were isolated from blood by standard density gradient separation using Ficoll density gradient (TBD Science, China). Each specimen is divided into five equal parts in testing $CD4^+$, $CD8^+$, Th1, Th2, Th17 and Treg cells. Isolated cells were washed three times with phosphate buffer saline and used for flow cytometry. A total of 1×10^5 PBMCs prepared for were acquired for each sample. Each sample was surface stained with CD3-PE, CD4-FITC plus PE-Cy7-labeled anti-rat CD8 (BD Bioscience, USA) to detect $CD4^+$T cells, $CD8^+$T cells at room temperature for 15 min (avoid light). The subsets detection needed analyze CD4 combined with specific cytokines such as $CD4^+IFN\text{-}\gamma^+$ for Th1, $CD4^+IL\text{-}4^+$for Th2, and $CD4^+IL\text{-}17^+$ for Th17. For the Th1, Th2, Th17, samples were surface stained with CD4-FITC at room temperature for 15 min (avoid light), and subsequently stimulated for the intracellular cytokines with PE-labeled anti-rat IFN-r, PE-labeled anti-rat IL-4, PE-labeled anti-rat IL-17A(BD Bioscience, USA) respectively according to the manufacturer's instructions. The $CD4^+Foxp3^+$ phenotype was recommended for identifying the Treg. Though, samples were surface stained with CD4-FITC at room temperature for 15 min (avoid light), and subsequently intracellularly stained with a PE anti-rat Foxp3 staining kit (BD Bioscience, USA) without stimulated according to the manufacturer's instructions. Cells were detected by flow cytometry using a FACSCalibur (BD Bioscience, USA), and data were analyzed by FlowJo VX (Treestar, USA).

Statistical analysis

Data are shown as mean ± SD for normally distributed data. Probability values< 0.05 were considered statistically significant. Then the data was transferred to the computer using SPSS Statistics 25.0(IBM, USA), normally distributed data were analyzed by using a one-way ANOVA followed by a post hoc S-N-K test (Equal variances assumed) and Tamhane T2 test (Equal variances not assumed) to compare the three groups at each time point. The descriptive findings were compared using Fisher's exact test with $P < 0.0001$.

Results

The food and water consumption, body weight, locomotor activity and the pain threshold in each group—The food consumption, water consumption, locomotor activity and MPT of Group C decline to a significantly lower degree than those of Group S and M on d1, d2, d3($P < 0.05$). The food consumption, water consumption, locomotor activity and pain threshold of Group S were similar with that of Group M at each time point. There were no significant differences of the body weight between the three groups (Fig. 1).

$CD4^+/CD8^+$ratio in blood of each group—Fig. 2. A shows the flow cytometric analysis of $CD4^+$ and $CD8^+$ cells. Figure 2. B shows the statistical analysis of $CD4^+/CD8^+$ ratio. The $CD4^+/CD8^+$ ratio of Group S and Group M were significantly higher than that of Group C on d3 and d7 ($P < 0.05$). The CD4+/CD8+ ratio of Group S was significantly higher than that of Group M on d3 ($P < 0.05$).

The proportion of Th1 and Th2 cellsin blood of each group—Fig. 3. A and C shows the flow cytometric analysis of Th1 ($CD4^+IFN\text{-}\gamma^+$) and Th2 ($CD4^+IL4^+$) cells. Figure 3. B and D shows the statistical analysis of Th1 and Th2 cells. The proportion of Th1 cells of Group S and Group M were significantly higher than that of Group C on d3 and d7 ($P < 0.05$, Fig. 3. B). The proportion of Th2 cells of Group S and Group M were significantly lower than that of Group C on d3 and d7 ($P < 0.05$, Fig. 3. D). There were no statistically significant differences in proportion of Th1 and Th2 cells between Group S and Group M on d3 and d7 (Fig. 3. B and D).

The proportion Th17 and Treg cells in blood of each group—Fig. 4. A and C shows the flow cytometric

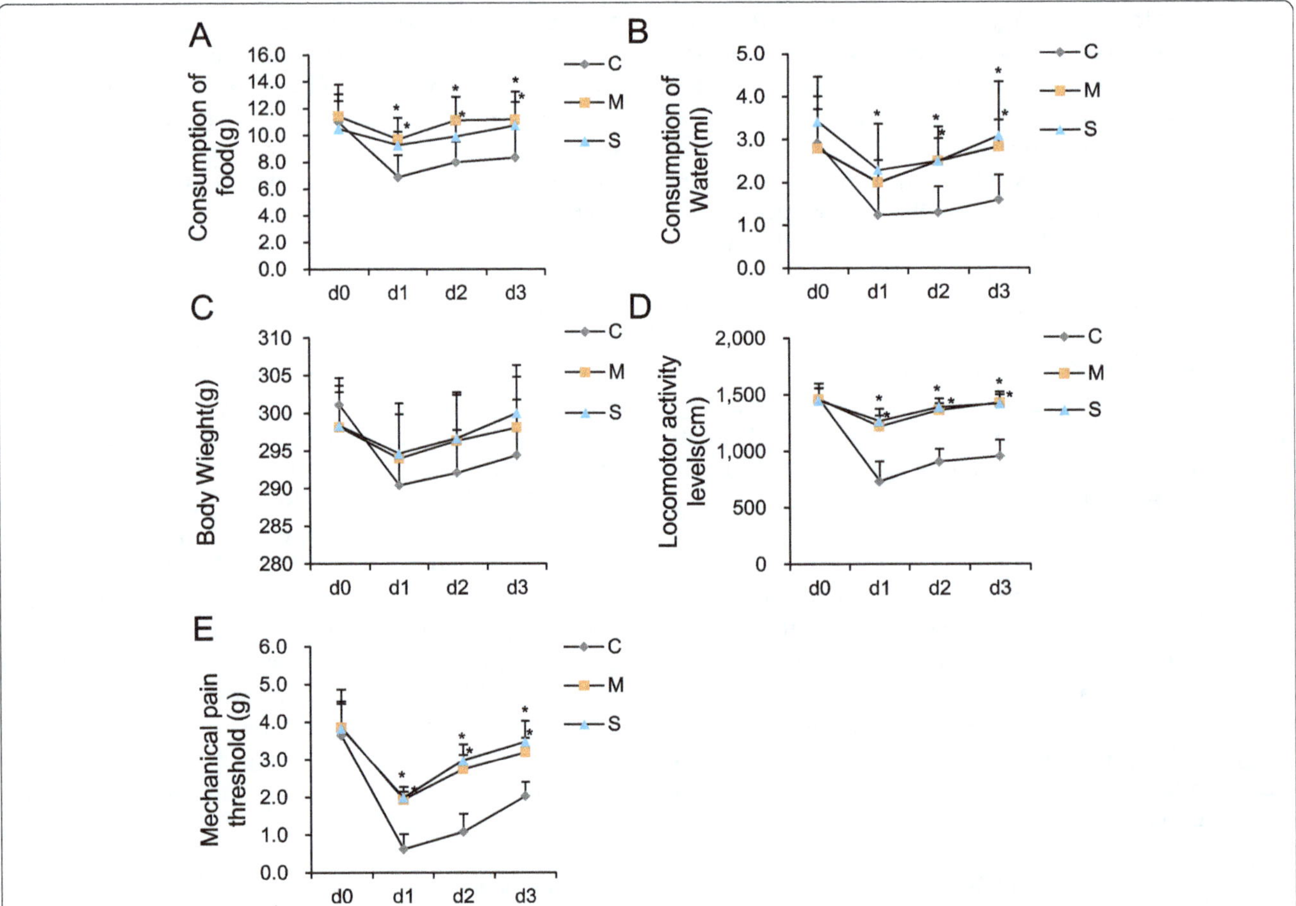

Fig. 1 The consumption of food and water, body weight, locomotor activity and the mechanical pain threshold for each of the 3 groups. **a** Statistical analysis of the consumption of food in each of the 3 groups. **b** Statistical analysis of the consumption of water in each of the 3 groups. **c** Statistical analysis of body weight in each of the 3 groups. **d** Statistical analysis of locomotor activity in each of the 3 groups. **e** Statistical analysis of the mechanical pain threshold in each of the 3 groups. The consumption of food and water, locomotor activity and mechanical pain threshold of Group C decline to a significantly lower degree than those of Group S and Group M on d1, d2, d3. *$P < 0.05$ vs Group C. d0, base line. d1, d2 and d3, first, second and third day after surgery

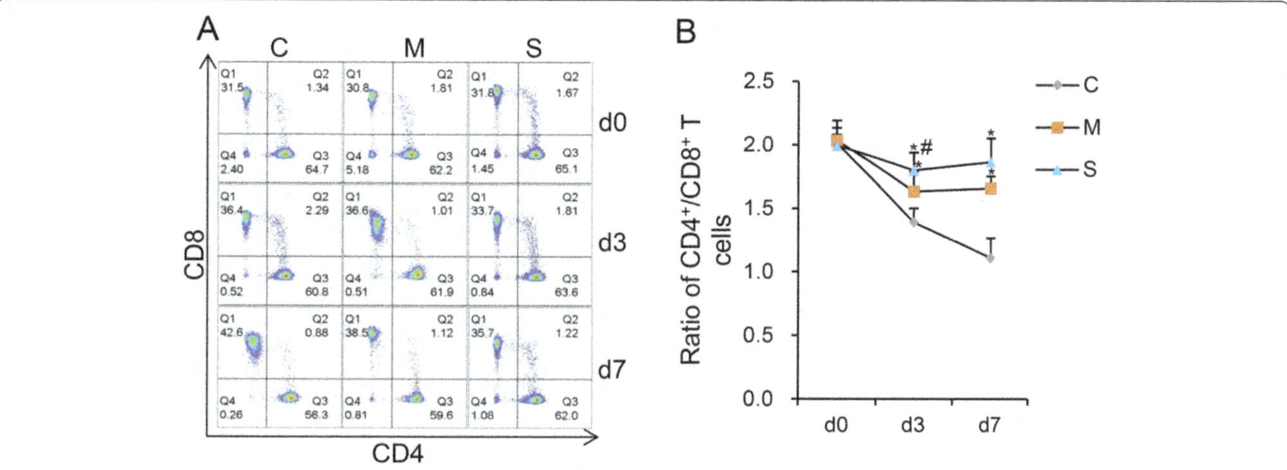

Fig. 2 The $CD4^+/CD8^+$ ratio in each of the 3 groups. **a** Flow cytometric analysis of $CD4^+$ and $CD8^+$ cells levels in the 3 groups. **b** Statistical analysis of $CD4^+/CD8^+$ ratio for each of the 3 groups. The ratio of $CD4^+/CD8^+$ in Group S and Group M was significantly higher than was noted in Group C on d3 and d7. The Group S had a higher ratio of $CD4^+/CD8^+$ than was noted in Group M on d3. *$P < 0.05$ vs Group C. # $P < 0.05$ Group S vs Group M. d0, base line, d3 and d7, third and 7th day after surgery

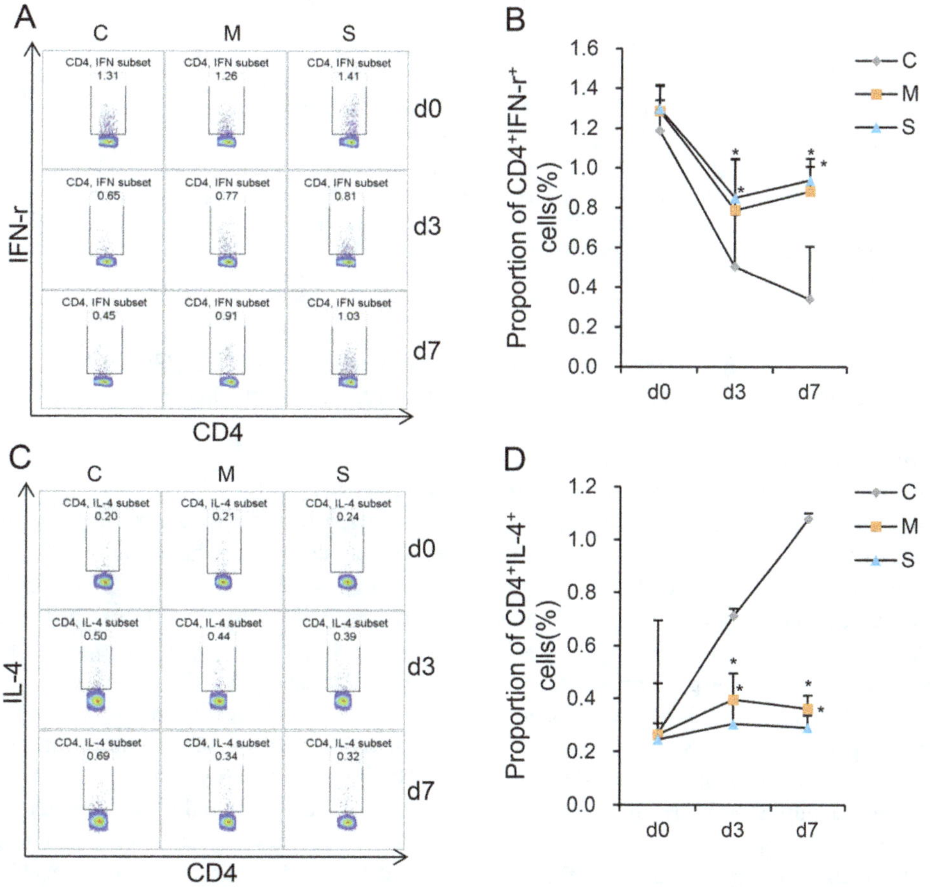

Fig. 3 Th1 and Th2 cells levels in the 3 groups. (**a** and **c**) Flow cytometric analysis of Th1 and Th2 cells levels in the 3 groups. (**b** and **d**) Statistical analysis of the proportion of Th1 and Th2 cells. The proportion of Th1 cells in Group S and Group M was significantly higher than was noted in Group C on d3 and d7. The proportion of Th2 cells in Group S and Group M, however, was significantly lower than was noted in Group C on d3 and d7. *$P < 0.05$ vs Group C. d0, base line; d3 and d7, third and 7th day after surgery

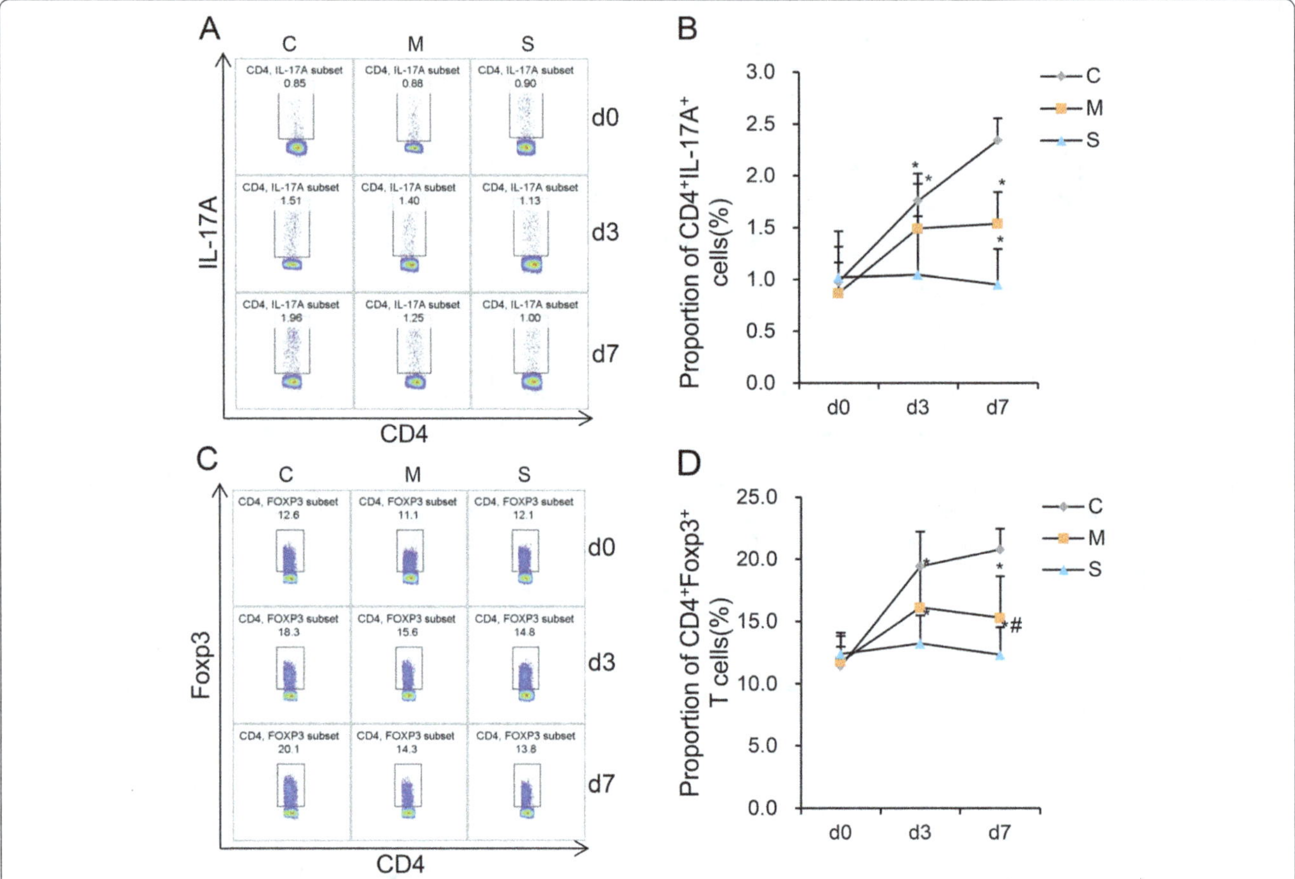

Fig. 4 Th17 and Treg cells levels in the 3 groups. (**a** and **c**) Flow cytometric analysis of Th17 and Treg cells levels in the 3 groups. (**b** and **d**) Statistical analysis of the proportion of Th17 and Treg cells. The proportion of Th17 and Treg cells in Group S and Group M was significantly lower than in Group C on d3 and d7. Compared to Group M, the proportion of Treg cells in Group S was significantly lower on d7. **P* < 0.05 vs Group C. d0, base line; d3 and d7, third and 7th day after surgery

analysis of Th17 ($CD4^+IL17\text{-}A^+$) cells and Treg ($CD4^+Foxp3^+$) cells. Figure 4. B and D shows the statistical analysis of Th17 and Treg cells. Rats showed lower proportion of Th17 and Treg cells in Group S and Group M than group C ($p < 0.05$, Fig. 4. B and D). There were no statistically significant differences in proportion of Th17 cells between Group S and Group M on d3 and d7, however, the proportion of Treg cells in Group S was significantly lower in comparison to Group M on d7 ($p < 0.05$, Fig. 4. D).

The liver function in each group after surgery—A significant increase of ALT and AST levels was observed in group C in comparison to Group S and Group M on d7($p < 0.05$). But no statistically significant difference was observed between Group S and Group M (Fig. 5. A and B).

The survival situation—Though we did not find statistically significant differences in mortality rate between postoperative analgesia rats and without analgesia rats ($P = 0.245$, Fisher's Exact Test). We did observe that two rats of Group C died respectively on fourth and fifth day after surgery, one rat of Group M died on sixth day after surgery, and no rat died in Group S.

Discussion

This study found that sufentanil and morphine postoperative analgesia rats have higher $CD4^+/CD8^+$ ratio, Th1 cells level while lower Th2, Th17 and Treg cells levels compared with that without postoperative analgesia. Sufentanil postoperative analgesia rats have higher $CD4^+/CD8^+$ratio on the third day after surgery while lower Treg cells level on the 7th day after surgery in comparison to morphine postoperative analgesia rats.

Acute postoperative pain can activate the hypothalamic–pituitary–adrenal axis, affect metabolism and cause neuroendocrine changes, which are strongly associated with postoperative outcome [12, 22, 23]. Postoperative pain relief can reduce surgery-associated cardiac, pulmonary, metabolic complications, and improve immune status which may improve the postoperative outcome [24].

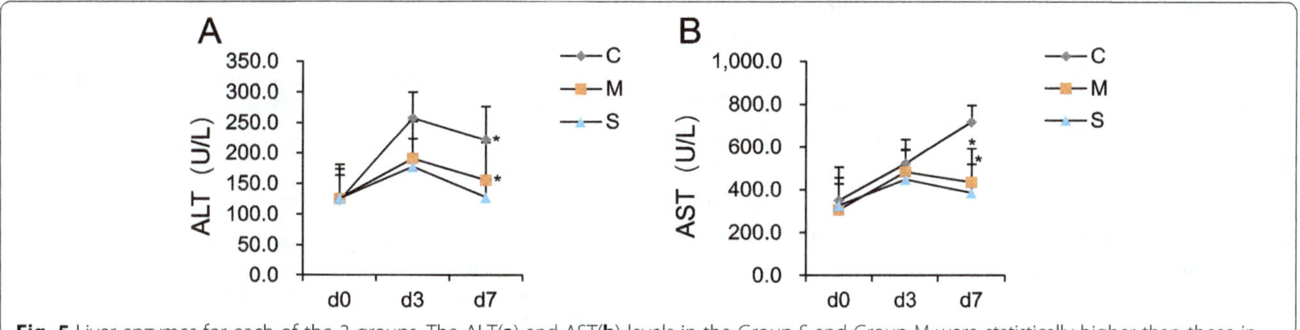

Fig. 5 Liver enzymes for each of the 3 groups. The ALT(**a**) and AST(**b**) levels in the Group S and Group M were statistically higher than those in the Group C at d7. *$P < 0.05$ vs Group C. # $P < 0.05$ Group S vs Group M. d0, base line, d3 and d7, third and 7th day after surgery

There is such a view that the interaction between $CD4^+$ and $CD8^+$ T lymphocyte mediates the control of tumor growth [25]. In a clinical study, the 5-year survival rate of cervical cancer patients with high $CD4^+$/ $CD8^+$ ratio was higher than that of patients with low $CD4^+$/ $CD8^+$ ratio, increasing the $CD4^+$/ $CD8^+$ ratio can slow the progression of cervical cancer and improve its prognosis [26]. It is generally believed that Th1 enhances tumor immune surveillance of tumor while Th2 associated with the tumor immune evasion can suppress the function of Th1 cells [27]. Th17 cells in peripheral blood are positively correlated with the progression of liver cancer [28]. Treg cells play a vital role in maintaining immunological homeostasis and exert major immunosuppressive activity [29]. A recent study has indicated that the percentages of $CD4^+CD25^+FOXP3^+$Treg cells and $CD4^+$IL-17^+Th17 cells were significantly higher in HCC patients than in the healthy individuals; Moreover, the increased percentages of Treg and Th17 cells were closely related to the tumor stage and tumor size of HCC [11]. Most published research have found that post-operative opioids inhibit cell-mediated immunity and promote tumor metastasis for both human and mouse [3]. Some patients choose to tolerate pain because of concerns about the immunosuppressive effect of analgesics. Is this appropriate? In our study, the $CD4^+/CD8^+$ratio, proportion of Th1 cells were obviously higher while proportion of Th2, Th17 and Treg cells were significantly lower in group S and group M compared with group C. Therefore, it seems that sufentanil and morphine postoperative analgesia can alleviate the immunosuppressive effect of HCC surgery and postoperative pain and is more conducive to postoperative recovery than tolerating pain.

In terms of analgesic effect, both of sufentanil and morphine can control postoperative pain. Which is better for sufentanil and *morphine* postoperative analgesia? Previous studies have demonstrated that morphine affect the signal transportation of activated T cells, thereby inhibiting T-cell activation. Morphine increases the ratio of $CD4^+/CD8^+$and Treg cells populations [15, 30, 31], shifts the balance of Th1/Th2 cells toward Th2 cells [32, 33], while in vivo studies, the ratio of $CD4^+/CD8^+$cells, the proportion of Th1 and Th17 T cell were not changed with the administration of morphine [30]. Sufentanil increased the quantity of the Tregs to a greater degree than fentanyl when the culturing was conducted in vitro, while there was no significant difference between them in vivo [34]. In a clinical trial, total $CD3^+$, $CD4^+$, $CD8^+$ cells and the ratio of $CD4^+/CD8^+$ cells in the sufentanil group were significant higher than that in the remifentanil group [35]. There are few direct comparative studies which involved in the effects of sufentanil and morphine on immunity. In our study, sufentanil and morphine have a similar effect on Th1, Th2, Th17 frequencies. Yet, the ratio of $CD4^+/CD8^+$ on d3 after surgery and the ratio of Treg cells on d7 after surgery in Group S is obviously less than that of Group S. This results indicate that sufentanil's inhibition on $CD4^+$ cells is lighter than morphine, but this inhibition may disappear with the withdrawal of the drugs. While the inhibition of sufentanil on Treg cells is less than that of morphine, but the inhibition of Treg cells may be manifested later. Recently, increasing studies have shown that there is a close positive correlation between recurrence and metastasis to the inhibition of immune system [36, 37]. Therefore, it seems that sufentanil is superior to morphine for postoperative anelgesia. The findings of the presented study provide help for the selection of postoperative analgesic drugs in clinic.

AST and ALT are important enzymes which represent liver cells function [38]. AST and ALT evidently increased can reflect severe liver cells necrosis. AST/ALT were the independent risk factors of overall survival [39]. Previous retrospective study indicated that hepatic cancer patients who underwent hepatectomy with higher ALT level had shorter mean recurrent interval than patients with lower ALT level [40]. In our study, we found that postoperative plasma ALT and AST values on the seventh day in Group S and Group M were significantly lower than in Group C. This suggests that postoperative analgesia can prevent liver function damage in HCC rats accepted hepatectomy.

There are some shortcomings in our experiment. First, we only measured the number of some T cell subsets without measuring important immune factors, such as TGF-beta, IL-6, IFN-gamma. Second, these rats' long-term survival, metastasis rates were not observed. We will evaluate these results in the future.

Conclusions

The current results have shown that sufentanil and morphine postoperative analgesia in HCC rats accepted hepatectomy can relieve postoperative pain, promote the recovery of liver function after surgery, alleviate the immunosuppressive effect of pain. Furthermore, Sufentanil postoperative analgesia is better than morphine resulted by the differences of $CD4^+/CD8^+$ ratio and Treg cells level after surgery.

Abbreviations

ALT: represent serum alanine aminotransferase; AST: represent aspartate transaminase; DENA: represent N-nitrosodiethylamine; USA: represent United States of America; HCC: represent hepatocellular carcinoma; Th: represent T helper cell; Thf: represent T follicular helper; Treg: represent regulatory T cells; MPT: represent Mechanical pain threshold; PBMCs: represent Peripheral Blood Mononuclear Cells

Acknowledgements

I would like to give my sincere gratitude to Prof. Jianbing Tong who with extraordinary patience and consistent encouragement gave me great help by providing me advice of great value and inspiration of new ideas. I would like to express my gratitude to all the other authors who helped me during the writing of this pater.

Authors' contributions

YP helped design and conduct the study, sought ethical approval, design and perform the research, acquisition, interpret, and analyze the data, write the manuscript, and revise the manuscript. DG helped perform the research and acquisition of data. CZ helped acquisition, interpret, and analyze the data. HS helped design and conduct the study; sought ethical approval; acquisition, interpret, and analyze the data; SZ and QZ helped perform the research and acquisition of data. YZ, KL and KC helped write and revise the manuscript. JY helped propose the study concept, design and conduct the study; sought ethical approval; design the research; write the manuscript; read and approved the final manuscript. All authors read and approved the final manuscript.

Author details

[1]Department of Anesthesiology, Hunan Cancer Hospital, The Affiliated Cancer Hospital of Xiangya School of Medicine, Central South University, Changsha 410013, Hunan, China. [2]Department of Anesthesiology, Perioperative Medicine and Pain Management, University of Miami-Miller School of Medicine, Miami, FL 33136, USA.

References

1. Njei B, Rotman Y, Ditah I, Lim JK. Emerging trends in hepatocellular carcinoma incidence and mortality. Hepatology. 2015;61(1):191–9.
2. Zarrinpar A, Busuttil RW. Liver transplantation: past, present and future. Nat Rev Gastroenterol Hepatol. 2013;10(7):434–40.
3. Plein LM, Rittner HL. Opioids and the immune system - friend or foe. Br J Pharmacol. 2017;175(14):2717–25.
4. Feng P, Yan R, Dai X, Xie X, Wen H, Yang S. The alteration and clinical significance of Th1/Th2/Th17/Treg cells in patients with multiple myeloma. Inflammation. 2015;38(2):705–9.
5. Geginat J, Paroni M, Maglie S, Alfen JS, Kastirr I, Gruarin P, et al. Plasticity of human CD4 T cell subsets. Front Immunol. 2014;5:630.
6. Asadzadeh Z, Mohammadi H, Safarzadeh E, Hemmatzadeh M, Mahdian-shakib A, Jadidi-Niaragh F, et al. The paradox of Th17 cell functions in tumor immunity. Cell Immunol. 2017;322:15–25.
7. Chung AS, Wu X, Zhuang G, Ngu H, Kasman I, Zhang J, et al. An interleukin-17-mediated paracrine network promotes tumor resistance to anti-angiogenic therapy. Nat Med. 2013;19(9):1114–23.
8. Liu H, Xu L, Wei JE, Xie MR, Wang SE, Zhou RX. Role of CD4+ CD25+ regulatory T cells in melatonin-mediated inhibition of murine gastric cancer cell growth in vivo and in vitro. Anat Rec (Hoboken). 2011;294(5):781–8.
9. Wu M, Chen X, Lou J, Zhang S, Zhang X, Huang L, et al. Changes in regulatory T cells in patients with ovarian cancer undergoing surgery: preliminary results. Int Immunopharmacol. 2017;47:244–50.
10. Dziobek K, Biedka M, Nowikiewicz T, Szymankiewicz M, Łukaszewska E, Dutsch-Wicherek M. Analysis of Treg cell population in patients with breast cancer with respect to progesterone receptor status. Contemp Oncol (Pozn). 2018;22(4):236–9.
11. Lan Y-T, Fan X-P, Fan Y-C, Zhao J, Wang K. Change in the Treg/Th17 cell imbalance in hepatocellular carcinoma patients and its clinical value. Medicine. 2017;96(32):e7704.
12. Boland JW, Pockley AG. Influence of opioids on immune function in patients with cancer pain: from bench to bedside. Br J Pharmacol. 2018; 175(14):2726–36.
13. Doulton B. Pharmacologic management of adult breakthrough cancer pain. Can Fam Physician. 2014;60(12):1111–4.
14. Bakr MA, Amr SA, Mohamed SA, Hamed HB, Abd El-Rahman AM, Mostafa MA, et al. Comparison between the effects of intravenous morphine, tramadol, and ketorolac on stress and immune responses in patients undergoing modified radical mastectomy. Clin J Pain. 2016;32(10):889–97.
15. Hou M, Zhou NB, Li H, Wang BS, Wang XQ, Wang XW, et al. Morphine and ketamine inhibit immune function of gastric cancer patients by increasing percentage of CD4(+)CD25(+)Foxp3(+) regulatory T cells in vitro. J Surg Res. 2016;203(2):306–12.
16. Volk T, Schenk M, Voigt K, Tohtz S, Putzier M, Kox WJ. Postoperative epidural anesthesia preserves lymphocyte, but not monocyte, immune function after major spine surgery. Anesth Analg. 2004;98:1086–92.
17. Yi X, Long L, Yang C, Lu Y, Cheng M. Maotai ameliorates diethylnitrosamine-initiated hepatocellular carcinoma formation in mice. PLoS One. 2014;9(4): e93599.
18. Filipczak-Bryniarska I, Nazimek K, Nowak B, Kozlowski M, Wasik M, Bryniarski K. In contrast to morphine, buprenorphine enhances macrophage-induced humoral immunity and, as oxycodone, slightly suppresses the effector phase of cell-mediated immune response in mice. Int Immunopharmacol. 2018;54:344–53.
19. Alexandre J, Parenta NB, Beaudrya H, Bergerona J, Patrick BGD, Sarreta P. Increased Anxiety-Like Behaviors in Rats Experiencing Chronic Inflammatory Pain. Behav Brain Res. 2012;229(1):160–7.
20. Offiah I, Didangelos A, O'Reilly BA, McMahon SB. Manipulating the extracellular matrix. Pain. 2017;158(1):161–70.
21. Chaplan SR, Bach FW, Pogrel JW, Chung JM, Yaksh TL. Quantitative assessment of tactile allodynia in the rat paw. J Neurosci Methods. 1994; 53(1):55–63.
22. Oswald N, Halle-Smith J, Kerr A, Webb J, Agostini P, Bishay E, et al. Perioperative immune function and pain control may underlie early hospital readmission and 90 day mortality following lung cancer resection: a prospective cohort study of 932 patients. Eur J Surg Oncol. 2019;45(5):863–9.
23. Shavit Y, Fridel K, Beilin B. Postoperative pain management and proinflammatory cytokines: animal and human studies. J NeuroImmune Pharmacol. 2006;1(4):443–51.
24. Page GG. The immune-suppressive effects of pain. Adv Exp Med Biol. 2003; 521:117–25.
25. Ostroumov D, Fekete-Drimusz N, Saborowski M, Kuhnel F, Woller N. CD4 and CD8 T lymphocyte interplay in controlling tumor growth. Cell Mol Life Sci. 2018;75(4):689–713.
26. Shah W, Yan X, Jing L, Zhou Y, Chen H, Wang Y. A reversed CD4/CD8 ratio of tumor-infiltrating lymphocytes and a high percentage of CD4(+)FOXP3(+

) regulatory T cells are significantly associated with clinical outcome in squamous cell carcinoma of the cervix. Cell Mol Immunol. 2011;8(1):59–66.
27. Hong M, Jiang Z, Zhou Y-F. Effects of thermotherapy on Th1/Th2 cells in esophageal Cancer patients treated with radiotherapy. Asian Pac J Cancer Prev. 2014;15(5):2359–62.
28. Liao Y, Wang B, Huang ZL, Shi M, Yu XJ, Zheng L, et al. Increased circulating Th17 cells after transarterial chemoembolization correlate with improved survival in stage III hepatocellular carcinoma: a prospective study. PLoS One. 2013;8(4):e60444.
29. Wing JB, Tanaka A, Sakaguchi S. Human FOXP3+ regulatory T cell heterogeneity and function in autoimmunity and Cancer. Immunity. 2019; 50(2):302–16.
30. Chen SH, Chen SS, Wang YP, Chen LK. Effects of systemic and neuraxial morphine on the immune system. Medicine (Baltimore). 2019;98(19):e15375.
31. Cornwell WD, Lewis MG, Fan X, Rappaport J, Rogers TJ. Effect of chronic morphine administration on circulating T cell population dynamics in rhesus macaques. J Neuroimmunol. 2013;265(1–2):43–50.
32. Mao M, Qian Y, Sun J. Morphine suppresses T helper lymphocyte differentiation to Th1 type through PI3K/AKT pathway. Inflammation. 2016; 39(2):813–21.
33. Zhou NB, Wang KG, Fu ZJ. Effect of morphine and a low dose of ketamine on the T cells of patients with refractory cancer pain in vitro. Oncol Lett. 2019;18(4):4230–6.
34. Gong L, Qian Qin, Zhou L, Ouyang W, Li Y, Wu Y, et al. Effects of fentanyl anesthesia and sufentanil anesthesia on regulatory T cells frequencies. Int J Clin Exp Pathol. 2014;7(11):7708–16.
35. Qi Y, Yao X, Zhang B, Du X. Comparison of recovery effect for sufentanil and remifentanil anesthesia with TCI in laparoscopic radical resection during colorectal cancer. Oncol Lett. 2016;11(5):3361–5.
36. Kuang DM, Zhao Q, Wu Y, Peng C, Wang J, Xu Z, et al. Peritumoral neutrophils link inflammatory response to disease progression by fostering angiogenesis in hepatocellular carcinoma. J Hepatol. 2011;54(5):948–55.
37. Amodeo G, Bugada D, Franchi S, Moschetti G, Grimaldi S, Panerai A, et al. Immune function after major surgical interventions: the effect of postoperative pain treatment. J Pain Res. 2018;11:1297–305.
38. Giannini EG, Testa R, Savarino V. Liver enzyme alteration: a guide for clinicians. CMAJ. 2005;172(3):367–79.
39. Zhang LX, Lv Y, Xu AM, Wang HZ. The prognostic significance of serum gamma-glutamyltransferase levels and AST/ALT in primary hepatic carcinoma. BMC Cancer. 2019;19(1):841.
40. Tarao K, Rino Y, Takemiya S, Tamai S, Ohkawa S, Sugimasa Y, et al. Close association between high serum ALT and more rapid recurrence of hepatocellular carcinoma in hepatectomized patients with HCV-associated liver cirrhosis and hepatocellular carcinoma. Intervirology. 2000;43(01):20–6.

The effect of intraoperative lidocaine versus esmolol infusion on postoperative analgesia in laparoscopic cholecystectomy

Joshan Lal Bajracharya[1], Asish Subedi[2*], Krishna Pokharel[3] and Balkrishna Bhattarai[4]

Abstract

Background: As a part of multimodal analgesia for laparoscopic cholecystectomy, both intraoperative lidocaine and esmolol facilitate postoperative analgesia. Our objective was to compare these two emerging strategies that challenge the use of intraoperative opioids. We aimed to assess if intraoperative esmolol infusion is not inferior to lidocaine infusion for opioid consumption after laparoscopic cholecystectomy.

Methods: In this prospective, randomized, double-blind, non-inferiority clinical trial, 90 female patients scheduled for elective laparoscopic cholecystectomy received either intravenous (IV) lidocaine bolus 1.5 mg/kg at induction followed by an infusion (1.5 mg/ kg/h) or IV bolus of esmolol 0.5 mg/kg at induction followed by an infusion (5–15 μg/kg/min) till the end of surgery. Remaining aspect of anesthesia followed a standard protocol apart from no intraoperative opioid supplementation. Postoperatively, patients received either morphine or tramadol IV to maintain visual analogue scale (VAS) scores ≤3. The primary outcome was opioid consumption (in morphine equivalents) during the first 24 postoperative hours. Pain and sedation scores, time to first perception of pain and void, and occurrence of nausea/vomiting were secondary outcomes measured up to 24 h postoperatively.

Results: Two patients in each group were excluded from the analysis. The postoperative median (IQR) morphine equivalent consumption in patients receiving esmolol was 1 (0–1.5) mg compared to 1.5 (1–2) mg in lidocaine group ($p = 0.27$). The median pain scores at various time points were similar between the two groups ($p > 0.05$). More patients receiving lidocaine were sedated in the post-anesthesia care unit (PACU) than those receiving esmolol ($p < 0.05$); however, no difference was detected later.

Conclusion: Infusion of esmolol is not inferior to lidocaine in terms of opioid requirement and pain severity in the first 24 h after surgery. Patients receiving lidocaine were more sedated during their stay in PACU than those receiving esmolol.

Keywords: Esmolol, Laparoscopic cholecystectomy, Lidocaine, Opioid analgesics, Postoperative pain

* Correspondence: ashish.subedi@bpkihs.edu; asishsubedi19@gmail.com
[2]Department of Anesthesiology & Critical Care Medicine, BP Koirala Institute of Health Sciences, BPKIHS, Dharan, Nepal

Introduction

Acute pain after laparoscopic cholecystectomy (LC) is complex in nature, and therefore, opioids alone might not be sufficient to achieve quality analgesia [1, 2]. Besides, usage of only opioids in perioperative settings is associated with undesirable effects [3–6]. In this regard, multimodal regimen (a combination of opioids and non-opioid drug) is recommended for LC, as it provides superior analgesia and improves quality of recovery after surgery [7].

Several strategies using intraoperative intravenous agents have been used for LC to improve the postoperative analgesic profile. Among these, systemic lidocaine is an extensively studied intervention due to its analgesic, anti-hyperalgesic and anti-inflammatory effects [8]. Moreover, doses of IV lidocaine ≤3 mg/kg/h is considered safe and is feasible to use in perioperative setting [8–10]. Surprisingly, the latest Cochrane systematic review demonstrated uncertaininty regarding the beneficial effects of IV perioperative lidocaine on postoperative pain outcomes [11].

In the last decade, intraoperative infusion of the short-acting betablocker esmolol has gained popularity as an alternative technique due to its antinoiceptive and opioid sparing effects [12–14]. A recent meta-analysis has revealed a significant reduction in perioperative opioid consumption with the use of intraoperative esmolol [15].

Although both lidocaine and esmolol are widely used for LC, studies comparing these agents are very few with conflicting results [16, 17]. Therefore, the primary objective of our study was to compare the effects of intraoperative lidocaine and esmolol infusion on postoperative opioid consumption and pain scores following LC. We hypothesized that esmolol infusion would be non-inferior to lidocaine infusion in terms of 24 h postoperative opioid requirement.

Methods

This prospective, randomized, double-blind, non-inferiority clinical trial was conducted at BP Koirala Institute of Health Sciences between January 2015 and April 2016. The study was approved by the Institutional Ethical Review Board (Ref: IERB 284/014) and the trial was registered prior to patient enrollment at clinicaltrials.gov (NCT02327923). The study was performed according to the Declaration of Helsinki and it adheres to the guidelines of the CONSORT statement.

Female patients aged 18 to 60 years, American society of Anesthesiologist physical status I and II, scheduled for general anesthesia for elective laparoscopic cholecystectomy were enrolled. Exclusion criteria included those with inability to comprehend VAS or severe mental impairment, difficult intubation, pregnancy, morbid obesity, history of epilepsy or allergy to any drugs used in the study, current use of opioids or beta-adrenergic receptor antagonists, baseline heart rate < 50 beats/min, acute cholecystitis, and chronic pain other than cholelithiasis.

Eligible participants were identified during the pre-anesthetic clinic visit. Informed written consent from the recruited patients was taken in the evening before surgery at the in-patient unit. Patients were also instructed about the use of the 10 cm VAS for pain where 0 was "no pain" and 10 was "worst pain". Oral diazepam (5 mg for ≤50 kg and 10 mg for > 50 kg) was given the night before and 2 h before surgery as premedication.

On the day of surgery at the preoperative holding area, patients were randomly assigned (allocation 1:1) into one of the two groups according to a computer generated random number table. Details of group assignment and case number were kept in a set of sealed opaque envelopes. The anesthesia staff opened the envelope and prepared drugs accordingly. Both the patient and the investigator observing the outcome were blinded to the patient group assignment. The attending anesthesiologist not involved in the study managed the case intraoperatively.

On arrival to the operating room, standard monitoring was applied and baseline heart rate (HR), non-invasive blood pressure, peripheral oxygen saturation and bispectral index (BIS) value (BIS® monitor; Covidien, Boulder, CO, USA) were recorded. General anesthesia was induced with IV fentanyl 1.5 μg/kg and propofol 2–2.5 mg/kg until the cessation of verbal response. Tracheal intubation was facilitated with vecuronium 0.1 mg/kg IV. The lungs were mechanically ventilated using the circle system with 50% mixture of oxygen with air to maintain end tidal carbon dioxide between 35 to 45 mmHg.

During induction, patients in the Lidocaine group received 1.5 mg/kg of lidocaine IV bolus followed by an infusion (Perfusor compact®, B-Braun, Melsungen, Germany) at 1.5 mg/kg/h. Patients in the Esmolol group received an IV bolus of esmolol (0.5 mg/kg) during induction followed by an infusion titrated between 5 and 15 μg/kg/min to maintain the HR within 25% of the baseline value. In both groups, 1 g of IV paracetamol was infused over 15 min after the induction of anesthesia. Anesthesia was maintained with isoflurane targeting mean arterial pressure (MAP) within 20% of baseline, and BIS value between 50 and 60 in both groups. Neuromuscular blockade was maintained with supplemental doses of IV vecuronium after observing the curare notch in capnogram. Hasson's surgical technique was used. Each port site was infiltrated with 3 ml of 2% lidocaine before incision. Pneumoperitoneum was achieved with carbon dioxide maintaining the intra-abdominal pressure below 15 mmHg. Episodes of intraoperative hypotension (MAP < 65 mmHg) and bradycardia (HR < 50 beats/min) were treated with IV ephedrine 5 mg and atropine 0.4 mg respectively.

No supplemental opioids were used during the surgery. All patients received 30 mg of IV ketorolac after the removal of the gall bladder. At the end of surgery, the carbon dioxide remaining in the peritoneal cavity was expelled by slow abdominal decompression. Both isoflurane and the study drug infusion were discontinued after the skin closure. Incision site was infiltrated with 10 ml of 0.25% bupivacaine. Residual neuromuscular block was reversed with IV neostigmine 0.05 mg/kg and glycopyrrolate 0.01 mg/kg. When the patients were conscious and had adequate muscle power, thorough oropharyngeal suctioning was done and endotracheal tube was removed. The investigator blinded to the group assignment now entered the operating room to collect data on intraoperative hemodynamics side effects. The patients were then transferred to the PACU after they followed verbal commands.

Postoperative pain management included 1 g of paracetamol and 30 mg of ketorolac IV at 6 h and 8 h respectively. The blinded investigator not involved in the anesthesia management assessed VAS pain scores at rest and during movement at the PACU (on arrival, 15 min, 30 min, 1 h) and surgical in-patient-unit (2 h, 6 h, 12 h and 24 h). If the VAS score for pain exceeded > 3 at rest, 1 mg of morphine IV was administered in the PACU, and repeated every five min until the VAS score was ≤3, or if any adverse effects were noticed. These included increased sleepiness (Ramsay sedation scale (RSS) score > 3), respiratory depression (SpO_2 < 90% in room air or respiratory rate < 8/min). The patients were transferred to the in-patient-unit after 1 h of stay in PACU. In the surgical unit, 50 mg of tramadol IV was administered and further doses of 50 mg was given every 10 min for maintaining VAS score for pain ≤3 (the maximum dose of tramadol was limited to 300 mg in the first 24 h). The tramadol used in surgical unit was converted to morphine equivalent using online calculator (http://clincalc.com/Opioids/).

The primary outcome was opioid consumption (in morphine equivalents) during the first 24 h after surgery. Secondary outcome measures included patient-reported VAS pain scores at rest and movement, postoperative nausea and vomiting (PONV) on a four point scale [18] (1 = no nausea, 2 = mild nausea, 3 = severe nausea, 4 = retching and/or vomiting), the 6-point RSS scores [19](1 = patient anxious and restless, 2 = cooperative and awake, 3 = responding to verbal commands, 4 = responding to mild stimulus, 5 = responding to deep stimulus, 6 = no response). These parameters were noted in PACU and at 2, 6, 12 and 24 h in the surgical unit. PONV grade 3 & 4 were treated with metoclopramide 10 mg IV. Time to first perception of pain and void, overall patient satisfaction from anesthesia at 24 h based on 5-point Likert scale (1 = highly satisfied, 2 = satisfied, 3 = neutral, 4 = dissatisfied, 5 = highly dissatisfied), and occurrence of lidocaine toxicity were also noted. The patients were discharged from the hospital at 24 h after surgery.

Sample size was determined with the aim to reject the inferiority of esmolol infusion compared with lidocaine for the primary outcome of 24 h morphine consumption after surgery. The non-inferiority margin was considered as 2 mg. A sample size of 78 patients (39 per arm) was required to achieve a power of 90%, a one-sided 95% confidence interval, assuming the standard deviation of 3. We finally enrolled 90 patients to allow for possible dropouts or protocol violators (https://www.sealedenvelope.com/power/continuous-noninferior/).

The data collected was entered into excel software and analyzed on STATA version 13.0 (Stata Corporation, College Station, TX, USA). Normality of data was checked using histograms, Skewness-Kurtosis test and Shapiro-Wilk test. Normally distributed data were compared between the two groups using the unpaired Student *t*-test. Mann-Whitney U-tests were used for continuous non-normally distributed data and ordinal data. Comparison of pain scores between the two groups was performed using a mixed effects model. Fixed effects were time of assessment of pain scores postoperatively (15 min to 24 h), study-group assignment (esmolol or lidocaine), and participants in the study as a random effect. Interaction between time of assessment of pain scores and study group was also included in the model and an unstructured covariance matrix was used. For categorical variables, Chi-square test was applied. Time to first perception of pain between the groups was plotted with Kaplan-Meier survival curves and compared with log-rank test. A p value < 0.05 was considered as statistically significant.

Results

Among the 104 consecutive patients assessed for eligibility, 90 met the inclusion criteria and they were randomly assigned to lidocaine or esmolol group. Two patients in each group needed conversion to open cholecystectomy, and eventually 86 patients were included in the analysis (Fig. 1). Both the groups were similar with respect to baseline demographic characteristics, duration of surgery and anesthesia time (Table 1).

In the PACU, median morphine consumption was 1 (0–1.5) mg in lidocaine group and 1(0–1.5) mg in esmolol group (p = 0.50). Similarly, in the surgical-unit, median tramadol needed was 0 (0–50) mg and 0 (0–50) mg in the lidocaine and esmolol groups, respectively (p = 0.65). The median 24 h total morphine equivalent consumed was 1 (0–1.5) mg in the esmolol group and 1.5 (1–2) mg in the lidocaine group (p = 0.27; Fig. 2).

There was no significant difference for the time until the first perception of pain in the two groups as

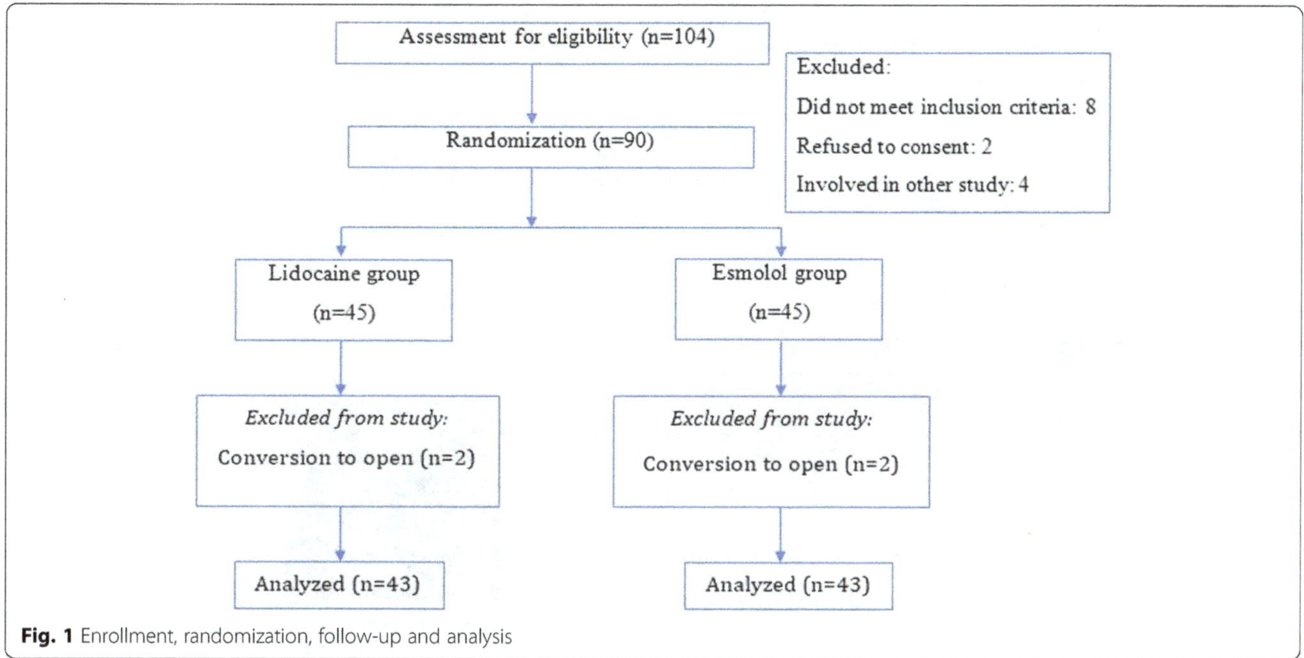

Fig. 1 Enrollment, randomization, follow-up and analysis

observed in the survival curve analysis (Fig. 3). Mixed model analysis revealed no difference in postoperative VAS scores for pain at rest (group time interaction effect, $p = 0.38$; Fig. 4) or with movement (group time interaction effect, $p = 0.25$; Fig. 5) between the two groups.

Postoperative sedation scores were comparable except in the PACU where more patients were sedated in lidocaine group (Table 2). Seven patients (16%) in lidocaine had PONV (score ≥ 2) compared to 6 patients (14%) in esmolol group ($p = 0.71$). Median (IQR) satisfaction scores with anesthesia were 2 (2-2) and 2 (2-2) in patients receiving lidocaine and esmolol respectively ($p = 0.40$). The time to first void was similar in the esmolol (2.60 ± 1.2 h) and the lidocaine group (2.67 ± 1.1 h, $p = 0.79$).

An abdominal drain was inserted in one patient in lidocaine and in 2 patients in esmolol group. Post-hoc analysis revealed that one patient in esmolol group manifested bradycardia intraoperatively, and it responded to IV atropine and pneumoperitoneum decompression. Likewise, one patient in both groups received IV ephedrine 5 mg for hypotensive episode. One patient in esmolol group manifested bronchospasm in PACU and it was managed successfully with salbutamol nebulization. No features of lidocaine toxicity were reported.

Table 1 Comparison of demographic and baseline characteristics of patients

Variables	Lidocaine group (*n* = 43)	Esmolol group (*n* = 43)
Age (y)	35 (30–49)	40 (27–48)
BMI (kg/m^2)	22.4 ± 3.1	22.5 ± 2.5
ASA PS I/II	35/8	34/9
Duration of anesthesia (min)	62 (51–77)	57 (48–64)
Duration of surgery (min)	55 (45–75)	50 (45–60)

Values are in median (IQR), mean ± SD, number. Abbreviations: *BMI* body mass index, *ASA PS* American society of Anesthesiologist physical status

Discussion

This study demonstrated that esmolol is not inferior to lidocaine in terms of postoperative opioid consumption when administered with multimodal analgesia for laparoscopic cholecystectomy. Likewise, pain scores in the first 24 h after surgery was not significantly different between the two groups. The time to first perception of pain, level of satisfaction with anesthesia and any occurrence of side effects were also similar. However, the level of sedation was significantly less in esmolol group than in lidocaine group until 1h in PACU, but no difference was detected thereafter.

Clinical studies investigating the effect of intraoperative IV lidocaine in comparison to esmolol on postoperative opioid and pain scores have shown conflicting results. Similar to our findings, Dogan et al. found no difference between the two groups in postoperative 24 h opioid consumption after laparoscopic cholecystectomy [16]. In contrast, Kavak Akelma et al. found significantly less fentanyl requirement in patients receiving esmolol than those receiving lidocaine infusion or placebo in the first 24 h of surgery [17]. This difference might be due to the higher dose of esmolol (fixed dose, 50 μg/kg/min) used in their patients in comparison to ours (esmolol infusion limited to 15 μg/kg/min). A recent meta-analysis focused on intraoperative use of esmolol on opioid

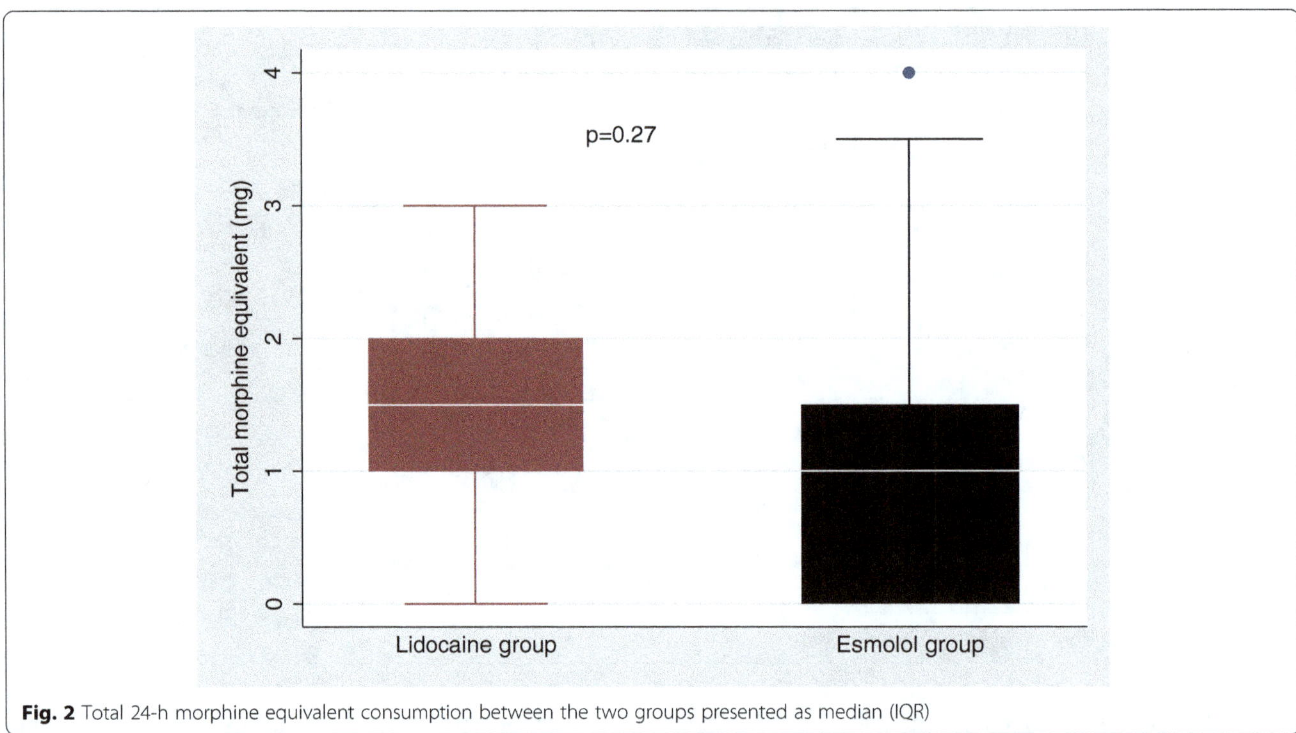

Fig. 2 Total 24-h morphine equivalent consumption between the two groups presented as median (IQR)

consumption or pain scores found high heterogeneity regarding esmolol dose [15]. Infusion rates varied from 5 to 500 µg/kg/min. Eleven studies had infusion rates ≤15 µg/ kg/min while other 11 studies had infusion rates > 15 µg/kg/min. However, this meta-analysis lacked meta-regression analysis on dose-response relationship. Another meta-analysis exploring the effect of intraoperative esmolol on haemodynamic profiles demonstrated dose-related significant increase in the incidence of hypotension [20]. The authors suggested that frequency of hypotension could be minimized by lowering the initial infusion dose and titrating it according to the hemodynamics response.

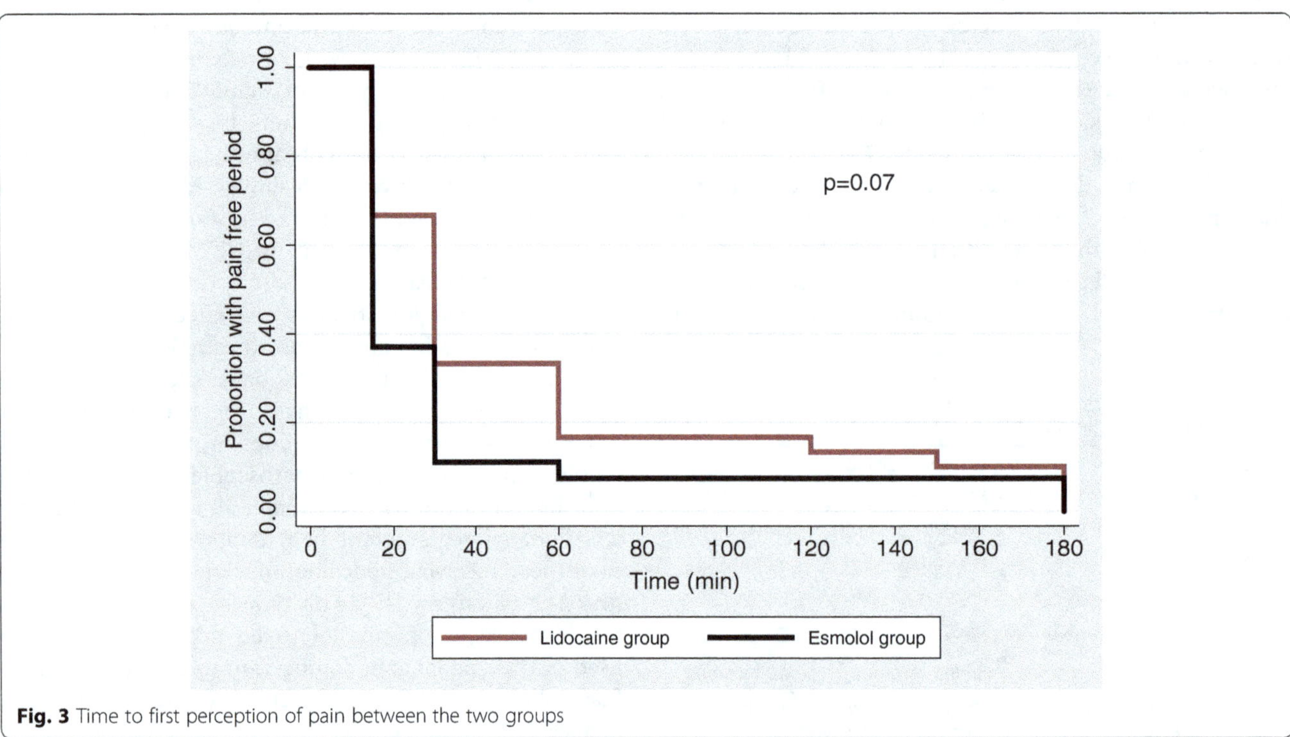

Fig. 3 Time to first perception of pain between the two groups

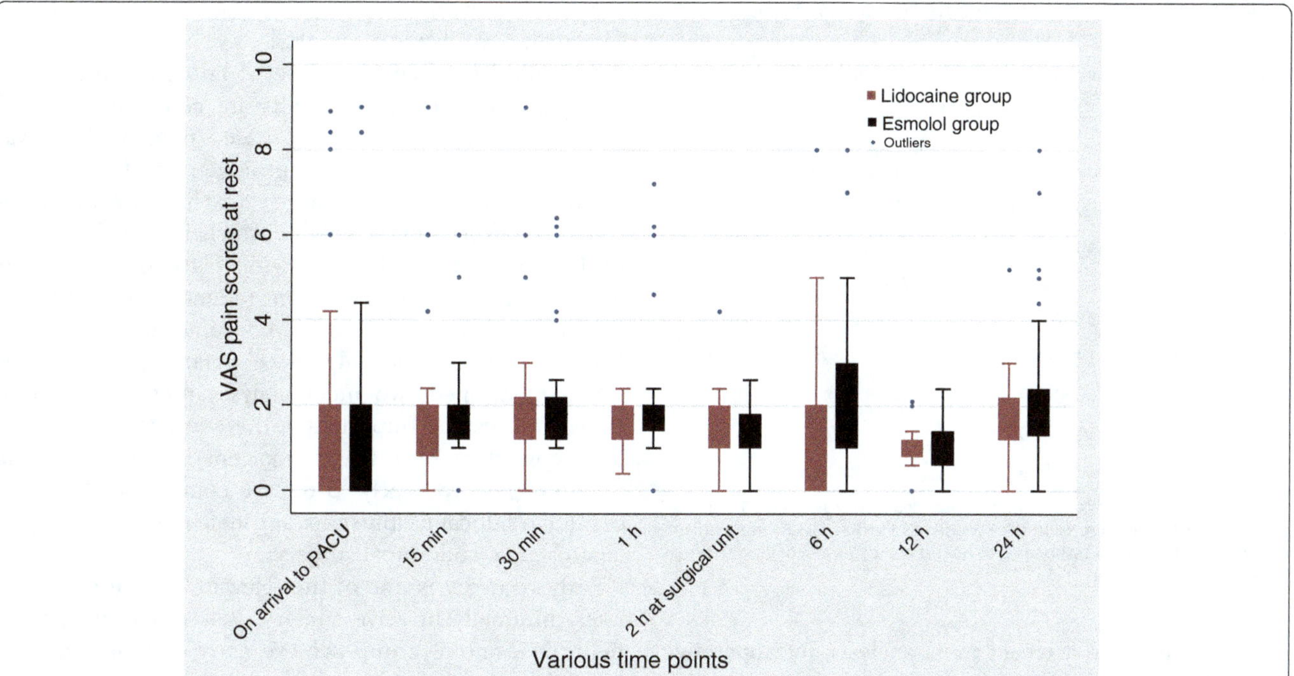

Fig. 4 Post-operative pain scores at rest during various time points. Mixed model analysis showed no significant difference in pain scores over times between lidocaine and esmolol group (group time interaction effect, $p = 0.38$). Data are presented as median (IQR)

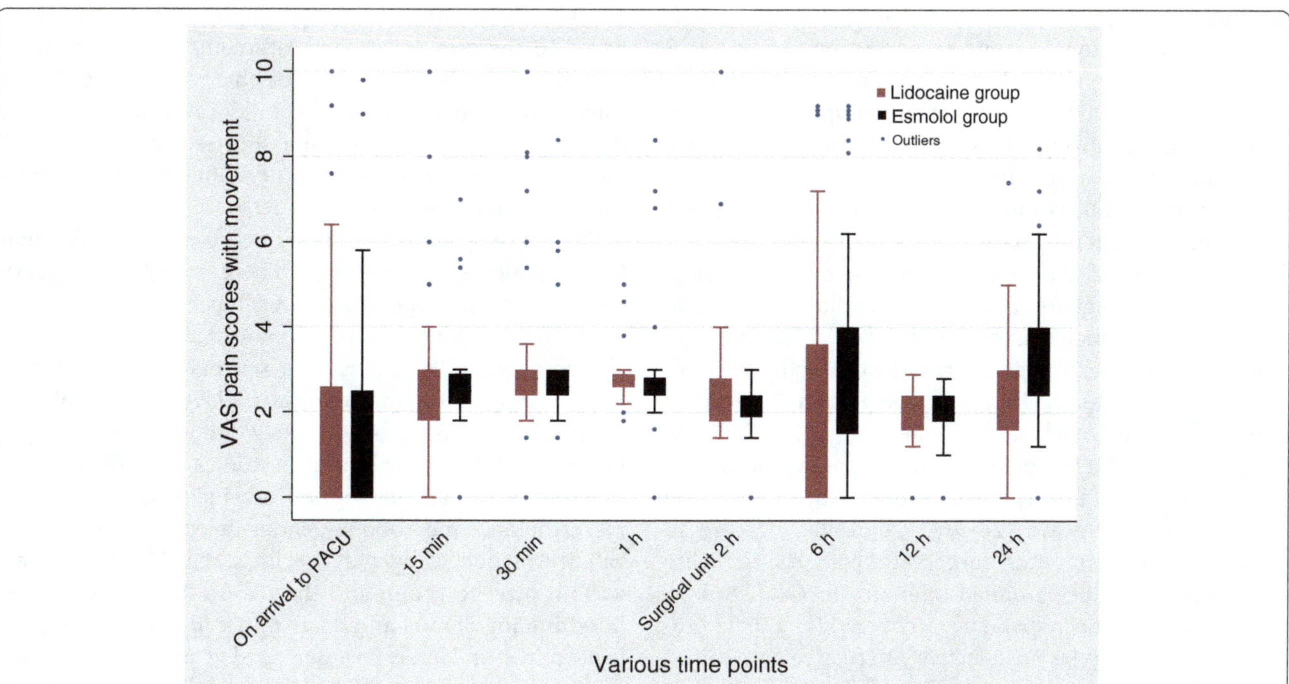

Fig. 5 Post-operative pain scores with movement at various time points. Mixed model analysis showed no significant difference in pain scores over times between lidocaine and esmolol group (group time interaction effect, $p = 0.25$). Data are presented as median (IQR)

Table 2 Comparison of postoperative sedation score at various time points

Time point	Lidocaine group ($n = 43$)	Esmolol group ($n = 43$)	*P* value
At PACU			
0 min	5/5/33/0/0/0	4/17/22/0/0/0	0.03
15 min	3/21/19/0/0/0	6/29/8/0/0/0	0.01
30 min	1/32/10/0/0/0	4/36/3/0/0/0	0.01
1 h	1/34/8/0/0/0	1/41/1/0/0/0	0.02
At Surgical unit			
2 h	1/39/3/0/0/0	0/41/2/0/0/0	0.98
6 h	0/41/2/0/0/0	1/40/2/0/0/0	0.66
12 h	0/43/0/0/0/0	0/42/1/0/0/0	0.32
24 h	0/43/0/0/0/0	0/43/0/0/0/0	1

Values are in number of patients with Ramsay sedation scale scores 1/2/3/4/5/6 (1 = patient anxious and restless, 2 = cooperative and awake, 3 = responding to verbal commands, 4 = responding to mild stimulus, 5 = responding to deep stimulus, 6 = no response)

As evident from a recent meta-analysis, intraoperative esmolol reduces both intraoperative and postoperative opioid requirement when compared to both remifentanil and non-remifentanil based controls [15]. However, the significant difference in postoperative opioid consumption was limited to the PACU stay only (standard mean difference, − 1.21; 95% CI, − 1.66 to − 0.77). Trials by Dogan et al. [16] and Kavak et al. [17] were not included, and perhaps inclusion of these studies might have further influenced the treatment effects. In a similar model to ours (laparoscopic cholecystectomy) [21], however, with a conventional control consisting of general anesthesia with opioids, the intraoperative fentanyl consumption was 200.5 μg in placebo group while it was null in esmolol group. This reflects that esmolol may have an opioid sparing effect.

Several mechanisms for esmolol antinociceptive effects or opioid-sparing role have been elucidated. These include blockade of the excitatory effects of norepinephrine on pain signals and/or modulation of central adrenergic (pronociceptive) activity [22, 23]. As beta-adrenergic receptors may potentiate the activity of N-methyl-d-aspartate (NMDA) subtype glutamate receptor and facilitate the mechanisms underlying opioid induced hyperalgesia (OIH), beta-adrenergic antagonists are likely to produce antihyperalgesic effects by at least one of these two pathways [24–26]. Clinically, increase in opioid requirement after surgery in patients receiving opioids is likely due to opioid tolerance or OIH, and, as a result it might delay patient's recovery [21, 27]. Therefore, esmolol may be an effective alternative to counter OIH. Although postoperative opioid sparing effect of esmolol seems promising, the question yet to be answered is whether it is caused directly by its intrinsic properties (anti-nociceptive, antihyperalgesic) and/or indirectly by avoidance of opioids.

Regarding the beneficial role of lidocaine infusion in perioperative setting, the results are confusing. The report from a recent Cochrane based meta-analysis was uncertain if lidocaine had any positive impact on postoperative outcomes [11]. Contrary to this; two other recently published meta-analyses which included only the RCTs comparing lidocaine with placebo in patients undergoing LC found significant reduction in postoperative pain related outcomes in lidocaine group [28, 29]. Perhaps, the use of only placebo comparator in the above mentioned two meta-analyses might have influenced the results. Importantly, there are several reasons for inconsistent results with lidocaine infusion [11], and therefore it is too early to draw a conclusion that perioperative lidocaine infusions are ineffective especially in laparoscopic abdominal surgery.

Early recovery is one of the relevant clinical outcomes after minimally invasive surgery. It is reported that patients in esmolol group achieve early discharge criteria from the PACU as compared to lidocaine group [16]. In the same study, patients receiving lidocaine had RSS scores higher than esmolol at 10 min post-extubation. Likewise, perioperative lidocaine failed to reduce the discharge time after ambulatory surgery compared to placebo when reported as a primary outcome [30]. This is likely due to mild sedative effect of lidocaine and therefore, it could have prolonged the PACU stay. This is in concordance with our results. Patients in the lidocaine group were more sedated up to 1 h after surgery compared to the esmolol group. Although, we did not compare the time to readiness to discharge from the PACU, esmolol has an advantage over lidocaine in relation to discharge time. Moreover, the shorter elimination half-life of esmolol as compared to lidocaine might be beneficial in ambulatory surgery [31, 32].

There are several limitations in our study. First, only female patients were enrolled. There is evidence suggesting that woman experience as well as express more pain after surgery and hence require an excess amount of analgesic agents [33–35]. Hence, sex may be a significant confounding factor in a clinical trial. Although, this difference in pain sensitivity is likely due to biopsychosocial factors/mechanism, laboratory studies investigating sex differences in pain perception are inconsistent [36, 37]. Nevertheless, due to one-gender selected, the external validity of our study may be impaired. Secondly, there was no placebo group and the reason for this is because lidocaine infusion is an effective therapy for laparoscopic procedures and therefore, we used it as an active comparator. Similarly, esmolol has already been shown to reduce opioids requirement after surgery when compared to placebo [15]. Importantly, had we used the placebo group the concern would have been more ethical with no intraoperative opioid supplementation. As evident from a previous study [21], the placebo group required significantly larger doses of opioids intraoperative than in esmolol group. Thirdly, we did not compare the intraoperative hemodynamic parameters. Although, reporting of intraoperative hemodynamic side-effects was not pre-specified, we did post-hoc analysis and found no difference. It is noteworthy that infusions of esmolol and lidocaine at lower doses are safe with no significant alteration in hemodynamics [11, 20]. Finally, the impact of these drugs on readiness to discharge the patients from hospital was not assessed since the patients were required to stay up to 24 h postoperatively following LC in our centre.

It would be interesting to explore the utility of lidocaine and esmolol with adequately powered future comparative studies with regard to PONV, early discharge from the PACU, quality of recovery and length of hospital stay. Also, future studies based on dose-response relationship of esmolol is required that would impact postoperative pain outcomes while lessen the side effects.

Conclusions

In conclusion, infusion of esmolol is not inferior to lidocaine for postoperative opioid consumption and pain scores following laparoscopic cholecystectomy. However, patients receiving esmolol were less sedated than those receiving lidocaine in the early period after surgery.

Abbreviations

BIS: Bispectral Index; CONSORT: Consolidated Standards of Reporting Trials; HR: Heart rate; IQR: Interquartile range; IV: Intravenous; MAP: Mean arterial pressure; OIH: Opioid induced hyperalgesia; PACU: Post anesthesia care unit; PONV: Postoperative nausea vomiting; RSS: Ramsay sedation scale; VAS: Visual analogue scale

Acknowledgements

Not applicable.

Authors' contributions

JLB: This author helped in study design, patient recruitment, data collection and writing up of the first draft of the paper. AS: This author helped in study design, patient recruitment, data collection, analysis and interpretation of data, manuscript revision and final draft. KP: This author helped in study design, analysis and interpretation of data, manuscript revision and final approval. BKB: This author helped in patient recruitment, data collection, manuscript first draft. All authors read and approved the manuscript.

Author details

[1]Department of Anesthesiology & Critical Care, Mechi Zonal Hospital, Bhadrapur, Nepal. [2]Department of Anesthesiology & Critical Care Medicine, BP Koirala Institute of Health Sciences, BPKIHS, Dharan, Nepal. [3]Department of Anesthesiology & Critical Care Medicine, BPKIHS, Dharan, Nepal. [4]Department of Anesthesiology & Critical Care Medicine, BPKIHS, Dharan, Nepal.

References

1. Bisgaard T. Analgesic treatment after laparoscopic cholecystectomy: a critical assessment of the evidence. Anesthesiology. 2006;104:835–46.
2. Joris J, Thiry E, Paris P, Weerts J, Lamy M. Pain after laparoscopic cholecystectomy: characteristics and effect of intraperitoneal bupivacaine. Anesth Analg. 1995;81:379–84.
3. Guignard B, Bossard AE, Coste C, et al. Acute opioid tolerance: intraoperative remifentanil increases postoperative pain and morphine requirement. Anesthesiology. 2000;93:409–17.
4. Lee LA, Caplan RA, Stephens LS, et al. Postoperative opioid induced respiratory depression: a closed claims analysis. Anesthesiology. 2015;122: 659–65.
5. Zhao SZ, Chung F, Hanna DB, Raymundo AL, Cheung RY, Chen C. Dose-response relationship between opioid use and adverse effects after ambulatory surgery. J Pain Symptom Manage. 2004;28:35–46.
6. White PF. The role of non-opioid analgesic techniques in the management of pain after ambulatory surgery. Anesth Analg. 2002;94:577–85.
7. Lau CS, Chamberlain RS. Enhanced recovery after surgery programs improve patient outcomes and recovery: a meta-analysis. World J Surg. 2017;41:899–913.
8. Marret E, Rolin M, Beaussier M, Bonnet F. Meta-analysis of intravenous lidocaine and postoperative recovery after abdominal surgery. Br J Surg. 2008;95:1331–8.
9. Sun Y, Li T, Wang N, Yun Y, Gan TJ. Perioperative systemic lidocaine for postoperative analgesia and recovery after abdominal surgery: A meta-analysis of randomized controlled trials. Dis Colon rectum. 2012;55:1183–94.
10. Kranke P, Jokinen J, Pace NL, et al. Continuous intravenous perioperative lidocaine infusion for postoperative pain and recovery. Cochrane Database Syst Rev. 2015;7:CD009642.
11. Weibel S, Jelting Y, Pace NL, et al. Continuous intravenous perioperative lidocaine infusion for postoperative pain and recovery in adults. Cochrane Database Syst Rev. 2018;6:CD009642.
12. Chia YY, Chan MH, Ko NH, Liu K. Role of beta-blockade in anaesthesia and postoperative pain management after hysterectomy. Br J Anaesth. 2004;93: 799–805.
13. Coloma M, Chiu JW, White PF, Armbruster SC. The use of esmolol as an alternative to remifentanil during desflurane anesthesia for fast-track outpatient gynecologic laparoscopic surgery. Anesth Analg. 2001;92:352–7.
14. White PF, Wang B, Tang J, Wender RH, Naruse R, Sloninsky A. The effect of intraoperative use of esmolol and nicardipine on recovery after ambulatory surgery. Anesth Analg. 2003;97:1633–8.
15. Gelineau AM, King MR, Ladha KS, Burns SM, Houle T, Anderson TA. Intraoperative esmolol as an adjunct for perioperative opioid and postoperative pain reduction: A systematic review, meta-analysis, and meta-regression. Anesth Analg. 2018;126:1035–49.
16. Dogan SD, Ustun FE, Sener EB, et al. Effects of lidocaine and esmolol infusions on hemodynamic changes, analgesic requirement, and recovery in laparoscopic cholecystectomy operations. Braz J Anesthesiol. 2016;66:145–50.
17. Kavak Akelma F, Ergıl J, Özkan D, Akinci M, Özmen M, Gümüs H. A comparison of the effects of intraoperative esmolol and lidocaine infusions on postoperative analgesia. Anestezi Dergisi. 2014;22:25–31.
18. Sonner JM, Hynson JM, Clark O, Katz JA. Nausea and vomiting following thyroid and parathyroid surgery. J Clin Anesth. 1997;9:398–402.
19. Ramsay MA, Savage TM, Simpson BR, Goodwin R. Controlled sedation with alphaxalone-alphadolone. Br Med J. 1974;2:656–9.
20. Yu SK, Tait G, Karkouti K, Wijeysundera D, McCluskey S, Beattie WS. The safety of perioperative esmolol: a systematic review and meta-analysis of randomized controlled trials. Anesth Analg. 2011;112:267–81.
21. Collard V, Mistraletti G, Taqi A, Asenjo JF, Feldman LS, Fried GM, Carli F. Intraoperative esmolol infusion in the absence of opioids spares postoperative fentanyl in patients undergoing ambulatory laparoscopic cholecystectomy. Anesth Analg. 2007;105:1255–62.
22. Pertovaara A. The noradrenergic pain regulation system: a potential target for pain therapy. Eur J Pharmacol. 2013;716:2–7.
23. Hagelüken A, Grünbaum L, Nürnberg B, Harhammer R, Schunack W, Seifert R. Lipophilic beta-adrenoceptor antagonists and local anesthetics are effective direct activators of G-proteins. Biochem Pharmacol. 1994;47:1789–95.
24. Barresi M, Grasso C, Licata F, Li VG. Noradrenergic modulation of neuronal responses to *N*-methyl-d-aspartate in the vestibular nuclei: an electrophysiological and immunohistochemical study. Neuroscience. 2014; 265:172–83.
25. Liang DY, Shi X, Li X, Li J, Clark JD. The β2-adrenergic receptor regulated morphine tolerance and physical dependence. Behav Brain Res. 2007;181: 118–26.
26. Chu LF, Cun T, Ngai LK, Kim JE, Zamora AK, Young CA, Angst MS, Clark DJ. Modulation of remifentanil-induced postinfusion hyperalgesia by the beta-blocker propranolol in humans. Pain. 2012;153:974 81.
27. Xuerong Y, Yuguang H, Xia J, Hailan W. Ketamine and lornoxicam for preventing a fentanyl-induced increase in postoperative morphine requirement. Anesth Analg. 2008;107:2032 7.

28. Zhao JB, Li YL, Wang YM, et al. Intravenous lidocaine infusion for pain control after laparoscopic cholecystectomy: A meta-analysis of randomized controlled trials. Medicine (Baltimore). 2018;97:e9771.
29. Li J, Wang G, Xu W, Ding M, Yu W. Efficacy of intravenous lidocaine on pain relief in patients undergoing laparoscopic cholecystectomy: A meta-analysis from randomized controlled trials. Int J Surg. 2018;50:137–45.
30. McKay A, Gottschalk A, Ploppa A, Durieux ME, Groves DS. Systemic lidocaine decreased the perioperative opioid analgesic requirements but failed to reduce discharge time after ambulatory surgery. Anesth Analg. 2009;109: 1805–8.
31. Wiest D. Esmolol. A review of its therapeutic efficacy and pharmacokinetic characteristics. Clin Pharmacokinet. 1995;28:190–202.
32. Rowland M, Thomson PD, Guichard A, Melmon KL. Disposition kinetics of lidocaine in normal subjects. Ann N Y Acad Sci. 1971;179:383–98.
33. Cepeda MS, Carr DB. Women experience more pain and require more morphine than men to achieve a similar degree of analgesia. Anesth Analg. 2003;97:1464–8.
34. Uchiyama K, Kawai M, Tani M, Ueno M, Hama T, Yamaue H. Gender differences in postoperative pain after laparoscopic cholecystectomy. Surg Endosc. 2006;20:448–51.
35. Taenzer AH, Clark C, Curry CS. Gender affects report of pain and function after arthroscopic anterior cruciate ligament reconstruction. Anesthesiology. 2000;93:670–5.
36. Racine M, Tousignant-Laflamme Y, Kloda LA, Dion D, Dupuis G, Choinière M. A systematic literature review of 10 years of research on sex/gender and pain perception - part 2: do biopsychosocial factors alter pain sensitivity differently in women and men? Pain. 2012;153:619–35.
37. Racine M, Tousignant-Laflamme Y, Kloda LA, Dion D, Dupuis G, Choinière M. A systematic literature review of 10 years of research on sex/gender and experimental pain perception - part 1: are there really differences between women and men? Pain. 2012;153:602–18.

Effect of postoperative Trendelenburg position on shoulder pain after gynecological laparoscopic procedures

Carine Zeeni[1†], Dina Chamsy[2†], Ali Khalil[2], Antoine Abu Musa[2], Majed Al Hassanieh[1], Fadia Shebbo[1] and Joseph Nassif[2*]

Abstract

Background: Laparoscopic surgery has become a standard of care for many gynecological surgeries due to its lower morbidity, pain and cost compared to open techniques. Unfortunately, the use of carbon dioxide (CO_2) to insufflate the abdomen is the main contributor to post-operative shoulder pain.

Methods: We aim to assess the effect of postoperative Trendelenburg position on shoulder pain after gynecological laparoscopic procedures. We hypothesize that maintaining the patient in Trendelenburg for 24 h postoperatively will significantly decrease postoperative shoulder pain and analgesic consumption. After obtaining written informed consent, 108 patients were prospectively randomized into two groups. In the control group, patients underwent standard gynecologic laparoscopic procedures; then after passive deflation of the pneumoperitoneum at the end of the surgery, the patients were placed in supine head up position in the post anesthesia care unit (PACU) and received our institution's common postoperative care. Patients in the intervention group were subjected to the same maneuver but were positioned in a Trendelenburg position (20 °) once fully awake and cooperative in the PACU and retained this position for the first 24 h. Numerical rating scale (NRS) was used to assess shoulder pain and nausea upon patient arrival to the PACU, at 4, 6, 12 (primary outcome) and 24 h postoperatively. Time to first rescue pain medication, total rescue pain medications and overall satisfaction with pain control were recorded. 101 patients were included in the final data analysis.

Results: Both groups were comparable in terms of baseline characteristics. NRS pain scores were significantly lower in the intervention group at 12 h compared to the control group (0 [0–1] versus 5 [1–4], $p < 0.001$), furthermore improvement in postoperative shoulder pain between time of arrival to PACU (time zero) and 12 h postoperatively was significantly higher in patients allocated to the experimental group compared to the control group. Pain scores were significantly lower in patients allocated to the experimental group versus the control group (0 [0–1] versus 5 [1–4], $p < 0.001$).

Conclusion: In conclusion, Trendelenburg position is an easy non-pharmacologic intervention that is beneficial in reducing postoperative shoulder pain following gynecologic laparoscopic surgery.

Keywords: Trendelenburg position, Shoulder pain, Laparoscopic surgery, Gynecological surgery

* Correspondence: jn25@aub.edu.lb
[†]Carine Zeeni and Dina Chamsy contributed equally to this work.
[2]Department of Obstetrics and Gynecology, American University of Beirut Medical Center, Beirut, Lebanon

Background

Laparoscopic gynecologic surgery has evolved from a limited surgical procedure used only for diagnostic purposes to a major surgical approach for treating a multitude of malignant and non-malignant pathologies. It is currently one of the most common surgical procedures performed by gynecologists [1]. Although laparoscopic surgery has proven its superiority over laparotomy in terms of improved post-operative pain scores, postoperative shoulder pain remains a major concern following laparoscopic surgeries. Shoulder pain is reported to occur in 35 to 70% of laparoscopic surgeries [2, 3]. The pain can be severe and is usually relieved in 24–48 h, but rarely persists for over 72 h after surgery [4]. The precise mechanism of this shoulder pain remains unclear. The main hypothesis is the presence of residual carbon dioxide (CO_2) in the abdominal cavity that causes irritation of the phrenic nerve and referred pain to the shoulders [5, 6]. Other theories include peritoneal stretching, diaphragmatic irritation or injury, and shoulder abduction during surgery [7–9].

Various preventative measures have been proposed intraoperatively to try to reduce residual CO_2 in the abdominal cavity including: low insufflation rate and pressure [10], Valsalva maneuvers [11, 12], filling the abdominal cavity with Lactated Ringers [13], and active deflation of the abdomen [14]. To our knowledge, there are no available published studies looking at the effect of postoperative Trendelenburg positioning on the incidence of shoulder pain after laparoscopic gynecologic surgery. The Trendelenburg position might decrease pain by reducing the mechanical pressure exerted by CO_2 on the diaphragm and the upper abdominal muscles. CO_2, known for its high solubility, would also be displaced to the pelvis that has a rich vasculature which in turn speeds up the resorption of pneumoperitoneum.

The purpose of this study is to assess the effect of postoperative Trendelenburg position on shoulder pain after gynecologic laparoscopic procedures. We hypothesize that maintaining the patient in Trendelenburg for 24 h postoperatively will significantly decrease postoperative shoulder pain.

Materials and methods

Subjects and study design

This is a prospective randomized controlled study that was conducted at the American University of Beirut Medical Center (AUBMC), on patients undergoing

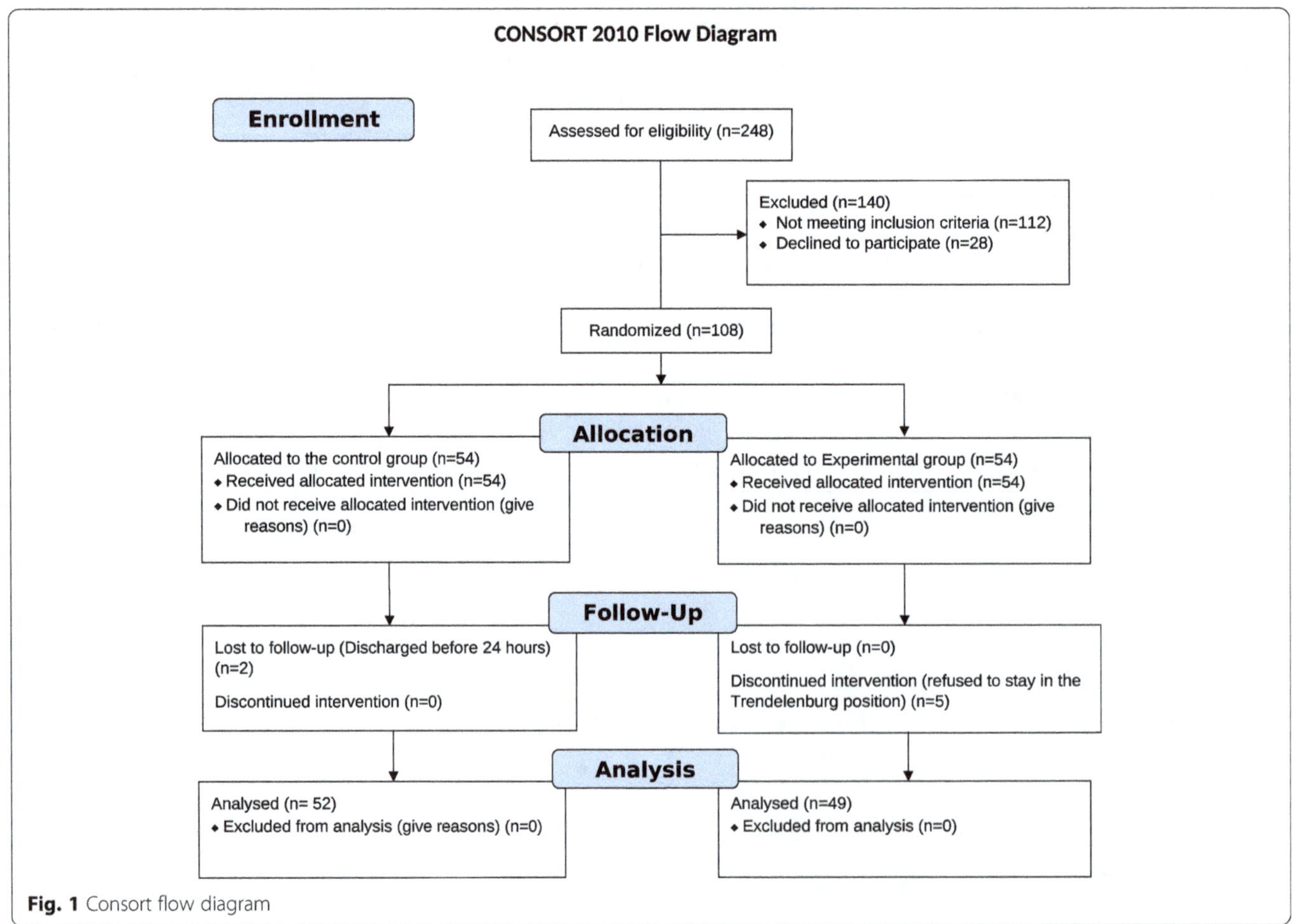

Fig. 1 Consort flow diagram

laparoscopic gynecologic surgeries. This study was approved by AUBMC's Institutional Review Board (IRB ID: OGY.JN.03) and written informed consent was obtained from all patients. The study adheres to the CONSORT guidelines (Fig. 1) and was retrospectively registered at clinicaltrials.gov (NCT04129385, principal investigator: Joseph Nassif, date of registration: June 28, 2019).

This study included female patients, aged between 18 and 60 years, with American Society of Anesthesiologist (ASA) physical status I or II scheduled for diagnostic or operative gynecological laparoscopic surgery of one to three-hour duration with abdominal incisions measuring less than 1.6 cm in size. Patients with the following criteria were excluded: conversion of the surgery to laparotomy, requirement of an abdominal insufflation pressure greater than 14 mmHg, history of gastroesophageal reflux, thrombophilia or high risk of deep vein thrombosis according to the ACOG 2007 practice bulletin, pregnancy, morbid obesity (BMI > 40), and 1 day surgery. Patients were randomly allocated to Groups 1 (Control) and 2 (Intervention) using a computer-generated randomization table. Blinding of the group allocation was not possible due to the design of the study.

Study design

All patients received Thrombo-Embolic-Deterrent (TED) stockings preoperatively. Intravenous (IV) access was established in the induction room then standard ASA monitoring devices were applied in the operating room. Induction of anesthesia was achieved using midazolam 1–2 mg fentanyl 1–2 μg/kg, lidocaine 1.5 mg/kg, and propofol 2 mg/kg IV. Rocuronium 0.6 mg/kg was administered to facilitate tracheal intubation. All patients received dexamethasone 8 mg IV after induction to prevent postoperative nausea and vomiting (PONV). Maintenance of anesthesia was provided using a mixture of oxygen and air ($FiO_2 = 50\%$), sevoflurane (1–1.2 MAC), fentanyl and rocuronium.

Upon deflation of abdomen, fentanyl 1 μg/kg was given for postoperative pain relief and ondansetron 4 mg for PONV prevention. At the end of surgery, muscle relaxation was reversed with a combination of glycopyrrolate/neostigmine or sugammadex.

In the control group, patients underwent the standard laparoscopic procedure. While still in Trendelenburg position and prior to wound closure and with the laparoscopic port valves open, the patients' abdomen was passively deflated. The patients were placed in supine head up position in the post anesthesia care unit (PACU) and postoperatively as is common practice at our institution. Patients in the intervention group were subjected to the same maneuver as the control group patients prior to wound closure but were positioned in a Trendelenburg position (20 °) once fully awake and cooperative in the PACU. They retained this posture for the first 24 h postoperatively. The maximum time allowed in a straight-up position was three 15-min intervals over a 24-h period (the first interval being at the time of clear fluid intake at 12 h postoperatively).

Incentive spirometry was mandatory for all patients postoperatively once fully awake.

Postoperative pain and nausea management was standardized and provided systematically for all patients. Starting in the PACU, medications included intravenous administration of 1 g acetaminophen IV and 100 mg ketoprofen IV every 6 and 8 h, respectively. Tramadol 100 mg IV was used as a rescue medication that was also given intravenously every 8 h upon demand. 4 mg of ondansetron and/or 10 mg of metoclopramide were given every 8 h as rescue medication for nausea and/or vomiting. Data collection of postoperative pain and nausea started at the arrival of patients to the PACU, then at 4, 6, 12 and 24 h postoperatively. Total amount of rescue pain and nausea medications used was recorded at all time-points.

Outcome measures

The primary outcome of this study was the presence and severity of shoulder pain 12 h after laparoscopic surgery. The numerical rating scale (NRS) was used to assess for pain measures on a 0 to 10-point scale; 0 representing "no pain" and 10 representing "worst pain". Secondary outcomes included the presence and severity of shoulder pain and nausea upon patient arrival to the PACU, then 4, 6, 12 and 24 h postoperatively using the NRS scale. Time to first rescue pain medication, total rescue pain medications during the first 24 h post-surgery, and the patients' pain scores (using the NRS) with the overall satisfaction from pain control were also recorded.

Statistical and power analysis

This is a two-sided randomized controlled study, with a proposed power of 80% and alpha = 0.05.

The sample size calculation was done by expecting a 30% reduction in shoulder pain in the interventional group compared to the control one at 12 h post operatively. Thus, a total sample size of 108 patients was obtained, divided into 54 patients in each group, taking into account a maximum dropout rate of 20%. The later rate is expected because of non-tolerance of the Trendelenburg position or to conversion to laparotomy if needed.

The Statistical Package for the Social Sciences Software (SPSS) and the Statistical Analysis System (SAS) were used for the data analysis. Data are presented as mean ± SD or median [IQR] for continuous data and frequency (percentage) for categorical data. Proc mixed test was used to the mixed group and time effect on pain and nausea scores post-operatively. Student's t-test was used to compare the normally distributed continuous data and Mann-Whitney test was used for ordinal data. Chi-square test or Fisher exact test was used for categorical data.

Results

A total of 248 patients were assessed for eligibility and 108 enrolled in the study between June 2016 and June 2018. Seven patients were excluded (five withdrew because they refused to stay in Trendelenburg position for the total duration of the study, and two were discharged before 24 h postoperatively). 101 patients were included in the final data analysis (52 patients in the control group and 49 patients in the experimental group).

Basic demographics, types of the surgical procedures, and procedural duration are presented in Table 1. Both were comparable with no significant differences between the two groups. We did not observe any hemodynamic or respiratory side effect that required any intervention in any of the patients throughout the study period and no patients were re-admitted due to any hemodynamic instability or respiratory adverse event.

Pain scores were significantly lower in the Trendelenburg group, and the trend was a decreasing pain score in both groups over time (Table 2). This effect was highly significant when taking into consideration the group allocation and different time points. Improvement in postoperative shoulder pain between time of arrival to PACU (time zero) and 12 h postoperatively was significantly higher in patients allocated to the experimental group compared to the control group with pain severity decreasing by 76% compared to 6.9% ($p < 0.001$) respectively (Fig. 2).

Time to first analgesic request was longer in the experimental group compared to the control group (111.39 ± 132.58 min vs. 85.86 ± 134.64 min, $p = 0.46$ respectively), yet the difference was not statistically significant.

Nausea scores significantly decreased with time in both groups, and was significantly higher in the experimental group (Table 2). Incidence of nausea at any time postop was not statistically different between the two groups (78% vs. 75% respectively with $p = 0.8$). However, the total PONV medications used were significantly lower in the experimental group, metoclopramide consumption (10.00 ± 14.95 mg vs. 4.08 ± 0.16, $p = 0.016$) and ondansetron consumption (0.85 ± 2.00 mg vs. 0.16 ± 0.80 mg, $p = 0.036$).

Non-opioid and opioid consumption showed statistically significant difference between both groups (Table 3). Patients allocated to the experimental group had lower postoperative analgesic consumption compared to the control group ($p < 0.001$).

Satisfaction score was significantly higher in patients who were randomized to the Trendelenburg position ($p < 0.001$). These patients had a median score of 9.5 compared to a score of 8 in the control patients (Fig. 3).

Discussion

As previously noted, shoulder pain is reported to occur in 35 to 70% of laparoscopic surgeries [2, 3], mostly to the patients' right side. The phrenic nerve originates from the C3 to C5 cervical nerves in the neck and descends through the thorax to innervate the diaphragm. A link between phrenic nerve irritation and this referred type of pain is suggested in the literature [15, 16]. Severe postoperative shoulder pain may lead to patient dissatisfaction but also to pulmonary complications such as atelectasis and pneumonia as patients are unable to take deep breaths. This study supports the theory that Trendelenburg position displaces retained CO_2 gas towards the pelvis and away from the diaphragm, thereby decreasing phrenic nerve irritation and hence shoulder

Table 1 Demographic Characteristics, Types of Surgical Procedures, and Procedural Durations

	Group 1, Control (*n* = 52)	Group 2, Trendelenburg (*n* = 49)	*p*-value
Age, years	38.42 ± 10.69	36.29 ± 8.67	0.27
Weight, kg	66.96 ± 12.66	61.98 ± 11.58	0.06
Surgery type			
Laparoscopic Hysterectomy	15 (28.8)	7 (14.3)	
Laparoscopic Adnexectomy	12 (23.1)	15 (30.6)	
Laparoscopic Endometriosis	3 (5.8)	6 (12.2)	
Laparoscopic Myomectomy	12 (23.1)	14 (28.6)	
Others	10 (19.2)	7 (14.3)	
Intraoperative time, minutes	105.5 (48.2)	92.37 (36.2)	0.23
Laparoscopic time, minutes	88 (47.4)	85.88 (54.5)	0.83
Total intra-op fentanyl, mcg	281 ± 88.9	283 ± 84.31	0.91

Values are mean ± SD, number (%)

Table 2 Postoperative Shoulder Pain Scores

	Group 1, Control ($n = 52$)	Group 2, Trendelenburg ($n = 49$)	p-value
NRS Pain Score			
PACU	6.00 [1.00–7.75]	2.00 [1.00–4.00]	0.003
4 h postop	6.00 [2.00–8.00]	2.00 [1.00–3.00]	< 0.001
6 h postop	6.00 [4.00–7.00]	1.00 [0.00–1.00]	< 0.001
12 h postop	5.00 [3.00–6.00]	0.00 [0.00–1.00]	< 0.001
24 h postop	3.00 [1.25–5.00]	0.00 [0.00–1.00]	< 0.001
NRS PONV Score			
PACU	2 [0.00–6.00]	1 [0.00–2.00]	0.033
4 h postop	2 [0.00–4.75]	1 [0.00–1.00]	< 0.001
6 h postop	1 [0.00–3.00]	0 [0.00–1.00]	0.001
12 h postop	1 [0.00–2.00]	0 [0.00–1.00]	< 0.001
24 h postop	1 [0.00–2.00]	0 [0.00–1.00]	< 0.001

PACU Post Anesthesia Care Unit, *PONV* Post-Operative Nausea and Vomiting
Values are medians and interquartile ranges

pain, as well as a quicker resorption of the soluble CO_2 gas in a highly vascular area which is the pelvis.

This study is the first to assess the effect of Trendelenburg position on postoperative shoulder pain following laparoscopic gynecologic surgery. Only one other study by Aydemir et al. [15] looked prospectively at the effect of Trendelenburg position on postoperative shoulder pain, however the study subjects were patients undergoing laparoscopic cholecystectomy.

It is difficult to compare both studies because they are not identically designed. This study is prospective and randomized while the other is non-randomized. Moreover, the duration of the study intervention (Trendelenburg positioning) as well as the study subjects and the nature and duration of the surgical procedures are different. While this study required that patients be placed in Trendelenburg position for 24 h postoperatively and measured the pain scores at 4, 6, 12 and 24 h, the study by Aydemir et al. placed patients in extreme Trendelenburg position upon reporting shoulder pain for only 10 min at a time, and recorded pain scores 10 min afterwards. The degree of Trendelenburg was not mentioned. Pain scores were statistically significantly improved thereby supporting the theory that Trendelenburg position decreases the phrenic nerve irritation caused by the CO_2 gas. Similar to this study results, total analgesic consumption over 24 h was statistically significantly improved in the experimental compared to the control group.

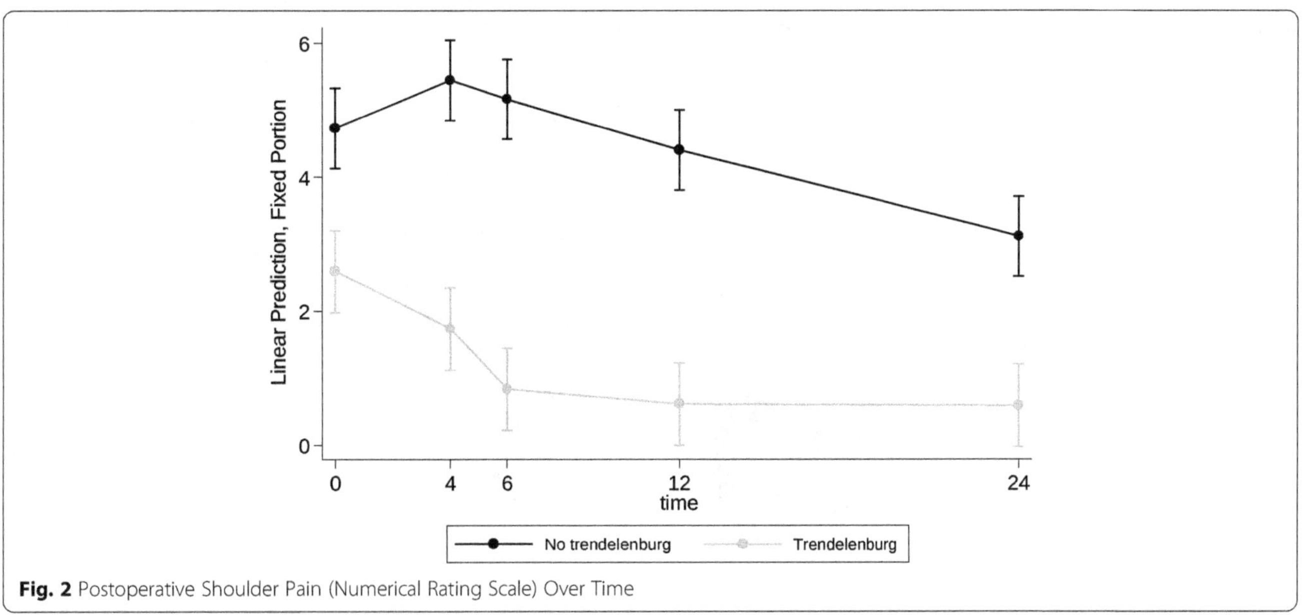

Fig. 2 Postoperative Shoulder Pain (Numerical Rating Scale) Over Time

Table 3 Opioid and Non-Opioid Postoperative Analgesic Consumption

	Group 1, Control	Group 2, Trendelenburg	*p*-value
Non-Opioid Consumption			
Acetaminophen, g	2 ± 1.4	0.99 ± 1.41	< 0.001
Ketoprofen, mg	146.15 ± 105.64	44.89 ± 86.75	< 0.001
Opioid consumption, mg	8.12 ± 7.07	0.82 ± 2.76	< 0.001
Time to first analgesic request, min	85.86 ± 134.64	111.39 ± 132.58	0.46

Values are mean ± SD
*total amount of opioids consumed (Tramadol and Morphine, where Tramadol was converted to morphine equivalent doses)

Aydemir et al. demonstrated that Trendelenburg position is both quick and effective, with improvement in pain scores as early as ten minutes after Trendelenburg positioning. Acute and fast improvement of shoulder pain was supported by our study as the most acute drop in shoulder pain score was noted from 0 to 6 h (Fig. 2). Beyond 6 h, the pain score was maintained more or less at the same level and did not improve further. Since some patients are unable to tolerate Trendelenburg position for a long time, adopting it for a shorter period of time may be enough to significantly improve shoulder pain scores. Further studies are needed to determine the optimal duration of this intervention for shoulder pain management.

Many other methods to decrease postoperative shoulder pain have been described in the literature. The most recent Cochrane review by Kaloo et al. [16] reviewed all interventions mentioned in the literature on shoulder pain following laparoscopic gynecologic surgery. Trendelenburg position is not listed as one the possible interventions in this review article. Among all the described methods, authors concluded that potentially beneficial interventions in the reduction of postoperative shoulder pain include: a specific technique for releasing the pneumoperitoneum (such as pulmonary recruitment maneuvers, extended assisted ventilation or active aspiration of intra-abdominal gas), intraperitoneal fluid instillation, placement of an intraperitoneal drain and local anesthetic application into the peritoneal cavity (not sub diaphragmatic). Comparing these interventions to postoperative Trendelenburg positioning through randomized controlled trials is important to evaluate which of them all is most beneficial, and which carries the lowest risk of adverse events.

This randomized study provides solid evidence that the intervention is beneficial in reducing shoulder pain. One limitation is that although all healthcare providers and patients were blinded to the study intraoperatively, they were not blinded to the patient postoperatively hence patients might have underreported pain when in the Trendelenburg position and there might have been a small bias due to a placebo effect. Another limitation is the duration of the study intervention: Although most patients tolerated Trendelenburg positioning for 24 h, six refused to stay in Trendelenburg for the entire 24 h and hence withdrew from the study, but the rate of dropout between the two groups was not significant and was below the 20% expected level. Moreover, among the advantages of laparoscopic surgery are early or immediate resumption of regular diet, early ambulation and

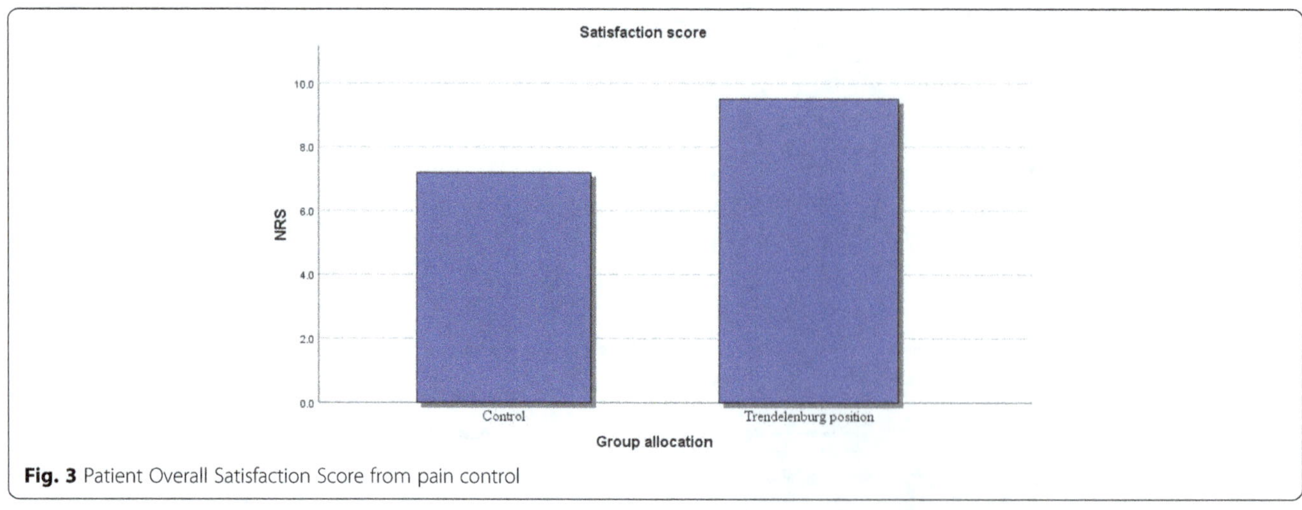

Fig. 3 Patient Overall Satisfaction Score from pain control

short hospital stay including same day discharge when applicable. Patients in the intervention arm were kept on a clear fluid diet for 12 h postoperatively, could not ambulate immediately postoperatively and were not discharged till after 24 h, thereby limiting some of the advantages of minimally invasive surgery. However, we can suggest to keep this position as much as feasible at home if an earlier discharge can be suggested in the future.

Conclusions

In conclusion, Trendelenburg position is an easy non-pharmacologic intervention that is beneficial in reducing postoperative shoulder pain following gynecologic laparoscopic surgery, decreasing the amount of analgesic consumption and improving patients' overall satisfaction with the surgical experience. Being non-pharmacologic, it can be administered by trained nursing staff and can even be taught to patients and implemented at home by simply elevating the pelvis with the use of pillows. Not only does it have zero cost, it can potentially decrease medical expenses as less analgesics are administered. More importantly, the smaller the amount of analgesic consumption, the lower the risk of medication adverse events such as respiratory depression, nausea, pruritus and ileus which are often encountered with the use of opioids [15]. Additional studies are required to determine whether Trendelenburg positioning improves postoperative shoulder pain following non-gynecologic procedures and to delineate the optimal duration of this intervention to maximally decrease shoulder pain scores.

Abbreviations

ASA: American Society of Anesthesiologists; NRS: Numerical Rating Scale; PACU: Post Anesthesia Care Unit; PONV: Postoperative Nausea and Vomiting; TED: Thrombo-Embolic-Deterrent

Acknowledgments

Not Applicable.

Authors' contributions

CZ and DC contributed equally to the study design, data analysis, and manuscript writing and review. AK, AAM, and MH helped in patient's recruitment and manuscript review. FS helped in patient recruitment, data analysis, and manuscript drafting. JN helped in the study design, patient recruitment, manuscript review, intervention, and data analysis. All authors have read and approved the manuscript.

Author details

[1]Department of Anesthesiology, American University of Beirut Medical Center, P.O. Box 11-0236, Beirut, Lebanon. [2]Department of Obstetrics and Gynecology, American University of Beirut Medical Center, Beirut, Lebanon.

References

1. Barnett JC, Hurd WW, Rogers RM Jr, Williams NL, Shapiro SA. Laparoscopic positioning and nerve injuries. J Minim Invasive Gynecol. 2007;14(5):664–72 quiz 73.
2. Dobbs F, Kumar V, Alexandar J, Hull M. Pain after laparoscopy related to posture and ring versus clip sterilization. Br J Gynaecol. 1987;94(3):262–6.
3. Ko-lam W, Paiboonworachat S, Pongchairerks P, Junrungsee S, Sandhu T. Combination of etoricoxib and low-pressure pneumoperitoneum versus standard treatment for the management of pain after laparoscopic cholecystectomy: a randomized controlled trial. Surg Endosc. 2016;30(11):4800–8.
4. Madsen MR, Jensen KE. Postoperative pain and nausea after laparoscopic cholecystectomy. Surg Laparosc Endosc. 1992;2:302–5.
5. Coventry D. Anaesthesia for laparoscopic surgery. J R Coll Surg Edinb. 1995;40:151–60.
6. Korell M, Schmaus F, Strowitzki T, Schneeweiss SG, Hepp H. Pain intensity following laparoscopy. Surg Laparosc Endosc. 1996;6:375–9.
7. Lepner U, Goroshina J, Samarütel J. Postoperative pain relief after laparoscopic cholecystectomy:a randomised prospective double-blind clinical trial. Scand J Surg. 2003;92:121–4.
8. Jackson SA, Laurence AS, Hill JC. Does post-laparoscopy pain relate to residual carbon dioxide? Anaesthesia. 1996;51:485–7.
9. Kojima Y, Yokota S, Ina H. Shoulder pain after gynaecological laparoscopy caused by arm abduction. Eur J Anaesthesiol. 2004;21:571–83.
10. Berberoglu M, Dilek O, Ercan F, Kati I, Özmen M. The effect of CO_2 insufflation rate on the Postlaparoscopic shoulder pain. J Laparoendosc Adv Surg Tech A. 1998;8:273–7.
11. Pergialiotis V, Vlachos DE, Kontzoglou K, Perrea D, Vlachos GD. Pulmonary recruitment maneuver to reduce pain after laparoscopy: a meta-analysis of randomized controlled trials. Surg Endosc. 2015;29(8):2101–8.
12. Sharami SH, Sharami MB, Abdollahzadeh M, Keyvan A. Randomised clinical trial of the influence of pulmonary recruitment manoeuvre on reducing shoulder pain after laparoscopy. J Obstet Gynaecol. 2010;30(5):505–10.
13. Nezhat C, Nezhat F, Nezhat C. Nezhat's operative gynecologic laparoscopy and hysteroscopy. Cambridge: Cambridge University press; 2008.
14. Suginami R, Taniguchi F, Suginami H. Prevention of Postlaparoscopic shoulder pain by forced evacuation of residual CO_2. JSLS. 2009;13:56–9.
15. Aydemir O, Aslan FE, Karabacak U, Akdas O. The effect of exaggerated lithotomy position on shoulder pain after laparoscopic cholecystectomy. Pain Manag Nurs. 2018;19(6):663–70.
16. Kaloo P, Hills R, Kaloo C, Whittaker M. Interventions for the reduction of shoulder pain following gynaecological laparoscopic procedures. Cochrane Database Syst Rev. 2014;6:CD011101.

22

The effect of intraoperative lidocaine infusion on opioid consumption and pain after totally extraperitoneal laparoscopic inguinal hernioplasty

Anup Ghimire[1], Asish Subedi[2*], Balkrishna Bhattarai[2] and Birendra Prasad Sah[2]

Abstract

Background: As a component of multimodal analgesia, the administration of systemic lidocaine is a well-known technique. We aimed to evaluate the efficacy of lidocaine infusion on postoperative pain-related outcomes in patients undergoing totally extraperitoneal (TEP) laparoscopies inguinal hernioplasty.

Methods: In this randomized controlled double-blind study, we recruited 64 patients to receive either lidocaine 2% (intravenous bolus 1.5 mg. kg^{-1} followed by an infusion of 2 mg. kg^{-1}. h^{-1}), or an equal volume of normal saline. The infusion was initiated just before the induction of anesthesia and discontinued after tracheal extubation. The primary outcome of the study was postoperative morphine equivalent consumption up to 24 h after surgery. Secondary outcomes included postoperative pain scores, nausea/vomiting (PONV), sedation, quality of recovery (scores based on QoR-40 questionnaire), patient satisfaction, and the incidence of chronic pain.

Results: The median (IQR) cumulative postoperative morphine equivalent consumption in the first 24 h was 0 (0–1) mg in the lidocaine group and 4 [1–8] mg in the saline group ($p < 0.001$). Postoperative pain intensity at rest and during movement at various time points in the first 24 h were significantly lower in the lidocaine group compared with the saline group ($p < 0.05$). Fewer patients reported PONV in the lidocaine group than in the saline group ($p < 0.05$). Median QoR scores at 24 h after surgery were significantly better in the lidocaine group (194 (194–196) than saline group 184 (183–186) ($p < 0.001$). Patients receiving lidocaine were more satisfied with postoperative analgesia than those receiving saline ($p = 0.02$). No difference was detected in terms of postoperative sedation and chronic pain after surgery.

Conclusions: Intraoperative lidocaine infusion for laparoscopic TEP inguinal hernioplasty reduces opioid consumption, pain intensity, PONV and improves the quality of recovery and patient satisfaction.

Keywords: Inguinal hernia, Laparoscopy, Lidocaine, Opioid analgesic, Postoperative pain

* Correspondence: asishsubedi19@gmail.com; ashish.subedi@bpkihs.edu
[2]Department of Anesthesiology & Critical Care Medicine, BP Koirala Institute of Health Sciences, Dharan, Nepal

Background

Inadequate pain relief after surgery causes undesirable effects. On the other hand, excessive use of opioids produces several adverse effects and might delay recovery [1, 2]. Therefore, a multimodal analgesia regimen is recommended in the perioperative setting as it provides superior analgesia and reduces opioid requirement [3]. Intravenous (IV) lidocaine is a widely studied drug for multimodal analgesia. IV lidocaine at the doses between 1.5–3 mg. kg^{-1}. h^{-1} produces analgesic, anti-hyperalgesic, and anti-inflammatory effects [4]. Besides, a low dose of lidocaine is relatively safe and more feasible for perioperative use [4–7]. Additional benefits of lidocaine infusion include a reduction in the incidence of postoperative nausea and vomiting, early return of bowel motility and improved quality of recovery [8].

Several studies have shown that perioperative lidocaine infusion reduces postoperative pain intensity and opioid consumption, while others have found lidocaine to be ineffective [8]. These inconsistent findings may be due to variation in surgical procedure, dose and duration of lidocaine infused. Interestingly, a current update from Cochrane based meta-analysis found a weak evidence for IV lidocaine compared to placebo on early postoperative pain scores and overall opioid requirements [9]. On the contrary, other recently published meta-analyses have shown improvement in postoperative pain-related outcomes with lidocaine infusion during laparoscopic clolecystectomy [10, 11].

Although lidocaine infusion was effective for postoperative analgesia in open inguinal hernia surgery [12], its use has not been reported in totally extraperitoneal (TEP) laparoscopic inguinal hernioplasty. Therefore, the primary objective of our study was to compare the effects of intraoperative lidocaine infusion on postoperative opioid consumption following TEP laparoscopic inguinal hernioplasty.

Methods

This prospective randomized double-blind clinical trial was conducted at the BP Koirala Institute of Health Sciences (BPKIHS) from December 2015 to March 2017. Ethical approval for this study (Ref No. IRC/520/015) was provided by the Institutional review committee of BPKIHS, Dharan, Nepal (Member secretary Dr. Ashish Shrestha) on 24 June 2015. Before enrollment of patients, the trial was registered by the principal investigator (AG) at clinicaltrials.gov (Ref No. NCT02601651). The trial was conducted according to Good Clinical Practice and the Consolidated Standards of Reporting Trials (CONSORT) guidelines.

Patients were screened for eligibility (AG) during the pre-anesthetic visit at the in-patient-unit, the night before surgery. Male patients aged between 18 and 65 years, of ASA physical status I–II, planned for laparoscopic TEP repair of the inguinal hernia were eligible. Patients were excluded if they were obese, unable to comprehend the pain assessment scale, allergic to local anesthetics, on pain medication or anti-arrhythmic drugs, or had, psychiatric disorders, cardiac arrhythmia, hepatorenal disease or epilepsy.

After obtaining written informed consent, all eligible participants were randomly assigned, in a 1:1 ratio, to receive either lidocaine (intervention) or normal saline (placebo comparator) infusion. The anesthesia supporting staff created the trial-group assignment from the computer-based randomization list, which remained secured in sequentially numbered sealed opaque envelopes and concealed until after enrollment.

On the day of surgery, an anesthesia assistant not involved in the study prepared the drug solution after breaking the codes. Patients received one of the two assigned study medications just before the induction of anesthesia: Lidocaine group received an IV bolus of 1.5 mg. kg^{-1} lidocaine (Lox 2%®, Neon pharmaceuticals limited, Mumbai, India) followed by a continuous infusion of 2 mg. kg^{-1}. h^{-1} until the tracheal extubation; The saline group received an equal volume of IV 0.9% normal saline (NS) bolus followed by a continuous infusion. Patients, attending anesthesiologists, and the investigator who collected the data and assessed the outcomes were unaware of the trial-group assignment.

Patients received no premedication. During the pre-anesthetic visit, they were educated on the numeric pain rating scale (NRS, 0–10 cm) for postoperative pain, where 0 is no pain and 10 is the worst imaginable excruciating pain. In the operating room, standard monitoring was applied. Just before the induction of anesthesia, patients received the study drug, according to the group allocation. Anesthesia was induced with IV fentanyl 1.5 μg. kg^{-1} and propofol 2–2.5 mg. kg^{-1} till the cessation of verbal response and the tracheal intubation was facilitated with vecuronium 0.1 mg. kg^{-1} IV. The lungs were mechanically ventilated in volume control mode, maintaining the end-tidal carbon dioxide ($ETCO_2$) between 35 and 45 mmHg.

Intravenous paracetamol 1 g was administered for 15 min after tracheal intubation. Pre-incisional infiltration in the three trocar sites was done with 2 ml of 0.25% bupivacaine. Anesthesia was maintained with an air / oxygen mixture (inspired oxygen fraction 0.40) and isoflurane, adjusting the end-tidal concentration of isoflurane to maintain mean arterial pressure (MAP) within 20% of the baseline. IV fentanyl 0.5 μg. kg^{-1} was supplemented intraoperatively if MAP and heart rate increased by 20% from the baseline after ensuring adequate end-tidal concentration of isoflurane, neuromuscular blockade and targeted range of $ETCO_2$. The adequate neuromuscular blockade was achieved with supplemental doses of vecuronium IV bolus after observing curare notch in capnograph. Any episode of intraoperative hypotension (MAP < 65 mmHg) and bradycardia (heart rate < 50 beats. min^{-1}) was treated with ephedrine 5 mg and atropine 0.4 mg IV respectively.

An experienced surgeon performed the TEP laparoscopic surgery for inguinal hernia repair as described elsewhere [13]. Ketorolac 30 mg IV was administered at the end of surgery and scheduled to be given at 8 h intervals. The residual neuromuscular block was reversed with IV neostigmine 0.05 mg. kg^{-1} and glycopyrrolate 0.01 mg. kg^{-1}. Following successful tracheal extubation, the study drug was discontinued and the patient was transferred to the postanesthesia care unit (PACU).

The blinded investigator assessed the postoperative outcomes. The primary outcome was total IV morphine equivalent consumed in the first 24 h. Secondary outcomes were postoperative pain scores (NRS) at rest and on movement, sedation scores recorded using a 5-point scale (0 = alert, 1 = arouses to voice, 2 = arouses with gentle tactile stimulation, 3 = arouses with vigorous tactile stimulation, 4 = lack of responsiveness) [14], the incidence of PONV using a 3-point scale (0 = none, 1 = nausea, 2 = vomiting), time to the first perception of pain (min), time to first void (h), adverse events (lightheadedness, tinnitus, perioral numbness, arrhythmia), quality of recovery based on QoR-40 questionnaire [15] at 24 h after surgery, patient satisfaction for postoperative pain relief using a five-point Likert scale at 24 h following surgery (1-highly satisfied, 2-satisfied, 3-neutral, 4-not satisfied, 5-strongly dissatisfied) and the incidence of chronic post-surgical pain (CPSP) at 3 months.

Pain and sedation scores were assessed at PACU (on arrival, 15 min, 30 min, 1 h, 2 h) and surgical unit (4 h, 6 h, 8 h, 12 h, 24 h). If the NRS score for pain was > 3 at rest, morphine 1 mg IV bolus was administered in the PACU, and repeated at 5 min interval until NRS was ≤3. After 2 h of the stay in the PACU, the patients were transferred to the ward. In the surgical unit, tramadol 50 mg IV was administered for NRS score > 3 and 50 mg was repeated at 10 min interval, up to a maximum dose of 300 mg in the first 24 h for maintaining VAS score for pain ≤3. The amount of tramadol consumed was converted to an equivalent dose of morphine from an online dose equivalent calculator (www.clincalc.com/Opioids). Ondansetron 4 mg IV was administered for persistent nausea (lasting > 5 min) or vomiting. CPSP was defined as pain that developed after a surgical procedure and persisted at least 3 months after surgery [16]. For this, the blinded investigator contacted the patients via telephone at 3 months after surgery. They were asked to answer the following question: Do you feel any pain in the operated area?

The sample size calculation was based on the study by H Kang on postoperative opioid consumption between the lidocaine infusion group and the placebo group in open inguinal hernia surgery [12]. Using an online statistical calculator (G power® version 3.0.1), an estimated sample size of 29 patients in each study group achieved a power of 80% to detect a Cohen's d effect size of 0.76 in the primary outcome measure of opioid consumption, assuming a type I error of 0.05. With an anticipated 10% drop-out, a total of 64 patients were enrolled.

The data were entered into excel software and analyzed using STATA version 13.0 (Stata Corporation, College Station, TX, USA). Histograms and the Shapiro-Wilk test was used to check the normality of the data. Normally distributed data were compared using a 2-tailed t-test for independent samples. Non-normally distributed data were analyzed using the Mann-Whitney U test. For ordinal data, the Kruskal-Wallis test was applied. Chi-square test or Fischer's exact test was used for analyzing the categorical variables as appropriate. The finding with an associated *p*-value less than 0.05 was considered as statistically significant.

Results

Of the 82 screened patients, 18 patients were excluded (Fig. 1). Two patients in each group could not be traced during follow-up in 3 months. All outcomes were analyzed with the intention-to-treat principle. The demographics and surgical characteristics between the two groups did not reveal any significant differences (Table 1). The median (IQR) intraoperative fentanyl consumption was significantly less in the lidocaine group 0(0–0) μg vs. 20 (0–30) μg in the saline group ($p < 0.001$).

The cumulative median IV morphine equivalent consumption at 24 h postoperatively was significantly reduced in the lidocaine group than in the saline group (Fig. 2). The median morphine requirement in PACU was 0 (0–1) mg in the lidocaine group compared with 2 (0–4) mg in the saline group ($p = 0.003$). In the surgical unit, patients consumed a lesser median (IQR) tramadol in the lidocaine group, 0 (0–0) mg compared with the saline group 0 (0–50) mg ($p < 0.001$). The median NRS scores at rest and during movement were significantly lower in the lidocaine group than in the saline group at all time points after surgery (Figs. 3 & 4). The time to the first perception of pain was longer in those receiving lidocaine (median 30 min (15–30) compared with those receiving NS (median 10 min (0–15); $p < 0.001$).

A significant number of patients in the saline group had PONV and needed antiemetic compared to the lidocaine group (Table 2). Postoperative sedation scores

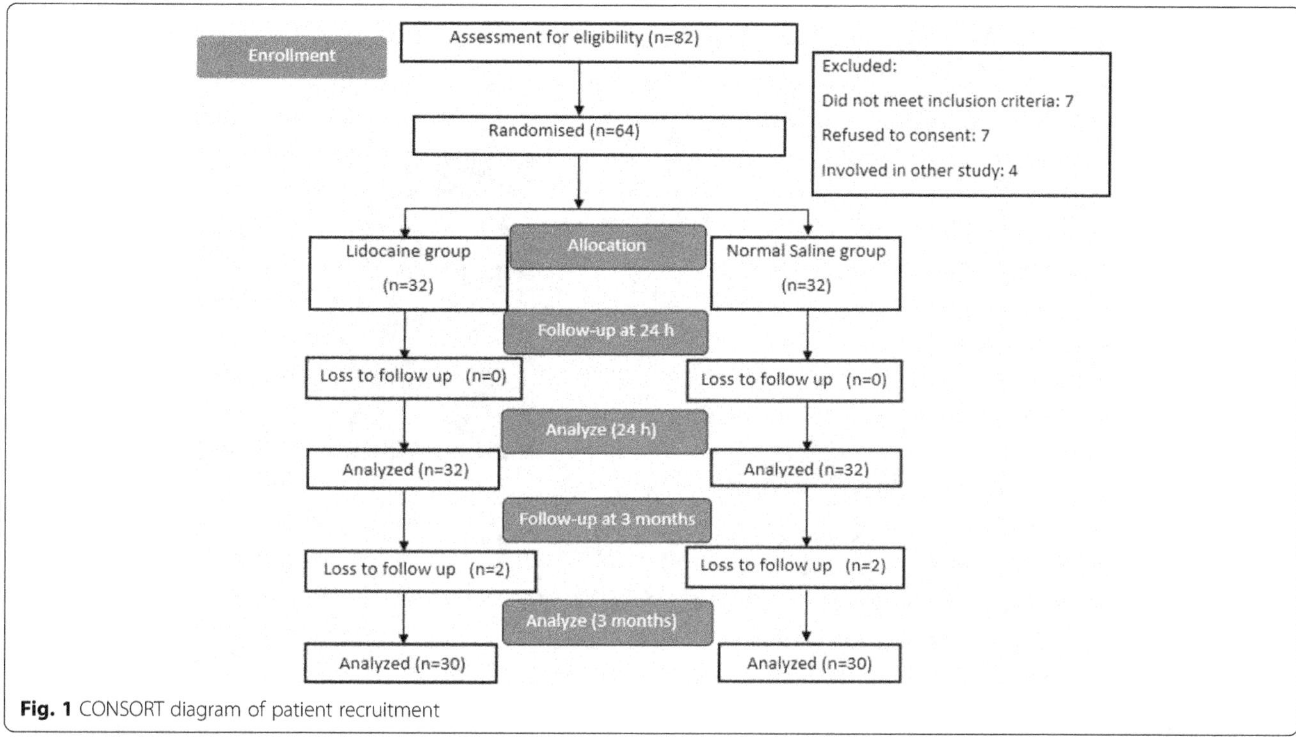

Fig. 1 CONSORT diagram of patient recruitment

were comparable between the two groups. Postoperative quality of recovery and patient satisfaction with postoperative pain relief was better in those receiving lidocaine (Table 2). No sign/symptoms related to lidocaine toxicity were observed. One patient in the lidocaine group developed intraoperative hypotension and bradycardia which was managed with ephedrine 5 mg and atropine 0.4 mg intravenously. When assessed in 3 months after surgery, two (7%) patients in the lidocaine group developed CPSP compared to four (13%) in the placebo group ($p = 0.67$).

Discussion

Our study showed that intraoperative infusion of low dose lidocaine decreased postoperative opioid requirement and pain intensity in comparison with normal saline in patients undergoing laparoscopic TEP inguinal hernia surgery. Patients receiving lidocaine had fewer occurrences of PONV, a better quality of recovery and were more satisfied with postoperative pain relief than those receiving saline. Patients complained of pain later in the lidocaine group than the saline group. No significant difference was observed for postoperative sedation and the incidence of chronic pain in 3 months.

It is well-established that lidocaine acts on voltage-gated sodium channels when administered locally for peripheral nerve block. However, at lower concentration systemic lidocaine is insufficient to produce direct analgesia solely by blocking the neuronal sodium channels [17]. Although it is not fully understood how intravenous lidocaine produces analgesia, several potential

Table 1 Patient characteristics and surgical profiles of patients

Variables	Lidocaine group ($n = 32$)	Normal saline group ($n = 32$)	P-value
Age (years)	40 (30–52)	43 (33–52)	0.61
ASA PS (1/2)	28/4	27/5	0.71
BMI (kg/m^2)	23.02 ± 2.85	22.01 ± 2.02	0.10
Surgical site: Unilateral/Bilateral	25/7	23/9	0.56
Mesh fixation (Yes/No)	31/1	32/0	0.50
Duration of surgery (min)	60 (48–90)	75 (60–90)	0.49
Intraoperative fentanyl supplement (μg)	0 (0–0)	20 (0–30)	< 0.001

Notes: Values are median (IQR), mean (SD), number.
Abbreviations: *BMI* body mass index; *ASA PS* American society of Anesthesiologist physical status

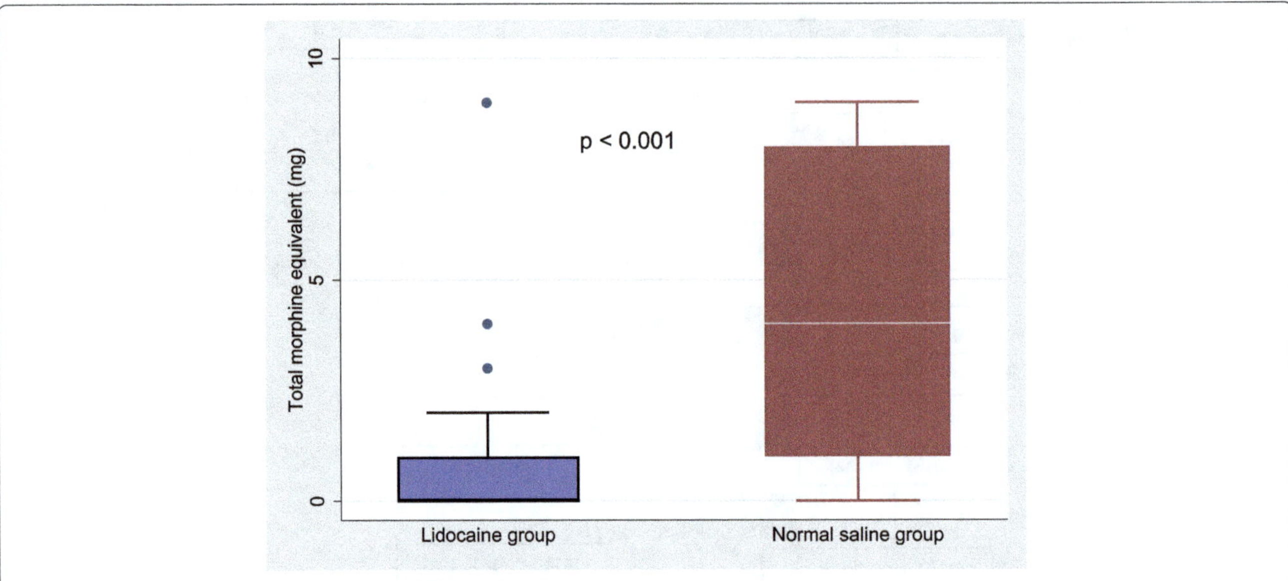

Fig. 2 Total morphine equivalent for 24 h postoperatively in patients receiving lidocaine and saline. Data are presented as median and interquartile range

mechanisms have been elucidated. Intravenous lidocaine increases acetylcholine concentration at the spinal level through an activation of both muscarinic and nicotinic receptors, and thereby prolongs the pain threshold [18]. Also, by activating central glycine (an inhibitory neurotransmitter) receptor, systemic lidocaine inhibits glutamate-induced excitatory response on the wide dynamic response in the spinal neurons [19]. The anti-hyperalgesic effect of IV lidocaine is due to blockade of NMDA receptor signaling and it is mediated indirectly by inhibition of the protein kinase C pathway [20]. In addition to this, systemic lidocaine has anti-inflammatory properties as a decline in pro-inflammatory cytokines is observed in patients receiving lidocaine infusion [21–23]. Because perioperative pain is linked to an inflammatory process, modulation of this phenomenon with the administration of systemic lidocaine could significantly reduce

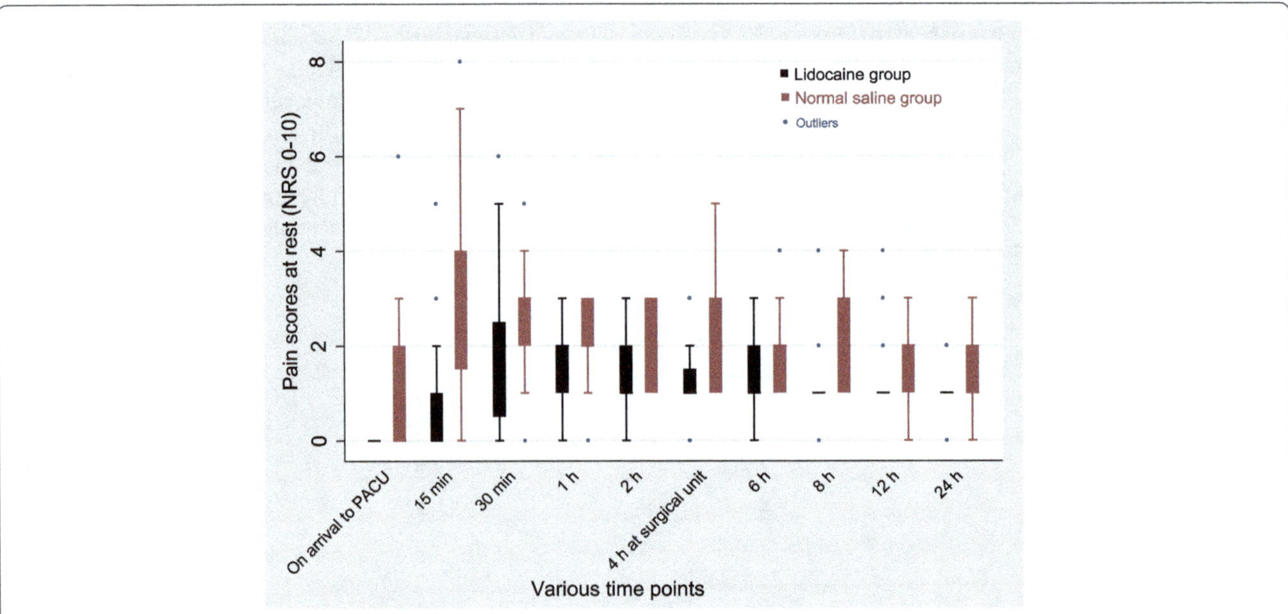

Fig. 3 Postoperative numerical rating pain (NRS) scores at various time points at rest. Data are median with error bars showing interquartile range. Significant difference between the groups was detected at all-time points ($p < 0.05$)

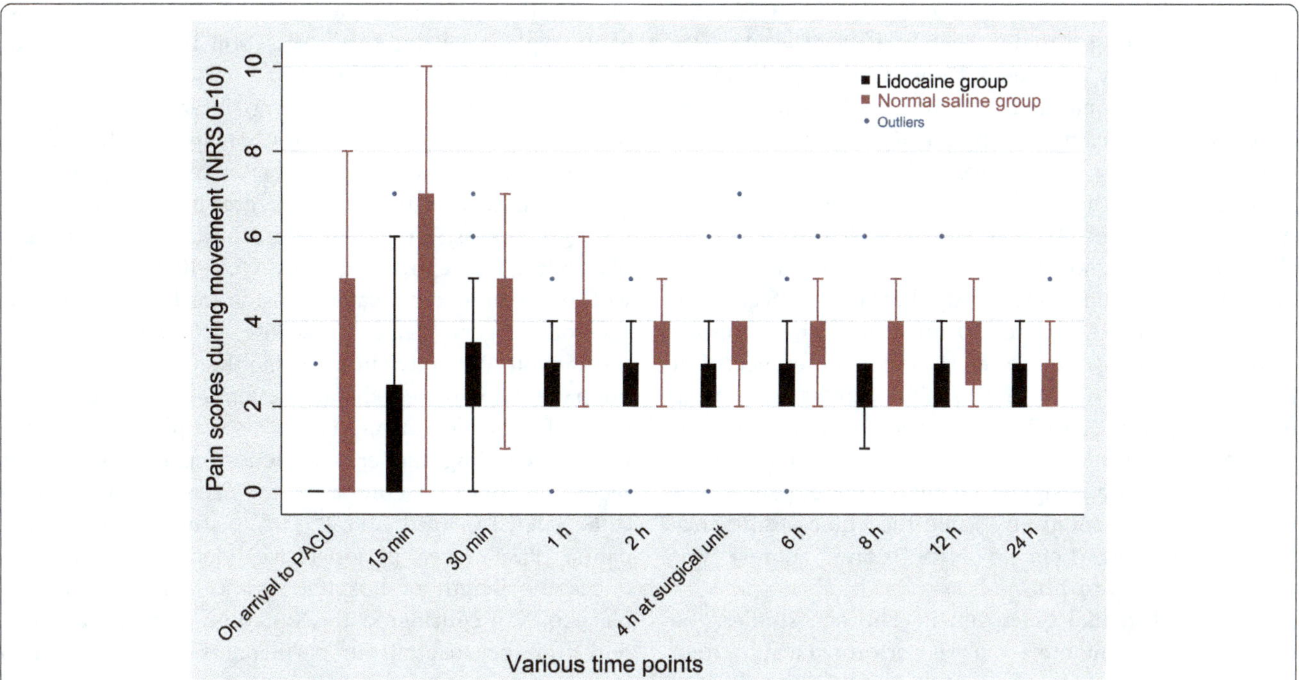

Fig. 4 Post-operative numerical rating pain scores (NRS) at various time points during movement. Data are median with error bars showing interquartile range. Significant difference between the groups was detected at all-time points ($p < 0.05$)

pain. Another relevant question is to explain how the intraoperative administration of IV lidocaine does reduces opioid and pain scores beyond its infusion period. This could be due to its action on various receptors and signal cascades that produces an anti-nociceptive, anti-hyperalgesia and anti-inflammatory effects [8].

Because of its influence in several pain pathways, systemic lidocaine is widely investigated adjuvant in the regimen of multimodal analgesia to reduce postoperative opioid consumption and pain. Although the majority of studies have demonstrated the analgesic effect of lidocaine, several other trials failed to confirm it. A recently updated Cochrane review in 2018 has provided a much-needed insight on the analgesic property of systemic lidocaine [9]. Random-effects meta-analysis from the same review on overall total postoperative opioid consumption favored lidocaine compared to the placebo (standardized mean difference (SMD) − 4.52 (mg, morphine equivalents (MEQ), 95%CI − 6.25 to− 2.79, $p < 0.001$; $I^2 = 73\%$; 40 studies, 2201 participants). The results of our study also indicated a similar reduction in total postoperative opioid consumption in the first 24 h after surgery in the lidocaine group compared to the saline group (median difference of − 4 mg morphine equivalents), despite using multimodal analgesia in both the groups.

Further, the aforementioned meta-analysis [9] demonstrated reduced pain scores at rest ("early time points"- in the PACU or 1 to 4 h postoperatively) in the lidocaine

Table 2 Postoperative outcomes

	Lidocaine group ($n = 32$)	Saline group ($n = 32$)	*p*-value
Nausea	5 (16%)	14 (44%)	0.01
Vomiting	2 (6%)	8 (25%)	0.04
Antiemetic needed	3 (9%)	11 (34%)	0.01
Time to first void; h	3 (2–4)	3 (3–4)	0.18
Quality of recovery;QoR-40 scores	194 (194–196)	184 (183–186)	< 0.001
Patients with satisfaction scores 1/2/3/4/5[a]	6/17/9/0/0	2/13/17/0/0	0.02

Notes: Values are number (proportion), or median (IQR)
[a]Satisfaction scores for postoperative pain relief, 1-Highly satisfied, 2-Satisfied, 3-Neutral, 4-Not satisfied, 5-Strongly dissatisfied

group compared to the control group (SMD − 0.50, 95% CI − 0.72 to− 0.28; Test for overall effect: Z = 4.41 ($P <$ 0.0001). This was equivalent to an average pain reduction between 0.37 cm and 2.48 cm on a VAS 0 to 10 cm scale in the lidocaine group. Likewise, at intermediate time points (24 h postoperatively) the standardized mean pain score at rest in the lidocaine group was 0.14 lower (95% CI − 0.25 to − 0.04; Test for overall effect: Z = 2.63 ($P = 0.0086$). This was equivalent to an average pain reduction in the lidocaine group between 0.48 cm and 0.10 cm on a VAS 0 to 10 cm scale. These results showed that lidocaine exerted a clinical difference of at least 1 cm on a 0–10 VAS scores for pain at rest during early time points (1 to 4 h); however, this difference was not observed at intermediate (24 h) time points. We too observed statistically significant difference in pain scores up to 24 h postoperatively, while the clinical difference of approximately 1 cm in NRS scores at rest was observed only up to 1 h.

Due to substantial heterogeneity between studies, the authors of the same meta-analysis performed a sub-group analysis based on type of surgery, duration and dose of lidocaine infusions [9]. In the older version (Cochrane review, 2015) there was a clear beneficial effect in terms of pain reduction in laparoscopic abdominal surgery compared to open abdominal surgery [6]. However, in the current updated version, no significant difference was observed, although the trend was towards a beneficial effect for abdominal laparoscopic surgery [9].

The optimal dose and time to terminate lidocaine infusion are still an unsolved issue. We had limited the duration of lidocaine infusion until the patients trachea was extubated due to a lack of dedicated infusion pumps and monitoring at the surgical unit. One might hypothesize that longer infusions would lead to more lasting analgesia but studies are yet to confirm this. The current meta-analysis (2018) had categorized the studies according to the usage of low ($< 2\ mg.kg^{-1}.\ h^{-1}$) and high ($\geq 2\ mg.kg^{-1} h^{-1}$) lidocaine doses in combination with either short (until the end of surgery or until PACU) or long (≥ 24 h postoperatively) duration of infusion [9]. However, they did not find any difference in outcomes when the dose or duration of the infusion was compared. A well designed randomized comparative study with a large sample size is needed to explore whether the continuation of systemic lidocaine infusion beyond the surgical period is effective.

In our study, fewer patients receiving lidocaine complained PONV compared to those receiving saline infusions. Similar to our finding, the Cochrane meta-analysis (2018) reported a significantly lower frequency of nausea in the lidocaine group than in the control group, but the vomiting rates did not differ [9]. Although, there is an association between lidocaine therapy and reduction in PONV, it may not reflect a causal relationship. The most likely explanation for this association is related to lidocaine's opioid-sparing effects.

Recently, there is a growing interest in patient-reported outcomes such as postoperative QoR and patient satisfaction. We observed better recovery profiles at 24 h of surgery in the lidocaine group as evident from the QoR scores. Similar to our study, De Oliveira and his colleagues reported greater QoR-40 scores at 24 h with perioperative lidocaine infusion for laparoscopic abdominal surgery [24, 25]. Likewise, in our study patient satisfaction was better in lidocaine than saline group and no patient expressed dissatisfaction over the intervention. The current meta-analysis also supports this finding by revealing higher satisfaction scores in patients receiving lidocaine compared to placebo group (SMD 0.76, 95% CI 0.46 to 1.06; $I^2 = 0\%$; 6 studies, 306 participants) [9]. Further, perioperative lidocaine infusion reduces the length of hospital stay as compared to the placebo. We considered this outcome as a limitation in our study because all our participants were required to stay in the hospital for 24 h after surgery. In terms of patient-reported outcomes, it would be interesting to explore the influence of perioperative lidocaine on the enhancement of recovery profiles, especially after major abdominal surgeries in future trials. A more recent meta-analysis focused on CPSP (total 6 trials included: 4 mastectomies, 1 thyroidectomy, 1 nephrectomy) found that systemic lidocaine administration reduces the development of CPSP [26]. As our study was not powered enough to detect the protective effect of lidocaine on CPSP after laparoscopic TEP, we would not like to draw any conclusion. This could be explored in a larger, multi-centric trial with CPSP as a primary outcome.

Conclusions

In summary, intraoperative lidocaine infusion decreases overall opioid requirement and postoperative pain intensity in patients undergoing laparoscopic TEP inguinal hernioplasty. It also lowers the incidence of PONV, improves the quality of recovery and patients satisfaction without any sedative effect.

Abbreviations

TEP: Totally extraperitoneal; PONV: Postoperative nausea and vomiting; QoR: Quality of recovery; IQR: Interquartile range; IV: Intravenous; BPKIHS: BP Koirala Institute of Health Sciences; ASA: American Society of Anesthesiologists; NS: Normal Saline; NRS: Numerical rating scale; $ETCO_2$: End-tidal carbondioxide concentration; MAP: Mean arterial pressure; PACU: Post anesthesia care unit; CPSP: Chronic post-surgical pain; SMD: Standardized mean difference; MEQ: Morphine equivalent; VAS: Visual analogue scale

Acknowledgements

Not applicable.

Authors' contributions

AG: This author helped in study design, patient recruitment, data collection and writing up of the first draft of the paper. AS: This author helped in study design, patient recruitment, data collection, analysis and interpretation of data, manuscript revision and final draft. BB: This author helped in study design, manuscript revision and final approval. BPS: This author helped in study design, manuscript first draft and final draft. All authors have read and approved the manuscript in its current state.

Author details

[1]Department of Anesthesiology, Nepal Mediciti Hospital, Lalitpur, Nepal. [2]Department of Anesthesiology & Critical Care Medicine, BP Koirala Institute of Health Sciences, Dharan, Nepal.

References

1. Gan TJ, Joshi GP, Zhao SZ, Hanna DB, Cheung RY, Chen C. Presurgical intravenous parecoxib sodium and follow-up oral valdecoxib for pain management after laparoscopic cholecystectomy surgery reduces opioid requirements and opioid-related adverse effects. Acta Anaesthesiol Scand. 2004;48:1194–207.
2. Magheli A, Knoll N, Lein M, Hinz S, Kempkensteffen C, Gralla O. Impact of fast-track postoperative care on intestinal function, pain, and length of hospital stay after laparoscopic radical prostatectomy. J Endourol. 2011;25: 1143–7.
3. Lau CS, Chamberlain RS. Enhanced recovery after surgery programs improve patient outcomes and recovery: a meta-analysis. World J Surg. 2017;41:899–913.
4. Marret E, Rolin M, Beaussier M, Bonnet F. Meta-analysis of intravenous lidocaine and postoperative recovery after abdominal surgery. Br J Surg. 2008;95:1331–8.
5. Sun Y, Li T, Wang N, Yun Y, Gan TJ. Perioperative systemic lidocaine for postoperative analgesia and recovery after abdominal surgery: a meta-analysis of randomized controlled trials. Dis Colon Rectum. 2012;55:1183–94.
6. Kranke P, Jokinen J, Pace NL, et al. Continuous intravenous perioperative lidocaine infusion for postoperative pain and recovery. Cochrane Database Syst Rev. 2015;7:CD009642.
7. Bajracharya JL, Subedi A, Pokharel K, Bhattarai B. The effect of intraoperative lidocaine versus esmolol infusion on postoperative analgesia in laparoscopic cholecystectomy: a randomized clinical trial. BMC Anesthesiol. 2019;19:198.
8. Dunn LK, Durieux ME. Perioperative use of intravenous lidocaine. Anesthesiology. 2017;126:729–37.
9. Weibel S, Jelting Y, Pace NL, et al. Continuous intravenous perioperative lidocaine infusion for postoperative pain and recovery in adults. Cochrane Database Syst Rev. 2018;6:CD009642.
10. Zhao JB, Li YL, Wang YM, Teng JL, Xia DY, Zhao JS, Li FL. Intravenous lidocaine infusion for pain control after laparoscopic cholecystectomy: a meta-analysis of randomized controlled trials. Medicine (Baltimore). 2018;97:e9771.
11. Li J, Wang G, Xu W, Ding M, Yu W. Efficacy of intravenous lidocaine on pain relief in patients undergoing laparoscopic cholecystectomy: a meta-analysis from randomized controlled trials. Int J Surg. 2018;50:137–45.
12. Kang H, Kim BG. Intravenous lidocaine for effective pain relief after inguinal herniorrhaphy: a prospective, randomized, double-blind, placebo-controlled study. J Int Med Res. 2011;39:435–45.
13. Liem MSL, van Steensel CJ, Boelhouwer RU, et al. The learning curve for totally extraperitoneal laparoscopic inguinal hernia repair. Am J Surg. 1996; 171:281–5.
14. De Witte JL, Alegret C, Sessler DI, Cammu G. Preoperative alprazolam reduces anxiety in ambulatory surgery patients: a comparison with oral midazolam. Anesth Analg. 2002;95:1601–6.
15. Myles PS, Weitkamp B, Jones K, Melick J, Hensen S. Validity and reliability of a postoperative quality of recovery score: the QoR-40. Br J Anaesth. 2000;84: 11–5.
16. Treede RD, Rief W, Barke A, Aziz Q, Bennett MI, Benoliel R, Cohen M, Evers S, Finnerup NB, First MB, Giamberardino MA, Kaasa S, Kosek E, Lavand'homme P, Nicholas M, Perrot S, Scholz J, Schug S, Smith BH, Svensson P, Vlaeyen JW, Wang SJ. A classification of chronic pain for ICD-11. Pain. 2015;156: 1003–7.
17. Brinkrolf P, Hahnenkamp K. Systemic lidocaine in surgical procedures: effects beyond sodium channel blockade. Curr Opin Anaesthesiol. 2014;27:420–5.
18. Abelson KS, Höglund AU. Intravenously administered lidocaine in therapeutic doses increases the intraspinal release of acetylcholine in rats. Neurosci Lett. 2002;317:93–6.
19. Biella G, Sotgiu ML. Central effects of systemic lidocaine mediated by glycine spinal receptors: an iontophoretic study in the rat spinal cord. Brain Res. 1993;603:201–6.
20. Hahnenkamp K, Durieux ME, Hahnenkamp A, Schauerte SK, Hoenemann CW, Vegh V, Theilmeier G, Hollmann MW. Local anaesthetics inhibit signalling of human NMDA receptors recombinantly expressed in Xenopus laevis oocytes: role of protein kinase C. Br J Anaesth. 2006;96:77–87.
21. Yardeni IZ, Beilin B, Mayburd E, Levinson Y, Bessler H. The effect of perioperative intravenous lidocaine on postoperative pain and immune function. Anesth Analg. 2009;109:1464–9.
22. Kuo CP, Jao SW, Chen KM, Wong CS, Yeh CC, Sheen MJ, Wu CT. Comparison of the effects of thoracic epidural analgesia and i.v. infusion with lidocaine on cytokine response, postoperative pain and bowel function in patients undergoing colonic surgery. Br J Anaesth. 2006;97:640–6.
23. Herroeder S, Pecher S, Schönherr ME, Kaulitz G, Hahnenkamp K, Friess H, Böttiger BW, Bauer H, Dijkgraaf MG, Durieux ME, Hollmann MW. Systemic lidocaine shortens length of hospital stay after colorectal surgery: a double-blinded, randomized, placebo-controlled trial. Ann Surg. 2007;246:192–200.
24. De Oliveira GS Jr, Fitzgerald P, Streicher LF, Marcus RJ, McCarthy RJ. Systemic lidocaine to improve postoperative quality of recovery after ambulatory laparoscopic surgery. Anesth Analg. 2012;115:262–7.
25. De Oliveira GS Jr, Duncan K, Fitzgerald P, Nader A, Gould RW, McCarthy RJ. Systemic lidocaine to improve quality of recovery after laparoscopic bariatric surgery: a randomized double-blinded placebo-controlled trial. Obes Surg. 2014;24:212–8.
26. Bailey M, Corcoran T, Schug S, Toner A. Perioperative lidocaine infusions for the prevention of chronic postsurgical pain: a systematic review and meta-analysis of efficacy and safety. Pain. 2018;159:1696–704.

Postoperative analgesia for pediatric craniotomy patients

Fei Xing[1,2], Li Xin An[1*], Fu Shan Xue[1], Chun Mei Zhao[2] and Ya Fan Bai[1]

Abstract

Background: Pain is often observed in pediatric patients after craniotomy procedures, which could lead to some serious postoperative complications. However, the optimal formula for postoperative analgesia for pediatric neurosurgery has not been well established. This study aimed to explore the optimal options and formulas for postoperative analgesia in pediatric neurosurgery.

Methods: Three hundred and twenty patients aged 1 to 12-years old who underwent craniotomy were randomly assigned to receive 4 different regimens of patient-controlled analgesia. The formulas used were as follows: Control group included normal saline 100 ml, with a background infusion of 2 ml/h, bolus 0.5 ml; Fentanyl group was used with a background infusion of 0.1–0.2 μg/k·h, bolus 0.1–0.2 μg/kg; Morphine group was used with a background infusion of 10–20 μg/kg·h, bolus 10–20 μg/kg; while Tramadol group was used with a background infusion of 100–400 μg/kg·h, bolus 100–200 μg/kg. Postoperative pain scores and analgesia-related complication were recorded respectively. Comparative analysis was performed between the four groups.

Results: In comparison of all groups with each other, lower pain scores were shown at 1 h and 8 h after surgery in Morphine group versus Tramadol, Fentanyl and Control groups ($P < 0.05$). Both Tramadol and Fentanyl groups showed lower pain scores in comparison to Control group ($P < 0.05$). Nausea and vomiting were observed more in Tramadol group in comparison to all other groups during the 48 h of PCIA usage after operation ($P = 0.020$). Much more rescue medicines including ibuprofen and morphine were used in Control group (CI = 0.000–0.019). Changes in consciousness and respiratory depression were not observed in study groups. Moderate-to-severe pain was observed in a total of 56 (17.5%) of the study population. Multiple regression analysis for identifying risk factors for moderate-to-severe pain revealed that, younger children (OR = 1.161, 1.027–1.312, $P = 0.017$), occipital craniotomy (OR = 0.374, 0.155–0.905, $P = 0.029$), and morphine treatment (OR = 0.077, 0.021–0.281, $P < 0.001$) are the relevant factors.

Conclusions: Compared with other analgesic projects, PCIA or NCIA analgesia with morphine appears to be the safest and most effective postoperative analgesia program for pediatric patients who underwent neurosurgical operations.

Keywords: Pain, Postoperative, Child, Craniotomy

* Correspondence: anlixin8120@163.com

[1]Department of Anesthesia, Beijing Friendship Hospital, Capital Medical University, No.95 Yongan Road, Xicheng District, Beijing 100050, China

Background

Pain after craniotomy is a frequent source of concern and controversy. Over the past decade, several studies—primarily in adult patients—have revealed that moderate-to-severe pain is common in patients after major craniotomy [1–4]. Furthermore, very few studies have assessed pain or analgesic requirements in pediatric patients following neurosurgery, primarily due to fear of opioid analgesics masking alterations in the postoperative neurological exam and delaying detection of intracranial postoperative complications [5–7]. Postoperative pain in pediatric neurosurgical patients appears to be underestimated often [6, 7]. Inadequate pain control in children after major craniotomy may contribute to significant anxiety, hypertension, shivering, and emesis, which may in turn increase intracranial pressure and cause bleeding [8, 9]. Therefore, although frequently overlooked, postoperative analgesia in children after craniotomy is important.

Opioids are the most frequently prescribed analgesics for moderate-severe pain. However, they may be associated with side effects such as nausea, vomiting, pruritus, respiratory depression, and neurological alterations [10–12]. In particular, treatment of postoperative pain after craniotomy without affecting neurological status remains a major clinical problem. Recent studies have reported neurosurgical postoperative pain in pediatric patients can be managed with opioids without neurologic deterioration [6, 7]. Nevertheless, these reports are mostly small cohort studies and reviews. So far, no prospective randomized controlled trial has been conducted on postoperative pain in pediatric neurosurgery.

Therefore, the aim of this prospective, randomized, controlled study is to assess the safety and efficacy of different postoperative pain treatment in pediatric craniotomy patients. We selected the most commonly used postoperative analgesic formulas in clinical practice in accordance with our previous research, and assumed that one of the postoperative pain treatment formulas has the best analgesic effect and no related side effect for 1–12 years old children undergoing craniotomy , so as to find an optimal formula for pediatric neurosurgery postoperative analgesia.

Methods

Study design and participants

This randomized controlled clinical trial was approved by the Institutional Review Board of Beijing Tiantan Hospital Affiliated to Capital Medical University (Beijing, China, KY2015–009-01). Written informed consent was obtained from all patients' parents. This study was conducted at a single tertiary medical center (Beijing Tiantan Hospital) and indexed in the Chinese Clinical Trial Registry (http://www.chictr.org.cn/index.aspx, ChiCTR-IOC-15007676).

The inclusion criteria were as follows: Patients aged 1–12 years, with American Society of Anesthesiologists physical status grades I–III undergoing open craniotomy procedures. Eligible subjects included patients undergoing surgery for brain tumors, craniofacial reconstruction and vascular malformations. Exclusion criteria included: Mental disorders; unsuitability for extubation; and development of hematomas or severe brain edema 3 days after surgery, requiring a subsequent operation. Additionally, we excluded patients with a history of allergy to opioids or other anesthetics, and those with a history of substance abuse. Patients were enrolled in this study only after obtaining written informed consent from their parents.

Anesthesia

Standard monitoring was implemented in the operating room. All children were monitored for non-invasive blood pressure (BP), heart rate (HR) and pulse oximetry (SpO_2); as well as invasive arterial pressure (ARP), end-tidal carbon dioxide partial pressure ($P_{ET}CO_2$), and minimum alveolar concentration (MAC). Midazolam 0.025–0.075 mg/kg and methylprednisolone sodium succinate 1–2 mg/kg were given before surgery. If necessary, patients were given oral midazolam 0.5 mg/kg to reduce anxiety before venous access.

Anesthesia was induced with the following approximate doses: Propofol (2 mg/kg), cisatracurium (0.2 mg/kg), and sufentanyl (0.3 μg/kg) or fentanyl (3 μg/kg). In patients aged < 5 years or those unable to cooperate with the anesthesiologist, tracheal intubation was performed under induction with 6–8% sevoflurane inhalation before peripheral venous access. Prior to surgical incision, local infiltration with 0.5% ropivacaine was performed at the surgical site, and surgical pin sites was placed. Anesthesia was maintained with 0.5 MAC sevoflurane at an inhalational concentration of 2–3%, and an intravenous infusion with remifentanil 0.1–0.2 μg/kg/min and propofol 3–5 mg/kg/h. Mean arterial blood pressure and heart rate were maintained within 20% of baseline measures. 30 min before the end of the operation, additional sufentanyl 5 μg or fentanyl 0.5–1 μg/kg was administered, while inhalation of sevoflurane and the infusion of remifentanil and propofol was stopped at the end of the operation. The parameters for mechanical ventilation were set to volume control with a tidal volume of 8–10 ml/kg and a respiratory rate of 14–20 times/min. Controlled mechanical ventilation maintained $P_{ET}CO_2$ of 30–35 mmHg using a 50% oxygen-air gas mixture. Additional rocuronium was administered, if needed, to maintain a train-of-four count of 2–3 intraoperatively. Whether patients received a central and arterial cannula after anesthesia induction was according to the needs of the operation.

Postoperative pain treatment protocol

After surgery, patients aged 1–6 years received a pump for nurse-controlled intravenous analgesia (NCIA), while those aged 7–12 received one for patient-controlled intravenous analgesia (PCIA). Based on our previous cohort study of pediatric postoperative analgesia, we found that only 12% in 1–6 years old and 58% in 7–12 years old patients used PCIA or NCIA after craniotomy [13]. Same results were obtained in another cohort study performed by Maxwell LG[7]. That means that single intravenous administration after operation is a common method of postoperative analgesia in pediatric neurosurgery. So in our study we used saline in PCIA/NCIA plus rescue medicine as our control group.

The regimens of PCIA or NCIA used the following formulas: Control (group C) included normal saline 100 ml, with a continuous background infusion of 2 ml/h, bolus 0.5 ml; Fentanyl (group F) was used with a loading dose of 0.5 μg/kg, a single bolus dose of 0.1–0.2 μg/kg, and a background dose 0.1–0.2 μg/k·h; Morphine (group M) was used with a loading dose of 50 μg/kg, a single bolus dose of 10–20 μg/kg, and a background dose of 10–20 μg/kg·h; while Tramadol (group T) was used with a loading dose of 500 μg/kg, a single bolus dose of 100–200 μg/kg, and a background dose of 100–400 μg/kg·h. The bolus locking time was 15 min. The total volume contained in the analgesia pump was adjusted to 100 ml with normal saline and 0.4 mg/kg of ondansetron. Patients would receive additional doses of ondansetron if they reported nausea or experienced vomiting. The type and dosed of medicines used in pump were converted to their respective milligram morphine equivalents (MME) using standardized conversion factors (1 mg of Fentanyl = 100 MME, 1 mg of tramadol = 0.1 MME) [14].

As a rescue medicine, ibuprofen suspension (20 mg/ml ibuprofen) was oral administered in the postoperative period in doses of 0.3 ml/kg for moderate pain (defined as a pain score ≥ 4 and < 7) within 48 postoperative hours. If the POPI is severe pain (defined as a pain score ≥ 7) or the first administration of ibuprofen couldn't comfort the patient within 30 min, another rescue medicine intravenous morphine 0.02 mg/kg would be administered through peri vein. All rescue medicines were recorded.

Evaluation of pain intensity

The primary outcome of this study was postoperative pain intensity (POPI). According to the particular characteristics of each patient, we adopted different evaluation methods for POPI. Patients aged 1–6 years were evaluated by the Faces, Legs, Activity, Cry and Consolability Scale (FLACC, 0–10 scores) and the Wong-Baker Faces Scale (WBFS). For patients aged 7–12 years, both the numeric rating scale (NRS) and the Wong-Baker Faces Scale (WBFS) were used. The FLACC is a behavioral pain assessment tool that was developed to provide a simple and consistent evaluation method for these cases [15], while the WBFS is a self-reported pain assessment tool, currently considered the preferred alternative for pain assessment in children [16]. The WBFS is comprised of a series of facial images, in which the face that depicts the most pain indicates the "worst pain imaginable" and the happiest face indicates "no pain" [15]. The numeric rating scale (NRS) is a self-reported measure of pain intensity comprised of a line marked with numbers 0–10, in which 0 is "no pain" and 10 is the "worst pain imaginable" [17]. POPI ratings were measured at 1, 2, 4, 16, 24, 36 and 48 h after surgery by the same observer. Moderate POPI was defined as a median pain score ≥ 4 and < 7 on the WBFS, FLACC or NRS scales. Severe pain was defined as a median pain score ≥ 7.

Randomization and blinding

Participants were randomly assigned 1:1:1:1 among four groups. The randomization schedule was generated by an independent investigator through a computerized random-number sequence. A specially selected nurse was informed of the group assignments and prepared the postoperative analgesia pumps according to the patients' weights. Anesthesiologists were blinded to grouping information. Physicians responsible for postoperative follow-up were also blinded to the grouping.

Data collection

Demographic data were recorded, including age, sex, height, weight, disease information, primary diagnosis, patients' medical history, and medications. Perioperative and anesthetic management information were also collected including: operation type; preoperative anesthetic medications; induction medications; intra-operative anesthetic medications; duration of surgery and anesthesia; and number of rescue medicine administrations.

The primary outcomes included pain scores at 1, 2, 4, 16, 24, 36 and 48 h after surgery. Secondary outcomes included the incidence of changes in consciousness, nausea, vomiting, pruritus, respiratory depression, and addition of perioperative acetaminophen. Nausea and vomiting were recorded if episodes of patient emesis were reported on nursing flow sheets, or if anti-emetic therapy was required. Respiratory depression was operationalized as a clinically significant decline in respiratory rate which required intervention, with SpO_2 < 92%.

Sample size and statistical analysis

Continuous variables were described as median and interquartile range (IQR) or mean and standard deviation (SD), as appropriate. Categorical variables (sex, site of craniotomy) were presented as frequencies and percentages. The chi-square test was used for comparing proportions, and one-way analysis of variance (ANOVA) was used for comparing continuous variables between groups. Because the POPI of patients was ranked data, we used Kruskal-Wallis H-test to compare the differences of POPI among all groups. If $P < 0.05$, Dunnett's T3 test was used to compare the differences of POPI between any two groups.

Our previous cohort study on POPI in pediatric craniotomy patients found that the incidence of moderate POPI in children to be approximately 45%. A final sample size was calculated based on the hypothesis that PCIA could reduce the incidence of moderate POPI at least 30%. A sample size of 36 patients was calculated to have a significance of 5% and a power of 80%, increased to 40 after considering a 10% maximal dropout rate.

Step-wise multivariate logistic regression was used to identify predictors for moderate POPI, with results presented as odds ratios (OR) and 95% confidence intervals (CI). Statistical analysis was performed using SPSS (version 22, BEIJING, Capital Medical University). All statistical tests were two-sided, and results were considered statistically significant when $P < 0.05$.

Results

Baseline characteristics

A total of 387 consecutive patients who underwent major craniotomy were screened for study participation between January 2016 and June 2018; 192 of which were in a younger group (aged 1–6 years) and 195 in an older group (aged 7–12 years). In the younger group, 12 cases refused informed consent, 18 children remained intubated for surgical reasons, and 2 children required a second operation due to postoperative hematoma. Therefore, 160 patients were ultimately included. In the older group, 11 cases refused informed consent, 21 children remained intubated for surgical reasons, and 3 children required a second operation within 48 h of surgery. Therefore, 160 patients (91 males and 69 females) were finally included. An explanatory flow chart is depicted in Fig. 1.

The baseline clinical characteristics in all pediatric patients are presented in Tables 1. No significant differences were found regarding these variables among the four PCIA regimens either in the younger or older pediatric patients.

Postoperative pain intensity

Pain intensity was evaluated at 1, 2, 4, 16, 24, 36 and 48 h after surgery (Table 2). In the younger patients, over time, the pain intensity gradually decreased, and increased slightly at 24 h after surgery (Additional file 1: Figure S1 and S2). The differences of WBFS/FLACC scores were significantly among all groups at 1–8 h ($P < 0.05$) by Kruskal-Wallis test. Through Dunnett's T3 test, lower pain scores (Both WBFS/FLACC Scores) were shown at 1 h and 8 h after surgery in Morphine Group versus Tramadol, Fentanyl and Control groups ($P < 0.05$). Both Fentanyl and Tramadol groups showed lower pain scores in comparison to Control group ($P < 0.05$), and there is no significant difference in pain scores between the Fentanyl and Tramadol groups ($P > 0.05$) (Table 2, Additional file 1: Table S1).

In the 7–12 years older patients, a similar trend was observed (Additional file 1: Figure S3 and S4), with WBFS/NRS scores being significantly lower at 1–16 h in Morphine group (Table 3, $P < 0.05$). There was no significant difference between Fentanyl and Tramadol groups (Additional file 1: Table S2, $P > 0.05$), but they were lower than Control group ($P < 0.05$).

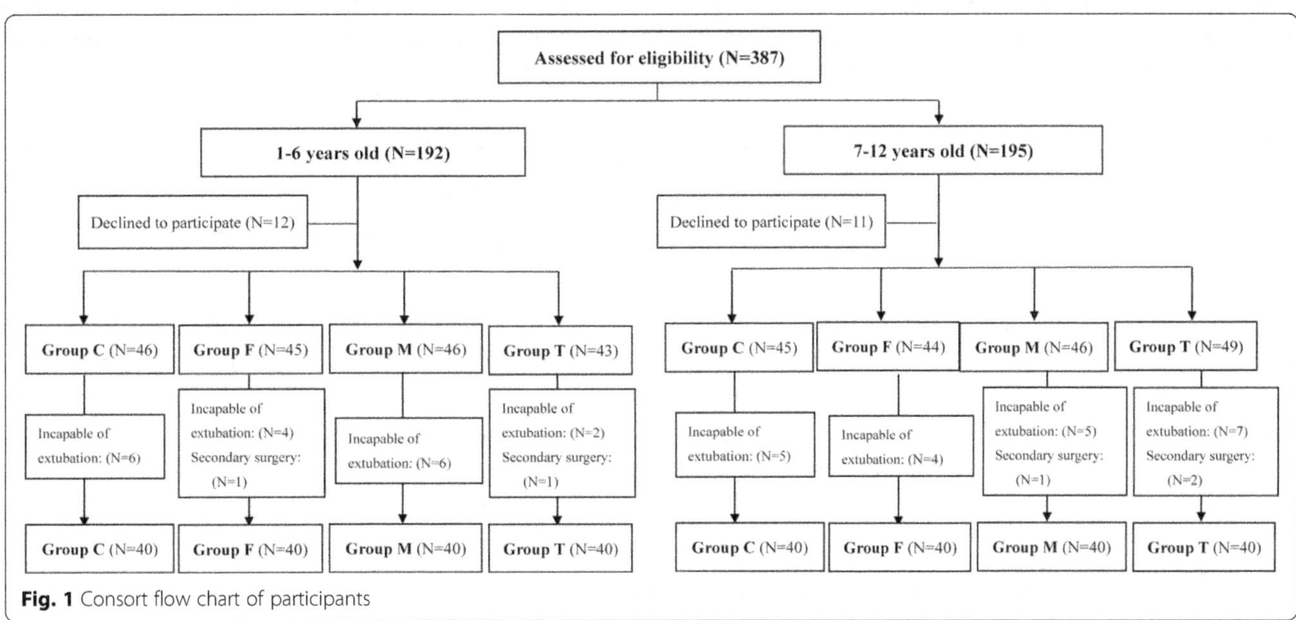

Fig. 1 Consort flow chart of participants

Table 1 Baseline Data For all Pediatric Patients (1–12 years old, $X \pm SD$)

	1–6 Years Old Patients				7–12 Years Old Patients			
	Group C	Group F	Group M	Group T	Group C	Group F	Group M	Group T
Age (yr)	4.00 ± 1.77	3.50 ± 1.54	4.05 ± 1.45	3.70 ± 1.64	8.97 ± 2.92	9.21 ± 1.68	8.51 ± 2.69	9.29 ± 1.60
Sex (male/female)	24/16	27/13	24/16	22/18	25/15	18/22	24/16	24/16
Height (m)	1.07 ± 0.16	1.03 ± 0.13	1.05 ± 0.11	1.06 ± 0.14	1.42 ± 0.15	1.33 ± 0.13	1.38 ± 0.14	1.40 ± 0.13
Weight (kg)	19.8 ± 5.4	17.4 ± 4.7	18.9 ± 6.0	18.3 ± 6.3	37.7 ± 15.5	32.6 ± 8.5	34.6 ± 10.9	36.12 ± 11.5
Craniotomy site(*n* / %)								
Forehead	24 (60)	19 (47.5)	18 (45)	17 (42.5)	22 (55.0)	23 (57.5)	21 (52.5)	19 (47.5)
Frontotemporal	2 (5)	6 (15)	9 (22.5)	3 (7.5)	4 (10.0)	3 (7.5)	7 (17.5)	5 (12.5)
Frontoparietal	1 (2.5)	1 (2.5)	2 (5)	2 (5)	3 (7.5)	2 (5.0)	2 (5.0)	3 (7.5)
Temporal occipital	1 (2.5)	0 (0)	1 (2.5)	2 (5)	1 (2.5)	0 (0.0)	1 (2.5)	1 (2.5)
Occipital	11 (27.5)	11 (27.5)	9 (22.5)	15 (37.5)	10 (25)	11 (27.5)	8 (20.0)	11 (27.5)
Temporal-parietal occipital	1 (2.5)	3 (7.5)	1 (2.5)	1 (2.5)	0 (0.0)	1 (2.5)	1 (2.5)	1 (2.5)
VP shunt surgery (Y/N)	5/35	8/32	7/33	7/33	7/33	4/36	1/39	7/33
Durations of surgery (min)	217 ± 81	229 ± 112	212 ± 67	215 ± 63	299 ± 59	205 ± 134	219 ± 49	229 ± 60
Durations of anesthesia (min)	320 ± 98	403 ± 73	310 ± 80	308 ± 74	331 ± 77	290 ± 81	311 ± 63	328 ± 66
Bleeding (ml)	161 ± 199	109 ± 72	136 ± 168	118 ± 93	133 ± 80	113 ± 95	163 ± 141	129 ± 80
Anesthesia maintenance phase								
Propofol (mg)	225 (155, 337)	190 (140, 367)	230 (160, 300)	220 (152, 340)	525 (292, 672)	350 (215, 555)	340 (200, 490)	280 (160, 480)
Remifentanil (mg)	0.63 ± 0.34	0.61 ± 0.46	0.49 ± 0.25	0.68 ± 0.36	1.07 ± 0.59	0.82 ± 0.45	0.91 ± 0.57	1.24 ± 1.44
Sevoflurane (ml)	30 ± 20	28 ± 22	28 ± 13	24 ± 13	29 ± 12	22 ± 12	26 ± 11	27 ± 11

No significant difference of baseline characteristics was observed

Total amount of medicines used in PCIA or NCIA or for remedy

Total amount of medicines used in the postoperative analgesia pump was calculated. After all kinds of medicines converted to their respective milligram morphine equivalents (MME) using standardized conversion factors, the average morphine equivalent amount in each day was similar between Fentanyl and Morphine groups, and in Tramadol group was a little bit higher (Table 4). As rescue medicines, the total amount and cases of ibuprofen and morphine used in Control group were much higher than that in Fentanyl, Morphine and Tramadol groups, this result was similar in both 1–6 years old patients and 7–12 years old patients.

Table 2 Postoperative Pain Scores For 1–6 Years Old Younger Pediatric Patients (median (interquartile range))

	Group C		Group F		Group M		Group T		95% CI	
	FLACC	WBFS	FLACC	WBFS	FLACC	WBFS	FLACC	WBFS	*CI 1*	*CI 2*
1 h	3 (2, 5)	4 (2, 6)	2 (1, 3.5) *	2 (2, 4) *	2 (1.25, 2) *Δ	2 (2, 2) *Δ	2 (2, 4) *	2 (2, 4) *	0.000–0.019	0.000–0.019
2 h	3 (2, 5)	4 (2, 6)	2 (0, 2) *	2 (1.5, 2) *	2 (1, 2) *Δ	2 (2, 2) *Δ	2 (2, 3) *	3 (2, 4) *	0.000–0.019	0.000–0.019
4 h	2 (0.5, 4)	2 (2, 4)	1.5 (0, 2) *	2 (0, 2) *	1 (0, 2) *Δ	0 (0, 2) *Δ	2 (0.25, 2) *	2 (0.5, 2) *	0.000–0.019	0.000–0.018
8 h	0 (0, 2.5)	0 (0, 3)	0 (0, 1.5) *	0 (0, 2) *	0 (0, 0.5) *Δ	0 (0, 0) *Δ	2 (0, 2) *	2 (0, 2) *	0.001–0.049	0.000–0.018
16 h	1 (0, 3.5)	2 (0, 4)	0 (0, 2)	0 (0, 2)	0 (0, 1)	0 (0, 2)	0.5 (0, 2)	1 (0, 2)	0.012–0.075	0.030–0.108
24 h	2 (2, 3)	2 (2, 4)	1.5 (0, 2)	2 (0, 2)	2 (0, 2)	2 (0, 3.5)	2 (0, 2)	2 (0, 2)	0.000–0.018	0.030–0.108
36 h	0 (0, 0.5)	0 (0, 1)	0 (0, 0)	0 (0, 0)	0 (0, 0)	0 (0, 0)	0 (0, 2)	0 (0, 2)	0.054–0.146	0.000–0.019
48 h	1.5 (0, 2)	2 (0, 2)	0 (0, 0.75)	0 (0, 2)	0 (0, 1)	0 (0, 2)	0 (0, 2)	0 (0, 2)	0.012–0.075	0.008–0.067

CI 1: 95% Confidence interval for FLACC score among four groups by Kruskal-Wallis H-test;
CI 2: 95% Confidence interval for WBFS score among four groups by Kruskal-Wallis H-test
*$P < 0.05$, the difference was significant compared with group C by Dunnett's T3 test;
Δ $P < 0.05$, compared with group F and M, the FLACC and WBFS in group M was significant lower through Dunnett's T3 test

Table 3 Postoperative Pain Scores For 7–12 Years Old Senior Pediatric Patients (median (interquartile range))

	Group C		Group F		Group M		Group T		95% CI	
	WBFS	NRS	WBFS	NRS	WBFS	NRS	WBFS	NRS	*CI 1*	*CI 2*
1 h	4 (2, 6)	4 (2, 5)	2 (2, 4) *	2 (2, 3.3) *	2 (2, 4) *Δ	2 (2, 3) *Δ	2 (2, 4) *	2 (2, 4) *	0.000–0.021	0.000–0.044
2 h	4 (2, 4)	3 (2, 4)	2 (2, 4) *	2 (2, 4) *	2 (2, 2) *Δ	2 (2, 3) *Δ	4 (2, 4) *	4 (2, 4) *	0.038–0.129	0.018–0.094
4 h	2 (0, 4)	2 (0, 4)	2 (0, 2.5) *	2 (0, 3) *	0 (0, 2) *Δ	0 (0, 2) *Δ	2 (2, 4) *	2 (2, 4) *	0.000–0.021	0.000–0.021
8 h	2 (0, 2)	2 (0, 2)	0 (0, 2) *	0 (0, 2) *	0 (0, 0) *Δ	0 (0, 0) *Δ	2 (0, 2) *	2 (0, 2) *	0.000–0.021	0.000–0.021
16 h	2 (0, 2)	2 (0, 2)	0 (0, 2) *	0 (0, 2) *	0 (0, 2) *Δ	0 (0, 2) *Δ	2 (0, 2) *	2 (0, 2) *	0.001–0.055	0.000–0.021
24 h	2 (2, 4)	2 (2, 4)	2 (2, 2)	2 (1, 2)	2 (0, 2)	2 (0, 2)	2 (1, 2)	2 (1, 2)	0.500–0.661	0.507–0.668
36 h	0 (0, 0)	0 (0, 1)	0 (0, 0)	0 (0, 0)	0 (0, 0)	0 (0, 0)	0 (0, 2)	0 (0, 1)	0.485–0.648	0.346–0.508
48 h	2 (0, 2)	2 (0, 2)	0 (0, 2)	0 (0, 2)	0 (0, 2)	0 (0, 2)	0 (0, 2)	0 (0, 2)	0.044–0.138	0.023–0.103

CI 1: 95% Confidence interval for WBFS score among four groups by Kruskal-Wallis H-test;
CI 2: 95% Confidence interval for NRS score among four groups by Kruskal-Wallis H-test
*$P < 0.05$, the difference was significant compared with group C by Dunnett's T3 test;
Δ $P < 0.05$, compared with group F and M, the WBFS and NRS in group M was significant lower through Dunnett's T3 test

Identical factors associated with moderate postoperative pain intensity

Moderate-to-severe pain was observed in a total of 56 (17.5%) of the all study population. There were 26 patients in 1–6 years old groups (26/160, 16.25%) and 30 patients in 7–12 years old groups (30/160, 18.75%). Only 3 children experienced severe pain in Control group and 1 child in Tramadol group among 1–6 years old patients. And there were 5 patients in Control Group experienced severe pain among 7–12 years old patients. Single regression analysis for identifying risk factors revealed that, older age, site of craniotomy, dose of remifentanil and PCIA group were associated with moderate-to-severe POPI (Table 5). Then, multiple factor regression analysis was conducted on factors with $P > 0.2$. Multiple regression analysis for identifying risk factors for moderate-to-severe pain revealed that, younger children (OR = 1.161, 1.027–1.312, $P = 0.017$), occipital craniotomy (OR = 0.374, 0.155–0.905, $P = 0.029$), and fentanyl treatment (OR = 0.355, 0.152–0.831, P = 0.017), or morphine treatment (OR = 0.077, 0.021–0.281, $P < 0.001$) are the relevant factors (Fig. 2).

Analgesia-related complications

There was no significant difference in complications during recovery among the four groups, either in the younger or older children. In Tramadol group, 11 children suffered nausea (27.5%) and 19 children suffered vomiting (47.5%) within 48 h after surgery, which were significantly higher than that in Fentanyl, Morphine and

Table 4 Total amount of medicines used in PCIA or NCIA or for remedy (1–12 years old, $\bar{X} \pm SD$)

	1–6 Years Old Patients				7–12 Years Old Patients			
	Group C	Group F	Group M	Group T	Group C	Group F	Group M	Group T
Average total medicines use in PCIA or NCIA pump (mcg/kg/d)								
1st day	0	5.23 ± 1.21	472 ± 85	7210 ± 1560	0	5.65 ± 1.54	504 ± 105	9010 ± 2060
2nd day	0	5.05 ± 1.04	495 ± 92	6780 ± 1050	0	5.54 ± 0.98	493 ± 118	8280 ± 1150
Morphine equivalents	0	514 ± 112	486 ± 90	699 ± 164	0	560 ± 112	502 ± 113	864 ± 154
Total amount of Rescue medicines used in each group (48 h)								
Ibuprofen (P.O., mg)	3120	920*	540*	1290*	6000	400*	840*	650*
Ibuprofen (cases / %)	26/65%	9/22.5%*	5/12.5%*	12/30%*	27/67.5%	2/5%*	4/10%*	3/7.5%*
Comparison of Ibuprofen	**X2 = 27.473**		**95%CI = 0.000–0.019**		**X2 = 54.504**		**95%CI = 0.000–0.019**	
Morphine (I.V., mg)	4.8	0.4*	0*	1.1*	11.1	0*	0*	2.2*
Morphine (cases / %)	12/30%	1/2.5%*	0*	3/7.5%*	15/37.5%	0*	0*	4/10%*
Comparison of Morphine	**X2 = 20.879**		**95%CI = 0.000–0.019**		**X2 = 31.848**		**95%CI = 0.000–0.019**	

Average total medicines use in PCIA or NCIA pump (mcg/kg/d):
1st day (2nd day), Group F = Total Fentanyl per kg used in pump during the first postoperative day (second day); Group M = Total Morphine per kg used in pump during the first postoperative day (second day); Group T = Total Tramadol per kg used in pump during the first postoperative day (second day)
Morphine equivalents: All medicines converted to their morphine equivalents, and the average total morphine per kg used in pump per day
Total amount of Rescue medicines used in each group (48 h): As rescue medicines, the total amount and cases(%) of ibuprofen or morphine used in one group; *$P < 0.001$ compared with Group C

Table 5 Univariate Logistic Regression Analysis Of Influencing Factors Of Pain Scores For 1–12 Years Old Patients

	WBFS< 4 (*n* = 264)	WBFS≥4 (*n* = 56)	OR	95%CI	*P*
Age (yr)	6.25 ± 3.16	7.08 ± 3.26	1.085	(0.988–1.192)	0.088
Sex (male/female)	151/113	37/19	1.455	(0.782–2.708)	0.237
Height (m)	1.20 ± 0.21	1.25 ± 0.23	0.981	(0.875–1.100)	0.741
Weight (kg)	26.1 ± 12.5	28.1 ± 11.7	1.013	(0.990–1.036)	0.275
Craniotomy site(*n* / %)					
Forehead	75 (28.4)	25 (45.3)	Ref	Ref	
Frontotemporal	93 (35.2)	13 (22.6)*	0.418	(0.200–0.877)	***0.021***
Frontoparietal	13 (4.8)	6 (11.3)	1.400	(0.475–4.127)	0.542
Temporal occipital	5 (2.0)	0 (0)	0.000	(0.000–0.000)	0.999
Occipital	74 (28.0)	11 (18.9)*	0.400	(0.179–0.894)	***0.026***
Temporal-parietal occipital	4 (1.6)	1 (1.9)	0.700	(0.075–6.565)	0.755
0.5% Ropivacaine for local anesthesia (Y/N)	14/250	3/53	0.914	(0.251–3.327)	0.892
VP shunt surgery (Y/N)	42/222	8/48	1.071	(0.470–2.444)	0.870
Durations of surgery (min)	222 ± 87	205 ± 62	0.997	(0.992–1.001)	0.174
Durations of anesthesia (min)	315 ± 80	300 ± 68	0.997	(0.993–1.001)	0.201
Bleeding (ml)	132 ± 117	134 ± 158	1.000	(0.998–1.002)	0.913
Anesthesia maintenance phase					
Propofol (mg)	315 ± 224	326 ± 242	1.000	(0.999–1.001)	0.747
Remifentanil (mg)	0.73 ± 0.47	0.84 ± 0.57*	1.644	(1.016–2.658)	***0.043***
Sevoflurane (ml)	23.3 ± 17.1	19.3 ± 14.9	0.983	(0.964–1.004)	0.106
Group (n / %)					
Placebo	55 (20.8)	24 (43.4)	Ref	Ref	
Fentanyl	71 (26.8)	12 (20.8)*	0.364	(0.167–0.793)	***0.011***
Morphine	75 (28.4)	4 (7.5)*	0.083	(0.024–0.291)	***< 0.001***
Tramadol	63 (24.0)	16 (28.3)	0.500	(0.238–1.050)	***0.067***

Control groups (Additional file 1: Table S3, $P < 0.05$). Changes in consciousness and respiratory depression were not observed in study groups ($P = 0.061$). In the younger patients, much children needed ibuprofen suspension and intravenous morphine as rescue medicine in the Tramadol and Control groups than that in the Fentanyl and Morphine groups ($P < 0.05$). In the 7–12 years old patients, the cases of used rescue medicine in the Control group were much higher than that in Fentanyl, Morphine and Tramadol groups (Additional file 1: Table S4, $P < 0.05$).

DISSCUSION

Although research has demonstrated 41–76% of adult patients experience moderate-severe pain within 48 h after craniotomy [18, 19], very few studies have focus specifically on the incidence and treatment of POPI in pediatric neurosurgery patients [20, 21]. In this prospective, randomized, controlled clinical study conducted at a single academic hospital, we found POPI could be well controlled with opioids administration by NCIA or PCIA. Compared to the opioid groups (Fentanyl and Morphine groups), the Control group needed more rescue medicine – ibuprofen suspension or morphine. In contrast, complications during recovery such as respiration depression and consciousness changes showed no significant difference among all groups. Finally, factors such as younger age, occipital site craniotomy, Fentanyl or Morphine treatment were the relevant factors.

To date, few studies have formally recommended postoperative pain treatment protocols in pediatric neurosurgery. A prospective cohort study conducted in three academic children's hospitals has previously reported POPI to be mild in children under various analgesic regimens [7]. However, this was a cohort study which only included where POPI was not accurately assessed. In contrast, Bronco [6]. found 16% of pediatric neurosurgical patients suffered moderate-severe pain in the recovery room, and 6% patients suffered moderate-severe pain in the first and second days after surgery despite application of multimodal analgesia [6]. The main analgesic methods advocated in current studies are multimodal analgesia and

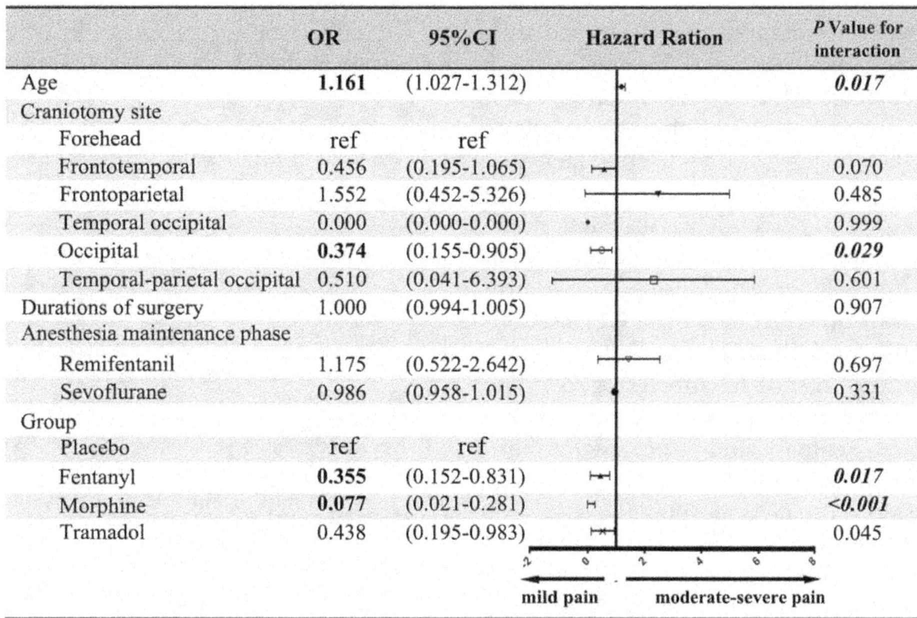

	OR	95%CI	Hazard Ration	P Value for interaction
Age	**1.161**	(1.027-1.312)		***0.017***
Craniotomy site				
Forehead	ref	ref		
Frontotemporal	0.456	(0.195-1.065)		0.070
Frontoparietal	1.552	(0.452-5.326)		0.485
Temporal occipital	0.000	(0.000-0.000)		0.999
Occipital	**0.374**	(0.155-0.905)		***0.029***
Temporal-parietal occipital	0.510	(0.041-6.393)		0.601
Durations of surgery	1.000	(0.994-1.005)		0.907
Anesthesia maintenance phase				
Remifentanil	1.175	(0.522-2.642)		0.697
Sevoflurane	0.986	(0.958-1.015)		0.331
Group				
Placebo	ref	ref		
Fentanyl	**0.355**	(0.152-0.831)		***0.017***
Morphine	**0.077**	(0.021-0.281)		***<0.001***
Tramadol	0.438	(0.195-0.983)		0.045

Fig. 2 OR (95% CI) for the associations between factors and moderate-severe POPI (≥4). A multiple factor regression analysis was conducted including all factors with $P < 0.2$ in univariate logistic regression analysis results. Craniotomy site expressed different craniotomy approaches. Durations of surgery meant the length of operation. Remifentanil means the total amount of the use of remifentanil during anesthesia. The total amount of sevoflurane use is calculated based on the patients' inhaled concentration and fresh gas flow and time. A total of 14 factors were included. For multiple groups of categorical variables, we chose one of them as the reference. So, we chose forehead in craniotomy site and placebo group in groups as reference. Age, occipital craniotomy, give fentanyl PCIA or NCIA, or give morphine PCIA or NCIA, were correlated risk factors of moderate-severe pain

PCIA or NCIA analgesia [5, 7]. Maxwell et al. [7] have demonstrated that PCIA or NCIA analgesia is an effective analgesia with a low incidence of opioid-related side effects; although it should be noted that the analgesic pump settings in their study were not standardized. Chiaretti [22] found PCIA with fentanyl plus midazolam could effectively relieve postoperative pain in pediatric neurosurgery. However, their study only included patients over the age of 6, all of whom were managed in an ICU setting. In this study, we enrolled pediatric patients in the range of 1–12 years of age. In addition, we have implemented three different methods of analgesia to compare with control group, in order to obtain the best analgesic regimen used in children.

Our study revealed that in both younger and older pediatric patients, morphine administration was the most effective regimen of PCIA or NCIA after neurosurgery. These results are consistent with those of Warren [23] who suggested continuous morphine infusions (CMI) had an analgesic effect comparable to that of acetaminophen and codeine; yet codeine phosphate alone is typically preferred as the standard treatment for pain after cranial surgery. The Fentanyl and Tramadol groups had similar analgesic effects; echoing results by Alencar [24] in neonates. Except for nausea and vomiting, no difference was observed in the incidence of side effects, and serious side effects such as respiratory depression and altered consciousness were not observed. Respiratory depression and excessive sedation are the two most feared adverse consequences of intravenous opioid use for postoperative pain in neurosurgery; as excessive sedation affects neurological status, and respiratory depression could cause negative physiological consequences such as elevated carbon dioxide levels and alterations of cerebral perfusion and intracranial pressure. In our study, these side effects were not observed. The incidence of nausea and vomiting was not significantly higher in the morphine or fentanyl groups, but was higher in the tramadol group. In a meta-analysis of postoperative PCIA in adults, Fentanyl has been ascertained to be as effective as Tramadol, but the incidence of nausea and vomiting is higher in the Tramadol group [25]. This is similar to our results in children.

Our study is a randomized controlled trial which balanced the confounding factors well. The assessment of pain in pediatric population presents a significant challenge. Children may often be unable to accurately describe the intensity of their pain. Thus, in our study, we used 2 different pain scales suitable for each age range. In order to avoid bias, research assistants who collected postoperative pain data in our study received subspecialty training in pediatric pain assessment. All patients were followed up by the same research assistants. We found pain scores gradually decreased with time, regardless age and treatment regimen, with a small ascent occurring at 24 h. In addition, pain scores at 8, 16 and 36 h were lower than their following time point; this might be due to the fact that children were asleep at night at these points, with lower responses to pain perception. Although much rescue medicines including oral ibuprofen suspension and intravenous morphine were used in Control group compared with other groups, the POPI in Control group was still much higher than other groups, especially within the first 8 h after surgery. The morphine equivalents amount in Tramadol group was higher than that in Fentanly and Morphine groups, which may be owned to the over-estimated tramadol MME (1 mg tramadol = 0.1 mcg morphine).

We also analyzed the factors affecting postoperative pain scores by multivariate logistic regression, proving the good control of confounding factors. We found age, craniotomy site and Fentanyl and Morphine treatment were predictors of POPI. Previous studies had described POPI to vary in different craniotomy sites due to the distribution of nerve endings [5, 17, 18]. Pain scores also varied with age, this may be owned to that older children describe pain intensity with increased accuracy.

There are several limitations to our study. First, we performed local anesthesia of the surgical incision with 0.5% ropivacaine instead of scalp nerve block, a more effective auxiliary analgesia. This method may provide longer lasting analgesia in comparison to local analgesia, perhaps decreasing POPI, especially in the early postoperative period. Secondly, in our multivariate logistic regression, we found the craniotomy site was associated with postoperative pain, but a sub-group analysis was not performed as the subsamples who underwent craniotomy at different sites were relatively small. Therefore, our next step is to find more individualized analgesia regimens for patients with different craniotomy sites, in combination with scalp nerve block [26, 27].

Conclusions

Our study indicates that factors such as younger age, occipital site craniotomy, use of fentanyl or morphine are the relevant factors for moderate-to-severe pain. PCIA or NCIA with morphine could significantly decrease postoperative pain scores without increasing the incidence of nausea, vomiting, respiratory depression and excessive sedation in pediatric patients after neurosurgery. These patients may benefit from application of our postoperative analgesia protocol.

Additional file

Additional file 1: Table S1. Supplementary details for Table 2 of POPI in 1–6 years old pediatric patients. The details including 95%CI and H(K) value for pain scores among four groups by Kruskal-Wallis H-test in 1–6 years old patients. **Table S2.** Supplementary details for Table 3 of POPI in 7–12 years old pediatric patients. The details including 95%CI and H(K) value for pain scores among four groups by Kruskal-Wallis H-test in 7–12 years old patients. **Table S3.** Supplementary details for Perioperative Events Experienced For 1–6 Years Old Younger Pediatric Patients. The results of perioperative events experienced for 1–6 years old patients. The cases suffered nausea and vomiting in Tramadol group were significantly higher than that in Fentanyl, Morphine and Control groups. **Table S4.** Supplementary details for Perioperative Events Experienced For 7–12 Years Old Senior Pediatric Patients. The results of perioperative events experienced for 7–12 years old patients. There was no different in pain intensity after the removal of intubation. But the incidence of nausea in Tramadol group were much higher than that in Fentanyl, Morphine and Control groups. **Figure S1.** Comparison of post-operative pain intensity of FLACC in patients aged 1–6 years among the four study groups. The FLACC in 1–6 years old pediatric patients, over time, the pain intensity gradually decreased, and increased slightly at 24 h after surgery. **Figure S2.** Comparison of post-operative pain intensity of WBFS in patients aged 1–6 years among the four study groups. The WBFS in 1–6 years old pediatric patients, the pain score gradually decreased within 8 h after surgery, and increased slightly at 24 h. Data are presented as the mean visual analog score. **Figure S3.** Comparison of post-operative pain intensity of NRS in patients aged 7–12 years among the four study groups. The NRS in 7–12 years old pediatric patients, over time, the pain intensity gradually decreased, and increased slightly at 24 h after surgery. Data are presented as the mean visual analog score. **Figure S4.** Comparison of post-operative pain intensity of WBFS in in patients aged 7–12 years among the four study groups. The WBFS in 7–12 years old pediatric patients, the pain score gradually decreased within 8 h after surgery, and increased slightly at 24 h. Data are presented as the mean visual analog score.

Abbreviations

ARP: Invasive arterial pressure; BP: Non-invasive blood pressure; FLACC: Faces, Legs, Activity, Cry and Consolability Scale; HR: Heart rate; MME: Milligram morphine equivalents; NCA: Nurse-controlled analgesia; NRS: Numeric rating scale; PCA: Patient-controlled analgesia; $P_{ET}CO_2$: End-tidal carbon dioxide partial pressure; POPI: Postoperative acute pain intensity; SpO_2: Pulse oximetry; WBFS: Wong-Baker Faces Scale

Acknowledgements

I would like to express my sincere thanks to all doctors and nurses in the department of neurosurgery, Beijing Tiantan Hospital, Capital Medical University.

Author's contributions

XF prepared the manuscript and implemented post-operative pain evaluation. ALX designed, interpreted the data and finally approved the version to be published. XFS assisted to prepare the draft and substantively revised it. BYF assisted to collect data and performed the statistical analysis. ZCM assisted in postoperative follow-up and the main data's acquisition. All authors had read and approved the final submitted version. All authors have agreed both to be personally accountable for their own contributions and to ensure that questions related to the accuracy or integrity of any part of the work.

Author details

[1]Department of Anesthesia, Beijing Friendship Hospital, Capital Medical University, No.95 Yongan Road, Xicheng District, Beijing 100050, China. [2]Department of Anesthesia, Beijing Tiantan Hospital, Capital Medical University, Beijing, China.

References

1. Tsaousi GG, Logan SW, Bilotta F. Postoperative pain control following craniotomy: a systematic review of recent clinical literature. Pain Pract. 2017; 17:968–81.
2. Suksompong S, Chaikittisilpa N, Rutchadawong T, Chankaew E, von Bormann B. Pain after major craniotomy in a university hospital: a prospective cohort study. J Med Assoc Thail. 2016;99:539–48.
3. Dilmen OK, Akcil EF, Tunali Y, Karabulut ES, Bahar M, Altindas F, et al. Postoperative analgesia for supratentorial craniotomy. Clin Neurol Neurosurg. 2016;146:90–5.
4. Peng Y, Zhang W, Kass IS, Han R. Lidocaine reduces acute postoperative pain after Supratentorial tumor surgery in the PACU: a secondary finding from a randomized, controlled trial. J Neurosurg Anesthesiol. 2016;28:309–15.
5. Teo JH, Palmer GM, Davidson AJ. Post-craniotomy pain in a paediatric population. Anaesth Intensive Care. 2011;39:89–94.
6. Bronco A, Pietrini D, Lamperti M, Somaini M, Tosi F, del Lungo LM, et al. Incidence of pain after craniotomy in children. Pediatr Anesth. 2014;24:781–7.
7. Maxwell LG, Buckley GM, Kudchadkar SR, Ely E, Stebbins EL, Dube C, et al. Pain management following major intracranial surgery in pediatric patients: a prospective cohort study in three academic children's hospitals. Pediatr Anesth. 2014;24:1132–40.
8. An LX, Chen X, Ren XJ, Wu HF. Electro-acupuncture decreases postoperative pain and improves recovery in patients undergoing a supratentorial craniotomy. Am J Chin Med. 2014;42:1099–109.
9. Hansen MS, Brennum J, Moltke FB, Dahl JB. Pain treatment after craniotomy: where is the (procedure-specific) evidence? A qualitative systematic review. Eur J Anaesthesiol. 2011;28:821–9.
10. Morad A, Winters B, Stevens R, White E, Weingart J, Yaster M, et al. The efficacy of intravenous patient-controlled analgesia after intracranial surgery of the posterior fossa: a prospective, randomized controlled trial. Anesth Analg. 2012;114:416–23.
11. Gottschalk A, Yaster M. The perioperative management of pain from intracranial surgery. Neurocrit Care. 2009;10:387–402.
12. Bauer DF, Waters AM, Tubbs RS, Rozzelle CJ, Wellons JC 3rd, Blount JP, et al. Safety and utility of scheduled nonnarcotic analgesic medications in children undergoing craniotomy for brain tumor. Neurosurgery. 2010;67: 353–5 discussion 355-356.
13. Ye H, Xie S, Li J, An LX. The observation of craniotomy postoperative pain in preschoolers (Chinese). Int J Anesth Resus. 2015;36(70):605–9.
14. Tan WH, Feaman S, Milam L, Garber V, McAllister J, Blatnik JA, et al. Postoperative opioid prescribing practices and the impact of the hydrocodone schedule change. Surgery. 2018;164:879–86.
15. Malviya S, Voepel-Lewis T, Burke C, Merkel S, Tait AR. The revised FLACC observational pain tool: improved reliability and validity for pain assessment in children with cognitive impairment. Peadiatr Anesth. 2006;16:258–65.
16. Garra G, Singer AJ, Taira BR, Chohan J, Cardoz H, Chisena E, et al. Validation of the Wong-baker FACES pain rating scale in pediatric emergency department patients. Acad Emerg Med. 2010;17:50–4.
17. Abu-Saad H. Assessing children's responses to pain. Pain. 1984;19:163–71.
18. Rocha-Filho PA. Post-craniotomy headache: a clinical view with a focus on the persistent form. Headache. 2015;55:733–8.
19. Haldar R, Kaushal A, Gupta D, Srivastava S, Singh PK. Pain following craniotomy: reassessment of the available options. Biomed Res Int. 2015;2015:509164.
20. Nelson KL, Yaster M, Kost-Byerly S, Monitto CL. A national survey of American pediatric anesthesiologists: patient- controlled analgesia and other intravenous opioid therapies in pediatric acute pain management. Anesth Analg. 2010;110:754–60.
21. Hummel P, Lawlor-Klean P, Weiss MG. Validity and reliability of the N-PASS assessment tool with acute pain. J Perinatol. 2010;30:474–8.
22. Chiaretti A, Viola L, Pietrini D, Piastra M, Savioli A, Tortorolo L, et al. Preemptive analgesia with tramadol and fentanyl in pediatric neurosurgery. Childs Nerv Syst. 2000;16:93–9 discussion 100.
23. Warren DT, Bowen-Roberts T, Ou C, Purdy R, Steinbok P. Safety and efficacy of continuous morphine infusions following pediatric cranial surgery in a surgical ward setting. Childs Nerv Syst. 2010;26:1535–41.
24. Alencar AJ, Sanudo A, Sampaio VM, Góis RP, Benevides FA, Guinsburg R. Efficacy of tramadol versus fentanyl for postoperative analgesia in neonates. Arch Dis Fetal Neonatal Ed. 2012;97:F24–9.
25. Murphy JD, Yan D, Hanna MN, Bravos ED, Isaac GR, Eng CA, et al. Comparison of the postoperative analgesic efficacy of intravenous patient-controlled analgesia with tramadol to intravenous patient-controlled analgesia with opioids. J Opioid Manag. 2010;6:141–7.
26. Guilfoyle MR, Helmy A, Duane D, Hutchinson PJ. Regional scalp block for postcraniotomy analgesia: a systematic review and meta-analysis. Anesth Analg. 2013;116:1093–102.
27. Jayaram K, Srilata M, Kulkarni D, Ramachandran G. Regional anesthesia to scalp for craniotomy: innovation with innervation. J Neurosurg Anesthesiol. 2016;28:32–7.

24

Effect of low dose naloxone on the immune system function of a patient undergoing video-assisted thoracoscopic resection of lung cancer with sufentanil controlled analgesia

Yun Lin[1], Zhuang Miao[1], Yue Wu[1], Fang-fang Ge[2] and Qing-ping Wen[1*]

Abstract

Background: Perioperative immune function plays an important role in the prognosis of patients. Several studies have indicated that low-dose opioid receptor blockers can improve immune function.

Methods: Sixty-nine patients undergoing video-assisted thoracoscopic resection of the lung cancer were randomly assigned to either the naloxone group ($n = 35$) or the non-naloxone group ($n = 34$) for postoperative analgesia during the first 48 h after the operation. Both groups received sufentanil and palonosetron via postoperative analgesia pump, while 0.05 μg·kg^{-1}·h^{-1} naloxone was added in naloxone group. The primary outcomes were the level of opioid growth factor (OGF) and immune function assessed by natural killer cells and CD4$^+$/CD8$^+$ T-cell ratio. Second outcomes were assessed by the intensity of postoperative pain, postoperative rescue analgesia dose, postoperative nausea and vomiting (PONV).

Results: The level of OGF in the naloxone group increased significantly at 24 h ($p<0.001$) and 48 h after the operation ($P < 0.01$). The natural killer cells ($P < 0.05$) and CD4$^+$/CD8$^+$ T-cell ratio ($P < 0.01$) in the naloxone group increased significantly at 48 h after the operation. The rest VAS scores were better with naloxone at 12 and 24 h after operation($P < 0.05$), and the coughing VAS scores were better with naloxone at 48 h after the operation($P <$ 0.05). The consumption of postoperative rescue analgesics in the naloxone group was lower (0.00(0.00–0.00) vs 25.00(0.00–62.50)), $P < 0.05$). Postoperative nausea scores at 24 h after operation decreased in naloxone group(0.00 (0.00–0.00) vs 1.00 (0.00–2.00), $P < 0.01$).

Conclusion: Infusion of 0.05 μg·kg^{-1}·h^{-1} naloxone for patients undergoing sufentanil-controlled analgesia for postoperative pain can significantly increase the level of OGF, natural killer cells, and CD4+/CD8+ T-cell ratio compared with non-naloxone group, and postoperative pain intensity, request for rescue analgesics, and opioid-related side effects can also be reduced.

Keywords: Low-dose naloxone, Opioid growth factor, Immune function, Postoperative pain, Nausea, Vomiting

* Correspondence: wqp.89@163.com
[1]Department of Anesthesiology, The First Affiliated Hospital of Dalian Medical University, No.193 Lian he Road, Xi gang District, Dalian City, Liaoning Province 116000, People's Republic of China

Background

Cancer has become a major public health concern all over the world, among which lung cancer is a prominent problem. Surgical resection is the principal treatment for tumors [1, 2]. Recurrence and metastasis of tumors are the main causes of death in patients with lung cancer [3]. The perioperative periods are a dangerous time points for tumor recurrence and metastasis. Immunosuppression plays a significantly important role in the development of tumors [4]. Improvement of postoperative immune function is vitally important for patients. In addition, appropriate postoperative pain control, and effective management of postoperative nausea and vomiting (PONV) lead to several benefits, including earlier restoration of mobility, shorter hospital stays, lower hospital costs and higher comfort and satisfaction of patients.

Opioid receptor antagonists such as naloxone are widely used in the clinical setting to treat opioid-induced respiratory depression and drug addiction. Regulation of endogenous opioids by opioid receptor antagonists may explain the role of opioid peptide-opioid receptor interactions in many biological processes and diseases [5]. One of the functions of endogenous opioids is the regulation of cell growth [6]. Studies have shown that one of the endogenous opioids called opioid growth factor (OGF, chemically termed [MET^5]-Enkephalins) enhances the immune function by increasing the number of natural killer cells (NK cells), T-cells and the levels of interleukin-2 [7–9].

Gans et al. were among the first to report that morphine requirement was significantly less in patients receiving low-dose naloxone, and the finding suggested that low-dose naloxone enhanced analgesia [10]. Moreover, several studies have shown that low-dose naloxone might enhance analgesia and reduce opioid-related adverse effects, such as nausea and vomiting and pruritus [11–13]. Studies showed that low-dose naloxone may enhance analgesic effects through increasing the release of endogenous opioids and up-regulating opioid receptor [14–16]. Some studies further suggested that low-dose naloxone may improve the analgesic effects by releasing enkephalin [13]. However, a survey of the literature shows that little is known about the effects of low dose naloxone on the immune system function of a patient undergoing video-assisted thoracoscopic resection of lung cancer with sufentanil-controlled analgesia. This study aimed to explore the effects of low dose infusion of naloxone 0.05 $\mu g \cdot kg^{-1} \cdot h^{-1}$ on a patient undergoing video-assisted thoracoscopic resection of lung cancer with sufentanil-controlled analgesia.

Methods

This randomized controlled trial was reported according to the Consolidated Standards of Reporting Trials (CONSORT) guidelines and conducted after the approval of the Ethics Committee of the First Affiliated Hospital of the Dalian Medical University on January 24, 2019 (protocol number: PJ-KY-2018-141(X)). Written informed consent was obtained from patients after providing them with adequate explanation regarding the aims of this study. The trial was registered at the Chinese Clinical Trial Registry before patients' enrolment (www.chictr.org.cn, number: ChiCTR1900021043) on January 26, 2019, with Lin Yun as principal investigator. The trial completed a pilot study of 20 patients to calculate the sample size of this trial. The pilot study was performed from February 1, 2019 to February 16, 2019, and the patient data were included in this trial. We enrolled 70 patients aged 18 to 65 with American Society of Anesthesiology physical status II to III undergoing video-assisted thoracoscopic resection of the lung cancer. Patients with severe cardiopulmonary, liver or kidney diseases, allergy to naloxone, opioid addiction or drug abuse, and vertigo were excluded.

Upon arrival in the operation room, standard monitoring was determined. Anesthesia was induced with midazolam, sufentanil, cisatracurium, and propofol, subsequently intubation with double lumen tube and location by fiber bronchoscope. Ventilator parameters were adjusted to maintain pulse saturation of oxygen (SpO_2) 95–100% and end-tidal carbon dioxide between 35 and 40 mmHg. Anesthesia was maintained with propofol, remifentanil and cisatracurium and the depth of anesthesia was maintained at a bispectral index value of 40 to 60. The postoperative analgesic pump was used at the end of the operation. Sufentanil 0.04 $\mu g \cdot kg^{-1} \cdot h^{-1}$ (calculated at 48 h), palonosetron 0.5 mg and saline diluted to 100 mL were used in a non-naloxone group, while 0.05 $\mu g \cdot kg^{-1} \cdot h^{-1}$ naloxone (calculated at 48 h) was added in naloxone group. PCA was set to administer a bolus dose of 2 mL with a lockout interval of 20 min and a background infusion rate of 2 mL/h. Patients were randomly allocated into 2 groups (1:1 allocation ratio) by a sequence generated from a pseudorandom number seed. Because other non-opioid drugs may have different effects on immune function, postoperative rescue analgesia was chosen to perform intramuscular injection with meperidine in both groups. All patients in both groups were instructed on how to use the PCA device and on how to use the visual analogue scale (VAS) to rate the intensity of the pain at rest or while coughing and nausea on a scale from 0 to 10 (with 0 denoting the lowest level of intensity of the symptom and 10, the worst imaginable intensity).

The primary outcomes of the study were the levels of OGF and postoperative immune function assessed by NK cells and $CD4^+/CD8^+$ T-cell ratio. Second outcomes were assessed by the VAS scores of postoperative pain, nausea and analgesic dose, inflammatory responses measured by white blood cell (WBC) count and neutrophil percentage, respiratory depression, and hospital stay. Immune function and inflammatory responses were measured before the surgery, at 24 and 48 h after surgery. Both groups of patients rated the intensity of their pain with VAS and respiratory depression 1, 6, 12, 24 and 48 h after the operation (respiratory depression: respiratory rate ≤ 8/min or SpO_2<90%). Both groups of patients rated the scale of nausea and the dose of Meperidine at 24 and 48 h after operation and hospital stay.

T lymphocyte subsets and natural killer cells assay

Venous blood samples were taken before the surgery, and 24 and 48 h after surgery. Moreover, flow cytometry (BD Company, USA) was applied to assess the changes in peripheral blood T lymphocyte subsets ($CD3^+$, $CD4^+$, $CD8^+$, and $CD4^+/CD8^+$ T-cell ratio) and NK cells.

OGF assay

Venous blood samples were taken before the surgery, 24 and 48 h after surgery. OGF was measured in serum using a commercial ELISA kit (MEK (Methionine-Enkephalin) ELISA kit; Elabscience.).

Statistical analysis

The primary aims of this study were to determine the differences in the levels of OGF, NK cells and $CD4^+/CD8^+$ T-cell ratio and the secondary outcomes including VAS scores of postoperative pain, nausea, postoperative rescue analgesia dose, WBC count, neutrophil percentage, respiratory depression and hospital stay in naloxone and control groups. Results were expressed as means ± SD, medians with interquartile range, or numbers and percentages of participants as appropriate. The demographics and intraoperative situations were compared by Student t test or χ^2 test. Fisher's exact test was used for small sample sizes (expected frequencies < 5). The levels of OGF, NK cells, $CD4^+/CD8^+$ T-cell ratio, WBC count, neutrophil percentage and hospital stay analyzed with a one-way ANOVA between the two groups, and non-normally distributed variables were analyzed with the Mann-Whitney U test. P values < 0.05 were considered significant. Statistical analysis was performed using SPSS version 22.0.

A pilot study was performed prior to patient recruitment to estimate an appropriate sample size. The pilot study included 20 subjects, 10 in each arm. We calculated the primary outcome of the study assessed by NK cells. The sample size of 32 participants each group provided $\alpha = 0.05$, 80% power, and an allocation ratio = 1.0. Accounting for loss of data, each group needed 35 patients. The sample calculation was performed with PASS version 11.0.

Results

Among the 81 patients assessed for eligibility, 70 patients were enrolled and randomly assigned to the groups, and 69 patients completed the study (Fig. 1). Data from one patient was excluded from the analysis due to early discharge (the next day after the operation). There were no significant differences in patient characteristics (Table 1).

The levels of OGF in the naloxone group were significantly higher at 24 h(p<0.001) and 48 h after the operation ($P < 0.01$) in Fig. 2. NK cells ($P < 0.05$) (Table 2) and $CD4^+/CD8^+$ T-cell ratio ($P < 0.01$) (Table 3) in patients from the naloxone group significantly increased compared with non-naloxone group at 48 h after the operation. There were no significant differences in the NK cells (Table 2) and $CD4^+/CD8^+$ T-cell ratio (Table 3) at 24 h after the operation. The rest VAS scores were better with naloxone at 12 and 24 h after the operation($P <$ 0.05) (Fig. 3). The coughing VAS scores were also better with naloxone at 48 h after the operation ($P < 0.05$) (Fig. 3). There were no significant differences at other time points in Fig. 3. The rescue postoperative analgesics dose injected in patients from the naloxone group was 0.00(0.00–0.00) mg lower compared with 25.00(0.00–62.50) mg injected in patients from the non-naloxone group ($P < 0.05$) (Table 4).

Table 4 showed that postoperative nausea scores significantly decreased in patients from the naloxone group(0.00 (0.00–0.00) vs. 1.00(0.00–2.00), $P < 0.01$) at 24 h after the operation. There were no significant differences in nausea scores between the groups at other time points (Table 4). There were no significant differences in the postoperative vomiting after the operation (Table 4). And there were no significant differences in the postoperative hospital stay (P>0.05) in Table 4. The data showed no significant differences in the postoperative inflammatory responses assessed by WBC count and the percentage of neutrophil between the two groups (P>0.05) in Table 5.

Discussion

In this study, we found that 0.05 $\mu g \cdot kg^{-1} \cdot h^{-1}$ naloxone for patients with sufentanil-controlled analgesia could increase the levels of OGF, NK cells and $CD4^+/CD8^+$ T-cell ratio compared with non-naloxone group. Studies have shown that OGF could increase the number of NK cells and T cells [7, 8]. NK cells have been showed to play an important role in effective immune responses and immunosurveillance. Cytolytic enzymes and cytokines produced by NK cells, like IFN-γ, are beneficial to inhibit cancer cells [17]. The survival of lung cancer patients was closely related to the level of NK cells [18], and patients' survival rates are bound up with the level of NK cells in primary squamous cell lung carcinoma

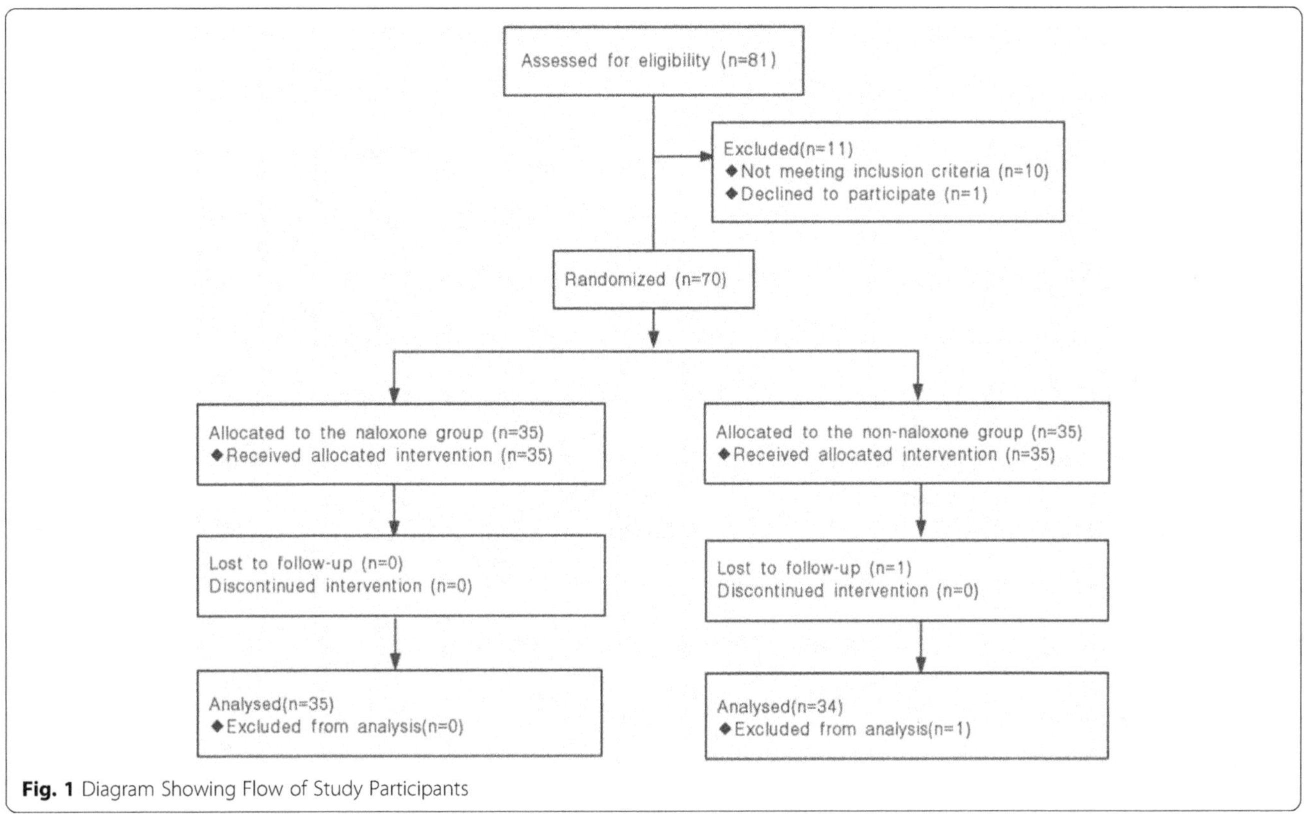

Fig. 1 Diagram Showing Flow of Study Participants

[19]. The decline of NK cells leads to the occurrence and development of tumors [20, 21] and the level of the NK cells is of great significance in judging clinical prognosis. Our results showed that low-dose naloxone may inhibit tumors by increasing the level of NK cells regulated by OGF.

T cell subsets play a major role in cellular immunity. The number of $CD3^+$ T cells represents the overall cellular immune status of the body. $CD8^+$ is a cytotoxic T lymphocyte, which can eradicate virally infected cells and cancer cells, trigger apoptosis by release of cytotoxins and directly contact with cells [22]. $CD4^+$ is a T helper cell with the function of immune regulation, which can recognize the antigens produced by tumor and inhibit cancer cells by activating other immune cells, such as NK cells and cytotoxic T lymphocyte, and NK cells also play a role in activation of cytotoxic T cell [23]. In addition, cytokines secreted by NK cells have effect on T helper cell polarization [17]. The maintenance of normal immune function depends on the cooperation or restriction between various immune cells (especially all kinds of T cell subsets and NK cells). $CD4^+/CD8^+$ T-cell ratio reflect the immune status of the body [24]. In physiological state, $CD4^+/CD8^+$ T-cell ratio is relatively constant. The decrease of $CD4^+/CD8^+$ T-cell ratio indicates the decrease of immune function and the severity of disease or poor prognosis [24]. The results showed that $CD4^+/CD8^+$ T-cell ratio in naloxone group was higher 48 h after the operation, suggesting that low dose naloxone may enhance cellular immunity and anti-tumor effects. Low-dose naloxone may enhance immune function by decreasing pain intensity, but whether the increase of $CD4^+/CD8^+$ T-cell ratio is related to OGF is uncertain.

The postoperative immune function may be related to operation, anesthesia, postoperative pain, body temperature and blood transfusion in the operation, etc [4, 25–27]. Some studies indicated that the operation itself and stress responses induced by operation could result in a reduction of the postoperative NK cells [28]. The effects of anesthesia on immune function have been widely discussed in recent years, but the result is still controversial. Opioid drugs may cause postoperative immunosuppression by reducing the number of NK cells [29, 30], but it is difficult to control the stress and pain caused by surgical stimulation without the use of opioids, and the acute pain could activate the hypothalamus-pituitary-adrenal (HPA) axis, which in turn has an effect on the number of NK cells [31]. And there are other non-opioid drugs that affect immune function [29]. The combination of these factors may result in our results that number of NK cells in the naloxone group was higher than that of non-naloxone group after operation, but the number of NK cells in the both

Table 1 Patient characteristics

	Naloxone($n = 35$)	Non-naloxone ($n = 34$)	*P* Value
Age(y)	55.46 ± 8.65	55.46 ± 8.65	0.378
Gender, N(%)			0.900
Male	17(48.57)	16(47.06)	
Female	18(51.43)	18(52.94)	
Body mass index (kg/m^2)	25.42 ± 4.19	24.52 ± 3.67	0.351
ASA physical status, N (%)			1.000
II	31(88.57)	30(11.76)	
III	4(11.43)	4(88.24)	
Type of operation, N (%)			0.777
Video-assisted thoracoscopic pulmonary lobectomy	25(71.43)	26(76.47)	
Video-assisted thoracoscopic pulmonary wedge resection	9(25.71)	8(23.93)	
Video-assisted thoracoscopic pulmonary segmentary	1(2.86)	0(0.00)	
Duration of operation (min)	150.00 (120.00–180.00)	180.00 (120.00–180.00)	0.339
Fluid intake (mL)	1000.00(1000.00–1000.00)	1000.00(1000.00–1000.00)	0.854
Blood loss (mL)	113.71 ± 38.278	106.76 ± 36.987	0.446
Type of cancer, N (%)			0.780
Carcinoma in situ	8(22.85)	6(17.65)	
Microinvasive adenocarcinoma	14(40.00)	11(32.35)	
infiltrating adenocarcinoma	12(34.29)	14(41.18)	
Mucinous adenocarcinoma	1(2.86)	2(5.88)	
Moderately differentiated adenocarcinoma	0(0.00)	1(2.94)	
Lymphatic metastasis			0.614
Yes	1(2.86)	2(5.88)	
No	34(97.14)	32(94.12)	

ASA American Society of Anesthesiologists

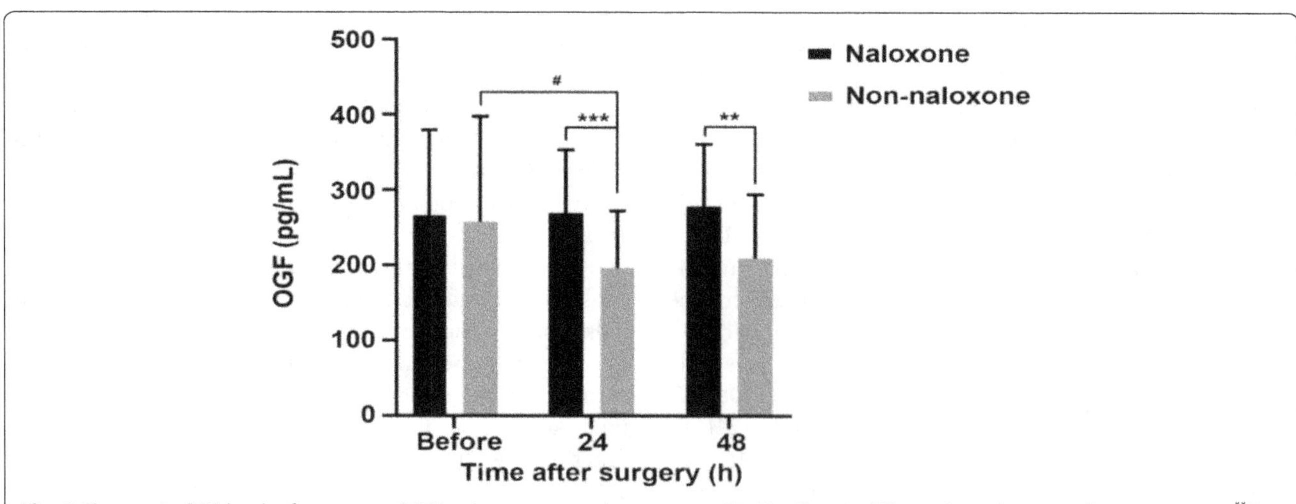

Fig. 2 Changes in OGF levels after surgery. OGF levels are presented as means ± SD. Significantly different from the non-naloxone group at $^{**}P<0.01$, $^{***}P<0.001$. $^{\#}P<0.05$ versus "before surgery" for each group

Table 2 Changes in NK Cells After Surgery

		Naloxone(n = 35)	Non-naloxone (n = 34)	P Value
NK cells(%)	Before surgery	16.14 ± 5.75	16.63 ± 6.40	0.519
	24 h after operation	14.13 ± 6.28	14.53 ± 5.85	0.918
	48 h after operation	15.97 ± 5.44	13.06 ± 5.47#	0.030

NK cells Natural Killer Cells. #P<0.05 versus "before surgery" for each group

of two groups were lower compared to the time before surgery.

Many experiments have been carried out to evaluate the effects of low-dose naloxone on postoperative analgesia and opioid-related side effects. The analgesic effects and adverse effects of opioids are dose-dependent. The dose of naloxone administration in the report provided highly variable ranging from 0.008 $\mu g \cdot kg^{-1} \cdot h^{-1}$ to 0.57 $\mu g \cdot kg^{-1} \cdot h^{-1}$ [32]. The reason why 0.05 $\mu g \cdot kg^{-1} \cdot h^{-1}$ naloxone was chosen in our study was that patient-controlled intravenous analgesia (PCIA) with this dose in YAO's experiment confirmed that low-dose naloxone increased the analgesic effects by increasing the levels of endogenous opioid peptides [16]. The data showed that the rest pain scores decreased significantly at 12 and 24 h after surgery and coughing pain scores decreased significantly at 48 h after surgery, and the rescue analgesic dose after surgery was lower in the naloxone group, indicating that low-dose naloxone could enhance the analgesic effects of sufentanil and reduce the dose of analgesic. Data showed that the coughing VAS scores were at a higher level than that of rest VAS scores after operation, and the patients in the two groups all showed low tolerance while coughing. It may be the reason for patients not to feel obviously relief at higher level of pain due to the subjectivity of VAS scores. This may explain why the difference happened at 48 h after surgery for the pain on coughing, but for the pain at rest, the difference happened at 12 and 24 h after surgery.

The VAS scores of postoperative nausea decreased significantly on the first day after the operation. The mechanism of the effects of low-dose naloxone on analgesic efficacy and opioid-related side effects is not clear. In addition to releasing enkephalins [33], it is believed that the functions of the μ-opioid receptor excitatory G-protein complexes (GS) are antagonized by naloxone at a low dose, triggering improvement of analgesic effects and reduction in adverse effects such as nausea and vomiting [13]. Some studies also indicated that low dose of naloxone could reduce neuropathic pain by lowering the levels of inflammatory factors [34]. Our study found that the levels of OGF increased significantly two days after the operation, suggesting that the mechanism of low-dose naloxone enhancing the analgesic effects of sufentanil, reducing opioids consumption and postoperative nausea may be related to the level of endogenous OGF.

We have always attached great importance to postoperative analgesia management. Our results showed that postoperative pain in rest can be well controlled, but the pain scores on coughing were overall on the high level. Patients were encouraged to mobilize out of bed early

Table 3 Changes in T cells After Surgery

		Naloxone(n = 35)	Non-naloxone(n = 34)	P Value
$CD3^+$T cells(%)	Before surgery	56.94 ± 9.01	56.95 ± 8.98	0.997
	24 h after operation	46.22 ± 12.67###	41.48 ± 9.99###	0.089
	48 h after operation	56.17 ± 8.96	53.36 ± 10.58	0.237
$CD4^+$T cells(%)	Before surgery	33.49 ± 6.92	32.61 ± 5.52	0.560
	24 h after operation	25.39 ± 8.55###	21.20 ± 7.81###	0.037
	48 h after operation	32.70 ± 6.39	28.91 ± 6.11#	0.014
$CD8^+$T cells(%)	Before surgery	23.45 ± 4.37	24.34 ± 5.09	0.437
	24 h after operation	20.83 ± 7.02#	20.28 ± 6.54##	0.734
	48 h after operation	23.47 ± 4.10	24.57 ± 6.21	0.391
$CD4^+/CD8^+$ T cell ratio	Before surgery	1.49 ± 0.36	1.39 ± 0.30	0.226
	24 h after operation	1.32 ± 0.51	1.15 ± 0.52#	0.163
	48 h after operation	1.41 ± 0.27	1.21 ± 0.29	0.003

CD Clusters of Differentiation

#P<0.05 versus "before surgery" for each group. ##P<0.01 versus "before surgery" for each group, ###P<0.001 versus "before surgery" for each group

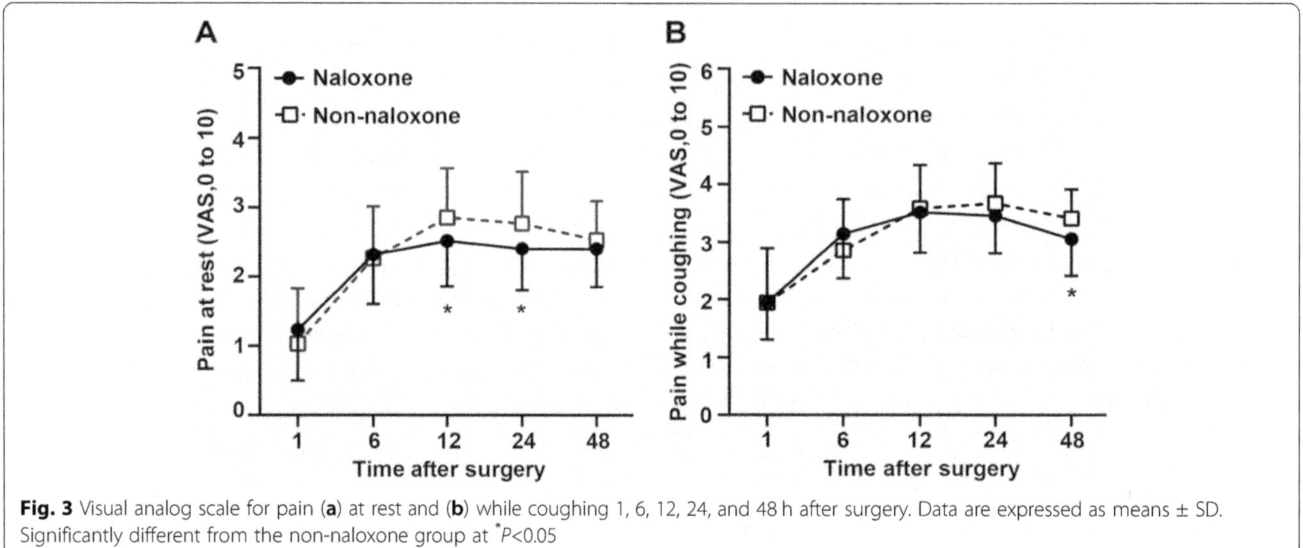

Fig. 3 Visual analog scale for pain (**a**) at rest and (**b**) while coughing 1, 6, 12, 24, and 48 h after surgery. Data are expressed as means ± SD. Significantly different from the non-naloxone group at $^{*}P<0.05$

and cough after the thoracoscopic surgery in order to reduce postoperative complications. This promote us to control the VAS scores at a lower level during coughing and activities to ensure patient's favorable prognosis and satisfaction. At the same time, we also found that opioids had effective analgesia on coughing but the frequency of postoperative nausea and vomiting after operation was higher. Hence, with respect to the better postoperative management, we would like to find a way to control the occurrence of postoperative nausea and vomiting in patients, not just the postoperative acute pain. And we hope to find a good balance between the control of postoperative nausea and pain. Low-dose naloxone may be a good choice from the experimental results, but more experiments are needed to prove this possibility.

We noticed the basic studies have shown that the regimen of short-term exposure to naltrexone appeared to lead to enhanced interaction of the up-regulated OGF [33]. Blockade of opioid peptides from opioid receptors for a short period each day (4–6 h), using a daily administration of low-dose naltrexone (LDH), provides an 18-20 h window wherein the elevated levels of endogenous opioids and opioid receptors can interact to elicit a response [33]. However, in this study, we used 0.05 $\mu g{\cdot}kg^{-1}{\cdot}h^{-1}$ naloxone continuous infusion along with sufentanil PCIA for about 48 h, and the levels of OGF increased significantly within 48 h. There may be two possibilities for this difference, one of which may be related to the difference of half-time of naloxone and naltrexone. Both naltrexone and naloxone are opioid receptor antagonists and have no intrinsic activity, but the duration of naltrexone blockade is about 3–4 times longer than that of naloxone. The other one may be associated with different dose. According to the potency relationship between naltrexone and naloxone, low dose naloxone (4.5 mg) [35] in the report was far more than 0.05 $\mu g{\cdot}kg^{-1}{\cdot}h^{-1}$ naloxone we used in this study.

Table 4 Rescue Analgesic Dose, Postoperative Nausea and Vomiting scores, Respiratory Depression and Hospital Stay

	Naloxone(*n* = 35)	Non-naloxone (*n* = 34)	*P* Value
Rescue analgesic dose (mg)	0.00(0.00–0.00)	25.0(0.00–62.50)	0.034
Nausea VAS score 24 h after operation	0.00(0.00–0.00)	1.00(0.00–2.00)	0.001
Vomiting 24 h after operation, n(%)	6(17.14)	11(32.35)	0.143
Nausea VAS score 48 h after operation	0.00(0.00–0.00)	0.00(0.00–0.00)	0.318
Vomiting 48 h after operation, n(%)	3(8.57)	5(14.71)	0.675
Respiratory depression 1 h after operation, n(%)	0.00(0.00)	0.00(0.00)	>0.99
Respiratory depression 6 h after operation, n(%)	0.00(0.00)	0.00(0.00)	>0.99
Respiratory depression 12 h after operation, n(%)	0.00(0.00)	0.00(0.00)	>0.99
Respiratory depression 24 h after operation, n(%)	0.00(0.00)	0.00(0.00)	>0.99
Respiratory depression 48 h after operation, n(%)	0.00(0.00)	0.00(0.00)	>0.99
Hospital stay (day)	4.66 ± 1.39	5.35 ± 1.77	0.074

Table 5 Changes in White Blood Cell Count and Neutrophil Percentage After Surgery

		Naloxone($n = 35$)	Non-naloxone ($n = 34$)	P Value
WBC count/uL	Before surgery	7.81 ± 1.23	7.78 ± 1.25	0.907
	24 h after operation	11.96 ± 3.13$^{###}$	13.21 ± 3.41$^{###}$	0.115
	48 h after operation	9.93 ± 2.86$^{##}$	10.79 ± 2.87$^{###}$	0.214
Neutrophil Percentage(%)	Before surgery	71.74 ± 7.06	72.49 ± 6.71	0.656
	24 h after operation	83.57 ± 5.71$^{###}$	85.48 ± 4.39$^{###}$	0.124
	48 h after operation	76.47 ± 8.55$^{##}$	79.41 ± 6.67$^{###}$	0.117

$^{##}P<0.01$ versus "before surgery" for each group. $^{###}P<0.001$ versus "before surgery" for each group

Although we used continuous naloxone infusion for 48 h, the shorter blockade duration and lower dose might not block all opioid receptors. These may be the reason why the elevated levels of OGF can still interact with its receptor to elicit a response. The mechanism of the increase in the levels of OGF is that low-dose naloxone may cause excessive release of endogenous opioids through blockade of presynaptic auto-inhibition of enkephalin release [13].

There are two limitations in this study. First, the duration of immune function detected was limited to 48 h after the operation, and we did not further observe changes of immune indexes. The experimental data showed that there were no significant changes in the immune function on the first day after the operation. The NK cells and CD4$^+$/CD8$^+$ T-cell ratio in naloxone group began to be higher on the second day after the operation. If we continue to test NK cells and T cells, we could explore the extent and duration of using low-dose naloxone to improve immune function with PCA after the operation. Second, the long-term prognosis of the patients was not observed. Studies have shown that OGF can not only enhance immune function but also directly inhibit tumors. OGF activates the Rb pathway by upregulating p16 and/p21, which are cyclin-dependent inhibitory kinases, with delayed cell replication and ultimate cell number resulting [36]. Thus, low-dose opioid receptor antagonists mediated modulation of the OGF-OGFr axis appears to account for the depressed DNA synthesis and proliferation of cancer cells [33]. OGF may inhibit the recurrence and metastasis of tumors after surgery. Since no further follow-up of the patients' OGF levels and recurrence or metastasis after surgery between the groups, it was not observed that whether low-dose naloxone could directly affect the occurrence and development of tumors through OGF-OGFr.

Conclusion

In conclusion, 0.05 $\mu g \cdot kg^{-1} \cdot h^{-1}$ naloxone increased the number of NK cells, CD4$^+$/CD8$^+$ T cell ratio and the analgesic effects after thoracoscopic resection of lung cancer on PCIA, meanwhile reduced analgesics dose and PONV after the operation. The enhancement of immune function and the analgesic effects of sufentanil and reduction of PONV may be related to the increased level of endogenous OGF.

Abbreviations

ASA: American Society of Anesthesiologists; CD: Clusters of Differentiation; GS: G-protein complexes; LDH: Low-dose naltrexone; NK cells: Natural killer cells; OGF: Opioid growth factor; PCA: Patient controlled analgesia; PCIA: Patient-controlled intravenous analgesia; PONV: Postoperative nausea, and vomiting; SpO_2: Pulse saturation of oxygen; T cells: T lymphocytes; VAS: Visual analogue scale; WBC: White blood cell

Acknowledgements

We would like to thank sincerely Dr. Qingping Wen and Dr. Zhuang Miao for their efforts and performance during this study.

Authors' contributions

LY designed the study, drafted and wrote the manuscript. LY and GFF implemented the trial and contributed samples collection.MZ and WY collected the data and did statistical analysis. WQP revised the manuscript critically and finally approved the manuscript. All authors gave intellectual input to the study and approved the final version of the manuscript.

Author details

[1]Department of Anesthesiology, The First Affiliated Hospital of Dalian Medical University, No.193 Lian he Road, Xi gang District, Dalian City, Liaoning Province 116000, People's Republic of China. [2]Dalian Medical of University, Dalian, China.

References

1. Pilleron S, Sarfati D, Janssen-Heijnen M, Vignat J, Ferlay J, Bray F, Soerjomataram I. Global cancer incidence in older adults, 2012 and 2035: a population-based study. Int J Cancer. 2019;144(1):49–58.
2. Bray F, Ferlay J, Soerjomataram I, Siegel RL, Torre LA, Jemal A. Global cancer statistics 2018: GLOBOCAN estimates of incidence and mortality worldwide for 36 cancers in 185 countries. CA Cancer J Clin. 2018;68(6):394–424.
3. Sullivan R, Alatise OI, Anderson BO, Audisio R, Autier P, Aggarwal A, et al. Global cancer surgery: delivering safe, affordable, and timely cancer surgery. Lancet Oncol. 2015;16(11):1193–224.
4. Snyder GL, Greenberg S. Effect of anaesthetic technique and other perioperative factors on cancer recurrence. Br J Anaesth. 2010;105(2):106–15.
5. Stagg NJ, Mata HP, Ibrahim MM, Henriksen EJ, Porreca F, Vanderah TW, Malan TP. Regular exercise reverses sensory hypersensitivity in a rat neuropathic pain modelrole of endogenous opioids. Anesthesiology. 2011; 114(4):940–8.
6. Zagon IS, Verderame MF, McLaughlin PJ. The biology of the opioid growth factor receptor (OGFr). Brain Res Rev. 2002;38(3):351–76.
7. Kowalski J. Immunologic action of [Met5] enkephalin fragments. Eur J Pharmacol. 1998;347(1):95–9.
8. Plotnikoff NP, Miller GC, Nimeh N, Faith RE, Murgo AJ, Wybran J. Enkephalins and T-cell enhancement in Normal volunteers and Cancer patients. Ann N Y Acad Sci. 1987;496(1):608–19.
9. Wybran J, Schandené L, Van Vooren JP, Vandermoten G, Latinne D, Sonnet J, et al. Immunologic properties of methionine-Enkephalin, and

therapeutic implications in AIDS, ARC, and Cancer. Ann N Y Acad Sci. 1987;496(1):108–14.

10. Gan TJ, Ginsberg B, Glass PS, Fortney J, Jhaveri R, Perno R. Opioid-sparing effects of a low-dose infusion of naloxone in patient-administered morphine sulfate. Anesthesiology. 1997;87(5):1075–81.
11. Maxwell LG, Kaufmann SC, Bitzer S, Jackson EV, McGready J, Kost-Byerly S, et al. The effects of a small-dose naloxone infusion on opioid-induced side effects and analgesia in children and adolescents treated with intravenous patient-controlled analgesia: a double-blind, prospective, randomized, controlled study. Anesth Analg. 2005;100(4):953–8.
12. Cepeda MS, Alvarez H, Morales O, Carr DB. Addition of ultralow dose naloxone to postoperative morphine PCA: unchanged analgesia and opioid requirement but decreased incidence of opioid side effects. Pain. 2004; 107(1–2):41–6.
13. Firouzian A, Gholipour Baradari A, Alipour A, Emami Zeydi A, Zamani Kiasari A, Emadi SA, et al. Ultra–low-dose naloxone as an adjuvant to patient controlled analgesia (PCA) with morphine for postoperative pain relief following lumber discectomy: a double-blind, randomized, placebo-controlled trial. J Neurosurg Anesthesiol. 2018;30(1):26–31.
14. Crain SM, Shen KF. Antagonists of excitatory opioid receptor functions enhance morphine's analgesic potency and attenuate opioid tolerance/dependence liability. Pain. 2000;84(2–3):121–31.
15. Yang CP, Cherng CH, Wu CT, Huang HY, Tao PL, Wong CS. Intrathecal ultra-low dose naloxone enhances the antinociceptive effect of morphine by enhancing the reuptake of excitatory amino acids from the synaptic cleft in the spinal cord of partial sciatic nerve–transected rats. Anesth Analg. 2011; 113(6):1490–500.
16. Yao P, Meng L, Gui J. Effects of low-dose naloxone on morphine analgesia and plasma leveb of opiold peptldes. Chinese J Anesthesiol. 1996;07.
17. Aktaş ON, Öztürk AB, Erman B, Erus S, Tanju S, Dilege Ş. Role of natural killer cells in lung cancer. J Cancer Res Clin Oncol. 2018;144(6):997–1003.
18. Jin S, Deng Y, Hao JW, Li Y, Liu B, Yu Y, et al. NK cell phenotypic modulation in lung cancer environment. PLoS One. 2014;9(10):e109976.
19. Villegas FR, Coca S, Villarrubia VG, Jiménez R, Chillón MJ, Jareño J, et al. Prognostic significance of tumor infiltrating natural killer cells subset CD57 in patients with squamous cell lung cancer. Lung Cancer. 2002;35(1):23–8.
20. Vivier E, Raulet DH, Moretta A, Caligiuri MA, Zitvogel L, Lanier LL, et al. Innate or adaptive immunity? The example of natural killer cells. Science. 2011;331(6013):44–9.
21. Zamai L, Ponti C, Mirandola P, Gobbi G, Papa S, Galeotti L, et al. NK cells and cancer. J Immunol. 2007;178(7):4011–6.
22. Boland JW, McWilliams K, Ahmedzai SH, Pockley AG. Effects of opioids on immunologic parameters that are relevant to anti-tumour immune potential in patients with cancer: a systematic literature review. Br J Cancer. 2014; 111(5):866.
23. Deniz G, van de Veen W, Akdis M. Natural killer cells in patients with allergic diseases. J Allergy Clin Immunol. 2013;132(3):527–35.
24. Dehghani M, Sharifpour S, Amirghofran Z, Zare HR. Prognostic significance of T cell subsets in peripheral blood of B cell non-Hodgkin's lymphoma patients. Med Oncol. 2012;29(4):2364–71.
25. Xu M, Bennett DL, Querol LA, Wu LJ, Irani SR, Watson JC, et al. Pain and the immune system: emerging concepts of IgG-mediated autoimmune pain and immunotherapies. J Neurol Neurosurg Psychiatry. 2018; jnnp-2018.
26. Cardone D, Klein AA. Perioperative blood conservation. Eur J Anaesthesiol. 2009;26(9):722–9.
27. Molenaar IQ, Warnaar N, Groen H, Tenvergert EM, Slooff MJH, Porte RJ. Efficacy and safety of antifibrinolytic drugs in liver transplantation: a systematic review and meta-analysis. Am J Transplant. 2007;7(1):185–94.
28. Ohira M, Ohdan H, Mitsuta H, Ishiyama K, Tanaka Y, Igarashi Y, Asahara T. Adoptive transfer of TRAIL-expressing natural killer cells prevents recurrence of hepatocellular carcinoma after partial hepatectomy. Transplantation. 2006;82(12):1712–9.
29. Gottschalk A, Sharma S, Ford J, Durieux ME, Tiouririne M. The role of the perioperative period in recurrence after cancer surgery. Anesth Analg. 2010; 110(6):1636–43.
30. Wei G, Moss J, Yuan CS. Opioid-induced immunosuppression: is it centrally mediated or peripherally mediated? Biochem Pharmacol. 2003; 65(11):1761–6.
31. Ge YL, Lv R, Zhou W, Ma XX, Zhong TD, Duan ML. Brain damage following severe acute normovolemic hemodilution in combination with controlled hypotension in rats. Acta Anaesthesiol Scand. 2007;51(10):1331–7.
32. Barrons RW, Woods JA. Low-dose naloxone for prophylaxis of postoperative nausea and vomiting: a systematic review and meta-analysis. Pharmacotherapy. 2017;37(5):546–54.
33. Donahue RN, McLaughlin PJ, Zagon IS. Low-dose naltrexone suppresses ovarian cancer and exhibits enhanced inhibition in combination with cisplatin. Exp Biol Med. 2011;236(7):883–95.
34. Yang CP, Cherng CH, Wu CT, Huang HY, Tao PL, Lee SO, Wong CS. Intrathecal ultra-low dose naloxone enhances the antihyperalgesic effects of morphine and attenuates tumor necrosis factor-α and tumor necrosis factor-α receptor 1 expression in the dorsal horn of rats with partial sciatic nerve transection. Anesth Analg. 2013;117(6):1493–502.
35. Donahue RN, McLaughlin PJ, Zagon IS. The opioid growth factor (OGF) and low dose naltrexone (LDN) suppress human ovarian cancer progression in mice. Gynecol Oncol. 2011;122(2):382–8.
36. McLaughlin PJ, Zagon IS. The opioid growth factor–opioid growth factor receptor axis: homeostatic regulator of cell proliferation and its implications for health and disease. Biochem Pharmacol. 2012;84(6):746–55.

25

Standardised concentrations of morphine infusions for nurse/patient-controlled analgesia use in children

Asia N Rashed[1,2*], Cate Whittlesea[3], Caroline Davies[4], Ben Forbes[1] and Stephen Tomlin[1,2*]

Abstract

Background: Standardizing concentrations of intravenous infusions enables pre-preparation and is effective in improving patient safety by avoiding large deviations from the prescribed concentration that can occur when infusions are made individually in wards and theatres. The use of pre-prepared morphine standardized concentration infusions for paediatric nurse/patient-controlled analgesia (N/PCA) has not been previously investigated. We aimed to establish, implement and evaluate standardized concentrations of morphine in pre-filled syringes (PFS) for use in paediatric N/PCA.

Methods: Concentrations of morphine in PFS for N/PCA were identified that accommodated dosage variation across a 1–50 kg weight range. The use of infusions in PFS was implemented and evaluated using mixed methods involved direct observation of healthcare professionals (HCPs), focus groups and failure mode and effects analysis, a HCP survey and medication incident reports analysis.

Results: Standardized concentrations, 3 mg, 10 mg and 50 mg morphine in 50 mL sodium chloride 0.9%, delivered prescribed continuous and bolus doses using programmable smart pumps with variable infusion rates. During the implementation, 175 morphine pre-prepared infusions were administered to 157 children (9.4 ± 5.1 years) in theatres and wards. Time taken to set up a N/PCA was 3.7 ± 1.7 min, a reduction of one third compared with the previous system. The number of incidents associated with N/PCA infusions was reduced by 41.2%, and preparation errors were eliminated. HCPs reported using morphine PFS was an easier and safer system.

Conclusion: A system using pre-prepared standardized concentrations of morphine for paediatric N/PCA was implemented successfully and sustainably.

Keywords: Standard infusion, Morphine, Ready-to-administer infusions, Children, Pre-filled syringe, Implementation, Nurse/patient-controlled analgesia

Background

Individually prepared morphine intravenous infusions have been associated with significant errors [1–3], leading to development of "ready-to-administer (RTA)" products [3–6]. Pre-prepared syringes containing standardized concentrations of drugs are recognized as important in improving patient safety by reducing medication errors [3–7]. A UK study reported aseptically prepared standardized dose-banded syringes, used with a pre-programmed safety pump was likely to reduce dosing errors in children [8].

Currently in European hospitals, morphine infusions are prepared for each paediatric patient based on their weight, using the "rule of six" formula [9]. This formula is described as: 6 x patient's weight (kg) equals the amount of drug in milligrams that should be added to 100 mL of so-

* Correspondence: asia.rashed@kcl.ac.uk; Stephen.tomlin@gstt.nhs.uk
[1]School of Cancer & Pharmaceutical Sciences, King's College London, 150 Stamford Street, London SE1 9NH, UK

lution. When administered at 1 mL/h will give an infusion rate of 1 microgram/kg/min (or 60 microgram/kg/h). This is error prone, which may lead to significant over or under dosing, resulting in adverse events, e.g. hypoventilation [10] or inadequate analgesia [11, 12].

At the study hospital, a morphine prefilled syringe (PFS) system is only used to deliver continuous infusions to critically ill children in the paediatric intensive care unit (PICU) [13]. This resulted in two systems within PICU; standard concentrations for continuous infusions and individually prepared infusions for nurse/patient--controlled analgesia (N/PCA), which contributed to medication errors [11, 12].

Pre-implementation studies involving direct observation of morphine infusion preparation, with morphine concentration quantification [11] and focus groups to assess the prescribing, preparing and administering of morphine infusion for paediatric N/PCA [12], identified risks in the established process, including significant deviations in the prepared infusions from the prescribed dose. Participants suggested providing standard concentration of morphine in a RTA form would improve current practice as identified in other studies to improve the safety [3, 4, 7, 12]. It has been reported that establishing standardized morphine concentration infusions for paediatric N/PCA is complex, as both bolus and continuous doses from the same solution need to be delivered [14]. Considering this challenge this study aimed to implement quality assured standardized concentrations of paediatric N/PCA morphine infusions, supplied as PFS, ready for administration via pre-programmed safety pumps (ALaris syringe Pumps) [15] to deliver accurate bolus and continuous doses.

Methods

This project was conducted in two stages. The pre-implementation which has previously been described [11, 12]. This paper presents the findings of the implementation stage.

Design: mixed methods approach.

Intervention development

Establishing standard concentration

Using Excel all possible morphine concentrations from 1 mg to 50 mg in 50 mL for all possible weight ranges in children from a lower weight limit of 1 kg upwards, were proposed (ANR) and reviewed by a Consultant Paediatric Pharmacist (ST). The criteria were:

- Total daily volume of morphine infusion should not account for more than 15% of child's total daily fluid allowance.
- Daily treatment delivered using no more than three syringes (ideally 1–2 syringes) per patient, to reduce risks and workload from multiple syringe changes;
- Manufacture a limited number of standard concentrations (safety and cost);
- Delivered by available infusion pumps for continuous infusion rate and bolus dose, with a minimum volume of 0.1 mL.

Proposed standard concentrations were reviewed and approved by the Lead Paediatric Acute Pain Consultant Anaesthetist (CD) and the Paediatric Clinical Nurse Specialist. Documentation, protocols, prescription labels (used on medication charts), and reprogramming of infusion pumps were approved (Paediatric Acute Pain Team, Paediatric Consultant Pharmacist, hospital Clinical Governance department).

The prefilled syringe containing morphine standard concentration infusions are being prepared by the centralised intravenous admixture service (CIVAS), which is a service run by the pharmacy department at our hospital.

Risk assessment

Failure mode and effects analysis (FMEA) was used to determine the risks/issues associated with changes to the process of delivering paediatric N/PCA infusions using morphine PFS containing standard concentration. Before implementation a multidisciplinary team (17 members; nurses, doctors and pharmacists) familiar with prescribing, preparing and administering morphine N/PCA undertook a FMEA.

The FMEA team met twice over two months (October–November 2013). Before the FMEA, the research team described the initial and final steps of the process of delivering morphine infusion for N/PCA, presented an overview of FMEA with a process scheme example [16].

Team members described the steps undertaken when prescribing, preparing, and administering morphine PFS for N/PCA use, identified potential process failures and determined severity, probability, and detectability scores for these failures. They also made recommendations to reduce the identified failures.

Education and training

Over three months (January–March 2014), in-house training on the use of standardized concentrations for paediatric N/PCA were provided (ANR, CD, ST) to all nurses and doctors in theatres and wards. Standard operating procedures (SOPs) for new documentation and pump programming were produced. Posters of the standard concentrations of morphine and SOPs were placed in all clinical areas.

Implementation

The implementation was conducted over eight months (March – November 2014):

- Stage I: dummy run of whole system on one day from theatre and transfer to a ward.
- Stage II: targeting one specific list of paediatric orthopaedic operations with the same designated consultant anaesthetist.
- Stage III: targeted lists extended to include spinal cases and cleft cases, with an increased number of anaesthetists and nursing staff participating.
- Stage IV: morphine PFS system was introduced across all clinical areas.

The staged implementation was designed to identify issues that arose when HCPs used the standardized morphine PFS for N/PCA. It also supported training of HCPs on the new system.

During implementation, all HCPs (doctors/nurses) prescribing/preparing morphine PFS for paediatric N/PCA, were observed (ANR). Data collected were patient demographics (age, sex, weight); morphine prescription details (PFS strength, N/PCA type); location; name of nurse or doctor programming and prescribing; and time spent prescribing, programming pump and administering a morphine PFS.

Sample size consideration for observation activity.

In 2011, 896 children were administered morphine for N/PCA at the study hospital (internal report), with the increase in surgery numbers, about 1000 children/year would benefit directly from standardized morphine concentration infusions for N/PCA. With RTA a 100% reduction in preparation errors was assumed because of the elimination of the individualized preparation stage by HCPs. Based on the reported medication error percentage (1%) (internal medication error report), a sample of 150 patients was required to provide a 95% confidence interval for the true mean rate of 0.6 to 2.6%.

Evaluation of the intervention

Focus groups

All HCPs (doctors/nurses) who prescribing and preparing/administering morphine N/PCA in paediatric theatres or wards were invited to attend focus groups. Signed informed consent was obtained from participants. Focus groups were conducted over 3–4 weeks (March 2015) following implementation and evaluation of the morphine PFS system post-implementation, to determine HCPs views, concerns and any aspects to improve the morphine PFS system.

Implementation across clinical areas

One week before the morphine PFS system's hospital-wide introduction date (1st April 2015), the new system was publicized by email to staff and posters displayed in all clinical areas. All previous protocols and paperwork were removed and replaced with the new documentation.

Self-administered questionnaire

All HCPs (doctors/nurses) within paediatric theatres and wards, who prepared/administered morphine N/PCA, were surveyed 12 months after the morphine PFS system implementation to determine staff views and satisfaction with the morphine PFS system compared with the previous system (individually prepared syringes based on patient's weight). The questionnaire was completed by HCPs over 6 weeks (April–May 2016). New staff were excluded because they had no experience of the previous system.

A structured anonymous questionnaire was developed based on previous studies [11, 12]. It included items assessing satisfaction, attitudes and views of HCPs on the recently implemented morphine PFS system together with demographic data (location and job title). This piloted questionnaire covered three themes: use; quality; and impact of the morphine PFS system on patient safety.

Hospital incident reports

Data of morphine N/PCA related incidents pre- and post-implementation of morphine PFS system for January 2013–December 2015 were extracted from the hospital electronic incident reporting system. Analysis of reported incidents was conducted to identify any medication related incidents and to assess the impact of implementing standard concentrations on reported error occurrence.

Data analysis

Data was analysed using Stata 11 (StataCorp, College Station, TX, USA). Descriptive statistics were performed on data from observations, questionnaire, and medication incident reports, and presented as number, percentages and mean ± standard deviation (SD), unless otherwise specified. Chi-squared test was used for statistical significant ($p < 0.05$) for categorical variables, between wards and theatres.

Each focus group was transcribed verbatim and the anonymized transcript uploaded to QSR NVivo (V.10) software for coding and categorization to identify themes. Qualitative content analysis was used with five main themes being set a priori and supplemented by emergent subthemes identified during analysis. An iterative approach involving constant comparison was employed where all data relating to each theme were constantly revisited after initial coding. Coding frames were prepared and framework analysis created by ANR and checked by ST independently.

Questionnaire data: the 5-point Likert questions were grouped to three groups; "strongly agree" and "agree" where considered as "agreement", likewise "strongly disagree" and "disagree" were considered "disagreement", and "neutral" (neither agree nor disagree).

Results

Intervention development

Establishing standard concentration

Three standard concentrations were established for paediatric N/PCA use (Table 1). Protocols and prescription labels were also developed (Additional file 1: Figure S1-S4).

Risk assessment

Seventeen (89.5%, 17/19) HCPs participated in the FMEA meetings (Additional file 1: Table S1). FMEA identified potential failures which might occur when using morphine PFS system for N/PCA as well as recommendations to address these aspects (Table 2).

The two aspects with the highest potential for failure were identified at ward level due to limited storage space and staff selection of the wrong strength. The risk assessment resulted in a staged implementation (I-IV).

Observation of HCP setting up N/PCA using morphine PFS

A total of 175 morphine PFS (theatres 157, wards 18) were administered to 157 children [mean (sd); age 9.4 years ±5.1, mean weight 32.4 kg ± 15.2, weight range 5–54 kg] were observed. Fig. 1 shows the pre- and post-implementation processes of setting up morphine PFS paediatric N/PCA. Using morphine PFS, resulted in fewer steps in the preparation process (5 compared to 9 steps). When programming the infusion pump, the infusion concentration was pre-set and fixed which reduced the values needed to be programmed (4 to 3 steps). Therefore, less time was required to set up each PFS.

Overall the total mean time required to set up N/PCA for a child (prescribing, programming pump/administering) was 3.7 ± 1.7 (sd) minutes. There was a significant difference between theatres and wards (theatre 3.6 ± 1.7; ward 4.7 ± 1.3 min, $p < 0.01$). This suggested that theatre staff might be faster in setting up a N/PCA for various reason; e.g. could be because of the theatre and ward's layout, i.e. theatre have the drug, paperwork and the patient in one place. While on the ward, nurses have to be between drug room and patient bedside.

Table 1 Weight bands and morphine standardized prefilled syringe strengths established for N/PCA[a]

Weight band	Protocol	Morphine PFS strength
Weight ≤ 3.9 kg	NCA	3 mg in 50 mL Glucose 5%
Weight ≥ 4 kg – 19.9 kg	NCA	10 mg in 50 mL Sodium Chloride 0.9%
Weight ≥ 20 kg	NCA	50 mg in 50 mL Sodium Chloride 0.9%
Weight ≥ 25 kg	PCA	

[a]N/PCA: Nurse- or/ Patient-Controlled Analgesia

The overall time spent by HCPs using the previous system to set up N/PCA for a child has been reported [11]. There was a significant difference between the morphine PFS system and previous system (3.7 ± 1.7 vs. 11.9 ± 4.1, $P < 0.001$ and between theatres (morphine PFS system 3.6 ± 1.7; previous system 10.5 ± 3.3, $p < 0.001$) and wards (morphine PFS system 4.7 ± 1.3; previous system14.5 ± 4.0, $p < 0.001$).

The majority of prescriptions were for NCA use (116/175, 66.3%), of which 69% (80/116) were for strength 50 mg/50 mL and 31% (36/116) for 10 mg/50 mL. Only 59 prescriptions were for PCA using 50 mg/50 mL PFS.

Evaluation of the intervention

Focus groups

Two focus groups were conducted with participants recruited from three different clinical areas; focus group 1 ward and recovery nurses ($n = 7$); focus group 2 paediatric anaesthetists ($n = 5$) from theatres.

Five main themes were identified: 1) the process of using morphine PFS system to set up N/PCA infusion; 2) impact of this system on the process of preparing/administering morphine N/PCA; 3) concerns about this system; 4) suggestions to address concerns with this system; 5) impact of this system on practice and patient care. Table 3 summarizes theme and subthemes identified.

All focus group participants preferred using the morphine PFS system and had positive comments. The morphine PFS system was described as easier and safer; because it eliminated errors with calculations, dose received by the patient, reduced infection risk and less time consuming. Example quotes from focus group participants;

One of the participated nurses commented that *"It* [morphine PFS system] *is much easier than starting that from the scratch ... time is less than* [it] *used to be."* While one of the anaesthetists said that morphine PFS system is *"Unquestionably quicker".*

The risk of selecting the wrong strength of morphine PFS was the main concern raised by participants. However, it was identified that it could be mitigated by enforcing the hospital policy of double-checking IV infusions by two people. Other measures suggested

Table 2 Potential failures of the morphine PFS system and recommendations identified by FMEA

Potential Failure	Causes	Effects	S	P	D	RPN	Recommendations
Staff prepare N/PCA infusion from ampoule using the previous system (based on patient weight)	PFSs stock not updated quickly or prefilled syringe expired.	Possible of delay in patient receiving morphine dose as individualized syringe can't be administered using the standard syringe programs on the pump, as protocols on the pump are for standard concentrations only.	2	8	1	16	– Nurse review stock levels – Protocols need to be clear about preparing standard concentrations from ampoules in ward in emergency (pharmacy)
Run out-of-stock quickly at ward level	No enough space to store PFSs and drug room temperature is above recommended temp, > 25 °C.	PFSs not available when required. Delays in patient receiving morphine injection	4	10	1	40	– Additional air conditioning in drug storage area (matrons) – Use Omnicell (electronic storage cabinets) for storage as temperature controlled (pharmacy)
Run out-of-stock in paediatric pharmacy dispensary area	No enough space in paediatric pharmacy dispensary area to accommodate large number of the three strengths.	Limited number of PFSs stored at wards level.	4	6	1	24	– Increase stock levels at paediatric Pharmacy – Consider using Omincell for CD storage in paediatric pharmacy dispensary area, wards, and theatres (Pharmacy)
Choosing the wrong strength of the PFS	Picking syringe by label, not by barcode.	Wrong dose given to patient	10	3	2	60	– Separate storage for each strength, with clear labelling, on the wards/theatre (Pharmacy) – Write weight between brackets in large font on the syringe label (pharmacy manufacture) – Introduce the use of barcodes for syringe's label, prescriptions' label.
Syringe Drive procedure incompatibility with manually made up solution in Emergency Department	Misinterpretation of fall-back case – Is manually mixing equivalent to PFSs, or follow previous procedure?	Would have to select standard concentrations	5	1	2	10	Protocols and SOPs on how to use standard concentrations should be made clear to all clinical areas, including Emergency Department. (Pharmacy)

FMEA: Failure Mode and Effects Analysis; N/PCA: Nurse- or/ Patient-Controlled Analgesia; PFS: prefilled syringe; SOPs: standard operating procedures; S=Severity; P=Probability; D = Detectability; RPN: risk priority number calculated as RPN = S x P x D; CD: controlled drug

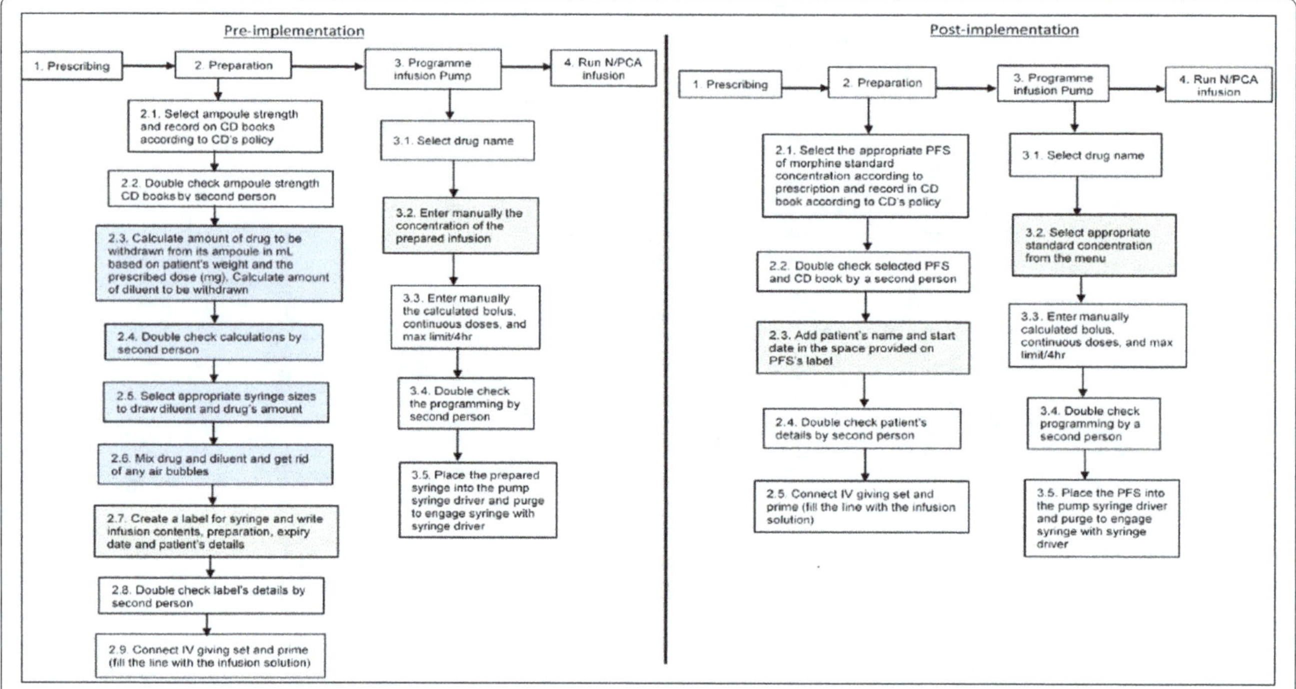

Fig. 1 Process of prescribing, preparing and administering morphine N/PCA pre- and post-implementation of PFS containing morphine standardised concentrations at the participated hospital. CD: controlled drug, IV: intravenous; PFS: prefilled syringe. Highlighted steps in blue in the preparation stage were eliminated after introducing PFS system. Green boxes show the changes in those steps pre- and post-implementation

were bar-coding and using electronic storage cabinets (Table 3).

Self-administered questionnaire

A total of 125 questionnaires (62.0%, 125/200) were completed (ward = 100, theatre = 25). Most respondents (90.4%, 113/125) were satisfied using the morphine PFS system and 8.8% (11/125) were neutral. Only one respondent (0.8%), who provided no explanation, was dissatisfied (Table 4).

Overall, most respondents (95.2%, 119/125) believed that using the PFS improved patient safety and 89.6% (112/125) indicated that the morphine PFS system minimized preparation/administration errors.

Majority of respondents (90.4%, 113/125: ward = 93, theatre = 20) reported that morphine PFS system decreased drug delivery time because set up time for an N/PCA infusion was quicker compared to the previous system; with 53.1% (60/113; ward = 51, Theatre = 9) reporting it took less than 5 min to set up a PFS. Most respondents (91.2%, 114/125) suggested that pre-programming of the infusion pumps was better compared to the previous system. Only one individual (ward nurse), reported the new system was much slower (> 25 min), however no explanation was provided. Four respondents from theatre did not answer this question as they had not set up a smart pump with a prefilled syringe.

Hospital incident reports

A total of 198 incident reports related to morphine reported pre-and post-implementation, were analysed, of which 54 (27.3%, 54/198) were related to N/PCA. Fig. 2 describes the reports (63%, 34/54) linked to the previous system (i.e. preparing individual syringe based on patient weight) and the reports (37%, 20/54) with the morphine PFS system.

Overall there was a 41.2% decrease in the occurrence of reported medication incidents following implementation of the standard concentrations for N/PCA use. Although this reduction was not statistically significant ($p = 0.115$), it is considered important, because incidents such as "wrong dose of medication administered to patient" and "dose or strength selected was wrong or unclear" were not reported in the morphine PFS system. They had been reported for the previous system [23.5% (8/34); 2.9% (1/34), respectively].

The incidence of "expiry date's wrong, omitted or passed" (25%, 5/20) was higher in the morphine PFS system compared to the previous system (5.9%, 2/34).

The majority of reported incidents were reported to have "no harm" (51/54). Only three were reported as "low harm", all related to the previous system (Fig. 2).

Discussion

The main finding of this study is that the established standardized concentrations of morphine provided in

Table 3 Summary of topic themes and subthemes identified from the focus groups

Theme	Subthemes
The process of setting up NCA/PCA infusion using morphine standardized concentration PFS	Prescribing - paper work Select PFS of the required standard concentration and check Programming the pump Double checking process Changing syringes on ward
Impact of the morphine PFS system on the process of preparing/administering morphine N/PCA	Faster – less time consuming Easier to set up No calculation of concentration Safer – less errors Eliminating any errors of how much patient is getting Less infection risks Paperwork and pump programming much easier to read Fixed standardized concentrations in all clinical areas Use same dose as previous system but volume vary for each patient Volume of continuous and bolus doses cannot be used as safety net as previous system
Concerns about the morphine PFS system	Risk of picking up the wrong PFS Out of stock - due to storage limit space or expiry Human error still same as previous system
Suggestions to overcome concerns and improve the morphine PFS system	Emphasize on the double checking as safety mechanism Possibility of introducing standard concentration in 50-ml vials to extend expiry and maximize stock storage Possibility of storing PFS in Omnicell to increase stock level Make up standard concentration in case of out-of-stock PFS Order before it ran-out or expired Look into using of barcoding syringe, label and prescription to avoid wrong selection of syringe
Impact of the morphine PFS system on practice and patient care	Time efficient Safer practice Less risk of errors - improve patient safety Allow focus on the patient rather than on paperwork and preparation Give more time for teaching trainee

N/PCA: Nurse- or/ Patient-Controlled Analgesia; PFS: pre-filled syringe; Omnicell: electronic storage cabinet

Table 4 Summary of the questionnaire results

Theme/Items	Disagree *n*(%)	Neutral *n*(%)	Agree *n*(%)
Evaluation of the morphine PFS system for N/PCA; n (%)			
Set up time is quicker (5–9 min)	1 (0.8)	11 (8.8)	113 (90.4)
New paperwork easier to use	2 (1.6)	26 (20.8)	97 (77.6)
If PFS out-of-stock; easier to prepare standard concentration than previous system (prepare individual syringe based on patient weight)	6 (4.8)	42 (33.6)	77 (61.6)
Little impact of distraction when setting up PFS compared to previous system	27 (21.6)	36 (28.8)	62 (49.6)
Satisfied with using morphine PFS on daily practice	1 (0.8)	11 (8.8)	113 (90.4)
Quality of the morphine PFS system			
Less time spend in setting up PFS is beneficial	0	5 (4.0)	120 (96)
Using PFS avoid waste of morphine ampoules	2 (1.6)	15 (12.0)	105 (84)
Prefer using aseptically prepared standard concentration to individualized preparation (mg/kg)	0	16 (12.8)	109 (87.2)
the morphine PFS system helped in making the process of administering N/PCA infusion safer	4 (3.2)	10 (8.0)	111 (88.8)
The morphine PFS system help to provide better quality of care to paediatric patients	2 (1.6)	35 (28.0)	88 (70.4)
Using PFS help in reducing incidents of injury might result from breaking ampoules	1 (0.8)	27 (21.6)	97 (77.6)
The morphine PFS system provide more accurate dosing	4 (3.2)	35 (28.0)	86 (68.8)
Impact of the morphine PFS system on patient safety			
Overall the morphine PFS system help to improve patient safety	0	6 (4.8)	119 (95.2)

Percentages (%) calculated out of the total number of respondents ($n = 125$)
N/PCA: Nurse- or/ Patient-Controlled Analgesia; PFS: pre-filled syringe

PFS were implemented successfully across all clinical areas in our hospital to deliver N/PCA infusion; both bolus and continuous doses from the same syringe, in children. While standard concentrations of some intravenous (IV) drugs have been widely used for IV infusions in various healthcare systems [4–7], this was the first study within a paediatric hospital where standardized morphine concentrations in "ready-to-administer (RTA)" infusions were implemented to deliver paediatric N/PCA infusions.

The data derived and feedback collected provided an evidence base that encouraged HCPs' acceptance of the change to standardized concentration infusions for paediatric N/PCA.

The new system eliminated the need to calculate the concentration and reducing the risk of microbial

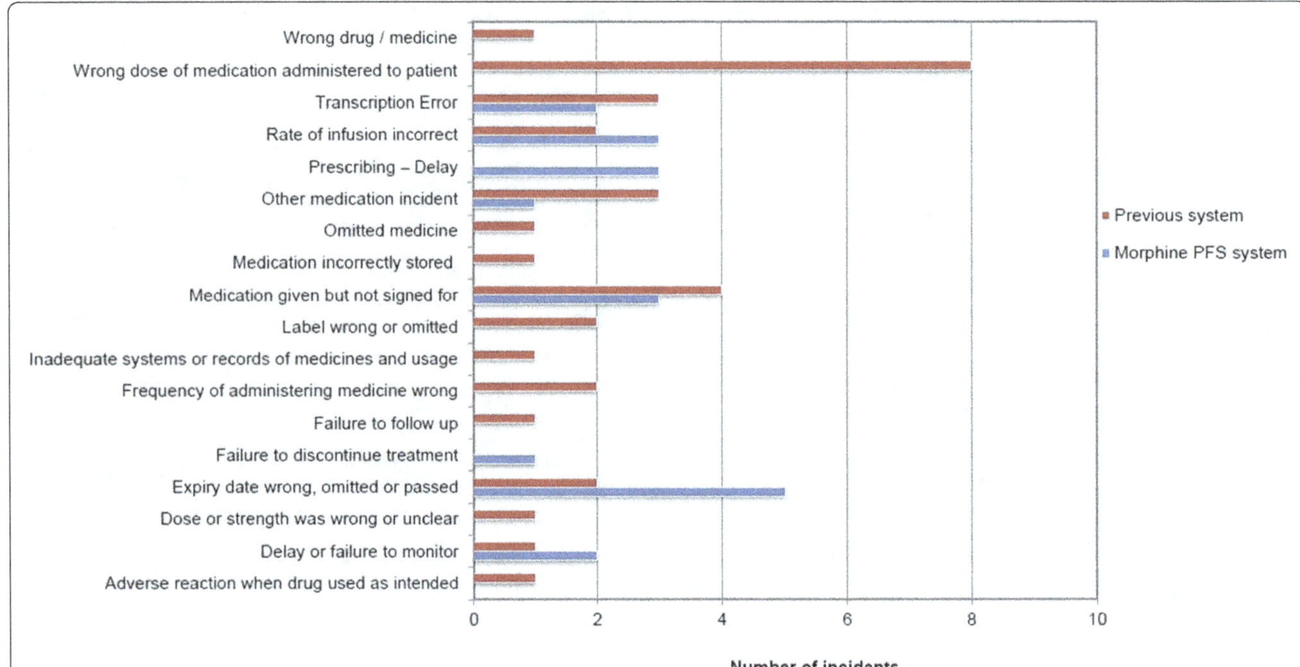

Fig. 2 Number of morphine N/PCA related errors reported pre- and post-implementation of morphine PFS system. Low harm incidents related to previous system; "adverse reaction when drug used as intended"; "wrong dose (concentration) of drug administered"; "medicine omitted" (i.e. PCA infusion discontinued without conversion to oral dose of opioid leaving the patient in pain)

contamination providing a safer and more time efficient system. This was evidenced by observation, findings from focus groups and survey questionnaire. Furthermore, the pre-implementation study [11] identified that 61.5% of individually prepared syringes deviated unacceptably from the intended morphine concentration. Infusions prepared on an individual patient basis in clinical areas are prone to such errors, which are classically 'unseen errors' because syringe content is not routinely analysed and therefore not captured by incident reporting systems. Such errors are eliminated in the new system through batch manufactured, quality assured morphine PFS.

The main goal in implementing morphine PFS containing standard concentrations was to improve paediatric patient safety by minimizing the risk of medication errors. Twelve months following implementation, there was a reduction in medication errors compared with the pre-implementation period. Although this was not statistically significant, from clinical perspective it was considered important because the newly implemented system eliminated errors associated with infusion preparation. Medication errors associated with intravenous infusion have previously been reduced using standard concentrations [4]. Importantly, the new system did not increase other types of medication error e.g. delivery of the wrong dose. The follow-up survey demonstrated that staff perceived that the morphine PFS improved medication safety and resulted in reduced set up time.

Limitations

The study has some limitations that need to be considered when interpreting our results. Observations of HCPs prescribing/preparing morphine PFS for N/PCA were conducted during day shifts (8 am - 5 pm) Monday to Friday. Therefore, any use of the morphine PFS system during other times was not undertaken. Whilst errors are generally under–reported [17], highlighting a process (positively or negatively) tends to lead to increased reporting [18]. Bias in reporting errors linked to the morphine PFS system might have occurred as it was well publicized. The incidents report data captured post-implementation might be relatively low due to the short period it was conducted within, therefore, it is recommended to re-analyse incidents reports over a longer period post-implementation.

The use of the lowest strength morphine PFS (3 mg/ 50 mL) was not observed. Finally, not all staff who participated in the implementation of the morphine PFS system attended focus groups; however, a follow-up self-administered survey, 12 months after implementation, was conducted to capture the impact of this system on HCPs practice and satisfaction.

Conclusions

The implementation of standardized concentration of morphine infusions for N/PCA was achieved in all clinical areas in our hospital and satisfied the requirements for delivering continuous infusions and bolus doses for children weighing 1–50 kg. This led to improved patient safety in the study hospital, by reducing medication errors reported post implementation of morphine PFS system. This system supported HCPs to more safely deliver a high-risk medicine to children, resulting in a quality improvement within the healthcare system in our hospital.

Abbreviations

FMEA: Failure Mode and Effects Analysis; HCPs: Healthcare professionals; N/PCA: Nurse- or/ Patient-Controlled Analgesia; NHS: National Health Service; PFS: Pre-filled syringe; PICU: Paediatric intensive care unit; RTA: Ready-to-administer; SOPs: Standard operating procedures

Acknowledgements

Authors wish to thank all the healthcare professionals who participated in the observations, FMEA, focus groups meeting, and survey questionnaire.

Authors' contributions

ANR ST BF CW contributed to the conception and design of the project. ANR, CW, ST conducted FMEA meetings. ANR and ST conducted the focus groups. ANR conducted direct observation, follow-up activities, performed data analysis and results interpretation, and wrote the first draft of the manuscript. CD contributed to the standard concentrations development and FMEA analysis. All authors contributed to the interpretation of the results, revised the manuscript and approved the final version.

Author details

[1]School of Cancer & Pharmaceutical Sciences, King's College London, 150 Stamford Street, London SE1 9NH, UK. [2]Pharmacy Department, Evelina London Children's Hospital, Guy's & St Thomas' NHS Foundation Trust, Westminster Bridge Road, London SE1 7EH, UK. [3]Research Department of Practice and Policy, UCL School of Pharmacy, London, UK. [4]Paediatric Anaesthetic Department, Evelina London Children's Hospital, Guy's & St Thomas' NHS Foundation Trust, London, UK.

References

1. Parshuram CS, Ng GY, Ho TK, Klein J, Moore AM, Bohn D, et al. Discrepancies between ordered and delivered concentrations of opiate infusions in critical care. Crit Care Med. 2003;31(10):2483–7.
2. Ross LM, Wallace J, Paton JY. Medication errors in a paediatric teaching hospital in the UK: five years operational experience. Arch Dis Child. 2000; 83(6):492–7.
3. Aguado-Lorenzo V, Weeks K, Tunstell P, Turnock K, Watts T, Arenas-Lopez S. Accuracy of the concentration of morphine infusions prepared for patients in a neonatal intensive care unit. Arch Dis Child. 2013;98:975–9.
4. Larsen GY, Parker HB, Cash J, O'Connell M, Grant MC. Standard drug concentrations and smart-pump technology reduce continuous-medication-infusion errors in pediatric patients. Pediatrics. 2005;116(1):e21–5.
5. Perkins J, Aguado-Lorenzo V, Arenas-Lopez S. Standard concentrations in paediatric intensive care: the clinical approach. J Pharm Pharmacol. 2017; 69(5):537–43.
6. Irwin D, Vaillancourt R, Dalgleish D, Thimas M, Grenier S, Wong E, et al. Standard concentrations of high-alert drug infusions across paediatric acute care. Paediatr Child Health. 2008;13(5):371–6.
7. Christie-Taylor SA, Tait PA. Implementation of standard concentration medication infusions for preterm infants. Infant. 2012;8(5):155–9.
8. Co-operative of Safety of Medicines in Children (COSMIC): Scoping study to identify and analyse interventions used to reduce errors in calculation of paediatric drug doses. Report to the Patient Safety Research Program, Department October 2007. http://www.birmingham.ac.uk/Documents/college-mds/haps/projects/cfhep/psrp/finalreports/PS026COSMICFinalReport.pdf. Accessed 11 Sept 2018.
9. Mcleroy PA. The rule of six: calculating intravenous infusions in a pediatric crisis situation. Hosp Pharm. 1994;29(10):939–40.
10. Rashed AN, Wong IC, Cranswick N, Hefele B, Tomlin S, Jackman J, et al. Adverse drug reactions in children--international surveillance and evaluation (ADVISE): a multicentre cohort study. Drug Saf. 2012;35(6):481–94.
11. Rashed AN, Tomlin S, Aguado V, Forbes B, Whittlesea C. Sources and magnitude of error in preparing morphine infusions for nurse-patient controlled analgesia in a UK paediatric hospital. Int J Clin Pharm. 2016;38(5): 1069–74.
12. Rashed AN, Tomlin S, Forbes B, Whittlesea C. Current practice of preparing morphine infusions for nurse/patient controlled analgesia in a UK paediatric hospital: healthcare professionals' views and experience. Eur J Hosp Pharm. 2016;0:1–4.
13. Arenas-Lopez S, Stanley IM, Tunstell P, Aguado-Lorenzo V, Philip J. Perkins J, et al. safe implementation of standard concentration infusions in paediatric intensive care. J Pharm Pharmacol. 2016;69(5):529–36.
14. Rashed AN, Whittlesea C, Forbes B, Tomlin S. The feasibility of using dose-banded syringes to improve the safety and availability of patient-controlled opioid analgesic infusions in children. Eur J Hosp Pharm Sci Pract 2014; 21: 306–308.
15. IVAC® PCAM® syringe pump. https://www.bd.com/en-uk/products/infusion/infusion-devices/anaesthesia-and-pain-management/ivac-pcam-syringe-pump. Accessed 11 Sept 2018.
16. Wetterneck TB, Skibinski KA, Roberts TL, Kleppin SM, Schroeder ME, Enloe M, et al. Using failure mode and effects analysis to plan implementation of smart i.V. Pump technology. Am J Health Syst Pharm. 2006;63(16):1528–38.
17. Olsen S, Neale G, Schwab K, Psaila B, Patel T, Chapman EJ, et al. Hospital staff should use more than one method to detect adverse events and potential adverse events: incident reporting, pharmacist surveillance and local real-time record review may all have a place. Qual Saf Health Care. 2007;16(1):40–4.
18. Woolever DR. The impact of a patient safety program on medical error reporting. In: Henriksen K, Battles JB, Marks ES, Lewin DI, editors. Advances in Patient Safety: From Research to Implementation (Volume 1: Research Findings). Rockville (MD): Agency for Healthcare Research and Quality (US); 2005.

Efficacy of continuous epidural infusion with epidural electric stimulation compared to that of conventional continuous epidural infusion for acute herpes zoster management

Chung Hun Lee, Sang Sik Choi*, Mi Kyoung Lee, Yeon Joo Lee and Jong Sun Park

Abstract

Background: Continuous epidural infusions are commonly used in clinical settings to reduce the likelihood of transition to postherpetic neuralgia via pain control. The purpose of this study was to compare the efficacy of conventional continuous epidural infusion to that of continuous epidural infusion in which the catheter is guided by electric stimulation to areas with neurological damage for the treatment of zoster-related pain and prevention of postherpetic neuralgia.

Methods: We analyzed the medical records of 114 patients in this study. The patients were divided into two groups: contrast (conventional continuous epidural infusion) and stimulation (continuous epidural infusion with epidural electric stimulation). In the contrast group, the position of the epidural catheter was confirmed using contrast medium alone, whereas in the stimulation group, the site of herpes zoster infection was identified through electric stimulation using a guidewire in the catheter. Clinical efficacy was assessed using a numerical rating scale (pain score) up to 6 months after the procedures. We compared the percentage of patients who showed complete remission (pain score less than 2 and no further medication) in each group. We also investigated whether the patients required additional interventional treatment due to insufficient pain control during the 6-month follow-up period after each procedure.

Results: After adjusting for confounding variables, the pain score was significantly lower in the stimulation group than in the contrast group for 6 months after the procedure. After adjustment, the odds of complete remission were 1.9-times higher in the stimulation group than in the contrast group (95% confidence interval [CI]: 0.81–4.44, $P = 0.14$). Patients in the contrast group were significantly more likely to require other interventions within 6 months of the procedure than patients in the stimulation group (odds ratio: 3.62, 95% CI: 1.17–11.19, $P = 0.03$).

Conclusion: Epidural drug administration to specific spinal segments using electric stimulation catheters may be more helpful than conventional continuous epidural infusion for improving pain and preventing postherpetic neuralgia in the acute phase of herpes zoster.

Keywords: Herpes zoster, Postherpetic neuralgia, Epidural analgesia, Continuous epidural infusion, Electric stimulation

* Correspondence: clonidine@empal.com
Department of Anesthesiology and Pain Medicine, Korea University Medical Center, Guro Hospital, Gurodong Road 148, Guro-Gu, Seoul 08308, Republic of Korea

Background

Herpes zoster is caused by reactivation of the latent varicella zoster virus (VZV), which persists in the dorsal root ganglion after the initial infection. It causes irritation along the nerve distribution, abnormal sensitization of nociceptive receptors, and induces hyperactivity of the central nerve [1]. The frequency of reactivation increases particularly in elderly patients and in patients with inhibited virus-specific cellular immunity [2, 3]. The acute phase of herpes zoster is defined as the period within 30 days of rash onset [4]. Postherpetic neuralgia (PHN) is the most common complication of herpes zoster and can occur if the patient is not properly treated during the acute phase; in elderly patients, it can be due to a weakened immune system, despite proper treatment [5]. PHN is a neuropathic condition associated with severe refractory pain, and it lowers the quality of life. Among patients with herpes zoster, 70% of those over 50 years of age complained of pain 1 month following the disappearance of the skin rash, whereas 50% of patients aged 70 years or older experienced pain 1 year following the disappearance of the rash [6, 7]. Patients at risk of developing PHN may therefore require aggressive treatment using appropriate drug therapies.

Epidural, sympathetic, and paravertebral blocks are considered active treatments for acute episodes of herpes zoster. For acute herpes zoster, continuous epidural infusion is commonly used in clinical settings and is reported to reduce the likelihood of transition to PHN via pain control [8–10]. For conventional continuous epidural infusion, the location of the epidural catheter is confirmed by injecting a contrast agent at the suspected epidural level, which is identified based on the site of rash or pain.

To improve the efficacy of continuous epidural infusion, it is important that the drug is administered precisely at the epidural level of the herpes zoster infection [11, 12], which is dependent on the proximity of the catheter to the affected nerve site. For this purpose, a continuous epidural infusion is administered utilizing epidural electric stimulation to confirm whether the catheter has accurately reached the site of infection. The present retrospective study was designed to assess the efficacy of continuous epidural infusion utilizing epidural electric stimulation, in comparison to that of conventional epidural infusion, for the control of acute herpes zoster pain and prevention of PHN.

Methods

Study design

Our retrospective observational study adhered to the STROBE checklist (S1 checklist) and was approved by the institutional review board of our hospital (No: 2019GR0073, March 11, 2019).

The medical records of patients who underwent continuous epidural infusion for herpes zoster-related pain from June 2010 to October 2017 were collected. Among these, only the medical records of patients who received continuous epidural infusion within 30 days of rash onset were included. The patients were divided into two groups depending on the type of epidural catheter used for continuous epidural infusion: the contrast group, which used standard epidural catheters, and the stimulation group, which used epidural catheters with electric stimulation. Patients had to meet the following criteria to be included in the present study: those older than 50 years of age with a numeric rating scale (NRS) score of 4 or greater; those who had only received standard drug therapy, including antiviral agents, until the administration of continuous epidural infusion; and those who underwent follow-up for a period of 6 months after continuous epidural infusion. The following criteria were used for exclusion: patients with insufficient medical records; patients who received other drugs (such as opioids) with epidural catheters; patients with immunosuppressed status; patients in whom the catheter was not maintained for more than 10 days after continuous epidural infusion; patients who did not receive standard medication (such as antiviral agents) until the procedure was performed; and patients who discontinued the prescribed standard medication (anticonvulsants and analgesics) because of adverse effects. Additionally, patients who had undergone other interventional procedures due to the exacerbation of herpes zoster-related pain within 6 months of continuous epidural infusion were excluded, and the requirement rates for interventional procedures were analyzed separately.

Procedure

Continuous epidural infusion: the contrast group

Patients were placed in the prone position, and an aseptic dressing was applied to the procedure site. An 18-gauge Tuohy needle was inserted into the interlaminar space three levels below the target level under the guidance of fluoroscopic imaging. The loss of resistance (LOR) technique was used to verify whether the Tuohy needle was placed in the epidural space. After confirming the epidural space, a 20-gauge epidural catheter (Perifix® Soft Tip epidural anesthesia catheter, B. Braun, Melsungen, Germany) was inserted through the Tuohy needle, and diffusion of the contrast agent was checked to ensure that the catheter was placed in the proper position (Fig. 1). Once the epidural catheters were confirmed to have been placed at the epidural levels identified based on the site of pain and rash, 0.187% ropivacaine and 1 mg dexamethasone (8 mL total) were administered via the epidural catheter.

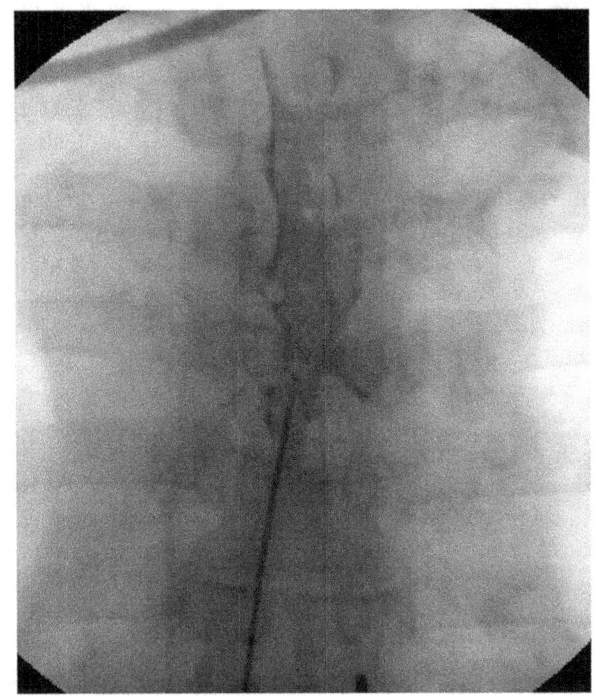

Fig. 1 Fluoroscopic images of conventional continuous epidural block. The position of the catheter tip was confirmed using a contrast agent

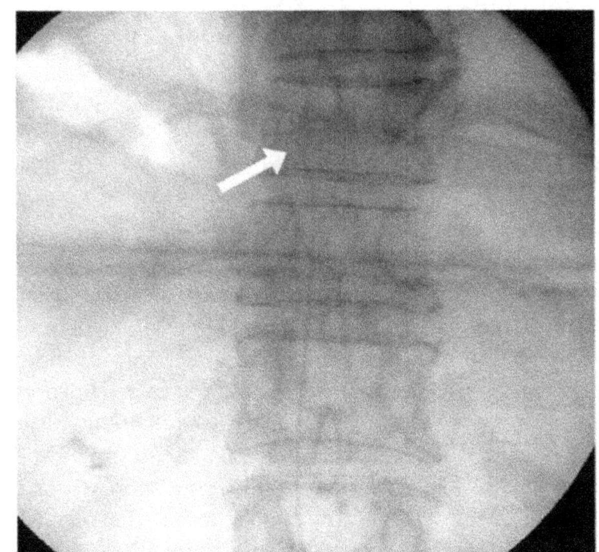

Fig. 2 Fluoroscopic images of continuous epidural block using the EpiStim catheter. This catheter has a built-in conductive guidewire that allows the detection of the location of the catheter tip using radiography along with electric stimulation. The arrow indicates the guidewire in the EpiStim catheter

Continuous epidural infusion: the stimulation group

Similar to that in the contrast group, after the epidural space was identified using the LOR technique, a 20-gauge epidural catheter (EpiStim™, length = 800 mm, Sewoon Medical Co., Ltd., Seoul, Korea) allowing radiographic confirmation was placed at the target level through the Tuohy needle (Fig. 2). This type of epidural catheter has a built-in conductive guidewire (Nitinol, length = 1100 mm) with 800 mm inside the catheter and 300 mm exposed for connection to an electric nerve-stimulator. The cathode of the electric nerve stimulator (Life-Tech EZstim, Stafford, TX, USA) was connected to the exposed guidewire, and the anode was attached to an electrode on the patient's calf. A 0–5 mA electric current was then delivered through the guidewire. Verbal communication with the patient confirmed that the electric stimulation had reached the herpes zoster-affected area. The catheter was placed in the appropriate epidural space, and once electric stimulation had been initiated, verbal communication with the patient confirmed the sensation. After patient confirmation, further communication established that the electric stimulus was following the herpes zoster dermatome. However, if electric stimulation was observed in a region other than the herpes zoster dermatome, the epidural catheter was adjusted under fluoroscopy, and electric stimulation was repeated to confirm localization to the herpes zoster-affected area. Once the stimulus effectively reached the herpes zoster-affected area, the guidewire was removed from the epidural catheter. The position of the epidural catheter tip was confirmed with a contrast agent under a fluoroscope. Subsequently, 0.187% ropivacaine and 1 mg of dexamethasone (8 mL total) were administered via the catheter.

In both groups, the epidural catheter was fixed by subcutaneous tunneling to decrease the risk of infection and catheter migration. The inserted catheter was maintained in its position for a minimum of 10 days and was removed after 2 weeks. While patients were undergoing catheterization as inpatients and outpatients, a physician changed dressings daily and monitored the procedure site.

After the initial drug injection, patients in both groups were administered a continuous epidural infusion (275 mL) of 0.11–15% ropivacaine at a rate of 4 mL/h using a portable balloon infusion device (AutoFuser pump, ACE Medical Co., Ltd., Seoul, Korea), for the entire duration of catheter insertion. Ropivacaine concentrations were adjusted according to the degree of pain relief or side effects. Additionally, anticonvulsants (pregabalin or gabapentin) and analgesics were administered to patients in both the groups. Anticonvulsants were prescribed by adjusting the drug dose according to age and renal function and were tapered according to symptoms. Oxycodone was administered as an analgesic starting with the minimum reported effective dose for PHN [13].

Data collection

Data on age, sex, involved dermatome, and days from the onset of rash to continuous epidural infusion, as well as history of hypertension, diabetes, liver disease, kidney disease, asthma, and amount of ropivacaine in the infusion device were collected. Pain was assessed with a pain score using an 11-point verbal NRS (0 = no pain, 10 = unbearable pain). Pain score data were collected from the patients' medical records at different time points: at baseline (immediately before the procedure) and immediately after, 14 days after, and 1, 3, and 6 months after the procedure. Complete remission was defined as a pain score of less than 2 with no further medication required. The number of patients included in this category during the 6-month follow-up period was also recorded. Finally, we also investigated whether other interventional treatments were required due to insufficient pain control during the 6-month follow-up period after each procedure.

Outcome measures

We compared the baseline pain scores of both groups and assessed whether they were significantly reduced during the 6-month post-procedure period. To assess analgesic effects, we compared the pain scores of the two groups at baseline and immediately after, 14 days after, and 1, 3, and 6 months after the procedure, following correction for confounding variables. Additionally, we compared the percentage of patients who achieved complete remission in each group and the proportion of patients requiring additional nerve block due to inadequate pain control after each procedure.

Statistical analysis

Demographic data were assessed for normality using the the Kolmogorov-Smirnov test. Comparisons between the groups were made using an independent t-test for normally distributed variables, and non-normally distributed variables were compared using the Mann-Whitney U test. A repeated measures analysis of variance with the Bonferroni post-hoc test was used to determine whether the pain score was significantly reduced at each time point after the procedure compared to that at the baseline within each treatment group. After correcting for various confounding variables (e.g. age, sex, site of herpes zoster infection, history of hypertension, diabetes mellitus, asthma, hepatic disease, and kidney disease), we analyzed the differences in pain scores between the groups using covariance analysis. Between the two groups, multivariable logistic regression analysis was used to compare the odds of achieving complete remission and the odds of undergoing other interventional procedures within 6 months of the procedure. Data were reported as mean ± standard deviation or median (interquartile range) and were analyzed with the Statistical Package for the Social Sciences software (version 17.0, IBM, Chicago, IL, USA). All statistical tests were two-tailed, and the threshold for statistical significance was set at $P < 0.05$.

Results

We reviewed 209 patient records. Nine patients missed follow-up appointments or had inadequate medical records for the 6 months following the procedure. Twenty-five patients underwent other interventional procedures within 6 months of continuous epidural infusion. In one patient, the catheter could not be maintained for more than 10 days due to side effects associated with continuous epidural infusion. Two patients did not receive antiviral drugs at the beginning of the herpes zoster episode. During the 6-month follow-up period, two patients reported other painful diseases. The medical records of these patients were excluded from the final analysis. Additionally, eight patients stopped using anticonvulsants and analgesics due to drug-associated side effects after the procedure, and 48 patients received other drugs, such as opioids, via the epidural catheter. To prevent drug-induced bias, these patients were also excluded from the final analysis. Finally, the medical records of 114 patients were analyzed, with 57 patients each in the contrast and stimulation groups (Fig. 3).

There were no significant differences in baseline demographics between the groups (Table 1). Bonferroni post-hoc tests revealed that the pain scores at each time point after the procedure were significantly lower than those at baseline in both groups (Table 2).

When the post-procedure pain scores of the two groups were compared, (after correcting for confounding variables), no significant differences were observed immediately after the procedure; however, there were significant differences in the post-procedure pain scores between the two groups after the 14th day and up to the 6th month (Table 3).

The difference between the post-procedure pain scores of the two groups was analyzed at each level. The cervical and thoracic level results were similar to those of the entire analysis, showing better pain control in the stimulation group than that in the contrast group. However, there was no significant difference between the two groups in the lumbar area, which was an affected site for a small number of patients (Table 4).

The odds of complete remission were 1.90-times higher in the stimulation group than in the contrast group (Table 5).

The odds of undergoing other interventional procedures within 6 months of continuous epidural infusion due to insufficient pain control were 3.62-times higher in the contrast group than in the stimulation group (Table 6).

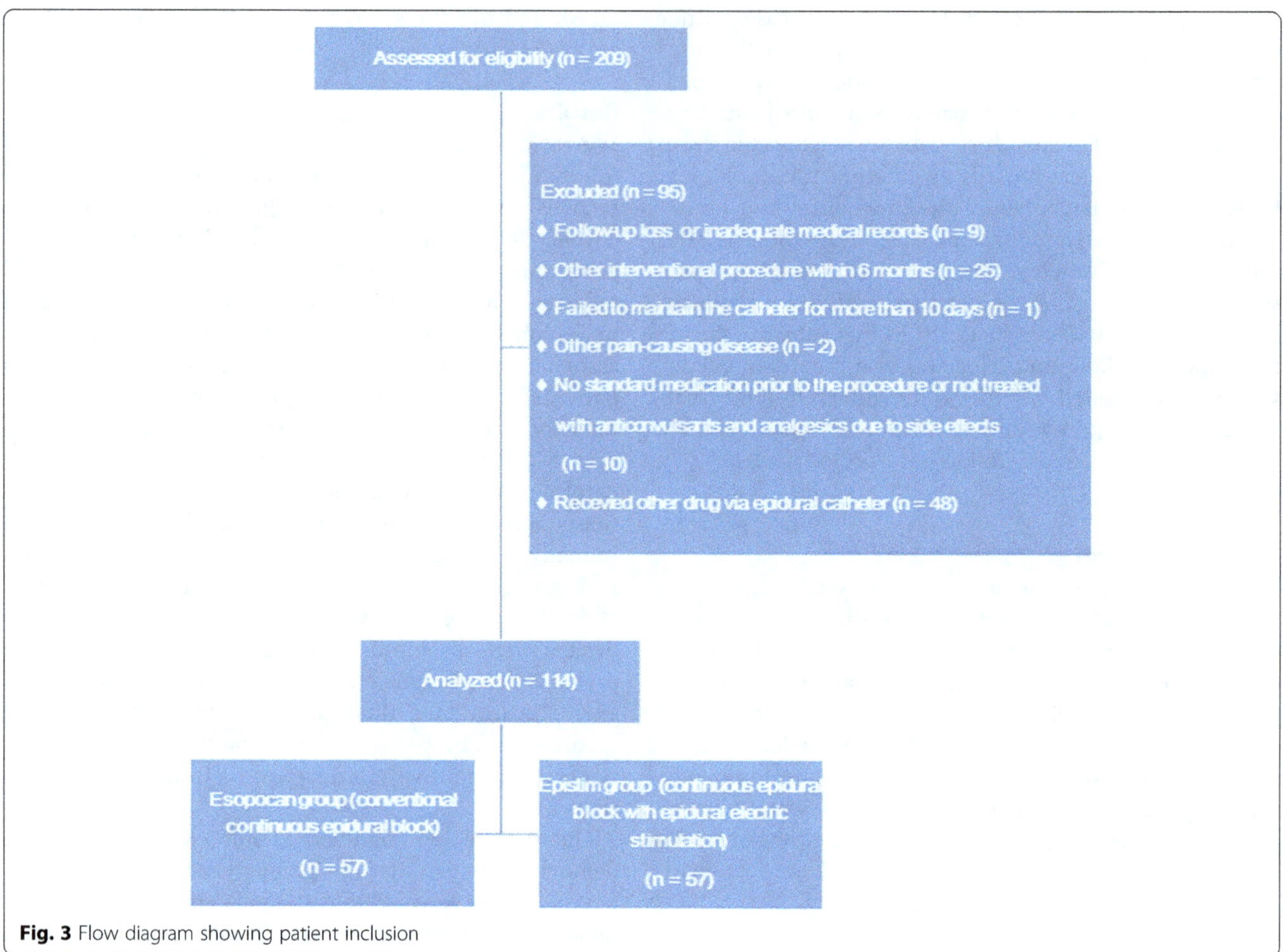

Fig. 3 Flow diagram showing patient inclusion

Table 1 Baseline characteristics of the patients

	Acute HZ (≤ 30 days)		*P* value
	Contrast group (*n* = 57)	Stimulation group (*n* = 57)	
Age (years)	67.0 ± 10.3	66.2 ± 11.7	*P* = 0.72
Sex (M/F)	25/32	16/41	*P* = 0.12
Site of HZ infection	C: 14	C: 13	*P* = 0.52
	T: 36	T: 33	
	L: 7	L: 11	
HTN	26 (46% [33, 58%])	21 (37% [26, 50%])	*P* = 0.45
DM	11 (19% [11, 31%])	16 (28% [18, 41%])	*P* = 0.38
Asthma	3 (5% [2, 14%])	1 (2% [0, 9%])	*P* = 0.62
Hepatic disease	5 (9% [4, 19%])	3 (5% [2, 14%])	*P* = 0.72
Kidney disease	2 (4% [1, 12%])	3 (5% [2, 14%])	*P* = 1.0
Avg. amount of ropivacaine in the infusion device (ml)	37.7 ± 3.8	37.5 ± 4.0	*P* = 0.79
Baseline pain score[a]	8 (7–8)	8 (7–8)	*P* = 0.22

Data are represented as mean ± standard deviation, median (interquartile range), or number (% [95% confidence interval])
HZ herpes zoster, *HTN* hypertension, *DM* diabetes mellitus, *Avg* average, [a]Pain score on an 11-point (0–10) numerical rating scale, *C* cervical, *T* thoracic, *L* lumbar

Table 2 Comparison with baseline pain scores at each time point

Group		Contrast group		Stimulation group	
Period A	Period B	Average difference (a – b)	*P* value	Average difference (a – b)	*P* value
Baseline pain score[a]	(1)	3.97	$P < 0.001$	4.25	$P < 0.001$
	(2)	4.62	$P < 0.001$	5.51	$P < 0.001$
	(3)	4.47	$P < 0.001$	5.21	$P < 0.001$
	(4)	4.88	$P < 0.001$	5.65	$P < 0.001$
	(5)	5.25	$P < 0.001$	5.88	$P < 0.001$

[a]Pain score on an 11-point (0–10) numerical rating scale. (1) Pain score immediately after epidural procedure, (2) Pain score 14 days after epidural procedure, (3) Pain score 1 month after epidural procedure, (4) Pain score 3 months after epidural procedure, (5) Pain score 6 months after epidural procedure. Data were analyzed using the Bonferroni post-hoc test. *P* value < 0.01 was considered statistically significant

Discussion

The purpose of the present study was to evaluate whether a procedure confirming a nerve block at the site of herpes zoster infection by application of epidural electric stimulation was more effective in reducing pain and preventing PHN than a procedure that identifies the location of epidural catheters with contrast agents alone.

In the present study, the pain scores of patients in both tested groups were significantly lower over the 6-month follow-up period than at the baseline. From 14 days to 6 months after the procedure (follow-up period), pain scores were significantly lower in the stimulation group than in the contrast group. The odds of complete remission of herpes zoster up to 6 months after the procedure was 1.9-times higher in the stimulation group than in the contrast group. This suggests that administering the drug after confirming the correct VZV-containing dorsal root ganglion using epidural electric stimulation may be more effective in treating herpes zoster than the conventional continuous epidural infusion. The proportion of patients who received other epidural blocks because of the lack of pain control within the 6 months following the procedure, was approximately one-third lower in the stimulation group than that in the contrast group.

There was also a difference in the drug injection site of the epidural catheter tip between the two groups. Reportedly, closed-tip, multi-orifice catheters are more effective for sensory blocks than open-tip, end-hole catheters. However, in our study, the stimulation group (in which open-tip, end-hole catheters were used) showed greater pain reduction than the contrast group (in which closed-tip multi-orifice catheters were used) [14, 15]. These results suggest that a continuous epidural infusion utilizing electric stimulation to confirm the location of herpes zoster is more effective in achieving pain relief than the conventional continuous epidural infusion. EpiStim™ epidural catheters have a bent tip and a flexible guidewire and use electric stimulation to identify the affected area, increasing the maneuverability of the catheter and making it easier to position the catheter at the target site [12]. These features yielded significant differences between the contrast and stimulation groups in our results.

In our study, there was no significant difference in pain reduction immediately after the procedure between the two groups. This is likely due to the spread of 8 mL of drug epidurally administered during the procedure. After administration, it is likely that the drug spread to adjacent dermatomes. Therefore, even if the epidural catheter was not precisely at the affected site, the drug may still have spread to the site of the herpes zoster infection, but this would occur only with a single epidural

Table 3 Comparison of pain scores between the groups after correction for confounding variables

	Acute HZ (≤ 30 days)		*P* value
	Contrast group ($n = 57$)	Stimulation group ($n = 57$)	
Baseline pain score	7.4 ± 1.5	7.2 ± 1.5	$P = 0.28$
Pain score[a] immediately after epidural procedure	3.5 ± 2.0	2.9 ± 1.8	$P = 0.25$
Pain score[a] 14 days after epidural procedure	2.8 ± 1.9	1.7 ± 0.8	$P = 0.001$
Pain score[a] 1 month after epidural procedure	3.0 ± 2.1	1.9 ± 1.1	$P = 0.01$
Pain score[a] 3 months after epidural procedure	2.6 ± 1.8	1.5 ± 1.2	$P = 0.001$
Pain score[a] 6 months after epidural procedure	2.2 ± 1.8	1.3 ± 1.1	$P = 0.01$

Data are reported as adjusted mean ± standard deviation. Data were analyzed for the difference in pain scores between the groups using covariance analysis. Adjustments were made for age, sex, timing from rash to epidural procedure, location of herpes zoster, hypertension, diabetes mellitus, asthma, hepatic disease, and kidney disease

HZ herpes zoster, [a]Pain score on an 11-point (0–10) numerical rating scale

Table 4 Comparison of pain scores between the groups for cervical, thoracic, and lumbar levels

	Cervical area			Thoracic area			Lumbar area		
	Acute HZ (≤ 30 days)		*P* value	Acute HZ (≤ 30 days)		*P* value	Acute HZ (≤ 30 days)		*P* value
	Contrast group ($n = 14$)	Stimulation group ($n = 13$)		Contrast group ($n = 36$)	Stimulation group ($n = 33$)		Contrast group ($n = 7$)	Stimulation group ($n = 11$)	
Baseline pain score	7.8 ± 1.4	6.9 ± 1.3	$P = 0.13$	7.4 ± 1.6	7.2 ± 1.5	$P = 0.85$	7.1 ± 1.7	7.3 ± 2.0	$P = 0.9$
Pain score[a] immediately after epidural procedure	3.8 ± 2.0	3.0 ± 2.1	$P = 0.44$	3.5 ± 2.0	3.1 ± 1.7	$P = 0.51$	3.0 ± 1.8	2.1 ± 1.8	$P = 0.58$
Pain score[a] 14 days after epidural procedure	3.2 ± 2.1	1.7 ± 0.8	$P = 0.02$	2.8 ± 1.9	1.7 ± 0.9	$P = 0.03$	2.3 ± 1.0	1.5 ± 0.8	$P = 0.08$
Pain score[a] 1 month after epidural procedure	3.4 ± 2.5	1.9 ± 1.2	$P = 0.06$	2.9 ± 2.1	2.0 ± 1.1	$P = 0.19$	2.7 ± 1.5	1.6 ± 1.1	$P = 0.12$
Pain score[a] 3 months after epidural procedure	2.3 ± 1.3	1.3 ± 1.3	$P = 0.04$	2.6 ± 2.0	1.6 ± 1.1	$P = 0.04$	2.9 ± 2.0	1.3 ± 1.2	$P = 0.07$
Pain score[a] 6 months after epidural procedure	2.2 ± 1.8	1.2 ± 1.1	$P = 0.03$	2.2 ± 1.8	1.3 ± 1.1	$P = 0.08$	2.3 ± 1.6	1.2 ± 1.2	$P = 0.46$

Data are represented as adjusted mean ± standard deviation. Data were analyzed for differences in pain score between the groups using covariance analysis. Adjustments were made for age, sex, timing from rash to epidural procedure, hypertension, diabetes mellitus, asthma, hepatic disease, and kidney disease

HZ herpes zoster, [a]Pain score on an 11-point (0–10) numerical rating scale

Table 5 Comparison of complete remission between the contrast and stimulation groups during the 6-month follow-up period after each procedure

	Contrast Group	Stimulation Group	Adjusted OR (95% CI) Reference: contrast group	*P* value
Acute HZ (≤3 0 days)	29/57 [51% (38, 63%)]	41/57 [72% (59, 82%)]	1.90 (0.81–4.44)	*P* = 0.14

Complete remission is defined as a pain score of less than 2 with no further medication. Data are represented as number (% [95% confidence interval]) and were analyzed by logistic regression analysis. Adjustments were made for age, sex, location of herpes zoster, days from the onset of rash to procedure, hypertension history, diabetes mellitus history, asthma history, hepatic disease history, kidney disease history, and baseline pain score
HZ herpes zoster, *OR* odds ratio, *CI* confidence interval

block. When the drug was administered continuously at the rate of 4 mL/h via a portable infusion pump, the spread of the drug decreased considerably. Therefore, precise administration of the drug to the correct site would have been possible only if the catheter was positioned in close proximity to the herpes zoster infection site. We suggest that the differences in pain scores at 14 days and 1, 3, and 6 months after the procedure were attributable to continued pain relief, despite reduced drug efficacy over the period of continuous administration, if the catheter was correctly placed in the target region.

Due to the complexity of the pathophysiological mechanisms that contribute to the progression of acute herpes zoster to PHN, various preventive strategies have been proposed, including vaccinations and the use of antiviral agents, anticonvulsants, and corticosteroids. However, according to a recent systematic review and meta-analysis, the efficacy of these treatments in preventing PHN is limited [16–21]. We focused on the nerve damage caused by VZV for the treatment of acute herpes zoster and PHN prevention. Reactivated VZV in the dorsal root ganglion, which manifests as herpes zoster, subsequently diffuses to the affected dermatome producing an inflammatory response and inducing nerve damage. Severe initial nerve damage or the inability to regain normal function after the loss of nerve function can lead to PHN [22]. Therefore, proactive treatment before nerve injury can help prevent PHN. According to a recent meta-analysis, continuous epidural infusion in acute herpes zoster is effective in preventing PHN [9]. The rationale behind the application of epidural blocks to control acute herpes zoster pain and prevent PHN is that the discontinued delivery of an invasive afferent stimulus to the central nervous system and improved flow of blood to the subjects' nerve tissue will minimize neural damage and reduce sensitization. In addition, it is possible that local anesthetics, along with the anti-inflammatory effects of corticosteroids, could be effective in areas corresponding to the affected nerves [23]. Epidural administration of steroids not only inhibits inflammation but also reduces deafferentation by decreasing any neural ischemia resulting from inflammatory swelling [21]. Local anesthetics administered epidurally control pain and interfere with sensitization by blocking sympathetic nerves; however, to maximize the effects of epidural steroids and local anesthetics on the affected site, it is important to administer the drug precisely to the site of nerve injury [24]. Therefore, we performed epidural electric stimulation to specifically identify the site sustaining the nerve injury caused by herpes zoster. This method allows for more accurate catheter placement than the conventional method, where the diffusion image of a contrast agent is used to confirm the location of the catheter.

In the current study, patients who could not maintain the inserted continuous epidural catheter for more than 10 days were excluded from the analysis because according to a previous study, a single epidural block may be effective in controlling herpes zoster-related pain, but it has limited efficacy in the prevention of PHN [25, 26].

All the patients included in our study underwent continuous epidural infusion and simultaneously took anticonvulsants and analgesics. To avoid bias due to drug treatments, patients who discontinued the drug due to side effects from other treatments and those who were administered drugs other than local anesthetics and steroids via the epidural catheter, such as opioids, were excluded from the analysis.

The complete remission rate in the present study was 51% in the contrast group and 72% in the stimulation group. Reportedly, the greater the severity of acute herpes zoster pain, the greater the likelihood of its progression to PHN [5, 27]. In our clinic, invasive treatments,

Table 6 Comparison of implemented procedures due to insufficient pain control during the 6-month follow-up period

	Contrast Group	Stimulation Group	Adjusted OR (95% CI) Reference: stimulation group	*P* value
Acute HZ (≤30 days)	20/77 [26% (17, 37%)]	5/62 [8% (3, 18%)]	3.62 (1.17–11.19)	*P* = 0.03

Data are reported as number [% (95% confidence interval)]. Data were analyzed by logistic regression analysis. Adjustments were made for age, sex, location of herpes zoster, days from the onset of rash to procedure, hypertension history, diabetes mellitus history, asthma history, hepatic disease history, kidney disease history, and baseline pain score
HZ herpes zoster, *OR* odds ratio, *CI* confidence interval

such as continuous epidural infusion, are not performed for less severe cases of herpes zoster (pain score, < 4). Consequently, all the participants in the present study had pain scores of 4 or higher (mean 7.5 ± 1.5 and 7.1 ± 1.4 in the control and stimulation groups, respectively), which may be one of the reasons for the lower rates of complete remission. Additionally, the definition we adopted for complete remission (pain score of ≤2, no further medication prescribed) is possibly another reason for lower remission rates, since other studies have defined a pain-free state with an NRS score of less than 3, or without discussion of medication withdrawal [8, 25].

Epidural hematoma, infection, and abscess are the complications that make continuous epidural catheterization difficult, but no infections were reported after continuous epidural infusion in this study. This is likely due to the involvement of well-trained physicians who changed dressings daily and well-educated patients and caregivers. The incidence of epidural hematoma is low and was not observed in the present study. However, one patient experienced severe urinary retention after the procedure, which was resolved after the epidural catheter was removed [1].

Limitations

First, this was a retrospective study, and there may be an influence of unmeasured confounding variables. Thus, we conducted a covariance analysis with the baseline demographics and underlying patient disease as covariates to control for potential disturbance factors. Additionally, only the patients who took both anticonvulsants and analgesics along with continuous epidural infusion were included in the study to ensure consistent drug use across the sample set.

Second, our research data were derived from electronic medical records, which may have led to an underestimation of the actual incidence of side effects. In the present study, continuous epidural infusion was discontinued in only one patient because of adverse effects, but side effects such as dysuria and motor weakness may not have been added to the medical record when the epidural block was maintained because of low symptom severity.

Third, we excluded patients who were treated with other interventional procedures within the 6-month period, and this could have caused a selection bias in the study. Nevertheless, if we had included patients who experienced other interventions in the analysis, there would have been uncertainty regarding whether the patient symptoms improved due to receiving a continuous epidural infusion for the first time, or because they had other interventions. Therefore, we excluded patients with other interventions when calculating complete remission and 6-month pain scores and analyzed the ratios separately.

Fourth, we investigated whether oral medications were administered simultaneously with continuous epidural infusion for herpes zoster, but the exact doses were not measured. The correct dose of oral medication may affect the incidence of PHN and pain in herpes zoster, which may limit the results of this study.

Conclusion

Continuous epidural catheterization combined with standard drug therapy in patients with acute herpes zoster may be effective in preventing the associated pain and development of PHN. Furthermore, using electric stimulation to identify the specific epidural location affected by the herpes zoster infection and administering the drug via an epidural catheter enables continuous drug administration to the exact site of neurological damage. A well-planned, prospective study comparing the methods for preventing herpes zoster-related pain and PHN is required to validate the results of the present study.

Abbreviations

NRS: Numeric rating scale; PHN: Postherpetic neuralgia; VZV: Varicella zoster virus

Acknowledgements

Statistical analysis was conducted after consulting Soon Young Hwang (Korea University Medical Center, Guro Hospital), a statistical expert. We would like to thank Editage (www.editage.co.kr) for English language editing.

Authors' contributions

All authors had full access to all the data and take responsibility for the integrity of the data and accuracy of the data analysis. CHL and SSC designed the experiments. CHL, SSC, MKL, YJL, and JSP were involved in recruiting patients and performed the experiments. CHL managed the literature searches and summaries of previous related work and wrote the first draft of the manuscript. CHL, MKL and SSC revised the intellectual content and finally approved the manuscript. All authors read and approved the final manuscript.

References

1. van Wijck AJ, Wallace M, Mekhail N, van Kleef M. Evidence-based interventional pain medicine according to clinical diagnoses. 17. Herpes zoster and post-herpetic neuralgia. Pain Pract. 2011;11(1):88–97. https://doi.org/10.1111/j.1533-2500.2010.00428.x Pubmed:21114617.
2. Sim WS, Choi JH, Han KR, Kim YC. Treatment of herpes zoster and postherpetic neuralgia. Korean J Pain. 2008;21(2):93–105. https://doi.org/10.3344/kjp.2008.21.2.93.
3. Werner RN, Nikkels AF, Marinović B, Schäfer M, Czarnecka-Operacz M, Agius AM, et al. European consensus-based (S2k) guideline on the management of herpes zoster - guided by the European dermatology forum (EDF) in cooperation with the European academy of dermatology and venereology (EADV), part 1: diagnosis. J Eur Acad Dermatol Venereol. 2017;31(1):9–19. https://doi.org/10.1111/jdv.13995 Pubmed:27804172.
4. Choudhary S, Dhande S, Kharat S, Singh AL. Safety and efficacy of different systemic treatment modalities for acute pain of herpes zoster: a pilot study. Indian Dermatol Online J. 2018;9(2):101–4. https://doi.org/10.4103/idoj.IDOJ_377_16 Pubmed:29644194.
5. Forbes HJ, Thomas SL, Smeeth L, Clayton T, Farmer R, Bhaskaran K, Langan SM. A systematic review and meta-analysis of risk factors for postherpetic neuralgia. Pain. 2016;157(1):30–54. https://doi.org/10.1097/j.pain.0000000000000307 Pubmed:26218719.
6. Harke H, Gretenkort P, Ladleif HU, Koester P, Rahman S. Spinal cord stimulation in postherpetic neuralgia and in acute herpes zoster pain. Anesth Analg. 2002;94(3):694–700. https://doi.org/10.1097/00000539-200203000-00040 Pubmed:11867400 table of contents.
7. Dworkin RH, Gnann JW Jr, Oaklander AL, Raja SN, Schmader KE, Whitley RJ. Diagnosis and assessment of pain associated with herpes zoster and

postherpetic neuralgia. J Pain. 2008;9(1 Suppl 1):S37–44. https://doi.org/10.1016/j.jpain.2007.10.008 Pubmed:18166464.

8. Pasqualucci A, Pasqualucci V, Galla F, De Angelis V, Marzocchi V, Colussi R, et al. Prevention of post-herpetic neuralgia: acyclovir and prednisolone versus epidural local anesthetic and methylprednisolone. Acta Anaesthesiol Scand. 2000;44(8):910–8. https://doi.org/10.1034/j.1399-6576.2000.440803.x Pubmed:10981565.
9. Kim HJ, Ahn HS, Lee JY, Choi SS, Cheong YS, Kwon K, et al. Effects of applying nerve blocks to prevent postherpetic neuralgia in patients with acute herpes zoster: a systematic review and meta-analysis. Korean J Pain. 2017;30(1):3–17. https://doi.org/10.3344/kjp.2017.30.1.3 Pubmed:28119767.
10. Kumar V, Krone K, Mathieu A. Neuraxial and sympathetic blocks in herpes zoster and postherpetic neuralgia: an appraisal of current evidence. Reg Anesth Pain Med. 2004;29(5):454–61. https://doi.org/10.1016/j.rapm.2004.04.010 Pubmed:15372391.
11. Manabe H, Dan K, Hirata K, Hori K, Shono S, Tateshi S, et al. Optimum pain relief with continuous epidural infusion of local anesthetics shortens the duration of zoster-associated pain. Clin J Pain. 2004;20(5):302–8. https://doi.org/10.1097/00002508-200409000-00004 Pubmed:15322436.
12. Kim JE, Lee MK, Lee CH, Kang HY, Choi SS. A novel treatment for herpes zoster pain using an electrical stimulating catheter with a steering guidewire. J Clin Anesth. 2017;41:46–7. https://doi.org/10.1016/j.jclinane.2017.05.016 Pubmed:28802604.
13. Watson CP, Babul N. Efficacy of oxycodone in neuropathic pain: a randomized trial in postherpetic neuralgia. Neurology. 1998;50(6):1837–41. https://doi.org/10.1212/wnl.50.6.1837 Pubmed:9633737.
14. Toledano RD, Tsen LC. Epidural catheter design: history, innovations, and clinical implications. Anesthesiology. 2014;121(1):9–17. https://doi.org/10.1097/ALN.0000000000000239 Pubmed:24681579.
15. Michael S, Richmond MN, Birks RJ. A comparison between open-end (single hole) and closed-end (three lateral holes) epidural catheters. Complications and quality of sensory blockade. Anaesthesia. 1989;44(7):578–80. https://doi.org/10.1111/j.1365-2044.1989.tb11446.x Pubmed:2774123.
16. Oxman MN, Levin MJ, Johnson GR, Schmader KE, Straus SE, Gelb LD, et al. A vaccine to prevent herpes zoster and postherpetic neuralgia in older adults. N Engl J Med. 2005;352(22):2271–84. https://doi.org/10.1056/NEJMoa051016 Pubmed:15930418.
17. Levin MJ, Gershon AA, Dworkin RH, Brisson M, Stanberry L. Prevention strategies for herpes zoster and post-herpetic neuralgia. J Clin Virol. 2010;48:S14–9. https://doi.org/10.1016/S1386-6532(10)70004-4 Pubmed:20510262.
18. Klenerman P, Luzzi GA. Acyclovir and postherpetic neuralgia. Biomed Pharmacother. 1990;44(9):455–9. https://doi.org/10.1016/0753-3322(90)90205-N Pubmed:2081273.
19. Chen N, Li Q, Yang J, Zhou M, Zhou D, He L. Antiviral treatment for preventing postherpetic neuralgia. Cochrane Database Syst Rev. 2014:CD006866. https://doi.org/10.1002/14651858.CD006866.pub3 Pubmed:24500927.
20. Chen N, Li Q, Zhang Y, Zhou M, Zhou D, He L. Vaccination for preventing postherpetic neuralgia. Cochrane Database Syst Rev. 2011:CD007795. https://doi.org/10.1002/14651858.CD007795.pub2 Pubmed:21412911.
21. Han Y, Zhang J, Chen N, He L, Zhou M, Zhu C. Corticosteroids for preventing postherpetic neuralgia. Cochrane Database Syst Rev. 2013:CD005582. https://doi.org/10.1002/14651858.CD005582.pub4 Pubmed:23543541.
22. Winnie AP, Hartwell PW. Relationship between time of treatment of acute herpes zoster with sympathetic blockade and prevention of postherpetic-neuralgia: clinical support for a new theory of the mechanism by which sympathetic blockade provides therapeutic benefit. Reg Anesth. 1993;18(5):277–82 Pubmed:8268115.
23. Doran C, Yi X. The anti-inflammatory effect of local anesthetics. Pain Clin. 2007;19(5):207–13. https://doi.org/10.1179/016911107X396943.
24. Opstelten W, van Wijck AJ, Stolker RJ. Interventions to prevent postherpetic neuralgia: cutaneous and percutaneous techniques. Pain. 2004;107(3):202–6. https://doi.org/10.1016/j.pain.2003.10.021 Pubmed:14736581.
25. van Wijck AJ, Opstelten W, Moons KG, van Essen GA, Stolker RJ, Kalkman CJ, et al. The PINE study of epidural steroids and local anaesthetics to prevent postherpetic neuralgia: a randomised controlled trial. Lancet. 2006;367(9506):219–24. https://doi.org/10.1016/S0140-6736(06)68032-X Pubmed:16427490.
26. Kikuchi A, Kotani N, Sato T, Takamura K, Sakai I, Matsuki A. Comparative therapeutic evaluation of intrathecal versus epidural methylprednisolone for long-term analgesia in patients with intractable postherpetic neuralgia. Reg Anesth Pain Med. 1999;24(4):287–93. https://doi.org/10.1016/S1098-7339(99)90101-3 Pubmed:10445766.
27. Kawai K, Rampakakis E, Tsai TF, Cheong HJ, Dhitavat J, Covarrubias AO, et al. Predictors of postherpetic neuralgia in patients with herpes zoster: a pooled analysis of prospective cohort studies from north and Latin America and Asia. Int J Infect Dis. 2015;34:126–31. https://doi.org/10.1016/j.ijid.2015.03.022 Pubmed:25841633.

Multimodal analgesia with ropivacaine wound infiltration and intravenous flurbiprofen axetil provides enhanced analgesic effects after radical thyroidectomy

Xiaoxi Li, Ling Yu, Jiaonan Yang and Hongyu Tan*

Abstract

Background: Thyroidectomy is a common procedure that causes mild trauma. Nevertheless, postoperative pain remains a major challenge in patient care. Multimodal analgesia comprising a combination of analgesics and analgesic techniques has become increasingly popular for the control of postoperative pain. The present study tested the hypothesis that multimodal analgesia with combined ropivacaine wound infiltration and intravenous flurbiprofen axetil after radical thyroidectomy provided better analgesia than a single dosage of tramadol.

Methods: This randomized controlled trial was conducted in a tertiary hospital. Forty-four patients (age, 18–75 years; American Society of Anesthesiologists status I or II; BMI < 32 kg/m^2) scheduled for radical thyroidectomy were randomly assigned to a multimodal analgesia group (Group M) or a control group (Group C) by random numbers assignments, and 40 patients completed the study. All participants and the nurse in charge of follow-up observations were blinded to group assignment. Anesthesia was induced with sufentanil, propofol, and cisatracurium. After tracheal intubation, Group M received pre-incision wound infiltration with 5 ml of 0.5% ropivacaine mixed with epinephrine at 1:200,000 (5 μg/ml); Group C received no wound infiltration. Anesthesia was maintained with target-controlled infusion of propofol, remifentanil, sevoflurane, and intermittent cisatracurium. Twenty minutes before the end of surgery, Group M received 100 mg flurbiprofen axetil while Group C received 100 mg tramadol. Postoperative pain was evaluated with the numerical rating scale (NRS) pain score. Remifentanil consumption, heart rate, and noninvasive blood pressure were recorded intraoperatively. Adverse events were documented. The primary outcome was analgesic effect according to NRS scores.

(Continued on next page)

* Correspondence: maggitan@163.com
Key Laboratory of Carcinogenesis and Translational Research (Ministry of Education/Beijing), Department of Anesthesiology, Peking University Cancer Hospital & Institute, #52 Fucheng Street, Haidian District, Beijing 100142, China

(Continued from previous page)

Results: NRS scores at rest were significantly lower in Group M than in Group C before discharge from the postoperative anesthetic care unit ($P = 0.003$) and at 2 ($P = 0.008$), 4 ($P = 0.020$), and 8 h ($P = 0.016$) postoperatively. Group M also had significantly lower NRS scores during coughing/swallowing at 5 min after extubation ($P = 0.017$), before discharge from the postoperative anesthetic care unit ($P = 0.001$), and at 2 ($P = 0.002$) and 4 h ($P = 0.013$) postoperatively. Compared with Group C, NRS scores were significantly lower throughout the first 24 h postoperatively in Group M at rest ($P = 0.008$) and during coughing/swallowing ($P = 0.003$). No serious adverse events were observed in either group.

Conclusion: Multimodal analgesia with ropivacaine wound infiltration and intravenous flurbiprofen axetil provided better analgesia than tramadol after radical thyroidectomy.

Keywords: Multimodal analgesia, Wound infiltration, Ropivacaine; flurbiprofen axetil, Postoperative analgesia, Thyroidectomy

Background

Thyroidectomy is a common procedure that causes mild trauma. Nevertheless, postoperative pain remains a major challenge in patient care. Optimizing postoperative pain management is an important goal in the perioperative period. Tramadol is a synthetic opioid frequently used to treat moderate pain. In contrast to pure opioid agonists, tramadol has a low risk of respiratory depression and sedative effects [1–4]. At our institution, tramadol is commonly prescribed to provide postoperative analgesia in patients undergoing thyroid surgery because it is effective in relieving mild to moderate pain, causes less respiratory depression and sedation than other opioids, and has a relatively low cost. However, tramadol has major adverse effects, including dizziness, nausea, and vomiting, which affect its clinical application and patient satisfaction [5]. Clinical research shows that postoperative nausea and vomiting (PONV) is primarily caused by the use of inhalational anesthesia and opioid analgesics [6]. Studies have shown that the incidence of PONV is reduced by the use of antiemetic drugs such as 5-HT3 receptor antagonists (e.g., dolasetron) and/or total intravenous anesthesia [7–9]. However, despite impressive advances in the field of anesthesia, PONV remains an unpleasant postoperative experience that must be considered.

Postoperative analgesia can be improved by combination therapies targeting different sites of the pain pathway. Moreover, multimodal analgesia can decrease opioid consumption and adverse effects. Therefore, multimodal analgesia using a combination of analgesics and analgesic techniques has become increasingly popular for the control of postoperative pain. Investigations on multimodal analgesia have been carried out in upper extremity surgery, hip and knee arthroplasty, cardiac surgery, and other major operations [10–14]. However, studies on multimodal analgesia in neck surgery remain limited.

Some inflammatory mediators released by damaged cells at the surgical site act directly on the nociceptor terminal to produce pain, while others lead to sensitization of the nociceptor terminal. Therefore, it has been proposed a multimodal analgesic regimen that includes anti-inflammatory drugs be used to control postoperative pain. Flurbiprofen axetil is a non-steroidal anti-inflammatory drug (NSAID) with a high affinity for inflamed tissues and a promising analgesic effect [15]. Local anesthetic wound infiltration has also been shown to reduce postoperative pain and opioid requirement in patients undergoing thyroid surgery [16, 17]. Ropivacaine is a popular long-acting local anesthetic that is widely used for local anesthesia due to its reduced toxic potential in comparison with other local anesthetic agents [18].

This prospective, randomized controlled trial aimed to evaluate the analgesic efficacy of multimodal analgesia with pre-incision ropivacaine wound infiltration and intravenous flurbiprofen axetil in patients undergoing radical thyroidectomy. The hypothesis was that multimodal analgesia benefits patients undergoing radical thyroidectomy by providing good analgesic effects with a low incidence of adverse effects. This is the first trial to compare a multimodal regimen consisting of pre-incision ropivacaine wound infiltration and intravenous flurbiprofen axetil versus a single dose of tramadol in patients undergoing thyroid surgery.

Methods

General information

This prospective, randomized controlled trial was designed in adherence to the CONSORT guidelines and was conducted in a tertiary hospital in Beijing, China. Ethics committee approval was obtained from the Institutional Review Board at Peking University Cancer Hospital (no. 2018YJZ74) and the study was registered on Chinese Clinical Trial Registry (no. ChiCTR1800020290). All participants provided written informed consent. Patients scheduled for elective radical thyroidectomy with an American Society of Anesthesiologists grade of I or II, aged 18–75 years, and a BMI < 32 kg/m^2 were enrolled. Random numbers generated by Statistical Package for Social Sciences version 17.0 (SPSS Inc., Chicago, IL, USA) were used to randomly assign patients to the multimodal analgesia group (Group M) or the control group (Group C) in a 1:1 ratio. Patients were blinded to group assignment. A research nurse placed the random numbers in sealed envelopes. A resident who was independent of the recruitment process opened each patient's envelope after all baseline assessments had been completed. Patients with the following conditions were excluded from the study: 1) history of chronic pain or chronic use of analgesics; 2) intake of NSAIDs, opioids, or other analgesics in the 24 h before surgery; 3) history of allergic reaction to NSAIDs; 4) any contraindications to flurbiprofen axetil, such as coagulation disorders, gastrointestinal ulceration, severe hypertension, severe cardiovascular or cerebrovascular disease, or renal dysfunction; 5) pregnancy or lactation; 6) inability to comprehend the concept of the numeric rating scale (NRS; 0, no pain; 10, worst pain imaginable); 7) lateral neck dissection during surgery; and 8) refusal to participate in the study.

Anesthesia

Patients were placed in supine position on the operating table, with the neck hyperextended. Standard monitoring, including electrocardiography, heart rate (HR), noninvasive blood pressure (NBP), pulse oximetry, and bispectral index to monitor depth of anesthesia, were established before anesthetic induction. Anesthesia was induced with intravenous sufentanil (0.3 μg/kg), propofol (2–2.5 mg/kg), and cisatracurium (0.2 mg/kg). Tracheal intubation was performed after sufficient muscle relaxation was achieved. Patients were mechanically ventilated to maintain end-tidal carbon dioxide between 35 and 45 mmHg. After tracheal intubation, patients in Group M received subcuticular wound infiltration with 5 ml of 0.5% ropivacaine mixed with epinephrine at a ratio of 1:200,000 (5 μg/ml) prior to skin incision. Group C received no wound infiltration. General anesthesia was maintained with target-controlled infusion (Graseby 3500; AstraZeneca, UK) of propofol (2.0 μg/ml, plasma concentration), remifentanil (3.0–4.0 ng/ml, plasma concentration), and sevoflurane (1.0–2.0%, end-tidal concentration) to maintain a spectral entropy value of 40 to 60. Muscle relaxation was achieved with intermittent cisatracurium. All patients received lactated Ringer's solution. If blood pressure fell to 30% below baseline for more than 1 min, fluid infusion was accelerated or 6 mg ephedrine was administered. Surgeries were performed by the same surgical team with the same standardized technique. At 20 min before the end of surgery, Group M received 100 mg flurbiprofen axetil (Beijing Taide Pharmaceutical Co., Ltd.) while Group C received 100 mg tramadol intravenously (slowly injected during a 5-min period), followed by injection of 12.5 mg dolasetron in both groups to prevent PONV. Sevoflurane was discontinued 15 min before the completion of surgery. Propofol/remifentanil infusion was terminated at the end of surgery. Muscle relaxation was antagonized with 1 mg intravenous atropine and 2 mg neostigmine. Patients were extubated after responding to verbal commands and achieving adequate spontaneous ventilation. Patients were then transferred to the postoperative anesthetic care unit (PACU) for further observation until they fulfilled discharge criteria.

Measurements

Hemodynamic parameters, including HR and NBP, were documented at specific timepoints: before induction (T1), 3 min after tracheal intubation (T2), at the beginning of surgery (T3), after 10 min of surgery (T4), after 30 min of surgery (T5), at the end of surgery (T6), immediately after extubation (T7), and before discharge from the PACU (T8).

Acute postoperative pain was assessed in accordance with the NRS score under two conditions (at rest and during coughing/swallowing) at 5 min after tracheal extubation, before patient discharge from the PACU, and at 2, 4, 8, 12, 24, and 48 h after surgery. If a patient had moderate pain (NRS score of 4–6), 50 mg flurbiprofen axetil was prescribed. If a patient had severe pain (NRS score above 6), 100 mg tramadol was administered as a rescue analgesic. All adverse events related to the administered agents, such as dizziness and PONV, were documented. If a patient experienced severe nausea or vomiting, metoclopramide was administered as a rescue antiemetic agent. Follow-up observations were performed by a nurse from the PACU who was not involved in the study and who was blinded to group assignment.

Outcomes

The primary outcome was analgesic effect in accordance with the NRS scores at specific timepoints. The secondary outcomes were intraoperative remifentanil consumption, the need for postoperative rescue analgesia, adverse effects, and hemodynamic response during surgery.

Sample size

A preliminary trial conducted by the authors found that the average NRS score within 48 h after surgery was 0.92 ± 0.53 in Group M and 1.48 ± 0.62 in Group C. With this information, a sample size of 15 patients per group was estimated to have at least 80.0% power at a significance level of 5%, according to Power Analysis and Sample Size software (version 11.0; NCSS, LLC, Kaysville, UT, USA).

Statistical analysis

SPSS was used for statistical analysis. Numerical variables are shown as mean ± standard deviation (SD) or median, in accordance with their distribution. Categorical variables were analyzed with the Pearson chi-squared test. Continuous variables were analyzed with independent-samples t-test or the rank sum test, in accordance with their distribution. Hemodynamic responses at different timepoints were compared with repeated-measures analysis of variance. A value of $P < 0.05$ was considered statistically significant.

Results

Forty-four patients were randomized from January to April 2019 (Fig. 1). Four patients were excluded due to missing data. Therefore, 40 patients were analyzed with 20 patients in each group. There were no significant differences between the groups in demographic characteristics or intraoperative data (Table 1). Compared with Group C, Group M had a lower mean blood pressure (MBP; $P = 0.019$) (Table 2). However, no significant differences were found between groups in HR ($P = 0.119$) or the use of vasoactive drugs ($P = 0.507$). In addition, the two groups did not differ in infusion volume ($P = 0.634$) or blood loss ($P = 0.515$).

Postoperative NRS scores are presented in Fig. 2 and Table 3. There was no significant difference between groups in the number of patients requiring additional analgesia postoperatively ($P = 1.000$).

No serious adverse events related to the agents used in the present study were observed. The incidence of adverse effects within the 48 h postoperative period was not significantly different between the groups (Table 4).

Discussion

Flurbiprofen axetil is an injectable non-selective cyclooxygenase inhibitor. It is a prodrug prepared by enveloping flurbiprofen ester in a drug carrier of lipid microspheres, which congregate selectively in inflammatory tissues with a high affinity and provide sustained drug release. A meta-analysis of randomized controlled trials showed that patients treated with preoperative flurbiprofen axetil had significantly lower postoperative pain scores than those who did not receive flurbiprofen axetil [15]. Regional techniques such as local anesthetic wound infiltration also reduce postoperative pain and opioid requirements [16, 17]. In thyroid surgery, local anesthetic wound infiltration is safe and easy to perform and has shown good analgesic effects in some studies [16, 19–22]; however, the results are controversial [23, 24]. In addition, the analgesic benefit of local wound infiltration seems to be maintained for only a short period of time after thyroid surgery [20, 25], and breast cancer surgery [26]; administration of local anesthetics significantly decreased pain only at 2 h postoperatively. Postoperative pain after total thyroidectomy reportedly reaches a maximum at 1 h postoperatively, and starts to decrease 3 h later [20]. Therefore, the first few hours following thyroidectomy are the most crucial for pain management.

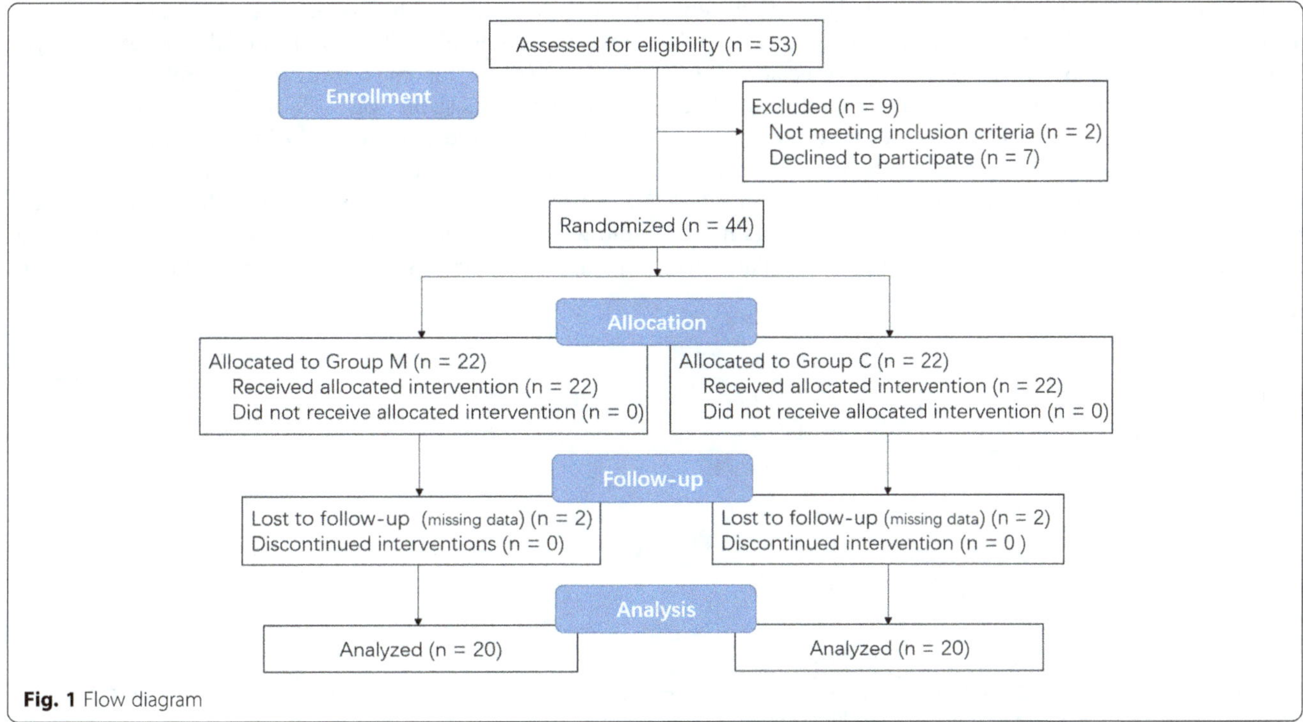

Fig. 1 Flow diagram

Table 1 Demographic characteristics and intraoperative data

	Group M (n = 20)	Group C (n = 20)	Statistics	P
Age (years)	42.4 ± 8.7	39.5 ± 8.4	1.066[a]	0.293
Sex (M/F)	4/16	6/14	0.533[b]	0.465
Weight (kg)	65.4 ± 10.3	63.6 ± 12.4	0.479[a]	0.635
BMI (kg/m^2)	24.2 ± 3.9	23.3 ± 3.6	0.801[a]	0.428
Type of operation, n (%)				
Hemithyroidectomy	13 (65.0%)	10 (50.0%)	0.921[b]	0.337
Total thyroidectomy	7 (35.0%)	10 (50.0%)		
Duration of surgery (s)	68.5 ± 32.2	66.7 ± 23.2	0.203[a]	0.840
Consciousness recovery time (s)	7.0 ± 4.1	6.4 ± 3.5	0.543[a]	0.590
Extubation time (s)	10.0 ± 5.5	11.1 ± 5.9	0.582[a]	0.564
Remifentanil (mg)	0.626 ± 0.268	0.645 ± 0.238	0.238[a]	0.813

Data are presented as mean ± SD or *n* (%). Group M, multimodal analgesia group who received ropivacaine locally plus intravenous flurbiprofen axetil; Group C, control group who received a single dose of tramadol; *BMI* Body mass index; [a], *t* value; [b], Chi-square value

To overcome the problems of the short duration of analgesia obtained with incisional infiltration and the insufficient analgesia provided by NSAIDs, we administered a combined analgesia protocol of ropivacaine wound infiltration plus intravenous flurbiprofen axetil. Ropivacaine was chosen for its longer block duration, lower toxicity, and greater safety compared with other local anesthetics; plasma levels and risks are associated with the total dose used and the extent of absorption [27]. According to previous studies, ropivacaine concentrations of 0.25, 0.5 and 0.75% provide adequate analgesia via wound infiltration [27–29]. Based on the literatures and our experiences, we chose to use 0.5% ropivacaine because it provides good analgesia with few adverse effects. To prolong local anesthetic action and reduce vascular absorption, epinephrine was added to the ropivacaine. However, epinephrine should be applied with caution in patients with severe hypertension, or cardiovascular and cerebrovascular diseases, as it may cause tachycardia and hypertension if absorbed intravascularly. In our study, postoperative pain reached its maximum at 2 h postoperatively in Group C, similarly to previous findings [20], and remained at a relatively high level until 8 h postoperatively. The pain scores of Group C at maximum (2 h postoperatively) were 1.6 at rest and 2.6 during coughing/swallowing. The average NRS pain scores of Group C were 1.4 at rest and 2.0 during coughing/swallowing during the 2–8 h postoperative period, whereas the average NRS pain scores of Group M were 0.6 at rest and 1.2 during coughing/swallowing. The postoperative pain score reached its maximum at 24 h postoperatively at rest and 8 h postoperatively during coughing/swallowing in Group M (0.6 at rest and 1.4 during coughing/swallowing). However, the maximum postoperative pain scores in Group M were still relatively low compared to that in Group C at the same observation timepoint. Thus, multimodal analgesia delayed the occurrence of maximum postoperative pain (the maximum pain score was still relatively low), and successfully achieved pain relief during the early postoperative period (2–8 h postoperatively). This is meaningful, as several studies have indicated that the first few hours following thyroidectomy are the most crucial for pain management because patients experienced maximum

Table 2 Mean blood pressure during surgery

	Group M (*n* = 20)	Group C (n = 20)	Statistic	P
Before induction (T1)	94.7 ± 13.5	95.0 ± 9.1	7.187	0.019*
3 min after induction (T2)	75.4 ± 15.3	74.7 ± 10.4		
At the beginning of surgery (T3)	66.9 ± 9.4	71.8 ± 7.0		
After 10 min of surgery (T4)	71.8 ± 5.8	78.6 ± 9.1		
After 30 min of surgery (T5)	69.1 ± 7.8	77.4 ± 10.6		
At the end of surgery (T6)	72.2 ± 11.5	83.8 ± 12.3		
Immediately after extubation (T7)	94.3 ± 11.7	99.2 ± 11.7		
Before discharge from the PACU (T8)	85.8 ± 8.1	91.5 ± 11.9		

Data are presented as mean ± SD. Group M, multimodal analgesia group who received ropivacaine locally plus intravenous flurbiprofen axetil; Group C, control group who received a single dose of tramadol; PACU, postoperative anesthetic care unit; *, $P < 0.05$

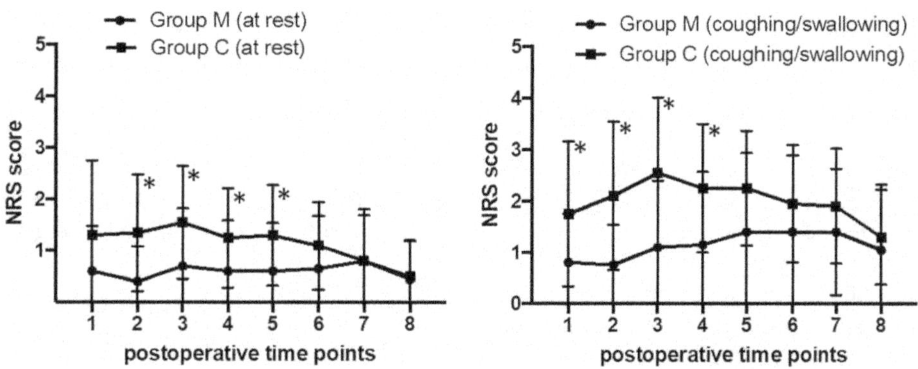

Fig. 2 Numerical rating scale (NRS) pain scores at various postoperative timepoints. NRS scores at rest were significantly lower in Group M than Group C before patient discharge from the PACU ($P = 0.003$), and at 2 ($P = 0.008$), 4 ($P = 0.020$), and 8 h ($P = 0.016$) postoperatively. NRS scores during coughing/swallowing were significantly lower in Group M than Group C at 5 min after tracheal extubation ($P = 0.017$), before patient discharge from the PACU ($P = 0.001$), and at 2 ($P = 0.002$) and 4 h ($P = 0.013$) postoperatively. Group M, multimodal analgesia group who received ropivacaine locally plus intravenous flurbiprofen axetil; Group C, control group who received a single dose of tramadol; PACU, postoperative anesthetic care unit; *$P < 0.05$

pain during this period. Our results also demonstrate that the analgesic effects in Group M were significantly better than those in Group C on the first postoperative day both at rest and during coughing/swallowing; the average NRS pain score in Group M was also significantly lower than that in Group C within the first 2 postoperative days. These results showed that multimodal analgesia enhanced postoperative pain relief not only during the early postoperative stage, but throughout the 48 h postoperative period. This is a meaningful improvement compared with several studies that reported insufficient maintenance of pain control after administration of local anesthesia [20, 25]. One of the adverse effects of tramadol is nausea, which may result in higher frequency of swallowing and could explain the higher NRS scores during coughing/swallowing in Group C versus Group M. However, the incidence of nausea did not significantly differ between the two groups, which means that the two groups had a similar frequency of swallowing. Therefore, we believe that the comparison between the two groups of pain scores during coughing/swallowing was not affected by nausea caused by tramadol.

Consistent with previous studies [30–33], 80.0% of patients had NRS scores lower than 4 (only one patient had a NRS score of greater than 6), indicating that thyroidectomy causes mild to moderate postoperative pain. Additional rescue analgesics were not usually required, and the need for additional rescue analgesics did not significantly differ between the groups. However, the intensity of postoperative pain may vary with surgical approach, anesthetic management, and pain-control protocols. In our study, the application of a small incision (approximately 4–7 cm) in thyroidectomy may have resulted in minimal pain in both groups. Our study showed that pain control after thyroid surgery can generally be accomplished with either a multimodal analgesia regimen of pre-incision wound infiltration and flurbiprofen axetil or with a single dose of tramadol, mostly without additional analgesics. Several previous studies suggested that local anesthetic wound infiltration decreases opioid consumption [16, 17, 34]. However, the present study found that intraoperative remifentanil use did not differ between the groups, consistent with a previous study [25].

Table 3 Average numerical rating scale (NRS) pain scores during the first 48 h postoperatively

	Group M ($n = 20$)	Group C ($n = 20$)	Statistics	P
During the first 24 h postoperatively				
At rest	0.614 ± 0.620	1.236 ± 0.777	2.795[a]	0.008*
During coughing or swallowing	1.143 ± 0.834	2.107 ± 1.057	3.203[a]	0.003*
During the first 24–48 h postoperatively				
At rest	0.000	0.500		0.662
During coughing or swallowing	1.225 ± 1.186	1.600 ± 0.968	1.095[a]	0.280
Average scores under both conditions within 48 h postoperatively	0.863 ± 0.647	1.575 ± 0.794	3.112[a]	0.004*

Data are presented as mean ± SD or median. Group M, multimodal analgesia group who received ropivacaine locally plus intravenous flurbiprofen axetil; Group C, control group who received a single dose of tramadol. [a], t value; *, $P < 0.05$

Table 4 Incidence of adverse effects

	Group M (n = 20)	Group C (*n* = 20)	χ^2	*P*
Dizziness	3 (15.0%)	3 (15.0%)	0.000	1.000
Nausea	4 (20.0%)	3 (15.0%)	0.000	1.000
Vomiting	1 (5.0%)	1 (5.0%)	0.000	1.000

Data are presented as *n* (%). Group M, multimodal analgesia group who received ropivacaine locally plus intravenous flurbiprofen axetil; Group C, control group who received a single dose of tramadol

Multimodal approaches to pain management have been shown to reduce adverse effects such as dizziness and PONV in patients undergoing surgical procedures [14, 35]. However, our results showed no significant differences in drug-associated adverse effects between the groups. In our study, the incidence of PONV was relatively low compared with data reported in a previous study [36]. PONV was only experienced by four (20.0%) patients in Group M and three (15.0%) in Group C. We assume that PONV was prevented by the combined use of dolasetron and propofol infusion (which allowed a lower concentration of sevoflurane during surgery). Furthermore, the relatively low incidence of PONV in Group C may be related to the slow injection of tramadol over a 5-min period. NSAIDs are associated with many adverse effects, including platelet aggregation inhibition, gastrointestinal mucosal injury, and renal failure. However, no adverse events were observed in our study. There were no significant differences between the two groups in intraoperative blood loss, and none of the patients experienced postoperative hemorrhage, probably because only a single dose of flurbiprofen axetil injection was administered. Similar data have been reported in other studies [37, 38]. Overall, our results demonstrated a low incidence of adverse effects due to multimodal analgesia with ropivacaine wound infiltration and intravenous flurbiprofen axetil (both administered within their recommended doses and volume) in patients undergoing thyroidectomy.

A previous study showed that patients treated with preoperative local infiltration exhibited lower MBP than other patients [25]. Similar changes were observed in our study, with a lower MBP in Group M than in Group C. In the previous study, the MBP reduction was explained as the result of preoperative local infiltration [25]. However, in our study, there were no significant differences between groups in vasoconstrictor requirement during surgery, indicating that the two groups had similar proportions of patients with hemodynamic changes within 30% of base line. Therefore, the differences in MBP may not be considered clinically significant.

The present study had some limitations. A sex ratio disparity existed among the participants, as 30 of the 40 patients analyzed were female. This distribution may be inevitable, as thyroid cancer is more common in women [39]. Nevertheless, these results need to be confirmed in a larger trial.

Conclusion

Multimodal analgesia with ropivacaine wound infiltration and intravenous flurbiprofen axetil improves the quality of postoperative analgesia in patients undergoing radical thyroidectomy, and has few adverse effects. This approach has advantages over tramadol for patients undergoing radical thyroidectomy. We recommend that this multimodal regimen be used in the clinical setting as described.

Abbreviations

HR: Heart rate; MBP: Mean blood pressure; NBP: Noninvasive blood pressure; NRS: Numerical rating scale; NSAID: Non-steroidal anti-inflammatory drug; PACU: Postoperative anesthetic care unit; PONV: Postoperative nausea and vomiting; SD: Standard deviation; SPSS: Statistical Package for Social Sciences

Acknowledgements

The authors would like to thank Mr. Zhendong Li from the postoperative anesthetic care unit for performing postoperative follow-up. We also thank Kelly Zammit, BVSc, and Rebecca Tollefson, DVM, from Liwen Bianji, Edanz Editing China (www.liwenbianji.cn/ac), for editing the English text of a draft of this manuscript.

Authors' contributions

XXL designed the study, performed the statistical analysis, and drafted the manuscript. LY interpreted the data and revised the manuscript. JNY collected the data and assisted in drafting the manuscript. HYT revised the manuscript and approved the version to be published. All authors read and approved the final submitted version of the manuscript.

References

1. le Roux PJ, Coetzee JF. Tramadol today. Curr Opin Anaesthesiol. 2000;13(4): 457–61.
2. Tas A, Mistanoqlu V, Kececioqlu M. Tramadol versus fentanyl during propofol-based deep sedation for uterine dilatation and curettage: a prospective study. J Obstet Gynaecol Res. 2014;40(3):749–53.
3. Tarkkila P, Tuominen M, Lindgren L. Comparison of respiratory effects of tramadol and oxycodone. J Clin Anesth. 1997;9(7):582–5.
4. Chu YC, Lin SM, Hsieh YC, Tsou MY. Intraoperative administration of tramadol for postoperative nurse-controlled analgesia resulted in earlier awakening and less sedation than morphine in children after cardiac surgery. Anesth Anal. 2006;102(6):1668–73.
5. Dejonckheere M, Desjeux L, Deneu S, Ewalenko P. Intravenous tramadol compared to propacetamol for postoperative analgesia following thyroidectomy. Acta Anaesthesiol Belg. 2001;52(1):29–33.
6. Horn CC, Wallisch WJ, Homanics GE, Williams JP. Pathophysiological and neurochemical mechanisms of postoperative nausea and vomiting. Eur J Pharmacol. 2014;722:55–66.
7. Roberts SM, Bezinover DS, Janicki PK. Reappraisal of the role of dolasetron in prevention and treatment of nausea and vomiting associated with surgery or chemotherapy. Cancer Manag Res. 2012;4:67–73.
8. Matsuura H, Inoue S, Kawaquchi M. The risk of postoperative nausea and vomiting between surgical patients received propofol and sevoflurane anesthesia: a matched study. Acta Anaesthesiol Taiwan. 2016;54(4):114–20.
9. Schraaq S, Pradelli L, AJO A, Bellone M, Ghetti G, Chung TL, et al. Propofol vs. inhalational agents to maintain general anaesthesia in ambulatory and in-patient surgery: a systematic review and meta-analysis. BMC Anesthesiol. 2018;18(1):162.
10. Lee SK, Lee JW, Choy WS. Is multimodal analgesia as effective as postoperative patient-controlled analgesia following upper extremity surgery? Orthop Traumatol Surg Res. 2013;99(8):895–901.
11. Parvizi J, Miller AG, Gandhi K. Multimodal pain management after total joint arthroplasty. J Bone Joint Surg Am. 2011;93(11):1075–84.
12. Parvizi J, Porat M, Gandhi K, Viscusi ER, Rothman RH. Postoperative pain management techniques in hip and knee arthroplasty. Instr Course Lect. 2009;58:769–79.
13. Rafiq S, Steinbruchel DA, Wanscher MJ, Andersen LW, Navne A, Lilleoer NB, et al. Multimodal analgesia versus traditional opiate based analgesia after cardiac surgery, a randomized controlled trial. J Cardiothorac Surg. 2014;9:52.
14. Gärtner R, Kroman N, Callesen T, Kehlet H. Multimodal prevention of pain, nausea and vomiting after breast cancer surgery. Minerva Anestesiol. 2010;

76(10):805–13.

15. Wang K, Luo J, Zheng L, Luo T. Preoperative flurbiprofen axetil administration for acute postoperative pain: a meta-analysis of randomized controlled trials. J Anesth. 2017;31(6):852–60.
16. Gozal Y, Shapira SC, Gozal D, Magora F. Bupivacaine wound infiltration in thyroid surgery reduces postoperative pain and opioid demand. Acta Anaesthesiol Scand. 1994;38(8):813–5.
17. Bagul A, Taha R, Metcalfe MS, Brook NR, Nicholson ML. Pre-incision infiltration of local anesthetic reduces postoperative pain with no effects on bruising and wound cosmesis after thyroid surgery. Thyroid. 2005;15(11):1245–8.
18. Leone S, Di Cianni S, Casati A, Fanelli G. Pharmacology, toxicology, and clinical use of new long acting local anesthetics, ropivacaine and levobupivacaine. Acta Biomed. 2008;79(2):92–105.
19. Lee JH, Suh YJ, Song RY, Yi JW, Yu HW, Kwon H, et al. Preoperative flap-site injection with ropivacaine and epinephrine in BABA robotic and endoscopic thyroidectomy safely reduces postoperative pain: a CONSORT-compliant double-blinded randomized controlled study (PAIN-BREKOR trial). Medicine (Baltimore). 2017;96(22):e6896.
20. Ayman M, Materazzi G, Bericotti M, Rago R, Nidal Y, Miccoli P. Bupivacaine 0.5% versus ropivacaine 0.75% wound infiltration to decrease postoperative pain in total thyroidectomy, a prospective controlled study. Minerva Chir. 2012;67(6):511–6.
21. Sellami M, Feki S, Triki Z, Zghal J, Zouche I, Hammami B, et al. Bupivacaine wound infiltration reduces postoperative pain and analgesic requirement after thyroid surgery. Eur Arch Otorhinolaryngol. 2018;275(5):1265–70.
22. Teksoz S, Arikan AE, Soylu S, Erbabacan SE, Ozcan M, Bukey Y. Bupivacaine application reduces post thyroidectomy pain: Cerrahpasa experience. Gland Surg. 2016;5(6):565–70.
23. Miu M, Royer C, Gaillat C, Schaup B, Meneqaux F, Langeron O, et al. Lack of analgesic effect induced by Ropivacaine wound infiltration in thyroid surgery: a randomized, double-blind, placebo-controlled trial. Anesth Analg. 2016;122(2):559–64.
24. Mismar AA, Mahseeri MI, Al-Ghazawi MA, Obeidat FW, Albsoul MN, Al-Qudah MS, et al. Wound infiltration with bupivacaine 0.5% with or without adrenaline does not decrease pain after thyroidectomy. A randomized controlled study. Saudi Med. 2017;38(10):994–9.
25. Shin S, Chung WY, Jeong JJ, Kang SW, Oh YJ. Analgesic efficacy of bilateral superficial cervical plexus block in robot-assisted endoscopic thyroidectomy using a transaxillary approach. World J Surg. 2012;36(12):2831–7.
26. Tam KW, Chen SY, Huang TW, Lin CC, Su CM, Li CL, et al. Effect of wound infiltration with ropivacaine or bupivacaine analgesia in breast cancer surgery: a meta-analysis of randomized controlled trials. Int J Surg. 2015;22:79–85.
27. Mulroy MF, Burgess FW, Emanuelsson BM. Ropivacaine 0.25 and 0.5%, but not 0.125%, provide effective wound infiltration analgesia after outpatient hernia repair, but with sustained plasma drug levels. Reg Anesth Pain Med. 1999;24(2):136–41.
28. Johansson B, Glise H, Hallerback B, Dalman P, Kristoffersson A. Preoperative local infiltration with ropivacaine for postoperative pain relief after cholecystectomy. Anesth Analg. 1994;78(2):210–4.
29. Zhu Z, Chen B, Ye W, Wang S, Xu G, Pan Z, et al. Clinical significance of wound infiltration with ropivacaine for elderly patients in China underwent total laparoscopic radical gastrectomy: a retrospective cohort study. Medicine. 2019;98(14):e15115.
30. Eti Z, Irmak P, Gulluoglu BM, Manukyan MN, Gogus FY. Does bilateral superficial cervical plexus block decrease analgesic requirement after thyroid surgery? Anesth Analg. 2006;102(4):1174–6.
31. Ma XD, Li BP, Wang DL, Yang WS. Postoperative benefits of dexmedetomidine combined with flurbiprofen axetil after thyroid surgery. Exp Ther Med. 2017;14(3):2148–52.
32. Kilbas Z, Mentes MO, Harlak A, Yigit T, Balkan SM, Cosar A, et al. Efficacy of wound infiltration with lornoxicam for postoperative analgesia following thyroidectomy: a prospective, randomized, double-blind study. Turk J Med Sci. 2015;45(3):700–5.
33. Yücel A, Yazıcı A, Müderris T, Gül F. Comparison of lornoxicam and low-dose tramadol for management of post-thyroidectomy pain. Agri. 2016;28(4):183–9.
34. Kang KH, Kim BS, Kang H. The benefits of preincision ropivacaine infiltration for reducing postoperative pain after robotic bilateral axillo-breast approach thyroidectomy: a prospective, randomized, double-blind, placebo-controlled study. Ann Surg Treat Res. 2015;88(4):193–9.
35. Chandrakantan A, Glass PS. Multimodal therapies for postoperative nausea and vomiting, and pain. Br J Anaesth. 2011;107(Suppl 1):i27–40.
36. Metaxari M, Papaioannou A, Petrou A, Chatzimichali A, Pharmakalidou E, Askitopoulou H. Antiemetic prophylaxis in thyroid surgery: a randomized, double-blind comparison of three 5-HT3 agents. J Anesth. 2011;25(3):356–62.
37. Zhang Z, Zhao H, Wang C, Han F, Wang G. Lack of preemptive analgesia by intravenous flurbiprofen in thyroid gland surgery: a randomized, double-blind and placebo-controlled clinical trial. Int J Med Sci. 2011;8(5):433–8.
38. Lin X, Zhang R, Xing J, Gao X, Chang P, Li W. Flurbiprofen axetil reduces postoperative sufentanil consumption and enhances postoperative analgesic effects in patients with colorectal cancer surgery. Int J Clin Exp Med. 2014;7(12):4887–96.
39. Cook MB, Dawsey SM, Freedman ND, Inskip PD, Wichner SM, Quraishi SM, et al. Sex disparities in cancer incidence by period and age. Cancer Epidemiol Biomarkers Prev. 2009;18(4):1174–82.

Permissions

All chapters in this book were first published by BioMed Central; hereby published with permission under the Creative Commons Attribution License or equivalent. Every chapter published in this book has been scrutinized by our experts. Their significance has been extensively debated. The topics covered herein carry significant findings which will fuel the growth of the discipline. They may even be implemented as practical applications or may be referred to as a beginning point for another development.

The contributors of this book come from diverse backgrounds, making this book a truly international effort. This book will bring forth new frontiers with its revolutionizing research information and detailed analysis of the nascent developments around the world.

We would like to thank all the contributing authors for lending their expertise to make the book truly unique. They have played a crucial role in the development of this book. Without their invaluable contributions this book wouldn't have been possible. They have made vital efforts to compile up to date information on the varied aspects of this subject to make this book a valuable addition to the collection of many professionals and students.

This book was conceptualized with the vision of imparting up-to-date information and advanced data in this field. To ensure the same, a matchless editorial board was set up. Every individual on the board went through rigorous rounds of assessment to prove their worth. After which they invested a large part of their time researching and compiling the most relevant data for our readers.

The editorial board has been involved in producing this book since its inception. They have spent rigorous hours researching and exploring the diverse topics which have resulted in the successful publishing of this book. They have passed on their knowledge of decades through this book. To expedite this challenging task, the publisher supported the team at every step. A small team of assistant editors was also appointed to further simplify the editing procedure and attain best results for the readers.

Apart from the editorial board, the designing team has also invested a significant amount of their time in understanding the subject and creating the most relevant covers. They scrutinized every image to scout for the most suitable representation of the subject and create an appropriate cover for the book.

The publishing team has been an ardent support to the editorial, designing and production team. Their endless efforts to recruit the best for this project, has resulted in the accomplishment of this book. They are a veteran in the field of academics and their pool of knowledge is as vast as their experience in printing. Their expertise and guidance has proved useful at every step. Their uncompromising quality standards have made this book an exceptional effort. Their encouragement from time to time has been an inspiration for everyone.

The publisher and the editorial board hope that this book will prove to be a valuable piece of knowledge for researchers, students, practitioners and scholars across the globe.

List of Contributors

Richard Wood, Richard Watts and John Currie
Department of Anaesthesia, The Queen Elizabeth Hospital, Woodville South 5011, South Australia, Australia

Venkatesan Thiruvenkatarajan and Roelof M. Van Wijk
Department of Anaesthesia, The Queen Elizabeth Hospital, Woodville South 5011, South Australia, Australia
The University of Adelaide, Adelaide 5000, South Australia, Australia

Medhat Wahba
Department of Anaesthesia, The Queen Elizabeth Hospital, Woodville South 5011, South Australia, Australia
Pain Management Unit, Flinders Medical Centre, Bedford Park 5042, South Australia, Australia

Fei Lan, Yanhui Ma, Ting Zhang and Tianlong Wang
Department of Anesthesiology Xuanwu Hospital, Capital Medical University, No.45, Changchun Street, Beijing 100053, China

Yanyan Shen
Department of Anesthesiology, Peking University International Hospital, Beijing, China

Guanglei Cao
Department of Orthopedics Xuanwu Hospital, Capital Medical University, Beijing, China

Nicole Philips
Department of Critical Care Medicine St. Michael's Hospital, University of Toronto, Toronto, Canada

Nantthasorn Zinboonyahgoon, Pawinee Pangthipampai, Choopong Luansritisakul, Sunsanee Mali-ong and Nawaporn Sateantantikul
Department of Anesthesiology, Siriraj Hospital, Mahidol University, 2 Phranok road, Bangkoknoi 10700, Thailand

Panya Luksanapruksa and Theera Chueaboonchai
Department of Orthopedic Surgery Siriraj Hospital, Mahidol University, 2 Phranok road, Bangkoknoi 10700, Thailand

Sitha Piyaselakul
Department of Anatomy, Siriraj Hospital, Mahidol University, 2 Phranok road, Bangkoknoi 10700, Thailand

Suphalerk Lohasammakul
Department of Surgery, Siriraj Hospital, Mahidol University, 2 Phranok road, Bangkoknoi 10700, Thailand

Kamen Vlassakov
Department of Anesthesiology, Perioperative and Pain Medicine, Brigham and Women's Hospital, Harvard Medical School, 75 Francis Street, Boston, MA 02115, USA

Frederick Sieber
Department of Anesthesiology and Critical Care Medicine, Johns Hopkins Bayview Medical Center, 4940 Eastern Avenue, Baltimore, MD 21224, USA

Karin Neufeld
Department of Psychiatry and Behavioral Sciences, Johns Hopkins University School of Medicine, A4Center Suite 457, 4940 Eastern Ave, Baltimore, USA

Esther S. Oh
Division of Geriatric Medicine and Gerontology, Psychiatry and Behavioral Sciences & Neuropathology, Johns Hopkins University School of Medicine, Mason F. Lord Building, Center Tower, 5200 Eastern Avenue, 7th Floor, Baltimore, MD 21224, USA

Allan Gottschalk
Departments of Anesthesiology and Critical Care Medicine and Neurosurgery, Johns Hopkins Hospital, 1800 Orleans St, Baltimore, MD 21287, USA

Nae-Yuh Wang
Medicine, Biostatistics and Epidemiology, The Johns Hopkins University, 2024 E. Monument Street, Suite 2-500, Baltimore, MD 21287, USA

John A. Carter
Blue Point LLC, 711 Warrenville Road, Wheaton, IL 60189, USA

Libby K. Black
Baudax Bio Inc, Malvern, PA, USA

Dolly Sharma and Tarun Bhagnani
EPI-Q, Inc, Oak Brook, IL, USA

Jonathan S. Jahr
Department of Anesthesiology and Perioperative Medicine, UCLA, Los Angeles, CA, USA

Kunpeng Li, Changbin Ji, Dawei Luo, Hongyong Feng, Keshi Yang and Hui Xu
Department of Orthopaedics, Liaocheng People's Hospital, No 67 Dongchang West Road, Liaocheng City 252000, Shandong Province, China

Bin Feng, Hui-Ming Peng, Yan-Yan Bian, Gui-Xing Qiu and Xisheng Weng
the Department of Orthopaedic Surgery, Peking Union Medical College Hospital, Beijing 100730, China

Kai-Yuan Cheng
the Department of Orthopaedic Surgery, Peking Union Medical College Hospital, Beijing 100730, China
Chinese Academy of Medical Sciences and Peking Union Medical College, Beijing 100730, China

Lin-Jie Zhang and Chang Han
Chinese Academy of Medical Sciences and Peking Union Medical College, Beijing 100730, China

Baona Wang, Tao Yan, Hui Zheng and Guohua Zhang
Department of Anesthesiology, National Cancer Center/National Clinical Research Center for Cancer/Cancer Hospital, Chinese Academy of Medical Sciences and Peking Union Medical College, Beijing 100021, China

Xiangyi Kong
Department of Breast Surgery, National Cancer Center/National Clinical Research Center for Cancer/Cancer Hospital, Chinese Academy of Medical Sciences and Peking Union Medical College, Beijing 100021, China

Li Sun
Department of Anesthesiology, National Cancer Center/National Clinical Research Center for Cancer/Cancer Hospital & Shenzhen Hospital, Chinese Academy of Medical Sciences and Peking Union Medical College, Shenzhen 518116, China

Mi K. Oh
Department of Anesthesiology and Pain Medicine, Hanyang University Guri Hospital, Guri-si, Gyeonggi-do, Republic of Korea

Jae H. Ryu
Department of Anesthesiology and Pain Medicine, Hanyang University Guri Hospital, Guri-si, Gyeonggi-do, Republic of Korea

Woo J. Jeon
Department of Anesthesiology and Pain Medicine, Hanyang University Guri Hospital, Guri-si, Gyeonggi-do, Republic of Korea

Chang W. Lee
Department of Anesthesiology and Pain Medicine, Hanyang University Guri Hospital, Guri-si, Gyeonggi-do, Republic of Korea

Sang Y. Cho
Department of Anesthesiology and Pain Medicine, Hanyang University Guri Hospital, 249-1, Gyomun-dong, Guri-si, Gyeonggi-do 471-701, Republic of Korea

Ming Jiang, Yu'e Sun, Yue Liu, Zhengliang Ma and Xiaoping Gu
Department of Anesthesiology, Affiliated Drum Tower Hospital of Nanjing University Medical School, Nanjing 210008, Jiangsu Province, China

Yishan Lei, Fan Hu and Zhengrong Xia
Analytical & Testing Center, Nanjing Medical University, Nanjing, Jiangsu Province, China

Rui Xu, Yi Lu, Wenxian Li and Jie Jia
Department of Anesthesiology, The Eye, Ear, Nose and Throat Hospital of Fudan University, Shanghai Medical College of Fudan University, Fenyang Road #83, Shanghai 200031, People's Republic of China

Yun Zhu
Department of Oro-maxillofacial Head and Neck Oncology, Shanghai Ninth People's Hospital, Shanghai Jiao Tong University School of Medicine, Shanghai Key Laboratory of Stomatology, Shanghai, China

Hang Chen, Fei Yang, Mao Ye, Hui Liu, Jing Zhang, Qin Tian, Ruiqi Liu, Qing Yu, Shangyingying Li and Shengfen Tu
Department of Anesthesiology, Children's Hospital of Chongqing Medical University, No.136 Zhongshan 2nd Road, Yuzhong District, Chongqing, People's Republic of China

Xiaona Zhu, Limei Chen, Shuang Zheng and Linmin Pan
Department of Anesthesiology, the First Affiliated Hospital, Wenzhou Medical University, Shangcai village, Nanbaixiang town, Ouhai District, Wenzhou City 325000, Zhejiang Province, China

Xiancun Liu, Tingting Song, Jingjing Zhang, Conghui Shan, Liangying Chang and Haiyang Xu
Department of Anesthesiology, The First Hospital of Jilin University, No.71 Xinmin street, Changchun, Jilin 130021, China

Xuejiao Chen
Department of Anesthesiology, China-Japan Friendship Hospital, Beijing 100029, China

Muzaffer Gencer
Department of Anesthesia, Istinye University Medical Faculty, Istanbul, Turkey

Ayşe Yeşim Göçmen
Department of Biochemistry, Bozok University Medical Faculty, Yozgat, Turkey

Yanqing Wang and Kexian Zhang
Department of Anesthesiology, Sichuan Cancer Hospital & Institute, Sichuan Cancer Center, School of Medicine, University of Electronic Science and Technology of China, No.55, Section 4, South Renmin Road, Chengdu 610041, People's Republic of China

Xiaojia Wang
Department of Pain management, West China Hospital, Sichuan University, Chengdu 610041, People's Republic of China

Gordan Mijovski, Matej Podbregar, Matej Jenko and Maja Šoštarič
Department of Anaesthesiology and Surgical Intensive Therapy, University Medical Centre Ljubljana, Faculty of Medicine, University of Ljubljana, Zaloška cesta 2, 1000 Ljubljana, Slovenia

Juš Kšela
Department of Cardiovascular Surgery, University Medical Centre Ljubljana, Faculty of Medicine, University of Ljubljana, Ljubljana, Slovenia

Magnus Olofsson, Bénédict Morin and Eric Albrecht
Department of Anaesthesia, Lausanne University Hospital, Rue du Bugnon 46, BH 05.311, 1011 Lausanne, Switzerland

Patrick Taffé
Institute of Social and Preventive Medicine (IUMSP), Lausanne University Hospital, Lausanne, Switzerland

Kyle Robert Kirkham
Department of Anaesthesia, Toronto Western Hospital, University of Toronto, Toronto, Canada

Frédéric Vauclair
Department of Orthopaedic, Lausanne University Hospital, Lausanne, Switzerland

Yanhua Peng, Jinfeng Yang, Duo Guo, Chumei Zheng, Huiping Sun, Qinya Zhang, Shuangfa Zou and Ke Luo
Department of Anesthesiology, Hunan Cancer Hospital, The Affiliated Cancer Hospital of Xiangya School of Medicine, Central South University, Changsha 410013, Hunan, China

Yanping Zhang and Keith A. Candiotti
Department of Anesthesiology, Perioperative Medicine and Pain Management, University of Miami-Miller School of Medicine, Miami, FL 33136, USA

Joshan Lal Bajracharya
Department of Anesthesiology & Critical Care, Mechi Zonal Hospital, Bhadrapur, Nepal

Krishna Pokharel
Department of Anesthesiology & Critical Care Medicine, BPKIHS, Dharan, Nepal

Balkrishna Bhattarai
Department of Anesthesiology & Critical Care Medicine, BPKIHS, Dharan, Nepal
Department of Anesthesiology & Critical Care Medicine, BP Koirala Institute of Health Sciences, Dharan, Nepal

Carine Zeeni, Majed Al Hassanieh and Fadia Shebbo
Department of Anesthesiology, American University of Beirut Medical Center, P.O. Box 11-0236, Beirut, Lebanon

Dina Chamsy, Ali Khalil, Antoine Abu Musa and Joseph Nassif
Department of Obstetrics and Gynecology, American University of Beirut Medical Center, Beirut, Lebanon

Anup Ghimire
Department of Anesthesiology, Nepal Mediciti Hospital, Lalitpur, Nepal

Asish Subedi and Birendra Prasad Sah
Department of Anesthesiology & Critical Care Medicine, BP Koirala Institute of Health Sciences, Dharan, Nepal

Li Xin An, Fu Shan Xue and Ya Fan Bai
Department of Anesthesia, Beijing Friendship Hospital, Capital Medical University, No.95 Yongan Road, Xicheng District, Beijing 100050, China

Chun Mei Zhao
Department of Anesthesia, Beijing Tiantan Hospital, Capital Medical University, Beijing, China

Fei Xing
Department of Anesthesia, Beijing Friendship Hospital, Capital Medical University, No.95 Yongan Road, Xicheng District, Beijing 100050, China
Department of Anesthesia, Beijing Tiantan Hospital, Capital Medical University, Beijing, China

Yun Lin, Zhuang Miao, Yue Wu and Qing-ping Wen
Department of Anesthesiology, The First Affiliated Hospital of Dalian Medical University, No.193 Lian he Road, Xi gang District, Dalian City, Liaoning Province 116000, People's Republic of China

Fang-fang Ge
Dalian Medical of University, Dalian, China

Ben Forbes
School of Cancer & Pharmaceutical Sciences, King's College London, 150 Stamford Street, London SE1 9NH, UK

Asia N Rashed and Stephen Tomlin
School of Cancer & Pharmaceutical Sciences, King's College London, 150 Stamford Street, London SE1 9NH, UK
Pharmacy Department, Evelina London Children's Hospital, Guy's & St Thomas' NHS Foundation Trust, Westminster Bridge Road, London SE1 7EH, UK

Cate Whittlesea
Research Department of Practice and Policy, UCL School of Pharmacy, London, UK

Caroline Davies
Paediatric Anaesthetic Department, Evelina London Children's Hospital, Guy's & St Thomas' NHS Foundation Trust, London, UK

Chung Hun Lee, Sang Sik Choi, Mi Kyoung Lee, Yeon Joo Lee and Jong Sun Park
Department of Anesthesiology and Pain Medicine, Korea University Medical Center, Guro Hospital, Gurodong Road 148, Guro-Gu, Seoul 08308, Republic of Korea

Xiaoxi Li, Ling Yu, Jiaonan Yang and Hongyu Tan
Key Laboratory of Carcinogenesis and Translational Research (Ministry of Education/Beijing), Department of Anesthesiology, Peking University Cancer Hospital & Institute, #52 Fucheng Street, Haidian District, Beijing 100142, China

Index

www.ingramcontent.com/pod-product-compliance
Lightning Source LLC
Chambersburg PA
CBHW080412190526
45161CB00003B/219

* 9 7 8 1 6 3 9 8 9 7 8 3 4 *